MEDICAL RADIOLOGY
Diagnostic Imaging

Softcover Edition

Editors:
A. L. Baert, Leuven
K. Sartor, Heidelberg

U. J. Schoepf (Ed.)

Multidetector-Row CT of the Thorax

With Contributions by

J. Aldrich · C. R. Becker · C. Beigelmann-Aubry · P. M. Boiselle · P. Costello · M. Das
R. Drosten · C. Fetita · R. Fischbach · E. K. Fishman · D. Fleischmann · T. Flohr
L. Gattinoni · B. Ghaye · L. R. Goodman · P. A. Grenier · C. I. Henschke · C. J. Herold
P. Herzog · A. R. Hunsacker · F. L. Jacobson · M. Kachelriess · W. A. Kalender
H.-U. Kauczor · J. P. Ko · W. Kostis · L. P. Lawler · A. N. Leung · R. Loose · J. M. Martensen
Y. Martin-Bouyer · J. R. Mayo · D. P. Naidich · A. Nchimi · M. U. Niethammer
B. Ohnesorge · M. Oldendorf · B. L. Partik · E. J. Potchen · M. F. Reiser · G. D. Rubin
S. Schaller · P. Schnyder · U. J. Schoepf · D. Shaham · S. Shankar · M. J. Siegel
H. C. Steinert · E. vanSonnenberg · M. Vazquez · J. Verschakelen · G. K. von Schulthess
J. E. Wildberger · M. Wintermark · S. A. Wood · D. F. Yankelevitz

Series Editor's Foreword by

A. L. Baert

Foreword by

M. F. Reiser

With 349 Figures in 641 Separate Illustrations, 100 in Color and 37 Tables

Springer

U. Joseph Schoepf, MD
Department of Radiology
Brigham and Women's Hospital
Harvard Medical School
75 Francis Street
Boston, MA 02115
USA

Medical Radiology · Diagnostic Imaging and Radiation Oncology
Series Editors: A. L. Baert · L. W. Brady · H.-P. Heilmann · M. Molls · K. Sartor

Continuation of Handbuch der medizinischen Radiologie
Encyclopedia of Medical Radiology

ISBN 3-540-26247-4 Springer-Verlag Berlin Heidelberg New York
ISBN 978 3-540-26247-3 Springer-Verlag Berlin Heidelberg New York

Library of Congress Cataloging-in-Publication Data

Multidtector-row CT of the thorax / U. J. Schoepf (ed.) ; with contributions by C. R.
Becker ... [et al.] ; foreword by A. L. Baert.
p. ; cm. -- (Medical radiology)
Includes bibliographical references and index.
ISBN 3540437746 (hardcover; alk. paper) ISBN 3540262474 (softcover; alk. paper)
1. Chest--Tomography. I. Schoepf, U. J. (U. Jeseph), 1969- II. Becker, C. R. (Christoph
R.) III Series.
[DNLM: 1. Radiography, Thoracic--methods. 2. Tomography, X-Ray
Computed--mehods. WF 975 M691 2004]
RC941.M76 2004
617.5'407572--dc21 2003052905

Springer-Verlag is part of Springer Science+Business Media

http//www.springeronline.com

Printed in Germany

Cover-Design and Typesetting: Verlagsservice Teichmann, 69256 Mauer

Printed on acid-free paper - 21/3151xq – 5 4 3 2 1

Für meine Eltern,

URSULA und
JOSEF SCHOEPF

Series Editor's Foreword

Almost 30 years after the clinical introduction of computed tomography revolutionised the practice of radiology, the development of multidetector-row CT (MDCT) marked another important step forward in this cross-sectional modality.

The correct application of MDCT for optimal clinical results requires from the radiologist a keen insight in the technical principles of this technique as well as specific knowledge and skills concerning the appropriate use of i.v. contrast media, workflow design and radiation dose.

This superb volume covers exhaustively all aspects of the clinical application of MDCT in the study of the lung, heart and great vessels The collaboration of many internationally renowned experts has resulted in top-quality up-to-date, well written and comprehensive chapters on all main topics. I would like to congratulate Dr. Schoepf and the authors most sincerely for producing this standard reference work on a very topical theme.

This outstanding book will certainly meet with great interest from general, chest and vascular radiologists but also from surgeons and medical specialists, whose management of patients with diseases of the chest will greatly benefit from its contents. I am confident that it will encounter the same success with readers as previous volumes published in this series.

Leuven

Albert L. Baert

Foreword

The introduction of computed tomography revolutionized diagnostic imaging in the thorax. Soon after the introduction of this technology first reports appeared showing for example that pulmonary metastases, especially those in a subpleural location, could be detected with greater sensitivity than with chest radiography. In addition, tumors of the lung and the mediastinum could be detected more easily and staged more precisely. It was also not long before reports began describing previously unknown diagnostic applications, especially pertaining to the use of CT for determining the nature of focal lung disease and its ability to differentiate between benign and malignant pulmonary lesions, based on measurements of density, calcium and contrast medium uptake. Early generation CT scanners with incremental image acquisition were, however, limited in their diagnostic capabilities by partial volume effects and motion artifacts, originating from the pulsation of the heart and great vessels.

High-resolution CT (HR-CT) enabled a very detailed assessment of normal and diseased lung, so that HR-CT justifiably became established as the method of choice for in-vivo assessment of the pulmonary parenchyma. Nevertheless, non-representative sections were often sampled due to the incremental nature of this scan technique, resulting in misdiagnosis.

The introduction of spiral CT made it possible for the first time to generate large-volume data sets during a single breath-hold. The scan range in z-direction, however, was still limited, and the slice thickness was too large to acquire isotropic data. A fundamental change came with the introduction of multidetector-row CT (MDCT), initially with 4, later 8, 10, and most recently 16 detector rows. This technology allows the entire thorax to be scanned with thin sections during a single breath-hold, making possible high-resolution, three-dimensional, artifact-free imaging. Even the structures of the heart can now be analyzed by CT, so that the "holy grail of imaging", namely non-invasive coronary arteriography, is within reach. These advantages have rendered CT a particularly useful and robust technique for diagnosing thoracic disease. This holds true for the accurate non-invasive display of the pulmonary vasculature and for the non-invasive assessment of the mediastinum including the heart. Three-dimensional imaging and other post-processing methods have added greatly to diagnosis and quantification.

Despite the breathtaking aesthetic beauty and clarity that can be achieved with current modalities, not all technical and diagnostic problems have been solved. With regard to radiation exposure, a suitable compromise between image quality, diagnostic accuracy and patient radiation dose still has to be found. Intelligent modifications of the scan technique already allow a significant reduction of radiation exposure to the patient. Contrast medium administration has to be optimized and individualized, if the best possible contrast enhancement of the vasculature and the cardiac cavities is to be obtained. Thus, it remains inevitable that a portrayal of the current state of technology and knowledge only captures a brief moment in time while technology continues to advance. This development, therefore, should be considered in relative terms as further progress of medical applications and technical improvements occurs.

Nevertheless, it is a great achievement of Dr. Schoepf to have summarized the current state of knowledge of CT in this highly interesting, cutting-edge contribution. In the preparation of this book he was able to secure the contributions of renowned international experts. The chapters are well written, comprehensive and up to date. Current techniques and future developments pertaining to diagnostic imaging of the airways, diffuse and focal lung disease, tumors of the lung and mediastinum, pulmonary embolism, and MDCT of the heart are all comprehensively discussed. Important topics that have emerged only recently with the introduction of novel imaging modalities, such as data management, computer aided diagnosis and medico-legal aspects, are also included. The selection of the contributing authors and the structure of each individual chapter and of the overall volume as an entity are compelling. The bibliography is extensive, yet relevant. The text is eminently readable and conveys modern CT applications in an interesting and enjoyable style.

Dr. Schoepf has succeeded in composing an important, timely contribution to the standard literature on a topic of exceeding clinical importance in concurrent imaging, which will be received with the greatest of interest by radiologists and those in other disciplines involved in the diagnosis and treatment of diseases of the chest. I wish this book, the publisher, and the authors the success that they deserve, and I have no doubt that "Multidetector-Row CT of the Thorax" will become a well-distributed, successful and widely read addition to the standard radiology literature.

Munich

Maximilian F. Reiser

Preface

Τα παντα ρει, παντα χωρει, και ουδεν μενει ...
Heraclitus

Change is a constant of medical imaging, more so than of any other medical specialty. Change, innovation and adaptation are the very essence of our profession, which ever since its sweeping entrance into the realm of medicine has constantly reinvented itself. Today more than ever, medical imaging is a thriving, exciting and expanding enterprise and is setting the pace for progress and innovation in medicine.

The subject matter of "Multidetector-Row CT of the Thorax" is the epitome of this paradigm. With the introduction of multidetector-row technology at the eve of the new millennium CT was reawakened from its dormant state as a mundane commodity and has since been transformed into a fascinating tool of exploration.

The chest is the site of the diseases of the greatest socioeconomic importance. Yet the organs of the chest have traditionally been most challenging to image because of their continuous motion and the need to acquire images in apnea. The unprecedented combination of speed and spatial resolution that suddenly became available with multidetector-row CT proved to be ideally suited for visualizing the minute but cardinal anatomy and pathology of the organs of the thorax.

So fundamental were the advantages of the new imaging modality that it was almost instantaneously embraced by the whole medical imaging community. Our new technical capabilities have since been used to enhance clarity, reduce diagnostic doubt and routinely render anatomy and pathology in almost breathtaking aesthetic appeal. More importantly, however, in sync with the very nature of our specialty we have instinctively availed ourselves of the new opportunities to successfully overcome vexing traditional limitations and to venture into uncharted territory in the exploration of the human body.

Our endeavors have come to great fruition, as expertly testified by the contributing authors for each of their respective fields. Equally in accordance with the nature of our profession, we did not succumb to the temptations of our newfound technical prowess but embraced new opportunities critically and responsibly and adequately addressed new challenges.

It lies in the ever-changing nature of our field, too, that the act of condensing expert knowledge and experience in the format of a book can only result in a snapshot of the status quo at a certain point in time. Novel iterations of existing technology and profoundly new concepts of medical imaging are already on the horizon.

What is timeless, though, is the diligence and ingenuity that so decisively hallmarked the introduction of this novel technology. The embrace and beneficial application of multidetector-row CT may thus serve as a blueprint for future change and development within our specialty.

This book is the work of many. I am grateful and indebted to Professor Albert L. Baert for entrusting me with the role as editor for "Multidetector-Row CT of the Thorax" and for his valuable guidance throughout this project. I feel very, very honored by all the kindness that my many friends in the cardiothoracic imaging community have shown me by volunteering their time, their knowledge, their experience and vision that went into their respective contributions. All authors are highly respected experts in their field and this book would never have come to pass without their incredible support, for which I am so grateful. Finally I would like to thank Ursula Davis and Kurt Teichmann of Springer for so efficiently and expertly steering the production of "Multidetector-Row CT of the Thorax".

Boston U. Joseph Schoepf

Contents

MDCT - Technical Background

1 Technical Bases of Multi-Slice CT

T. Flohr, B. Ohnesorge, S. Schaller

CONTENTS

1.1 Introduction

The introduction of spiral CT in the early 1990s resulted in a fundamental and far-reaching improvement of CT imaging (Kalender et al. 1990; Crawford and King 1990). For the first time volume data could be acquired without mis-registration of anatomical details, which initiated the development of three-dimensional image processing techniques such as multi-planar reformations (MPRs), maximum intensity projections (MIPs), surface-shaded displays (SSDs) or volume renderings. As an important application CT angiography (CTA) has been established in clinical practice. As a consequence of increasing clinical demands, single-slice spiral CT with 1-s gantry rotation time soon encountered its limitations. To avoid motion artefacts and to optimally use the contrast bolus, spiral examinations of the thorax and of the abdomen have to be completed within the time of one held breath of the patient, typically within 25–30 s. If a larger scan range, such as the entire thorax or abdomen (30 cm), has to be covered within this time frame, a collimation of 5–8 mm must be chosen. The result is a considerable mis-match of transverse resolution, which is determined by the width of the collimated slice, and in-plane resolution, which is approximately 0.5–0.7 mm using a standard body kernel. Approaching the ideal of isotropic resolution – of acquiring image voxels with comparable sizes in all three dimensions – is only possible with single-slice CT by a substantial reduction of the scan range (Kalender 1995).

Larger volume coverage and improved transverse resolution can be achieved by simultaneous acquisition of more than one slice and by a shorter gantry rotation time. The first step towards multi-slice acquisition was a two-slice CT scanner introduced in 1993 (Elscint Twin). In 1998 all major CT manufacturers introduced multi-slice CT systems which brought about considerable improvements of scan speed, transverse resolution and utilization of the tube output (Klingenbeck-Regn et al. 1999; Hu et al. 2000; Ohnesorge et al. 1999). These systems typically offer simultaneous acquisition of four slices at 0.5-s rotation time. The increased performance compared with single-slice CT allowed for the optimization of a variety of clinical protocols: simulta-

T. Flohr, PhD; B. Ohnesorge, PhD; S. Schaller, PhD
CT Division, Siemens Medical Solutions, Siemensstrasse 1, 91301 Forchheim, Germany

neous acquisition of *M* slices results in an *M*-fold increase in speed if all other parameters, such as slice thickness, are unchanged; hence, the examination time for standard protocols could be significantly reduced, which is clinically important for trauma victims and non-cooperative patients. Alternatively, the scan range that could be covered within a certain scan time was extended by a factor of *M*, relevant for oncological screening or for CTAs of the extremities. The most important clinical benefit, however, turned out to be the possibility to scan a given volume in a given time with substantially smaller slice width, at a transverse resolution *M* times higher, to approach the goal of isotropic resolution. Thorax and abdomen examinations could now routinely be performed with 1- or 1.25-mm collimated slice width. As a consequence, volumetric viewing and diagnosis in a volumetric mode have become integrated elements of the routine work flow. New applications have been introduced in clinical practice, the most important application being cardiac CT. With a gantry rotation time of 0.5 s and dedicated image reconstruction approaches, the temporal resolution of an image could be reduced to 250 ms or less (Kachelriess et al. 2000b; Ohnesorge et al. 2000), which proved to be sufficient for motion-free imaging of the heart in the mid- to end-diastolic phase at low to moderate heart rates. Due to the increased scan speed with four simultaneously acquired slices, coverage of the entire heart volume with thin slices (down to 4×1-mm collimation) within the time of one held breath became feasible. The improved transverse resolution in combination with the excellent low-contrast detectability of modern CT systems allowed for high-resolution CTAs of the coronary arteries (Achenbach et al. 2000; Becker et al. 2000; Knez et al. 2000; Nieman et al. 2001). In the meantime, first clinical studies have demonstrated the potential of multi-slice CT to not only detect but characterize lipid, fibrous and calcified plaques in the coronary arteries according to their CT density (Schroeder et al. 2001).

Despite all promising advances, clinical challenges and limitations remain for 4-slice CT systems. True isotropic resolution for routine applications has not yet been reached, since the transverse resolution of approximately 1 mm does not fully match the in-plane resolution of approximately 0.5 mm. For long-term studies, such as peripheral CTAs, even thicker slices (2.5-mm collimated slice width) have to be chosen for acceptable scan times. Scan times are often still too long to allow for CTAs in the purely arterial phase. For a CTA of the circle of Willis, for instance, a scan range of approximately 100 mm has to be covered. With 4-slice scanning at 1-mm collimated slice width using a pitch of 1.5 (for the pitch definition with multi-slice CT refer to section 1.3.1) and 0.5-s gantry rotation time this takes approximately 9 s, not fast enough to avoid venous overlay assuming a cerebral circulation time of less than 5 s. In cardiac examinations, stents or severely calcified arteries cannot yet be adequately visualized and suffer from "blooming", mainly due to partial-volume artefacts as a consequence of the still not fully sufficient transverse resolution (Nieman et al. 2001). For patients with higher heart rates, careful selection of separate reconstruction intervals for left and right coronary artery becomes mandatory (Kopp et al. 2001), yet a diagnostic outcome cannot be guaranteed in this case. The scan time of approximately 40 s required to cover the entire heart volume (~12 cm) with 4×1-mm collimation is at the limit for a single breath-hold scan, and it may be problematic for patients who cannot adequately cooperate.

Consequently, more than four simultaneously acquired slices combined with sub-millimeter collimation for routine clinical applications have been the next step on the way towards true isotropic scanning with multi-slice CT, leading to the introduction of 16-slice CT systems in 2001 (Flohr et al. 2002a). To improve the temporal resolution of cardiac imaging in a clinically stable way, gantry rotation times have been further reduced to 0.42 s (Flohr et al. 2002b).

In this overview chapter, we concentrate on the technical bases of multi-slice CT, as they apply to established 4-slice systems as well as to the new generation of 16-slice scanners. We give an overview on system properties and on the detector design, distinguishing between fixed-array and adaptive-array detectors. We discuss dose efficiency and briefly examine dose reduction techniques. We describe multi-slice spiral scan- and image reconstruction techniques. We show that the cone-angle of the measurement rays can be neglected for established 4-slice CT systems. We introduce a new type of multi-slice spiral reconstruction, the z-filtering approach, which is now standard in most 4-slice scanners, though in manufacturer-dependent realizations (Taguchi and Aradate 1998; Schaller et al. 2000a). We demonstrate that the cone-beam geometry has to be considered for 16-slice systems, leading to novel image reconstruction approaches such as advanced single-slice rebinning (ASSR; Larson et al. 1998; Kachelriess et al. 2000a), adaptive multiple plane reconstruction (AMPR; Schaller et al. 2001; Flohr et al. 2003) or 3D backprojection. We elaborate on ECG-gated spiral scanning with increased gantry rotation speed. We briefly discuss clinical applications and end with an outlook on the potential further road map of medical CT.

1.2 Detector Design, Dose and Dose Efficiency, Dose Reduction Concepts

In the following sub-sections we give an overview on the relevant system parameters for volumetric scanning with multi-slice CT. We discuss detector design, dose and dose efficiency, and give a short overview on dose reduction techniques.

1.2.1 Detector Design

For clinical purposes different slice widths must be available to adjust the optimum compromise between scan speed, transverse resolution and image noise for each application. With a single-slice CT detector, different collimated slice widths are obtained by pre-patient collimation of the X-ray beam. A very elementary model of an *M*-slice CT detector consists of *M* detector rows: only for $M = 2$, however, can different slice widths be realized by pre-patient collimation. For $M > 2$ this simple design principle encounters its limitations. It has to be replaced by more flexible concepts requiring more than *M* detector rows to simultaneously acquire *M* slices. The signals of these detector rows are combined differently according to the selected beam collimation. For established 4-slice CT systems, two different detector types are commonly used. The fixed-array detector consists of detector elements with equal sizes in the transverse direction. A representative example (GE Lightspeed) has 16 detector rows, each of them defining 1.25-mm collimated slice width in the centre of rotation (Hu et al. 2000). The total coverage in the transverse direction is 20 mm at iso-centre; due to geometrical magnification, the actual detector is approximately twice as wide. By pre-patient collimation and combination of the signals of the individual detector rows, the following slice widths (measured at iso-centre) can be realized: 4×1.25 mm; 4×2.5 mm; 4×3.75 mm; and 4×5 mm (see Fig. 1.1a). The adaptive array detector consists of detector rows with different sizes in the transverse direction. A representative example (Siemens SOMATOM Sensation 4) has 8 detector rows (Klingenbeck-Regn et al. 1999; Ohnesorge et al. 1999). Their widths in the transverse direction range from 1 to 5 mm (at iso-centre) and allow for the following collimated slice widths: 2×0.5 mm; 4×1 mm; 4×2.5 mm; 4×5mm; 2×8 mm; and 2×10 mm (see Fig. 1.1b). The adaptive-array detector is designed for optimum dose efficiency, as the width of the detector rows is tailored to the available beam collimations and unnecessary cuts and dead zones are avoided. The selection of the collimated slice width determines the intrinsic transverse resolution of a scan. In a "step-and-shoot" axial mode, any multiple of the collimated width of one detector slice can be obtained by adding the detector signals during image reconstruction. In a spiral mode, the effective slice width, which is defined as the full width at half maximum (FWHM) of the spiral slice sensitivity profile (SSP), is adjusted independently in the spiral interpolation process during image recon-

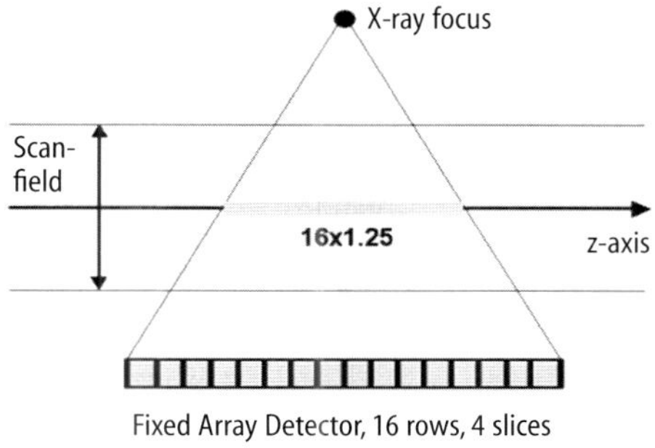

a

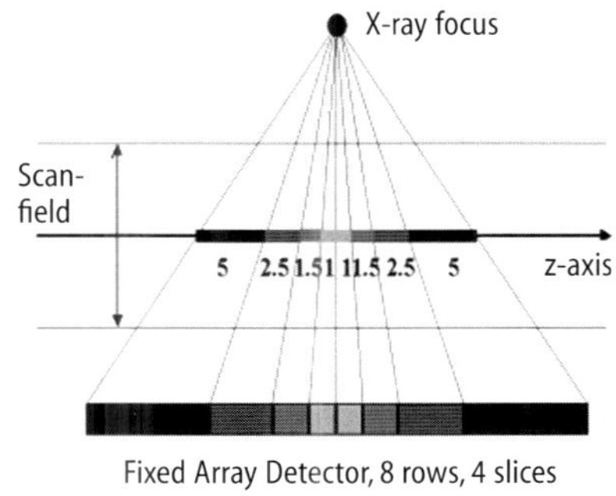

b

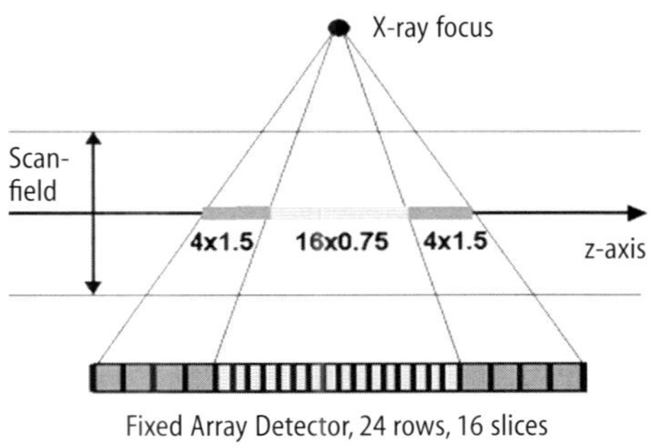

c

Fig. 1.1. Examples of fixed-array detectors and adaptive-array detectors used in commercially available 4-slice and 16-slice CT systems struction (see below); hence, from the same data set both narrow slices for high-contrast details or as an input to 3D postprocessing and wide slices for low contrast information and/or overview and filming may be derived.

The recently introduced 16-slice CT systems have adaptive-array detectors in general. A representative example (Siemens SOMATOM Sensation 16) uses 24 detector rows (Flohr et al. 2002a). The 16 central rows define 0.75-mm collimated slice width at iso-centre, and the 4 outer rows on both sides define 1.5-mm collimated slice width (see Fig. 1.1c). The total coverage in the transverse direction is 24 mm at iso-centre. By appropriate combination of the signals of the individual detector rows, either 12 or 16 slices with 0.75- or 1.5-mm collimated slice width can be acquired simultaneously. A similar design (GE Lightspeed 16) provides 16 slices with either 0.625 mm or 1.25 mm collimated slice width (Hsieh 2003).

1.2.2
Dose and Dose Efficiency

For multi-slice CT scanning a certain dose increase compared with single-slice CT is unavoidable due to the underlying physical principles. The collimated dose profile is a trapezoid in the transverse direction. This is a consequence of the finite length of the focal spot and the pre-patient collimation. In the plateau region of the trapezoid, X-rays emitted from the entire area of the focal spot illuminate the detector. In the penumbra regions only a part of the focal spot illuminates the detector while other parts are blocked off by the pre-patient collimator. With single-slice CT, the entire trapezoidal dose profile can contribute to the detector signal and the collimated slice width is determined as the FWHM of this trapezoid. With multi-slice CT, only the plateau region of the dose profile may be used to ensure equal signal level for all detector slices. The penumbra region has to be discarded, either by a post-patient collimator or by the intrinsic self-collimation of the multi-slice detector, and represents "wasted" dose. The relative contribution of the penumbra region increases with decreasing slice width, and it decreases with increasing number of simultaneously acquired slices. This is demonstrated by Fig. 1.2, which compares the "minimum width" dose profiles for a 4-slice CT system and a corresponding 16-slice CT system with equal collimated width of one detector slice. Correspondingly, the relative dose utilization of a representative 4-slice CT scanner (SOMATOM Sensation 4, Siemens, Forchheim, Germany) is 70% for 4×1-mm

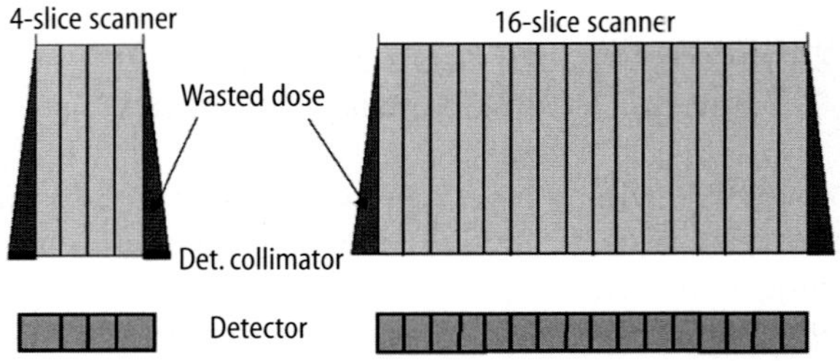

Fig. 1.2. Dose profiles for a 4-slice CT system and a 16-slice CT system with equal collimated width of one detector slice. The relative contribution of the penumbra region, which represents wasted dose, decreases with increasing number of simultaneously acquired slices

collimation and 85% for 4×2.5-mm collimation. A comparable 16-slice CT system (SOMATOM Sensation 16) has an improved dose utilization of 76 and 82%, respectively, for 16×0.75-mm collimation, and 85 and 89%, respectively, for 16×1.5-mm collimation, depending on the size of the focal spot (large and small, respectively). A clinically appropriate measure for dose is the weighted computerized tomographic dose index ($CTDI_w$), which is measured using a 16-cm Lucite phantom for head and a 32-cm Lucite phantom for body. The $CTDI_w$ is determined as one-third of the CTDI value in the centre plus two-thirds of the CTDI value at the periphery of the phantom. Figure 1.3 shows $CTDI_w$ for the 32-cm body phantom as a function of the total collimated width of the detector for the 4-slice CT system and the 16-slice CT system. With 16 simultaneously acquired slices, sub-millimeter collimation is available at reasonable dose efficiency and is therefore ready for routine scanning.

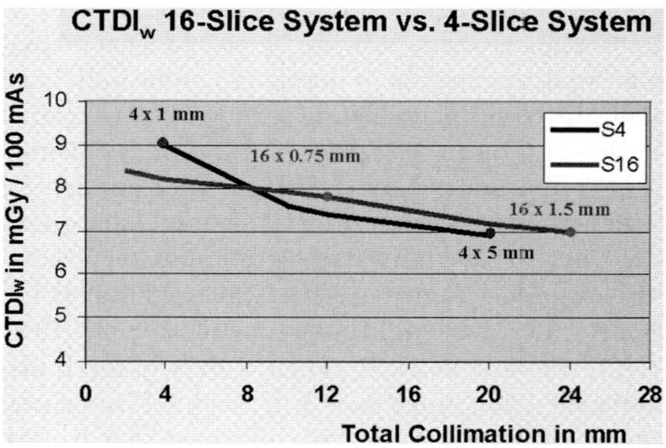

Fig. 1.3. $CTDI_W$ for the 32 cm body phantom as a function of the total collimated width of the detector for the 4-slice CT system and the 16-slice CT system

1.2.3 Dose Reduction Concepts

The most important potential for dose reduction is an adaptation of the dose to the patient size (Donelly et al. 2001; Frush et al. 2002). As a rule of thumb, the dose necessary to maintain constant image noise has to be increased by a factor of 2 if the patient diameter is increased by 4 cm. Correspondingly, for patients 4 cm smaller than the average, half the standard dose is sufficient for adequate image quality, which is of tremendous importance in paediatric scanning. Most CT-manufacturers therefore offer dedicated paediatric protocols, e.g. with dose recommendations according to the weights of the children. For contrast-enhanced examinations, such as CTA, lowering the tube voltage to 80 or 100 kV results in an increased contrast-to-noise ratio if the dose is maintained. Correspondingly, for equivalent contrast-to-noise ratio the patient dose can be decreased. Clinical studies have demonstrated a dose reduction potential of approximately 50% when using 80 kV instead of 120 kV for CTA (Schaller et al. 2001b). Practically, the maximum tube current available at 80 kV, which is generally not sufficient to scan obese patients, limits the application spectrum. In that case an intermediate X-ray voltage, e.g. 100 kV, is helpful in applications such as thoracic CTA or cardiac CTA. In anatomical dose modulation approaches the tube output is adapted to the patient geometry during each rotation of the scanner to compensate for strongly varying X-ray attenuations in asymmetrical body regions such as shoulder and pelvis. Depending on the body region, dose can be reduced by 15–35% without degradation of image quality (Greess et al. 2000). In more elaborate approaches, the tube output is modified according to the patient geometry in the transverse direction to maintain adequate dose when moving to different body regions, e.g. from thorax to abdomen (automatic exposure control). In the special case of ECG-gated spiral scanning for cardiac applications, dose can be reduced by 30–50% using ECG-controlled dose modulation (Jakobs et al. 2002). During the spiral scan, the output of the X-ray tube is modulated according to the patient's ECG. It is kept at its nominal value during a user-defined phase of the cardiac cycle, in general the mid- to end-diastolic phase. During the rest of the cardiac cycle, the tube output is reduced to 20% of its nominal value. The tube current is not switched off but kept at 20% of its nominal value to allow for image reconstruction throughout the entire cardiac cycle. Even though their signal-to-noise ratio is decreased, the low-dose images are sufficient for functional evaluation.

1.3 General-Purpose Multi-Slice Spiral CT

1.3.1 Definition of the Spiral Pitch

An important parameter to characterize a spiral scan is the pitch. According to IEC specifications the pitch p is given by

$$p = \text{table feed per rotation/total width of the collimated beam} \qquad (1)$$

This definition holds for single-slice CT as well as for multi-slice CT. It shows whether data acquisition occurs with gaps ($p>1$) or with overlap in the transverse direction ($p<1$). With 16×0.75-mm collimation and a table feed of 18 mm/rotation, the pitch is $p=18/12=1.5$. With 4×1-mm collimation and a table feed of 6 mm/rotation, the pitch is $p=6/4=1.5$, too. In the early days of 4-slice CT, the term volume pitch has been additionally introduced, which uses the width of one single slice in the denominator. For a beam collimation of 16×0.75 mm, the beam consists of 16 sub-beams, each 0.75 mm wide at the centre of rotation. With 18-mm table feed per rotation, the volume pitch is $p_{vol}=18/0.75=24$. For the sake of clarity, the volume pitch should no longer be used.

1.3.2 The Cone-Angle Problem and Multi-Slice Spiral Reconstruction Approaches

Two-dimensional image reconstruction approaches used in commercially available single-slice CT scanners, such as the convolution-backprojection reconstruction, require all measurement rays contributing to an image to run in a plane perpendicular to the patient's transverse axis (the z-axis). In multi-slice CT systems this condition is violated. Figure 1.4 shows the geometry of a 4-slice scanner: the measurement rays are tilted by the so-called cone-angle relative to a plane perpendicular to the z-axis. The cone-angle is largest for the slices at the outer edges of the detector and it increases with increasing number of detector rows. As a first approximation, the cone-angle of the measurement rays is neglected in multi-slice CT reconstruction approaches: the rays are treated as if they travelled perpendicular to the z-axis, and modified two-dimensional image reconstruction algorithms are used. The data, however, are then inconsistent. This gives rise to cone-beam artefacts at high-contrast objects such

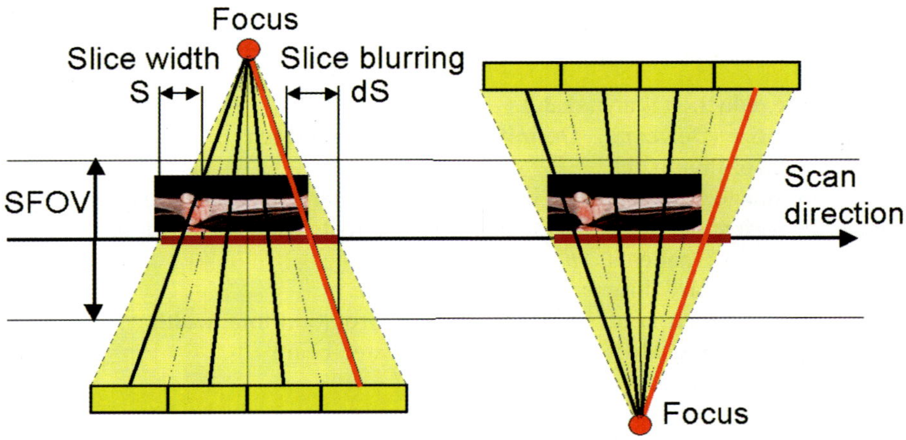

Fig. 1.4. Geometry of a 4-slice scanner illustrating the cone-angle problem: the measurement rays are tilted by the so-called cone-angle with respect to the center plane. If the positions of X-ray tube and detector are interchanged, different measurement values are acquired

as bones: if the positions of X-ray tube and detector are interchanged, the same measurement values are acquired with a single-slice CT system, but they are not with a multi-slice CT system due to the cone-angle of the measurement rays. The slices with nominal slice width s, defined as the FWHM of the SSP at iso-centre, suffer from widening and a degradation of the SSP (see Fig. 1.4). The slice broadening δs is a good indicator whether it is justified to neglect the cone angle of the measurement rays for a given scanner geometry. For the outmost detector row of a multi-slice CT scanner δs is given by

$$\frac{\delta s}{s} = (M-1)\frac{R_{FOV}}{R_F} \qquad (2)$$

where R_F is the focus-iso-centre distance, R_{FOV} is the diameter of the scan field of view.

It has been demonstrated (Saito and Suzuki 1998) that the ratio $\delta s/s$ should not exceed 1 to keep cone-beam artefacts at a level tolerable for medical CT. Using the typical geometry of a medical CT system (R_{FOV} = 250 mm and $R_F \approx$ 600 mm) we obtain for the maximum number of simultaneously acquired slices ≤4. As a consequence, the image reconstruction approaches of all commercially available 4-slice CT systems and of some with even more slices neglect the cone-angle of the measurement rays and either extend 180 or 360° single-slice spiral interpolation techniques to multi-slice spiral scanning (180° or 360° MLI; see Hu 1999), or they introduce generalized z-filtering approaches (Taguchi and Aradate 1998, Schaller et al. 2000a). An example for a z-filter approach is the adaptive axial interpolation of the SOMATOM Sensation 4 (Siemens, Forchheim, Germany; Schaller et al. 2000a). While these approaches are adequate for 4 slices, they will lead to artefacts and image quality degradation if applied to spiral scanning with 8 slices and more. This can be demonstrated by simulating and reconstructing CT data for virtual scanner geometries with 4×1, 8×1, 12×1 and 16×1-mm collimation. Calculated CT data of a mathematical thorax phantom, all at pitch 1.5 for the respective geometry, have been reconstructed using 180° MLI. Figure 1.5 shows oblique multiplanar reformations (MPRs) of the images. The image quality of the virtual 4-slice system is the clinically accepted standard. Compared with that, the MPRs of the 8-slice scanner show streak artefacts and geometrical deformations of the ribs. For the 16-slice scanner, the image quality is no longer clinically acceptable. For CT systems with 8, 12 or 16 slices, the cone angle of the measurement rays can no longer be neglected, and modified reconstruction approaches are required. Two different types of cone-beam reconstruction algorithms are currently implemented in state-of-the art 16-slice CT systems. The first one uses 3D backprojection and generalizes the Feldkamp algorithm (Feldkamp et al. 1984), which was originally introduced for sequential cone-beam scanning, to spiral scanning. The second reconstruction approach is based on nutating-slice algorithms, which split up the 3D reconstruction into a series of 2D reconstructions on tilted intermediate image planes individually adapted to the local curvature of the spiral path. An example is the AMPR implemented in the Somatom Sensation 16 (Schaller et al. 2001a, Flohr et al. 2003).

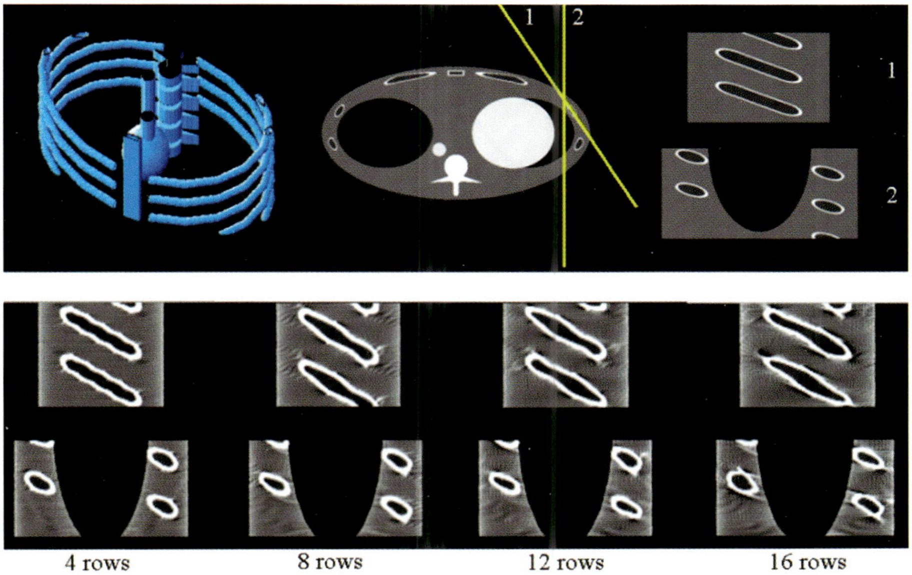

Fig. 1.5. *Top:* Mathematical model of an anthropomorphic thorax phantom. *Bottom:* Multiplanar reformations (MPRs) for virtual CT scanners with 4×1, 8×1, 12×1 and 16×1-mm collimation. The 180° MLI neglecting the cone angle of the measurement rays has been used for image reconstruction of the multi-slice spiral CT data at pitch 1.5

1.3.3 Four-Slice Spiral CT: 180° and 360° Multi-Slice Linear Interpolation

1.3.3.1 Theory

The 360° and 180° LI single-slice spiral reconstruction approaches can be extended to multi-slice spiral scanning in a straightforward way (Schaller et al. 2000b, Hu 1999). Both 360° and 180° MLI are characterized by a projection-wise linear interpolation between two rays on either side of the image plane at z_{ima}. The cone angle of the measurement rays is not taken into account, and the rays are treated as if they travelled perpendicular to the patient axis. To account for the multi-slice geometry, the interpolation is not restricted to data from the same detector slice. Instead, the interpolation may also be performed between two rays of different slices, if those rays are closest to the image plane for the projection angle under consideration.

In the 360° MLI spiral reconstruction approach, rays measured at the same projection angle in consecutive rotations of the scanner (i.e. 360° apart) are used for spiral interpolation. Mathematically, for each projection angle α_n only rays measured at $\alpha_n \pm 2\pi k$, k integer, may contribute to the image. k=0 means that the interpolation is performed between two rays of different detector slices measured simultaneously at the same projection angle.

In the 180° MLI spiral reconstruction approach, both direct and complementary rays are used for spiral interpolation. After half a rotation of the scanner (i.e. after 180°), X-ray tube and detector have interchanged their positions, and the central ray, which is now the so-called complementary ray, is measured along the same direction as the corresponding direct ray. Due to the fan-beam geometry, this correlation is only valid for the central ray. For off-center rays at fan angle β the complementary ray is not obtained after exactly half a rotation of the scanner, but after $180° + 2\beta$. Mathematically, for each projection angle α_n, all rays measured at $\alpha_n \pm 2\pi k$ and at

$$\alpha_n(\beta) = \alpha_n + 2\beta \pm (2k-1)\,\pi, \tag{3}$$

k integer, are potential interpolation partners. From all these rays, those two are selected which lie closest to the image plane. In contrast to 180° LI single-slice spiral interpolation, where interpolation partners are always measured at opposite projection angles, interpolation partners in 180° MLI multi-slice spiral interpolation can be measured at opposite or corresponding projection angles. As a consequence of the complicated z-sampling schemes and deviating from single-slice spiral CT, the spiral SSPs for 180° MLI are not necessarily smaller than those for 360° MLI. The 180 and 360° MLI for a 4-slice spiral are schematically illustrated in Fig. 1.6.

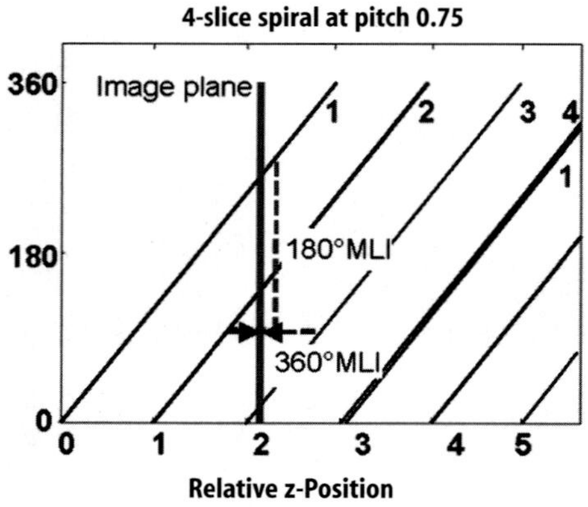

Fig. 1.6. The 180° and 360° MLI for the example of a 4-slice CT system at pitch 0.75. The projection angle of the 4 detector slices is indicated as a function of their relative z-position. For 360° MLI rays measured at the same projection angle are used, which may be either taken from subsequent rotations or from different detector slices in the same rotation. For 180° MLI rays from opposite directions are used, which are shifted by 180° in the center of rotation

1.3.3.2 Properties

In summary, 180° and 360° MLI are characterized by the following properties.

1. The effective slice width d (FWHM of the spiral SSP) is a complicated function of the spiral pitch, varying between d=1.27 s at even pitch and somewhat smaller values in-between (minimum d=s). s is the collimated slice width of the detector (Hu 1999, Schaller et al. 2000a).
2. The image noise for fixed milliampere value (fixed tube current) is a complicated function of the spiral pitch. All even pitch values show low image noise; in between, noise is considerably increased (Hu 1999).
3. Similar to single-slice CT, the dose for fixed tube current decreases monotonously with increasing pitch.
4. Spiral artefacts gradually increase with increasing pitch.

As a consequence of this behaviour, 4-slice CT scanners relying on 180° or 360° MLI techniques generally offer few discrete pitch values to the user, such as 0.75 and 1.5 (Hu 1999, Hu et al. 2000). These pitch values are intended to provide optimized sampling schemes in the transverse direction and hence optimized image quality.

1.3.4 Four-Slice Spiral CT: z-Filter Approaches

1.3.4.1 Theory

To maintain free selection of the pitch, more versatile multi-slice spiral reconstruction approaches are necessary. In a z-filter multi-slice spiral reconstruction (Taguchi and Aradate 1998; Schaller et al. 2000a), the spiral interpolation for each projection angle is no longer restricted to the two rays in closest proximity to the image plane. Instead, all rays within a selectable distance $|z_{max}|$ from the image plane contribute to the image. Still, the cone angle of the measurement rays is neglected. A 2D raw data set in parallel geometry at the desired image z-position z_{ima} is generated by adding up contributions from all projections at corresponding or opposite projection angles. The weight of contribution depends on the distance of the respective measurement ray from the image plane. The weighting function is selectable, which allows to adjust both the functional form and the FWHM of the spiral SSP. A representative example for a z-filter approach is the adaptive axial interpolation implemented in the SOMATOM Sensation 4 (Siemens, Forchheim, Germany; Schaller et al. 2000a), which is illustrated in Fig. 1.7. The

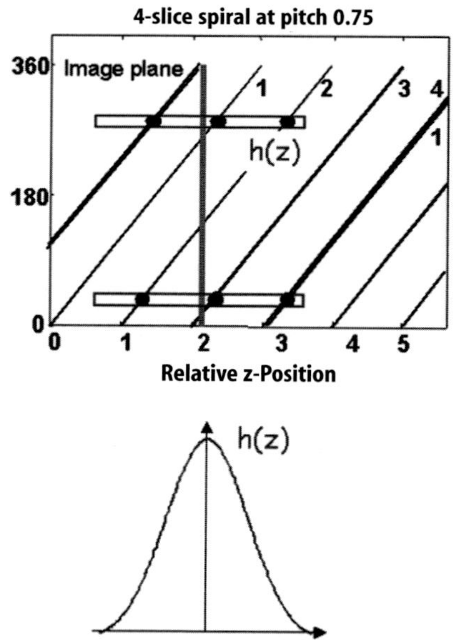

Fig. 1.7. A z-filtering reconstruction (adaptive axial interpolation) for the example of a 4-slice CT system at pitch 0.75. Contributions from all projections at corresponding or opposite projection angles are used. The weight of contribution depends on the distance of the respective measurement ray from the image plane. The weighting function $h(z)$ is selectable

larger $|z_{max}|$ is, the more the spiral SSP widens. The functional form of the SSP can be modified by the use of appropriate linear and non-linear weighting functions, which are stored in tables and are therefore easily exchangeable. With the adaptive axial interpolation, a new concept of multi-slice spiral scanning has been introduced (Klingenbeck-Regn et al. 1999; Schaller et al. 2000a): the spiral pitch is freely selectable, the functional form of the SSP and consequently the slice width, which is the FWHM of the spiral SSP, are independent of the pitch. A major reason why a pitch-independent SSP can be realized is the sampling scheme with multiple slices along the z-direction. Although both sampling pattern and sampling density vary with the pitch, the sampling distance in the center of rotation is never larger than the sub-beam collimation for any pitch up to 2. To achieve a constant SSP, the functional forms and the widths of the spiral weighting functions are automatically adapted to the pitch. Figure 1.8 shows the SSPs of the 2-mm slice (for 4×1-mm collimation) for selected pitch values. As a consequence of the pitch-independent spiral slice width, the image noise for fixed tube current would decrease with decreasing pitch due to the increasingly overlapping spiral acquisition. Instead wih the SOMATOM Sensation 4, the tube current (mA) is automatically adapted to the pitch of the spiral scan to compensate for dose accumulation and to maintain constant image noise. The user selects an effective milliampere-time product (effective mAs), which is also called "volume mAs". The tube current is then automatically adjusted to pitch and rotation time according to

$$\text{mA} = \text{eff. mAs} \times 1/T_{rot} \times p \qquad (4)$$

As a consequence of Eq. (4) the patient dose is independent of the pitch p. The weighted computerized tomographic dose index CTDI_w of an examination is given by

$$\text{CTDI}_w = (\text{CTDI}_w)_n \times \text{eff. mAs} \qquad (5)$$

with $(\text{CTDI}_w)_n$ in mGy/mAs. The n in the subscript stands for normalized. The spiral dose is therefore constant and equal to the dose of a sequential scan with the same mAs. CTDI_w according to Eq. (5) is also called "volume CTDI".

1.3.4.2 Properties

In summary, multi-slice spiral scanning using adaptive axial interpolation is characterized by the following properties:

1. The effective slice width d (FWHM of the spiral SSP) is independent of the spiral pitch, which is continuously selectable in the range 0.5–2. For each collimation (e.g. 4×1 or 4×2.5 mm) a range of different slice widths is available for retrospective reconstruction (Schaller et al. 2000a, Fuchs et al. 2000).
2. The image noise for fixed effective mAs is independent of the spiral pitch (Fuchs et al. 2000).
3. The dose for fixed effective mAs is independent of the spiral pitch and equals the dose of a sequential scan with the same mAs.
4. Spiral artefacts gradually increase with increasing pitch.

The intrinsic resolution of a multi-slice spiral scan is determined by the choice of collimation, e.g. 4×1 or 4×2.5 mm. Only slice widths equal to or larger than the sub-beam collimation can be reconstructed retrospectively. For instance, the spiral slice widths 1, 1.25, 1.5, 2, 3, 4, 5, 6, 7, 8 and 10 mm are available for 4×1-mm collimation. Images with different slice

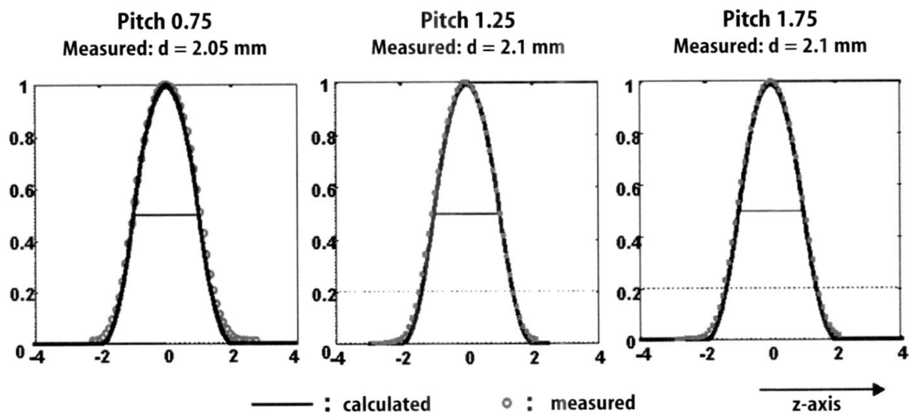

Fig. 1.8. Slice sensitivity profiles (SSPs) of the 2-mm slice (for 4×1-mm collimation) for selected pitch values using adaptive axial interpolation

widths can be obtained from the same CT raw data set, which has been widely used in clinical practice. In many cases, both thick slices for initial viewing and filming and thin slices as an input for advanced 3D post-processing are routinely reconstructed. On the other hand, a given slice width, e.g. 3 mm, can be obtained from different collimations, e.g. 4×1 and 4×2.5 mm. Narrow collimation is preferable for optimum image quality owing to a better suppression of partial-volume artifacts. Furthermore, a more rectangular SSP can be established. Figure 1.9a shows the SSPs of the 3-mm slice both for 4×1- and 4×2.5-mm collimation. Figure 1.9b shows 3-mm axial slices of a thorax-phantom scanned with 4×2.5-mm collimation and with 4×1-mm collimation. Despite higher pitch, the images obtained from 4×1-mm collimation show fewer artefacts. Similar to single-slice spiral CT, narrow collimation at high pitch is preferable to wide collimation at low pitch for artefact reduction. Best suppression of spiral artifacts is achieved by using both narrow collimation relative to the desired slice-width and reducing the spiral pitch. In general, demanding clinical protocols such as spine- and base-of-the-skull examinations rely on a combination of narrow collimation and low pitch. Some manufacturers using z-filter approaches do not provide completely free selection of the spiral pitch, but recommend a selection of fixed pitch values which are supposed to result in optimized z-sampling schemes and reduced spiral artifacts (Taguchi and Aradate 1998)

1.3.5 Overview on Cone-Beam Reconstruction Approaches

For a general-purpose CT scanner with 8 or more slices, modified reconstruction approaches taking into account the cone-beam geometry of the measurement rays should be considered. A variety of cone-beam reconstruction algorithms for axial and spiral scanning have been published thus far (e.g. Larson et al. 1998; Kachelriess et al. 2000; Feldkamp et al. 1984; Kudo et al. 1998; Schaller et al. 2000b; Turbell and Danielsson 1999; Proksa et al. 2000; Bruder et al. 2000; Katsevich 2002; Wang et al. 1993; Schaller 1998). Most of them, however, are not easily applicable to medical CT. Exact spiral reconstruction approaches (Kudo et al. 1998; Schaller et al. 2000b), relying on a 3D Radon inversion, offer a theoretically exact solution of the cone-beam reconstruction problem. They are

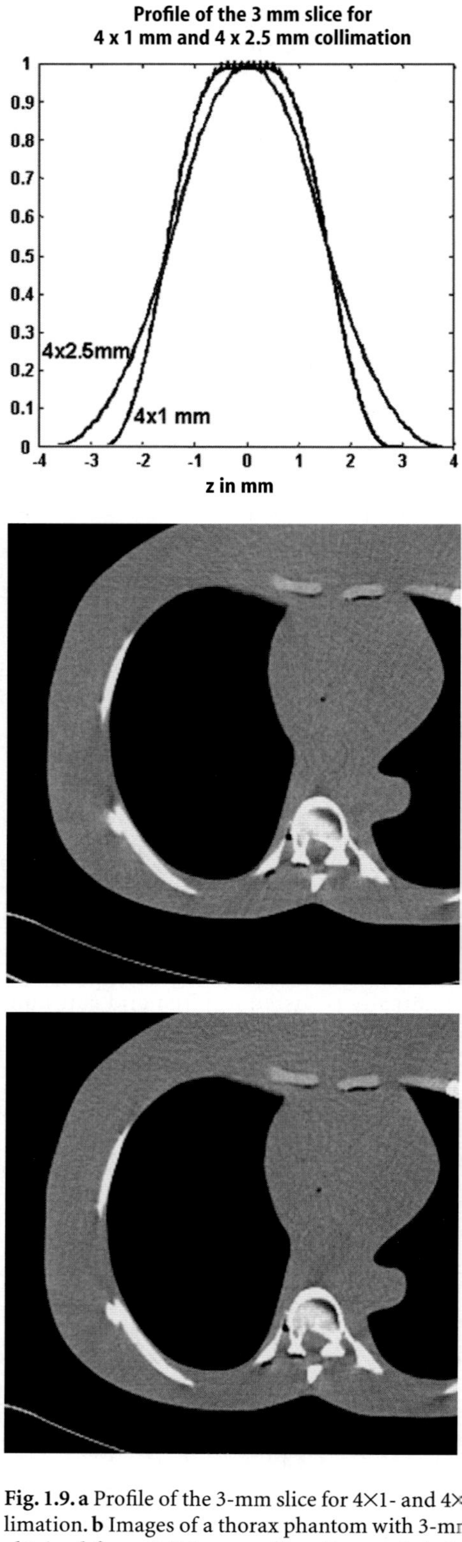

a

b

Fig. 1.9. a Profile of the 3-mm slice for 4×1- and 4×2.5-mm collimation. b Images of a thorax phantom with 3-mm slice width obtained from 4×2.5-mm collimation at pitch 0.75 (*top*) and 4×1-mm collimation at pitch 1.75 (*bottom*). Despite higher pitch, the images acquired with 4×1-mm collimation show fewer artefacts at the ribs computationally very expensive and result in image reconstruction times far away from being acceptable in a clinical environment. Recently, an exact multi-slice spiral reconstruction algorithm which is not based on 3D Radon inversion has been proposed by KATSEVICH (2002). This approach shows promising properties concerning computational complexity, yet it is in research state thus far. In the field of approximate multi-slice spiral algorithms, approximations are used to handle the cone-beam geometry. Although these algorithms are theoretically not exact, image artefacts may be controlled for a moderate number of simultaneously acquired slices and kept at a level tolerable for medical CT. The Feldkamp algorithm (FELDKAMP et al. 1984), a convolution/back-projection reconstruction which was originally introduced for axial scanning, can be extended to multi-slice spiral scanning (WANG et al. 1993; SCHALLER 1998). Using this approach, the measurement rays are back-projected into a 3D volume along the lines of measurement, in this way accounting for their cone-beam geometry. The 3D back-projection is computationally demanding and requires dedicated hardware to achieve acceptable image reconstruction times. The π methods (TURBELL and DANIELSSON 1999; PROKSA et al. 2000) or nutating slice algorithms, such as advanced single-slice rebinning (ASSR; LARSON et al. 1998; KACHELRIESS et al. 2000a), show promising properties with regard to image quality. The ASSR in particular is an effective approach to split up the 3D reconstruction into a series of conventional 2D reconstructions on tilted image planes, in this way benefiting from established and very fast 2D reconstruction techniques. Unfortunately, the π methods as well as ASSR suffer from two drawbacks: they do not provide free selection of the spiral pitch according to the clinical needs of an examination; instead, they are optimized for a fixed pitch of approximately 1.5. Even at this optimum pitch dose utilization is limited to approximately 70% for a standard fan-beam CT detector, which is problematic for medical CT. The ASSR algorithm, however, is an important intermediate step on the way towards the adaptive multiple plane reconstruction (AMPR; SCHALLER et al. 2001a; FLOHR et al. 2003), which overcomes these limitations and has been implemented in a recently introduced 16-slice CT system (SOMATOM Sensation 16, Siemens, Forchheim, Germany).

1.3.6 Sixteen-Slice Spiral CT: Adaptive Multiple Plane Reconstruction

1.3.6.1 Theory

In the ASSR, a partial scan interval (~240°) is used for image reconstruction. The image planes are no longer perpendicular to the patient axis; instead, they are tilted to match the spiral path of the focal spot (see Fig. 1.10 for a 16-slice scanner at pitch 1.5). For every viewing angle in this partial scan interval, the focal spot lies in or nearby the image plane, i.e. measurement rays running in or very close to the image plane are available for image reconstruction. These are the conditions required for a standard 2D convolution/back-projection reconstruction. In a final z-reforma-

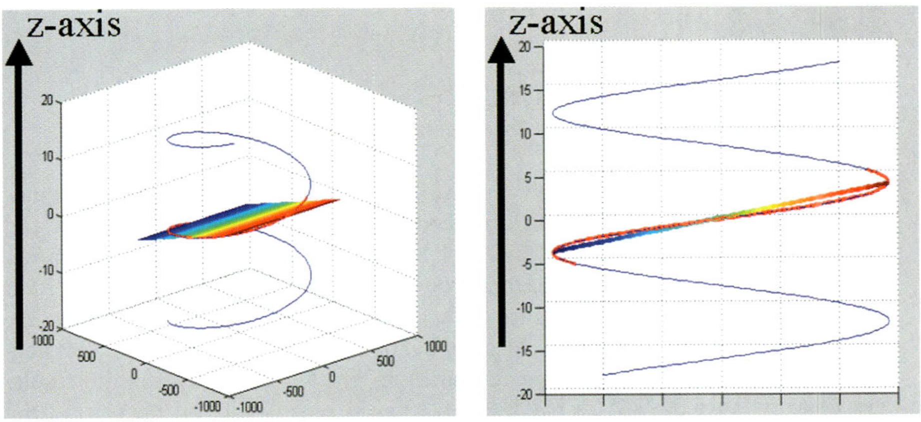

Fig. 1.10. The ASSR approach for a 16 slice CT-scanner at pitch 1.5. The *blue line* represents the spiral path of the focal spot. On the right side a projection into a plane containing the z-axis is shown, where the spiral path is represented as a *sinusoidal line*. A partial scan interval (~240° , marked in *red*) is used for image reconstruction. The intermediate image planes are no longer perpendicular to the patient axis; instead, they are tilted to match the spiral path of the focal spot

tion step, the traditional axial images are calculated by an interpolation between the tilted intermediate image planes. The ASSR has been compared with several other approximate image reconstruction approaches (Bruder et al. 2000; Koehler et al. 2002), and it has been demonstrated to provide good image quality at reasonable computational expenses. The ASSR encounters its limitations when the spiral pitch is reduced to make use of the overlapping spiral acquisition and the resulting dose accumulation. For a 16-slice scanner at pitch 0.5 two full rotations (720°) of multi-slice spiral data have to be used for every image to ensure complete dose utilization, and there is no way of tilting a single image plane to match the spiral path. A solution for this problem has been found in the adaptive multiple plane reconstruction (AMPR) algorithm (Schaller et al. 2001a; Flohr et al. 2003): instead of using all available data for one single image, it is distributed to several partial images on double oblique image planes, which are individually adapted to the spiral path. Each of these partial images has the same reference projection angle, i.e. they fan out like the pages of a book (see Fig. 1.11). To ensure full dose utilization the number of images per reference projection angle (the number of "pages" in the book) as well as the length of the data interval per image depend on the spiral pitch. The number of images varies from five, each using 360° of multi-slice spiral data, at very low pitch values, to two, each using 240° of multi-slice spiral data, at high pitch values >1. The final images with full dose utilization are calculated by a z-interpolation between the tilted partial image planes (see Fig. 1.12). Similar to the adaptive axial interpolation approach (section 1.3.4), the

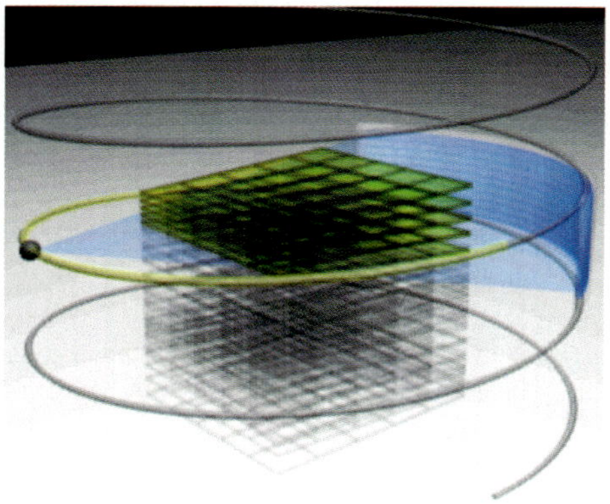

Fig. 1.11. The adaptive multiple plane reconstruction (AMPR) approach. As a first step the multi-slice spiral data are used to reconstruct several partial images on double oblique image planes, which are individually adapted to the spiral path. Each of these partial images has the same reference projection angle, i.e. they fan out like the pages of a book

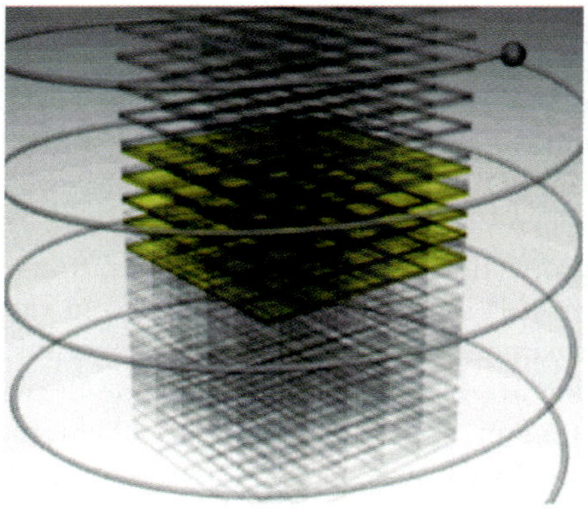

Fig. 1.12. The AMPR approach. As a second step the final images with full-dose utilization are calculated by a z-interpolation between the tilted partial image planes

shape and the width of the interpolation functions are selectable, and different SSPs and different slice widths can therefore easily be adjusted in this z-reformation step. Furthermore, by automatically adapting the functional form of the interpolation functions to the pitch, the spiral concept introduced with adaptive axial interpolation can be maintained with AMPR: the spiral pitch is continuously selectable, the slice width is independent of the pitch. Similar to adaptive axial interpolation the image noise for fixed tube current would decrease with decreasing pitch due to the increasingly overlapping spiral acquisition. Instead, the tube current (mA) is automatically adapted to the pitch of the spiral scan according to Eq. (4) to compensate for dose accumulation and to maintain constant image noise. The concept of "effective mAs" or "volume mAs" introduced in section 1.3.4.1 is also valid for AMPR.

1.3.6.2
Image Quality, Slice Sensitivity Profiles and Transverse Resolution

With the AMPR approach, excellent image quality is obtained for all pitch values between 0.5 and 1.5. In Fig. 1.13, MPRs of the mathematical thorax phantom reconstructed with AMPR are shown for a 16-slice CT scanner at pitch 1 and pitch 1.5. They are free of cone-beam artefacts and geometrical distortions, (compare to Fig. 1.5, which shows the results of a 180°-MLI spiral reconstruction neglecting the cone-angle of the measurement rays). The results of the simulation study are confirmed by phantom and patient scans. Figure 1.14 shows an axial slice and a MPR of a pelvis phantom scanned with 16×1.5-mm

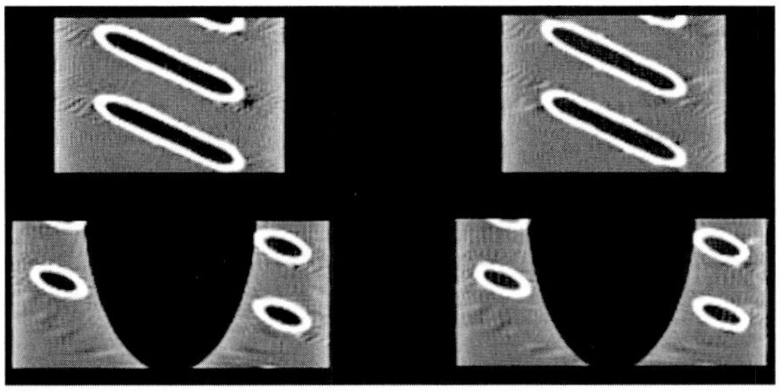

16 rows pitch 1.0 16 rows pitch 1.5

Fig. 1.13. The multi-planar reformations (MPRs) of the mathematical thorax phantom for a 16-slice CT scanner at pitch 1 and pitch 1.5, reconstructed with AMPR

collimation, 0.5-s gantry rotation time, pitch p=1, corresponding to a table feed of 48 mm/s. Scan data was reconstructed at 2-mm nominal slice width, both with the AMPR algorithm (right) and with z-filtering (left). Neglecting the cone-angle leads to severe artefacts at high-contrast objects (left). Cone artefacts are reduced with the AMPR algorithm, and the spatial integrity of the objects is restored (right). Recent studies have demonstrated the applicability of extended versions of AMPR for medical CT systems with up to 64 rows (Stierstorfer et al. 2002).

For the 16-slice CT scanner under consideration, a variety of different slice widths can be selected for retrospective reconstruction. For 16×0.75-mm collimation, the nominal slice widths 0.75, 1, 1.5, 2, 3, 4, 5, 6, 7, 8 and 10 mm are available. Using 0.5-s rotation time the table feed is adjustable between 12 and 36 mm/s. For 16×1.5-mm collimation, the nominal slice widths 2, 3, 4, 5, 6, 7, 8 and 10 mm can be selected, and the table feed is adjustable between 24 and 72 mm/s. Figure 1.15a shows measured SSPs in the iso-center at different pitch values together with calculated curves, for 16×0.75-mm collimation and 1-mm and 2-mm nominal slice width. The SSPs show only slight variations as a function of the spiral pitch. This was intended in the design of the image z-reformation step. Figure 1.15b demonstrates that the measured FWHMs of the spiral SSPs deviate less than 0.2 mm from the corresponding nominal slice widths for all pitch values. Figure 1.16 shows MPRs of a z-resolution phantom scanned with 16×0.75-mm collimation at pitch 0.75, 1.0, 1.25 and 1.5. The phantom consists of a lucite plate with rows of cylindrical holes (diameters 0.5, 0.6, 0.7, 0.8, 1.0, 1.2, 1.5, 2 and 3 mm) aligned in the transverse direction. Overlapping images with 0.75-mm nominal slice width (measured FWHM ~0.9 mm) and 0.4-mm increment were reconstructed, and MPRs in the transverse direction were calculated. Independent of the pitch all cylinders down to 0.6-mm diameter can be resolved and the MPRs are free of geometric distortions, thus proving the spatial integrity of the 3D image. With an in-plane resolution of approximately 0.5 mm using a standard body kernel and a transverse resolution of

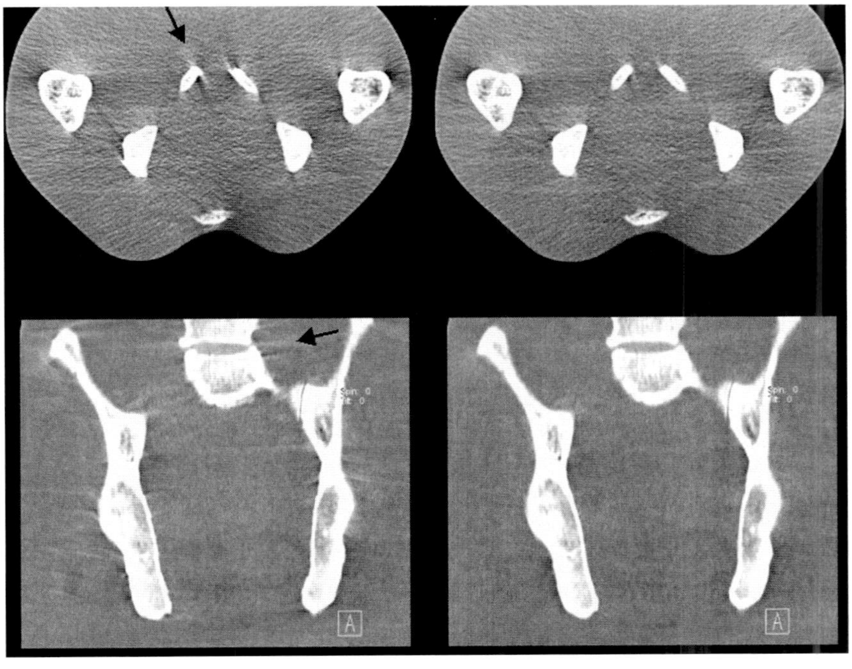

Fig. 1.14. Axial slice (*top*) and MPR (*bottom*) of the pelvis phantom, 16×1.5-mm collimation, 2-mm reconstructed slice width, 0.5-s rotation time, pitch 1.0, i.e. table feed 48 mm/s. *Left:* z-filtering multi-slice spiral reconstruction neglecting the cone-angle of the measurement rays. Cone beam-artefacts are indicated by *arrows*. *Right:* AMPR. Cone-beam artefacts are suppressed

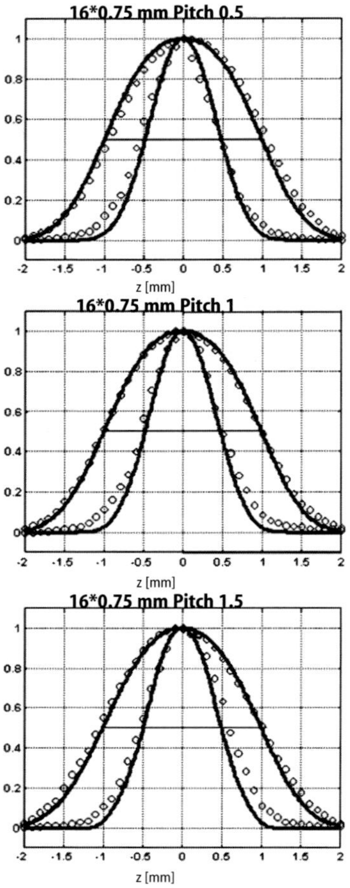

a

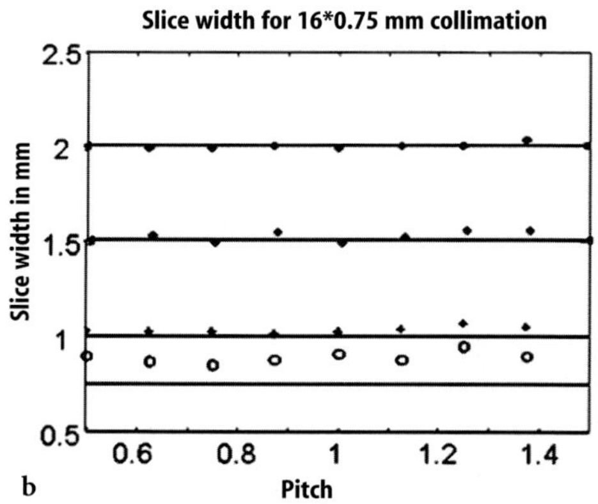

b

Fig. 1.15. a The SSPs for 1- and 2-mm slice width obtained from a scan with 16×0.75-mm collimation at pitch p=0.5 (table feed 12 mm/s), p=1 (table feed 24 mm/s) and p =1.5 (table feed 36 mm/s). *Lines* are calculated, *circles* are measured. **b** The FWHM for the nominal 0.75-, 1-, 1.5- and 2-mm slice, measured as a function of the spiral pitch. For the evaluated CT scanner, the slice width shows only minor variations as a function of the pitch.

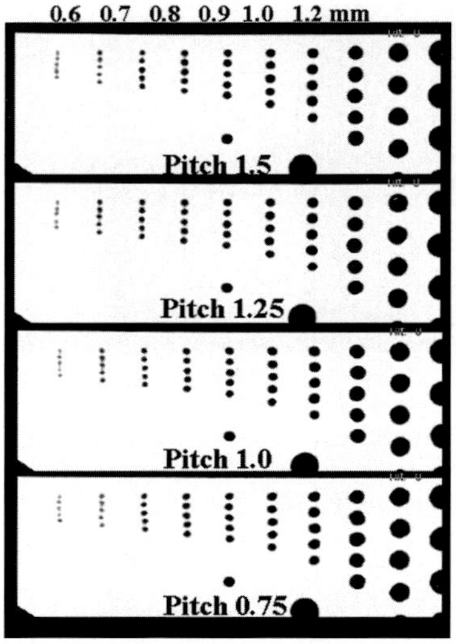

Fig. 1.16. The MPRs of a z-resolution phantom at iso-center, scanned with 16×0.75-mm collimation at pitch 0.75, 1.0, 1.25 and 1.5, reconstruction slice width 0.75 mm. Independent of the pitch, all cylinders down to 0.6-mm diameter can be resolved and the MPRs are free of geometric distortions, thus proving the spatial integrity of the 3D image

0.6 mm due to overlapping image reconstruction, the ideal of isotropic resolution for routine applications has been reached with state-of-the-art 16-slice CT systems.

1.3.6.3
Properties

In summary, multi-slice spiral scanning using AMPR is characterized by the following properties:

1. The cone-beam geometry of the measurement rays is taken into account, cone-beam artefacts are effectively suppressed. The AMPR can be expanded to medical CT systems with up to 64 rows (Stierstorfer et al. 2002).
2. The effective slice width d (FWHM of the spiral SSP) is independent of the spiral pitch, which is continuously selectable in the range 0.5–1.5. For each collimation (e.g. 16×0.75 or 16×1.5 mm) a range of different slice widths is available for retrospective reconstruction (Flohr et al. 2003).
3. The image noise for fixed effective mAs is independent of the spiral pitch.
4. The dose for fixed effective mAs is independent of the spiral pitch and equals the dose of a sequential scan with the same mAs.

1.4 ECG-Synchronized Multi-Slice CT for Cardio-Thoracic Applications

1.4.1 ECG Triggering and ECG Gating

One of the most exciting new applications of multi-slice CT is the ability to image the heart and the cardio-thoracic anatomy without motion artefacts. For ECG-synchronized examinations of the cardio-thoracic anatomy, either ECG-triggered axial scanning or ECG-gated spiral scanning can be used. In ECG-triggered axial scanning, the heart volume is covered by subsequent axial scans in a "step-and-shoot" technique. For each axial scan, the number of images corresponds to the number of active detector slices. A partial scan data interval is acquired with a pre-defined temporal offset relative to the R-waves of the patient's ECG signal which can be either relative (given as a certain percentage of the RR interval time) or absolute (given in milliseconds) and either forward or reverse (Ohnesorge et al. 2000; Flohr and Ohnesorge 2001). With retrospective ECG gating, the heart volume is covered continuously by a spiral scan. The patient's ECG signal is recorded simultaneously to allow for a retrospective selection of the data segments used for image reconstruction. Only scan data acquired in a pre-defined cardiac phase, usually the diastolic phase, is used for image reconstruction (Kachelriess et al. 2000b; Ohnesorge et al. 2000). The data segments contributing to an image start with a user-defined offset relative to the onset of the R-waves, similar to ECG-triggered axial scanning. The temporal resolution of an image can be improved up to $T_{rot}/(2\,N)$ by using scan data of N subsequent heart cycles for image reconstruction (Kachelriess et al. 2000b; Flohr and Ohnesorge 2001; Bruder et al. 1999). T_{rot} is the gantry rotation time of the CT scanner. Image reconstruction during different heart phases is feasible by shifting the start points of the data segments used for image reconstruction relative to the R-waves. For a given start position, a stack of images at different z-positions covering a small sub-volume of the heart can be reconstructed thanks to the multi-slice data acquisition (Kachelriess et al. 2000b; Ohnesorge et al. 2000; Flohr and Ohnesorge 2001). Prospective ECG triggering has the benefit of a smaller effective patient dose, since scan data is acquired in the previously selected heart phases only. It is, however, more sensitive to arrhythmia than ECG gating. Furthermore, it does not provide continuous volume coverage with overlapping slices or reconstruction of images in different phases of the cardiac cycle for functional evaluation.

1.4.2 ECG-Gated Four-Slice Spiral CT: Adaptive Cardio-Volume Reconstruction

A variety of dedicated reconstruction approaches for ECG-gated multi-slice spiral CT has been introduced with 4-slice CT scanners (Kachelriess et al. 2000b; Ohnesorge et al. 2000; Flohr and Ohnesorge 2001; Taguchi and Anno 2000). A representative example is the adaptive cardio-volume (ACV) algorithm (Flohr and Ohnesorge 2001) used in the 4-slice CT scanner SOMATOM Sensation 4 (Siemens, Forchheim, Germany). The adaptive cardio-volume reconstruction (ACV) consists of two major steps and combines a partial scan reconstruction optimized for temporal resolution with multi-slice spiral weighting to compensate for the z-movement of the patient table during the spiral scan and to provide a well-defined SSP. During multi-slice spiral weighting – the first reconstruction step – a "single-slice" partial scan data segment is generated for each image using a partial rotation of the multi-slice spiral scan data. Multi-slice spiral weighting is illustrated in Fig. 1.17. The scan data segments start with a user-defined offset relative to the

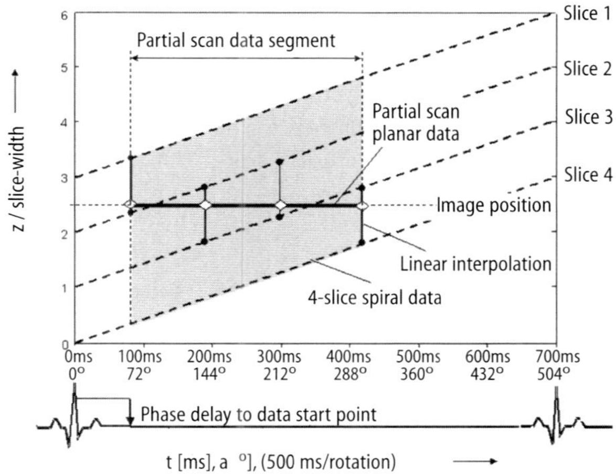

Fig. 1.17. The ECG-gated spiral interpolation scheme for a 4-slice scanner using one segment of multi-slice data for image reconstruction. The z-position of the 4 detector slices changes linearly relative to the patient due to the constant spiral feed. For each projection angle within the partial scan data segment a linear interpolation is performed between the data of those two detector slices that are in closest proximity to the desired image plane. The spiral interpolation is indicated for some representative projection angles α. On the bottom, the ECG signal is shown schematically

onset of the R-waves. For each projection angle within the data segment a linear interpolation is performed between the data of those two detector slices that are in closest proximity to the desired image plane. The cone angle of the measurement rays is neglected, and the rays are treated as if they travelled in planes perpendicular to the z-axis. Depending on the patient's heart rate during the examination, the partial scan data segment is automatically divided into one or two sub-segments. At heart rates below a certain threshold, one sub-segment of consecutive multi-slice spiral data from the same heart period is used, resulting in a constant temporal resolution of half the gantry rotation time ($T_{rot}/2$) for sufficiently centred objects. At higher heart rates, two sub-segments from adjacent heart cycles contribute to the partial scan data segment. In that case, the temporal resolution varies between $T_{rot}/4$ and $T_{rot}/2$ depending on the patient's heart rate, since the heart cycle time and the gantry rotation time have to be de-synchronized (Flohr and Ohnesorge 2001). For T_{rot}=0.5 s the threshold for two-segment reconstruction is 65 bpm, for higher heart rates the temporal resolution varies between 125 and 250 ms. Improved temporal resolution at the expense of reduced transverse resolution by the use of multi-segment reconstruction approaches can degrade the image quality of cardiac examinations by blurring coronary plaques and stenoses (Flohr and Ohnesorge 2001). In addition, multi-segment approaches encounter their limitations if the patient's heart rate is arrhythmic during examination. As a consequence, the ACV approach is limited to two segments as a maximum. Using ACV, well-defined narrow SSPs are maintained for all clinically relevant heart rates (Flohr and Ohnesorge 2001).

1.4.3 ECG-Gated Sixteen-Slice Spiral CT: Extended ACV

The ACV reconstruction as well as all other ECG-gated multi-slice spiral reconstruction approaches used so far neglect the cone-angle of the measurement rays. In section 1.3.2 we demonstrate that a cone correction becomes mandatory for general-purpose CT scanning with 8 or more slices; hence, with increasing number of simultaneously acquired slices, the question of cone correction also arises for cardiac CT. Cone artefacts are most pronounced at high contrast structures and they increase with increasing distance of the object from the iso-center. Since the heart is usually sufficiently centred and does not contain extended high-contrast structures, severe cone artefacts are not expected even for a larger number of slices. Simulated CT data of an anthropomorphic heart phantom with contrast-enhanced coronary arteries containing atherosclerotic plaques and stents was used to investigate the limits of the ACV approach for scanning with significantly more than 4 slices. Figure 1.18 shows two cross sections along the right and the left coronary artery (RCA and LAD) of the mathematical heart phantom: this is the "ideal image" which serves as a quality benchmark. Figure 1.19a shows MPRs along RCA and LAD, which are the outcome of an ACV reconstruction for a virtual CT scanner geometry with 4×1-mm collimation, 0.5-s rotation time and pitch p=0.375 (table feed 3 mm/s). Realistic noise has been added to the simulated CT data, and images with effective slice width 1.3 mm and increment 0.6 mm have been reconstructed using a standard body kernel and a fictive ECG signal with 55 bpm. The MPRs demonstrate the clinical image quality typical for established 4-slice CT systems and illustrate their performance limits: coronary plaques can be differentiated and classified according to their CT density (Hounsfield units, HU), stents suffer from blooming and artefacts. For the MPRs shown in Fig. 1.17b the ACV approach has been applied to scan data simulated for a virtual CT scanner geometry with 16×0.75-mm collimation, 0.42-s rotation time and pitch p=0.28 (table feed 8 mm/s). Images with effective slice width 1.0 mm and increment 0.5 mm have been reconstructed using an artificial ECG signal with 55 bpm. The MPRs are free of cone-beam artefacts, thus demonstrating that a cone correction is not required. Instead, due to the smaller slice width and the improved axial sampling compared with a scan with 4×1-mm collimation, the stents show fewer geometric distortions and a reduction of the blooming artefact. An extended version of ACV has therefore been

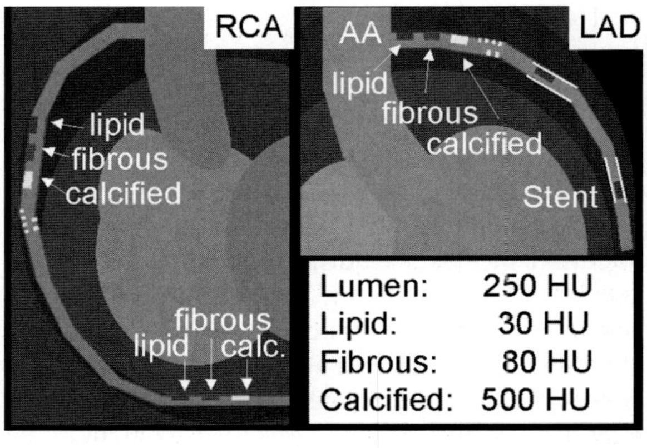

Fig. 1.18. Two cross sections along the right and the left coronary artery (*RCA, LAD*) of the mathematical heart phantom

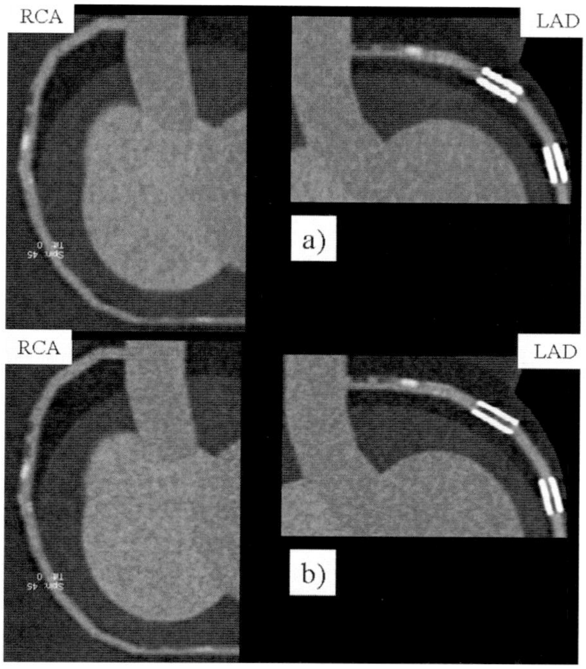

Fig. 1.19. The MPRs along RCA and LAD of the mathematical heart phantom for virtual CT scanners with **a** 4×1-mm collimation and with **b** 16×0.75-mm collimation. The ACV reconstruction of simulated CT data neglecting the cone angle of the measurement rays

implemented in the 16-slice CT scanner SOMATOM Sensation 16 (Siemens, Forchheim, Germany). Modifications of the ACV approach providing cone correction, which are currently being investigated (FLOHR et al. 2001; BRUDER et al. 2001), will be reserved to future CT systems with more than 16 slices.

Some 16-slice CT systems offer reduced gantry rotation times down to 0.4 s to improve the temporal resolution in cardiac applications. Using ACV with T_{rot}=0.42 s the threshold for two-segment reconstruction is 71 bpm. Below 71 bpm the temporal resolution is 210 ms, for higher heart rates it varies between 105 and 210 ms (see Fig. 1.20). A final z-filtering step (the z-direction is the transverse direction) is applied to the original ACV images. Shape and width of the filter functions are selectable; different SSPs and different slice widths can therefore be adjusted similar to general purpose spiral scanning. For 16×0.75-mm collimation, which is the standard protocol for ECG-gated coronary CTAs, the nominal slice widths 0.75, 1, 1.5, 2 and 3 mm are available for retrospective reconstruction. For 16×1.5-mm collimation, which is recommended for ECG-gated Ca scoring, the nominal slice widths 2, 3, 4 and 5 mm can be selected.

1.4.4 Pitch Limitations

For each heart period, a stack of images at different z-positions covering a small sub-volume of the heart is reconstructed, which is indicated as a box in Fig. 1.17. To maintain complete volume coverage, image sub-volumes reconstructed in consecutive heart cycles have to fit together in the transverse direction. As a consequence, the spiral pitch has to be limited for ECG-gated multi-slice CT examinations of the heart (OHNESORGE et al. 2000). If the table moves too fast, gaps between the image sub-volumes occur, which have to be closed by far-reaching interpolations at the expense of a loss of transverse resolution and a degradation of the SSPs. In theory, the spiral pitch could be adapted to the patient's heart rate. For maximum ease of use and clinical stability, however, one fixed pitch value for all examinations is preferable. It has been demonstrated that a table feed of 3 mm/s must not be exceeded for cardiac scanning with the ACV approach and 4×1-mm collimation (FLOHR and OHNESORGE 2001). The time to cover the entire heart volume (~12 cm) is approximately 40 s, which is at the limit for a scan within one held breath of the patient. The ECG-gated scanning of the entire thorax or the aorta with 4×1-mm collimation is not possible within reasonable scan times. For a 16-slice CT system, a table feed of 8 mm/s should not be exceeded for 16×0.75-mm collimation, both for 0.5-s and for 0.42-s gantry rotation time. Scans of a z-resolution phantom (see section 1.3.6.2) with 0.42-s rotation time, 0.75-mm reconstructed slice

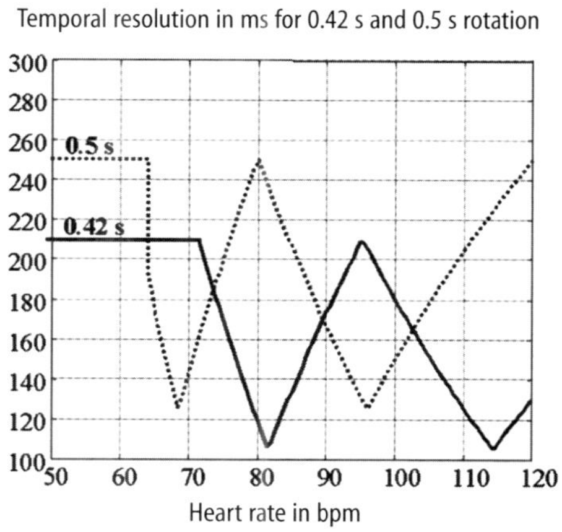

Fig. 1.20. Temporal resolution for sufficiently centred objects as a function of the heart rate for the ACV approach using 0.5- and 0.42-s gantry rotation time. For 0.42-s rotation time, the temporal resolution reaches its optimum (105 ms) at 81 bpm. This is clinically important, since without administration of beta-blockers the majority of heart rates are in the range 75–85 bpm

width and table feed 8 mm/s using artificial ECG signals with 55, 70, 80 and 90 bpm demonstrate that independent of the heart rate all cylinders down to 0.6- to 0.7-mm diameter can be resolved. The MPRs of this phantom are shown in Fig. 1.21. With an in-plane resolution of approximately 0.5 mm and a transverse resolution of 0.6 mm, the goal of isotropic resolution has also been reached for cardiac scanning with state-of-the-art 16-slice technology. The time to cover the entire heart volume (~12 cm) with 16×0.75-mm collimation is approximately 15 s. Covering the entire thorax (30 cm) with 16×0.75-mm collimation takes approximately 38 s, with 16×1.5-mm collimation it takes approximately 19 s. The ECG-gated examinations of extended cardio-thoracic morphology become feasible with 16-slice CT systems, opening a spectrum of applications which benefit from a suppression of cardiac pulsation. Typical diagnostic pitfalls caused by transmitted cardiac pulsation can be avoided, such as an artefactual intimal flap resembling dissection in the ascending aorta (Loubeyre et al. 1997). Suppression of cardiac pulsation improves the assessment of paracardiac lung segments and allows for a confident exclusion of small peripheral pulmonary emboli in segmental and subsegmental arteries (Schoepf et al. 2000) and an accurate assessment of pulmonary nodules. On routine thoracic studies that are not synchronized to the patient's ECG, cardiac motion usually precludes the assessment of coronary bypasses.

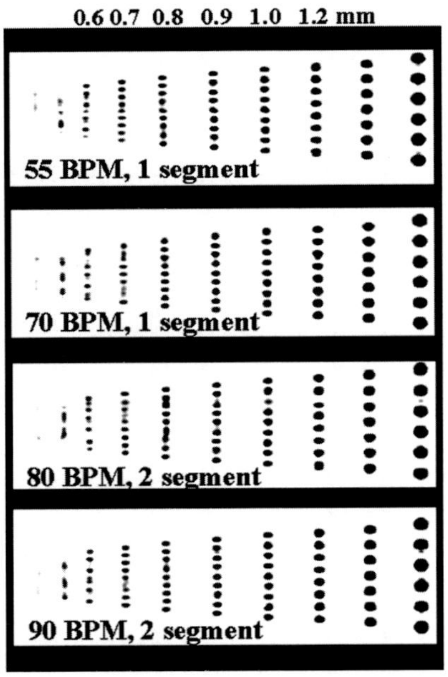

Fig. 1.21. The MPRs of a z-resolution phantom scanned with 16×0.75-mm collimation, 0.42-s rotation time and table feed 8 mm/s. Overlapping images with 0.75-mm slice width and 0.4-mm increment were reconstructed using the ACV approach and artificial ECG signals with 55, 70, 80 and 90 bpm. Independent of the heart rate, all cylinders down to 0.6- to 0.7-mm diameter can be resolved

1.5 Outlook: Future Direction of Medical CT

The latest generation of 16-slice CT systems allows for truly isotropic imaging in virtually any application. As a consequence, the distinction between transverse and in-plane resolution is gradually becoming a historical remnant, and the traditional axial slice is losing its clinical predominance. It is replaced by interactive viewing and manipulation of isotropic volume images, with only the key slices or views in arbitrary directions used for filming or stored for a demonstration of the diagnosis. Improved transverse resolution goes hand in hand with considerably reduced scan times, facilitating the examination of un-cooperative patients and reducing the amount of contrast agent needed, but also requiring optimized contrast agent protocols. New clinical applications are evolving as a result of the tremendously increased volume scan speed, such as CT angiographic examinations in the pure arterial phase. A CTA of the Circle of Willis with 16×0.75-mm collimation, 0.5-s rotation time and pitch 1.5 requires only 3.5 s for a scan range of 100 mm (table feed 36 mm/s). A thorax–abdomen CTA with sub-millimeter collimation takes approximately 17 s for a scan range of 600 mm (see Fig. 1.22 for the example of a patient who presented with Leriche syndrome; courtesy of Tübingen University, Germany). For a CTA of the renal arteries, the table feed can be reduced to 24 mm/s (pitch 1) to make better use of the tube output for obese patients (see Eq. (4)); nevertheless, the total scan time for 250 mm scan range with 16×0.75-mm collimation is not longer than 11 s. Examining the entire thorax (350 mm) with 16×0.75-mm collimation, 0.5-s rotation time and pitch 1.375 (table feed 33 mm/s) can be done in 11 s; hence, both a native and a contrast-enhanced scan can be obtained within the same breath-hold period for optimum matching of both image volumes. The ECG-gated cardiac scanning benefits both from improved temporal resolution and improved spatial resolution. Characterization and classification of coronary plaques even in the presence of severe calcifications is entering clinical routine as a consequence of the increased clinical

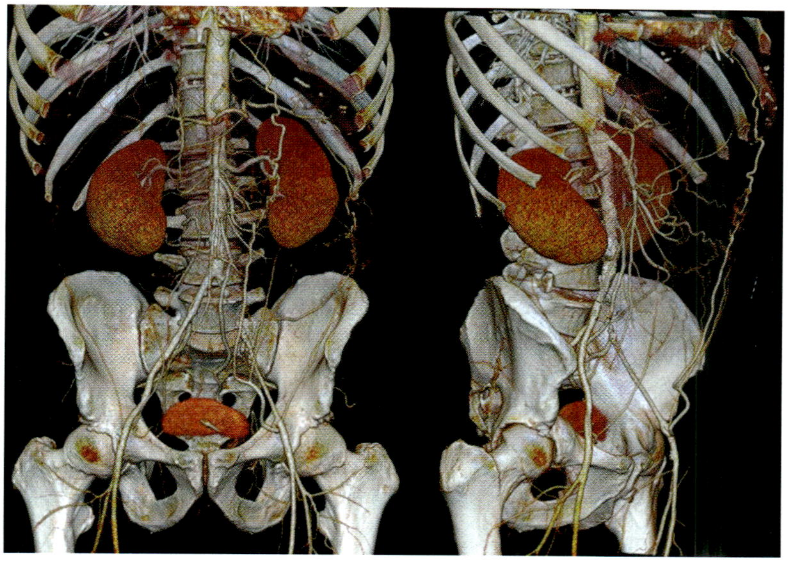

Fig. 1.22. Patient example: Leriche syndrome, scanned with 16×0.75-mm collimation (courtesy of Tübingen University, Germany)

robustness of the method. A recent study for coronary CTA with a 16-slice system on 59 patients demonstrated 86% specificity and 95% sensitivity. None of the patients had to be excluded (Nieman et al. 2002). Figure 1.23 shows the example of a patient with severe coronary artery disease and a heart rate of approximately 60 bpm during the scan (courtesy of Groningen University, The Netherlands).

With a spatial resolution of $0.5 \times 0.5 \times 0.6\ mm^3$ 16-slice CT sets the present benchmark in spatial resolution for non-invasive coronary artery imaging. Motion artefacts in patients with higher heart rates remain the most important challenge for multi-slice coronary CTA, although diagnostic image quality can be achieved in most cases by administration of beta blockers. Improved temporal resolution is desirable in the future to avoid patient preparation, requiring increased gantry rotation speed rather than multi-segment reconstruction approaches for robust clinical performance. Obviously, significant development efforts will be needed to handle the substantial increase of mechanical forces (~17 G for 0.42-s rotation time, >33 G for 0.3-s rotation time) and increased data transmission rates. Rotation times of less than 0.2 s (mechanical forces >75 G) required to provide a temporal resolution of less than 100 ms independent of the heart rate appear to be beyond the present mechanical limits. An alternative to further increased rotation speed is the re-consideration of a scanner concept with multiple tubes and multiple detectors that has been described for the first time in the early times of CT (Robb and Ritman 1979). For general-purpose CT, we will see a further increase of the number of simultaneously

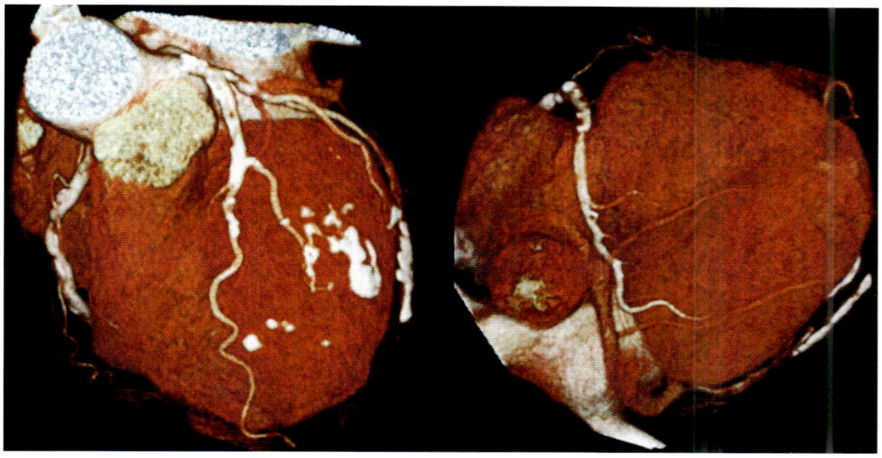

Fig. 1.23. Patient example: severe coronary artery disease (courtesy of Groningen University, The Netherlands)

acquired slices. The resulting clinical benefits, however, may not be substantial and have to be carefully considered in the light of the necessary technical efforts. Potential further improvement of the spatial resolution will have to be reserved to special applications due to the inevitable increase of dose that has to be applied for adequate signal-to-noise ratio. It will have to go along with the development of more powerful X-ray tubes and generators. Instead of a mere quantitative enhancement of scan parameters with doubtful clinical relevance, the introduction of area detectors large enough to cover the entire heart or the entire brain in one axial scan (~120 mm scan range) could bring a new quality to medical CT. With these systems dynamic volume scanning would become possible, and a whole spectrum of new applications, such as functional or volume-perfusion studies, could arise. Area detector technology is currently under development, yet no commercially available solution thus far fulfils the high requirements of medical CT concerning dynamic range of the acquisition system and fast data readout. Initial experience with the present CsJ-aSi flat panel detector technology originally used for conventional catheter angiography is limited in low contrast resolution and scan speed. Due to the intrinsic slow signal decay of flat panel detectors, rotation times of at least 20 s are needed to acquire a sufficient number of projections (600). On the other hand, high-contrast resolution is excellent due to the small detector pixel size, yet dose requirements preclude the examination of larger objects. Initial experimental results are limited to small high-contrast objects such as joints, inner ear or contrast-filled vessel specimens. Figure 1.24 shows a prototype set-up incorporating a flat panel detector into a standard CT gantry (SOMATOM Sensation 16, Forchheim, Germany). The detector covers 25×25×18 cm^3 scan field of view, and the pixel size is 250×250 μm^2, both measured in the center of rotation.

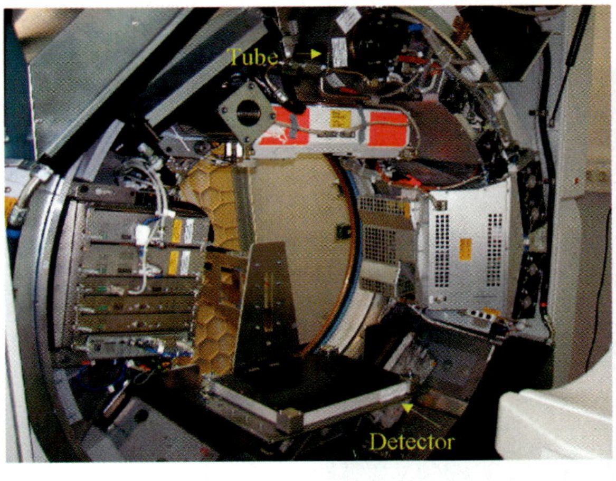

Fig. 1.24. Prototype set-up incorporating a flat-panel detector into a standard CT gantry (SOMATOM Sensation 16)

Figure 1.25 shows MPRs and VRTs of a hand specimen, demonstrating excellent spatial resolution. The combination of area detectors with sufficient quality with fast gantry rotation speeds will be a promising technical concept for medical CT systems. Due to the present technical restrictions, however, these systems will probably not be available in the near future.

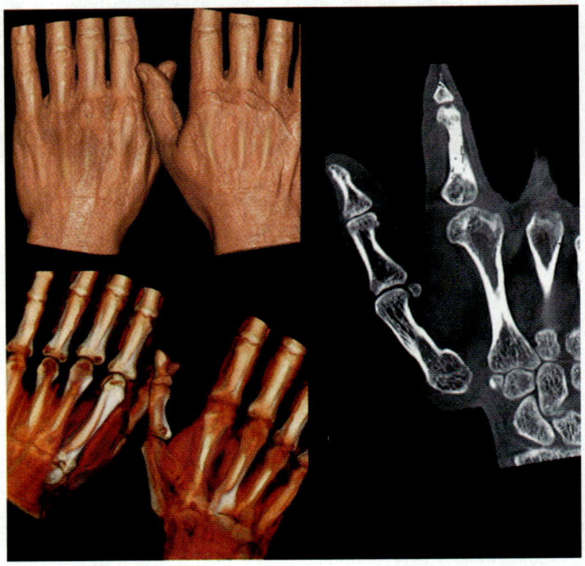

Fig. 1.25. The MPRs and VRTs of a hand specimen, scanned with a CT prototype with flat-panel detector

References

Achenbach S, Ulzheimer S, Baum U et al. (2000) Noninvasive coronary angiography by retrospectively ECG-gated multislice spiral CT. Circulation 102:2823–2828

Becker C, Knez A, Ohnesorge B, Schöpf U, Reiser M (2000) Imaging of non calcified coronary plaques using helical CT with retrospective EKG gating. AJR 175:423–424

Bruder H, Schaller S, Ohnesorge B, Mertelmeier T (1999) High temporal resolution volume heart imaging with multirow computed tomography. SPIE 3661:420–432

Bruder H, Kachelriess M, Schaller S, Stierstorfer K, Flohr T (2000) Single-slice rebinning reconstruction in spiral cone-beam computed tomography. IEEE Trans Med Imag 19:873–887

Bruder H, Stierstorfer K, Ohnesorge B, Schaller S, Flohr T (2001) Segmented cardiac volume reconstruction: a novel reconstruction scheme for multi-slice cardiac spiral CT. The 6th international meeting on fully three-dimensional image reconstruction in radiology and nuclear medicine, Pacific Grove, California

Crawford CR, King KF (1990) Computed tomography scanning with simultaneous patient translation. Med Phys 17:967–982
Donelly LF, Emery KH, Brody AS et al. (2001) Minimizing radiation dose for pediatric body applications of single-detector helical CT: strategies at a large children's hospital. AJR 176: 303–306
Feldkamp LA, Davis LC, Kress JW (1984) Practical cone-beam algorithm. J Opt Soc Am A 1:612–619
Flohr T, Ohnesorge B (2001) Heart-rate adaptive optimization of spatial and temporal resolution for ECG-gated multi-slice spiral CT of the heart. J Comput Assist Tomogr 25:907–923
Flohr T, Bruder H, Stierstorfer K, Schaller S, Ohnesorge B (2001) Cone-beam reconstruction for ECG-gated multislice spiral CT of the heart with optimized temporal resolution. Abstract book of the 87th Scientific Assembly and Annual Meeting of the RSNA
Flohr T, Stierstorfer K, Bruder H, Simon J, Schaller S (2002a) New technical developments in multislice CT. Part 1: Approaching isotropic resolution with sub-millimeter 16-slice scanning. Fortschr Röntgenstr 174:839–845
Flohr T, Bruder H, Stierstorfer K, Simon J, Schaller S, Ohnesorge B (2002b) New technical developments in multislice CT. Part 2: Sub-millimeter 16-slice scanning and increased gantry rotation speed for cardiac imaging. Fortschr Röntgenstr 174:1022–1027
Flohr T, Stierstorfer K, Bruder H, Simon S, Polacin A, Schaller S (2003) Image reconstruction and image quality evaluation for a 16-slice CT-scanner. Med Phys 30(5):832–845
Frush DP, Soden B, Frush KS, Lowry C (2002) Improved pediatric multidetector body CT using a size-based color-coded format. AJR 178:721–726
Fuchs T, Krause S, Schaller S, Flohr T, Kalender WA (2000) Spiral interpolation algorithm for multi-slice spiral CT. Part 2: Measurement and evaluation of slice sensitivity profiles and noise at a clinical multi-slice system. IEEE Trans Med Imag 19(9):835–847
Greess H, Wolf H, Baum U et al. (2000) Dose reduction in computed tomography by attenuation-based on-line modulation of the tube current: evaluation of six anatomical regions. Eur Radiol 10:391–394
Hsieh J (2003) Analytical models for multi-slice helical CT performance parameters. Med Phys 30(2):169–178
Hu H (1999) Multi-slice helical CT: scan and reconstruction. Med Phys 26:5–18
Hu H, He HD, Foley WD, Fox SH (2000) Four multidetector-row helical CT: image quality and volume coverage speed. Radiology 215:55–62
Jakobs TF, Becker CR, Ohnesorge B, Flohr T, Suess C, Schoepf UJ, Reiser MF (2002) Multislice helical CT of the heart with retrospective ECG gating: reduction of radiation exposure by ECG-controlled tube current modulation. Eur Radiol 12:1081–1086
Kachelriess M, Schaller S, Kalender WA (2000a) Advanced single-slice rebinning in cone-beam spiral CT. Med Phys 27: 754–772
Kachelriess M, Ulzheimer S, Kalender W (2000b) ECG-correlated image reconstruction from subsecond multi-slice spiral CT scans of the heart. Med Phys 27:1881–1902
Kalender W (1995) Thin-section three-dimensional spiral CT: Is isotropic imaging possible? Radiology 197:578–580
Kalender W, Seissler W, Klotz E, Vock P (1990) Spiral volumetric CT with single-breath-hold technique, continuous transport and continuous scanner rotation. Radiology 176: 181–183
Katsevich A (2002) Theoretically exact filtered backprojection-type inversion algorithm for spiral CT. SIAM J Appl Math 62:2012–2026
Klingenbeck-Regn K, Schaller S, Flohr T, Ohnesorge B, Kopp AF, Baum U (1999) Subsecond multi-slice computed tomography: basics and applications. Eur J Radiol 31:110–124
Knez A, Becker C, Leber A, Ohnesorge B, Reiser M, Haberl R (2000) Non-invasive assessment of coronary artery stenoses with multidetector helical computed tomography. Circulation 101:e221–e222
Koehler T, Proksa R, Bontus C, Grass M, Timmer J (2002) Artifact analysis of approximate helical cone-beam CT reconstruction algorithms. Med Phys 29:51–64
Kopp A, Schröder S, Küttner A et al. (2001) Coronary arteries: retrospectively ECG-gated multi-detector row CT angiography with selective optimization of the image reconstruction window. Radiology:683–688
Kudo H, Noo F, Defrise M (1998) Cone-beam filtered-back-projection algorithm for truncated helical data. Phys Med Biol 43:2885–2909
Larson G, Ruth C, Crawford C (1998) Nutating slice CT image reconstruction, patent application WO 98/44847, filed 8 April 1998
Loubeyre P, Angelie E, Grozel F, Abidi H, Minh VA (1997) Spiral CT artifact that simulates aortic dissection: image reconstruction with use of 180 degrees and 360 degrees linear-interpolation algorithms. Radiology 205:153–157
Nieman K, Oudkerk M, Rensing B, van Oijen P, Munne A, van Geuns R, de Feyter P (2001) Coronary angiography with multi-slice computed tomography. Lancet 357:599–603
Nieman K, Cademartiri F, Lemos PA, Raaijmakers R, Pattynama PMT, de Feyter PJ (2002) Reliable noninvasive coronary angiography with fast submillimeter multislice spiral computed tomography. Circulation 106:2051–2054
Ohnesorge B, Flohr T, Schaller S, Klingenbeck-Regn K, Becker C, Schöpf UJ, Brüning R, Reiser MF (1999) Technische Grundlagen und Anwendungen der Mehrschicht-CT. Radiologe 39:923–931
Ohnesorge B, Flohr T, Becker C, Kopp A, Schoepf U, Baum U, Knez A, Klingenbeck Regn K, Reiser M (2000) Cardiac imaging by means of electro-cardiographically gated multisection spiral CT: initial experience. Radiology 217:564–571
Proksa R, Koehler T, Grass M, Timmer J (2000) The n-PI method for helical cone-beam CT. IEEE Trans Med Imaging 19:848–863
Robb R, Rietman E (1979) High speed synchronous volume computed tomography of the heart. Radiology 133: 655–661
Saito Y, Suzuki T (1998) Evaluation of the performance of multi-slice CT system in non-helical scanning. Abstract book of the 84th Scientific Assembly and Annual Meeting of the RSNA, p 578
Schaller S (1998) Practical image reconstruction for cone-beam computed tomography. PhD thesis, University Erlangen Nürnberg, Germany
Schaller S, Flohr T, Klingenbeck K, Krause J, Fuchs T, Kalender W A (2000a) Spiral interpolation algorithm for multi-slice spiral CT. Part I: Theory. IEEE Trans Med Imaging 19:822–834
Schaller S, Noo F, Sauer F, Tam KC, Lauritsch G, Flohr T (2000b) Exact radon rebinning algorithm for the long object problem in helical cone-beam CT. IEEE Trans Med Imaging 19: 361–375
Schaller S, Stierstorfer K, Bruder H, Kachelriess M, Flohr T (2001a) Novel approximate approach for high-quality

image reconstruction in helical cone beam CT at arbitrary pitch. Proc SPIE Int Symp Med Imaging 4322:113–127

Schaller S, Niethammer MU, Chen X, Klotz E, Wildberger JE, Flohr T (2001b) Comparison of signal-to-noise and dose values at different tube voltages for protocol optimization in pediatric CT. Abstract book of the 87th Scientific Assembly and Annual Meeting of the RSNA, 366

Schoepf U, Helmberger T, Holzknecht N, Kang DS, Bruening RD, Aydemir S, Becker CR, Muehling O, Knez A, Haberl R, Reiser MF (2000) Segmental and subsegmental pulmonary arteries: evaluation with electron beam CT versus spiral CT. Radiology 214:433–439

Schroeder S, Kopp A, Baumbach A, Meisner C, Kuettner A, Georg C, Ohnesorge B, Herdeg C, Claussen C, Karsch K (2001) Noninvasive detection and evaluation of atherosclerotic coronary plaques with multi-slice computed tomography. JACC 37:1430–1435

Stierstorfer K, Flohr T, Bruder H (2002) Segmented multiple plane reconstruction: a novel approximate reconstruction scheme for multi-slice spiral CT. Phys Med Biol 47: 2571–2581

Taguchi K, Anno H (2000) High temporal resolution for multislice helical computed tomography. Med Phys 27:861–872

Taguchi T, Aradate H (1998) Algorithm for image reconstruction in multi-slice helical CT. Med Phys 25:550–561

Turbell H, Danielsson PE (1999) An improved PI-method for reconstruction from helical cone beam projections. IEEE Medical Imaging Conference, Seattle

Wang G, Lin T, Cheng P (1993) A general cone-beam reconstruction algorithm. IEEE Trans Med Imaging 12:486–496

2 Radiation Exposure in Thoracic CT

J. R. Mayo and J. Aldrich

CONTENTS

2.1 Introduction

Helical or spiral CT has revolutionized X-ray-based diagnostic medical imaging in the past 15 years (Berland and Smith 1998; Kalender and Polacin 1991; Kalender et al. 1990; Remy-Jardin et al. 2001). Introduced in the late 1980s, single and, more recently, multidetector-row CT scanners have greatly expanded the clinical indications and demand for CT scans of the thorax. This has led to a considerable increase in the number of examinations and in the average scanned volume obtained per examination. This has inevitably led to an increase in the radiation exposure delivered by these studies. The increased utilization of CT has been documented by studies in the USA and UK that have found approximately a twofold increase in the number of CT examinations between the late 1980s and the late 1990s (Mettler et al. 2000; Shrimpton and Edyvean 1998; Shrimpton et al. 1991). A recent report from an American academic institution showed that CT scans formed 11.1% of diagnostic radiologic procedures in 1999 compared with 6.1% in 1990 (Mettler et al. 2000). Because CT is a relatively high-radiation-dose technique, these authors reported that CT delivered approximately 67% of the total effective dose from diagnostic radiology in 1999. This study also noted that 11% of the CT scans were performed in the pediatric population, which was higher than previously estimated (Mettler et al. 2000). The relatively high dose of CT examinations was also noted in a radiation dose survey performed in the UK in 1989 which showed CT studies accounted for 2% of radiographic examinations and 20% of the effective dose (Shrimpton et al. 1991). A follow-up survey in 1995 showed that CT now accounted for 4% of all radiographic examinations (Shrimpton and Edyvean 1998) and for 40% of the medical effective dose.

The increase in population radiation exposure from CT examinations, particularly in children, has been of concern to radiologists, medical physicists, government regulators, and the media (Sternberg 2001). The suggestion that excessive radiation doses are being prescribed for CT examinations has appropriately aroused the attention of the radiology community (Rogers 2001). We must be attentive to our responsibility to maintain an appropriate balance between diagnostic image quality and radiation dose (Nickoloff and Alderson 2001). It has been suggested that the rapid expansion of clinical indications for spiral thoracic CT examinations radiation dose issues may have not received adequate attention (Golding and Shrimpton 2002).

This chapter reviews (a) measurement units used to quantify radiation exposure, (b) parameters that affect CT radiation dose and efficiency, and (c) advances in dose reduction in chest CT. Radiation dosimetry and bioeffects are not addressed in detail and interested readers are referred to more complete works in these areas (Golding and Shrimpton 2002; Huda and Atherton 1995; Jones et al. 1992; Mettler and Upton 1995; Metz et al. 1995).

J. R. Mayo, MD
Department of Radiology, Vancouver General Hospital, University of British Columbia, 899 W. 12th Ave, Vancouver, BC, V5Z 1M9 Canada
J. Aldrich, PhD
Department of Radiology, Vancouver General Hospital, University of British Columbia, 899 W. 12th Ave, Vancouver, BC, V5Z 1M9 Canada

2.2 Radiation Dose Measurement

Many measures of ionizing radiation exist (Table 2.1; Huda 1997) which attests to the complexity of this issue. Unfortunately, the plethora of measures can be confusing to the diagnostic radiologist with a limited grasp of the subtlety of the measurement differences. This may contribute to difficulty with radiation dose issues at the clinical level.

The simplest parameter, radiation exposure, measures ionization in air caused by the X-ray beam. The measurement unit is coulombs per kilogram. It has limited clinical value, as it does not take into account the area irradiated, the penetrating power of the radiation, or the radiation sensitivity of the irradiated organ; however, this quantity can be accurately and easily measured using ionization chambers. From radiation exposure we can calculate skin entrance dose, which is of importance for deterministic effects such as skin erythema; however, deterministic effects are not encountered in routine CT exams, although they are of potential concern in CT fluoroscopy (Golding and Shrimpton 2002).

Absorbed dose measures the energy absorbed per unit mass within an object. The measurement unit is the gray (Gy). Unlike radiation exposure, it is dependent upon the composition of the object or subject placed in the radiation beam. However, absorbed dose does not account for the differing radiation sensitivity of organs and cannot provide a whole-body risk estimate or be used to facilitate comparisons between examinations in different parts of the body. Equivalent dose is a modification of absorbed dose that incorporates weighting factors to account for the different biologic effect of various sources of radiation. For X-rays the radiation-weighting factor is 1 and the equivalent dose has the same numerical value as absorbed dose (ICRP-60 1991).

Effective dose is an estimate of the whole-body dose that would be required to produce the same stochastic (mainly cancer risk) as the partial-body dose that was actually delivered in a localized radiologic procedure. Effective dose is useful because it allows comparison with other types of radiation exposure such as whole-body radiation exposure secondary to natural background radiation. Effective dose is calculated by summing the absorbed doses to individual organs weighted for their radiation sensitivity (ICRP-60 1991). The measurement unit is the sievert (Sv). Effective dose has limitations, as we cannot obtain accurate measures of all pertinent organ doses and the risk coefficients specific to the age, gender, and organ of the subject being irradiated (McCollough and Schueler 2000; Sinclair 1994). Therefore, the estimated dose is calculated for an idealized 70-kg, 30-year-old subject; however, despite these limitations, it is currently the best quantity available for comparison between radiologic and nuclear medicine procedures.

Once the effective dose has been calculated, risk estimates for stochastic effects can be produced using a linear extrapolation of radiation exposure data from Japanese atomic bomb survivors (National Council on Radiation Protection and Measurements 1993; Beir 1990; ICRP-60 1991). While the stochastic risk depends upon such factors as age at exposure and nationality, ICRP have recommended the use of a conservative risk of 50 additional fatal cancers induced per million people of the general population exposed to 1 mSv of medical radiation (ICRP-60 1991). A more detailed discussion of the assessment of stochastic risk is given in ICRP60 (ICRP-60 1991).

Effective dose can be calculated for thoracic CT examinations using dose distributions pre-calculated for specific CT scanner geometry and beam-filtration quality (Atherton and Huda 1996; Jones and Shrimpton 1993; McCollough and Schueler 2000; Shrimpton and Edyvean 1998; Zankl et al. 1991). These pre-calculated distributions can be modified for the specific technical parameters of the scan by entering the mA, kVp, scanned volume, and pitch values to calculate effective dose. There are several commercial and free programs which can be used to facilitate this calculation (e.g., CT Dose from www.impactscan.org; WinDose from www.wellhofer.de)

Table 2.1. Radiation dose quantities

Quantity	Old	International system (SI)
Exposure	Roentgen (R)	Coulombs per kilogram
Absorbed dose (D)	Rad	Gray (Gy)
Equivalent dose		D multiplied by ICRP radiation-weighting factor w_R. The w_R for X-rays is 1
Effective dose (E)	Effective dose equivalent Sv 1977 tissue-weighting factors	Sievert (Sv) 1990 tissue-weighting factors

The computed tomography dose index (CTDI) is commonly used to describe the radiation output of CT scanners. First introduced by SHOPE et al. (1981), the CTDI is now commonly measured from one axial rotation of the scanner using a 100-mm pencil ionization chamber. This chamber is inserted into a standardized plastic phantom designed to simulate either a head (16-cm) or a body (32-cm diameter) object. The 100-mm chamber length accounts for the imperfect collimation of the X-ray beam and measures radiation scattered from the slice. Measurements are made in the center of the phantom and close to the periphery as attenuation of the X-ray beam within the phantom causes the dose to change with depth. An average or weighted CTDI is calculated by adding one-third of the central and two-thirds of the peripheral values together and is known as $CTDI_w$.

Dose-length product (DLP) is a quantity that has been developed to describe the amount of radiation used to perform a complete series of slices or exam. The DLP depends upon the $CTDI_w$, the pitch, and the length of the scan. Current scanners come equipped with tables of $CTDI_w$ values for the scan parameters specified. The scan length is calculated from the start and end locations identified on the pre-scan image. The pitch value of the scan is added to the calculation and the DLP calculated. The effective dose of the scan can then be calculated by multiplying the DLP by the effective dose coefficients for the region scanned (Fig. 2.1; Table 2.2; JESSEN et al. 1999). Once the effective dose is calculated, the risk of cancer induction can be estimated using the population average risk of 50 induced cancers per mSv effective dose per million people exposed (ICRP-60 1991). The DLP is especially useful because it can be calculated from the pre-scan image, prior to obtaining the CT examination. Automated calculation of the DLP from the pre-scan information is now available on all current CT scanners.

Calculation of the effective dose for pediatric patients has been difficult until recently. A complete set of dose coefficients for a wide range of ages has only recently been published (KHURSHEED et al. 2002). The mathematical phantoms used for these calculations were different from those used to calculate the dose distributions for adults, so it may not be possible to incorporate them directly into the dose calculation programs mentioned previously; however, it may be possible to use a simple effective dose-modifying factor to account for age. Further research into this approach is required.

As for adults, the DLP can be used to estimate the effective dose to the pediatric population (CHAPPLE et al. 2002; SHRIMPTON and WALL 2000; ZANKL et al. 1993). It is noted that there is a pronounced age effect on the cancer risk from ionizing radiation (BRENNER et al. 2001; PIERCE et al. 1996). Children may be an order of magnitude more sensitive than adults to the risk of cancer induction from the same effective dose of ionizing radiation (Fig. 2.2). This arises from the fact that they have more time to express the cancer and they have more rapidly dividing cells than do adults.

Table 2.2. Normalized effective dose coefficients. (From JESSEN et al. 1999)

Body part	$mSv \times mGy^{-1} \times cm^{-1}$
Head	0.0021
Neck	0.0048
Chest	0.014
Abdomen	0.012
Pelvis	0.016

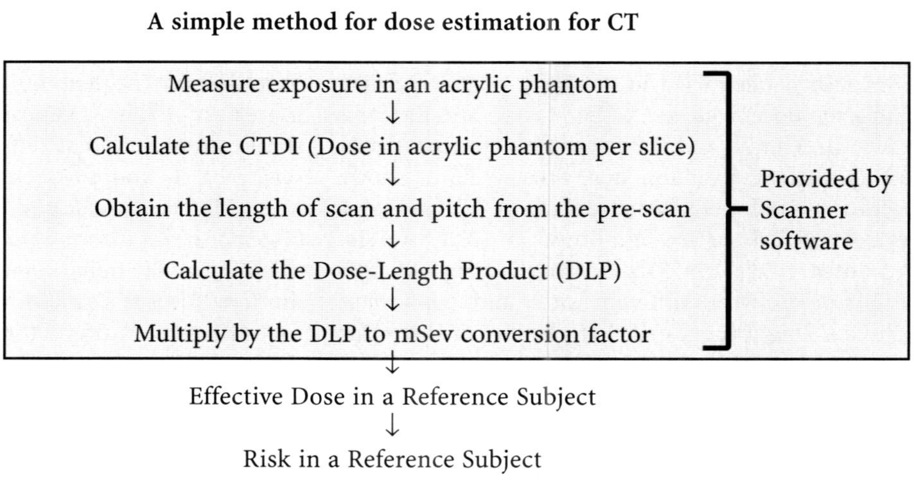

Fig. 2.1. Algorithm for the simple estimation of risk from CT examinations

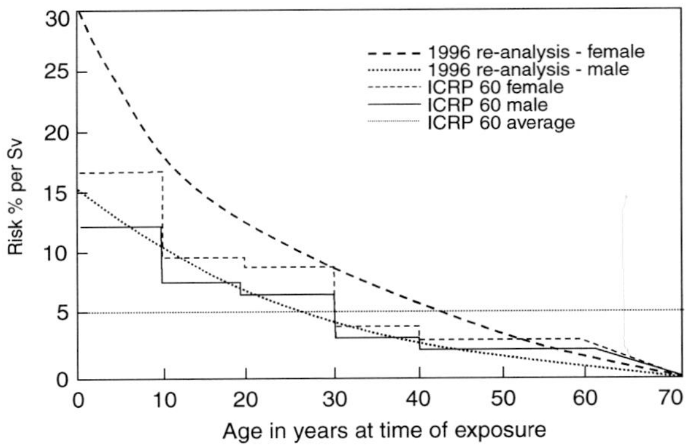

Fig. 2.2. Lifetime mortality risk from cancer per Sievert to age at the time of exposure. (Adapted from BRENNER et al. 2002)

2.3 CT Radiation Exposure

The relatively high radiation dose associated with CT results from two properties of the technique (SPRAWLS 1992). Firstly, unlike analogue film radiography, where the image receptor and display are both performed by the film, CT is a digital technique where image acquisition and display can be independently manipulated; therefore, unlike plain-film radiography, when CT dose is excessive, the image does not become too dark but merely improves because of decreased image noise (ROTHENBERG and PENTLOW 1992). Secondly, the ability to window or map the entire gray scale onto selected segments of the CT-number scale enhances visualization of image noise. As a result, image degradation due to quantum noise (mottle) is easily recognized and may interfere with image analysis. As a result of these two effects and the overwhelming drive of radiologists for the very best image quality to support high levels of diagnostic accuracy, CT images are often obtained using high patient radiation exposure, which may not be recognized by the radiologist.

Concern was raised in the early 1990s regarding radiation dose in chest CT (DI MARCO and BRIONES 1993; DI MARCO and RENSTON 1994; NAIDICH et al. 1994). Patient radiation dose surveys have shown (CONWAY et al. 1992; NISHIZAWA et al. 1991; PANZER et al. 1989; SHRIMPTON and EDYVEAN 1998; SHRIMPTON et al. 1991a, 1991b) wide variations in radiation exposure between different sites and equipment. These CT data suggested that greater consideration needed to be given to the optimization chest CT exposures; however, the current data concerning CT radiation dose indicate that insufficient progress has been made.

2.4 Scanner Radiation Efficiency

Several physical aspects of CT scanners result in wasted radiation dose; these include the shielding effect of the post patient collimator, imperfect collimation of the X-ray beam, and movement of the X-ray focal spot. The sum of all these effects is measured by the geometric efficiency of the CT scanner.

Single-detector-row CT scanners, with their wide single-detector-row configuration, have higher geometric efficiency than multidetector-row CT scanners. The decreased geometric efficiency of multidetector-row CT scanners arises from three major factors: gaps between detector elements in the array; the effect of focal spot penumbra; and motion of the focal spot. Since the focal spot of the X-ray tube is not a point, the collimator cannot perfectly collimate the beam; therefore, the edge of the beam or penumbra has spatially varying X-ray intensity. On single-detector helical scanners this portion of the beam can be detected and utilized in the reconstruction process; however, on multislice scanners, utilization of the penumbra would result in different readings from detectors in this region compared with those in the central or umbra portion of the beam. Since all detector rows contribute data to each reconstructed image, the amount of radiation that each detector row receives must be the same. To achieve this, the active detectors in multidetector-row CT scanners only measure the umbra of the X-ray beam. Radiation in the penumbra falls on inactive detectors and is discarded, although it contributes to patient radiation dose. In addition, thermal and mechanical stresses within the X-ray tube cause the focal spot to move. This motion causes the X-ray beam to wander over the detector array during the scan. Again, to exclude penumbra radiation from striking the active detectors, the X-ray beam is widened, further decreasing geometric efficiency and increasing wasted radiation dose. Because the penumbra is a fixed size, this effect is greatest on four-slice scanners operating with thin slice collimation. The effect is progressively less severe on 8- and 16-track multidetector-row scanners. Manufacturers have devised beam-tracking systems to stabilize the position of the X-ray beam to minimize the radiation wasting effect of focal spot motion (TOTH et al. 2000).

Scattered radiation is formed by the interaction of the primary beam with the patient. Scattered radiation exits in all directions and, if detected, reduces contrast and generates artifacts. In plain chest radiography, depending on the technique chosen, between 50 and 90% of film darkening is due to scattered radiation, contributing to the low soft tissue contrast of this technique (Curry et al. 1984). The extensive collimation in CT reverses this ratio, with 90% of detected X-rays being primary image photons. This partially accounts for the improved soft tissue contrast of CT.

Because of scatter and imperfect collimation, the radiation intensity profile does not fall to zero at the edge of the nominal slice width. It has been shown using a single-slice scanner that contiguous slices generate a peak radiation dose approximately 50% over that of a single slice (10-mm collimation, 10-mm table increment, measured at the surface of a 15-cm Lucite head phantom (Pentlow et al. 1977). The increase in radiation dose associated with multiple adjacent CT slices has been measured and is characterized by the multiple slice average dose (MSAD) parameter (Jucius and Kambic 1977; Shope et al. 1981). Helical scanning with a pitch of 1 results in a dose distribution essentially equivalent to contiguous single-slice imaging (McGee and Humphreys 1994). Overlapping slices or helical scanning with pitch less than 1 can result in even higher doses if techniques are not adjusted. Radiation dose can be reduced if gaps are introduced between scanned sections (Evans et al. 1989; Mayo et al. 1993); however, diagnostic information can be lost using gapped slices as only a portion of the chest is imaged. For this reason, gaps between sections are only practical when imaging diffuse processes such as interstitial lung disease (Lee et al. 1994).

The CT detectors vary in their efficiency. Ideally, a detector should count all incident beam X-ray photons; however, depending on the technology used, detectors will record only from 60% (high-pressure xenon) to 95% (solid state) of the incident X-ray photons. Most current detectors are solid state. The accuracy of conversion of the absorbed X-ray signal into an electrical signal is known as the conversion efficiency. The overall dose efficiency of the scanner is the product of the geometric efficiency, the quantum detection efficiency, and the conversion efficiency (Cunningham 1995). This can vary substantially between scanners. Noise is also introduced by the electronics of the scanner data acquisition system. The sum of quantum noise and electronic noise results in differences in image quality between scanners at the same radiation dose.

Similar to other radiological techniques, the primary X-ray beam in CT is filtered to eliminate low-energy photons, which would be preferentially absorbed relative to high-energy photons and only contribute to radiation dose. In CT additional spatially varying filtration is often placed in the primary beam. These filters reduce both the necessary dynamic range of the detector system in the periphery of the detector array and the radiation dose for larger fields of view (FOV). They are often referred to as "bow tie" filters because of their shape, and they create variations in entrance radiation exposure depending on both the size of the object and its position in the FOV. In some scanners multiple filters of varying shapes are moved into place depending on the specified scan FOV. In other scanners these filters are permanently positioned. These filters substantially reduce radiation dose in adult body CT scans, but they are less effective in pediatric patients.

2.5 User-Specified Scan Parameters

Reduction in radiation dose results in increased image noise and may result in decreased image quality. Studies assessing subjective evaluation of CT scans of the chest by radiologists have shown consistently higher subjective image quality scores when images were obtained using higher radiation dose (Haaga et al. 1981; Mayo et al. 1995). Image noise can be measured by placing a region of interest (ROI >100 pixels) over an area of uniform density in the body (e.g., the thoracic aorta; Sprawls 1992). The standard deviation of the pixel values represents image noise. It is noted that the choice of reconstruction algorithm influences image noise, with higher noise obtained using high spatial frequency reconstruction algorithms (e.g., bone, lung) compared with low spatial frequency algorithms (e.g., standard, soft tissue algorithm). High spatial frequency reconstruction algorithms are most commonly used when searching for fine structures within bones or lung tissue. The increase in image noise associated with the high spatial frequency algorithm is not a problem in these applications because of the high radiographic contrast of these tissues.

Radiation dose and image noise can be modified by adjusting the tube current (mA), scan time, tube voltage (kVp), slice width, and reconstruction algorithm. Most of these parameters affect noise in a non-linear way. In practice, the tube current is usually adjusted to change the radiation dose and image noise. On most scanners, the tube current is adjustable in steps from 20 to approximately 400 mA. Scan time also linearly affects the radiation dose, but it is usually minimized in the chest to reduce the effect of patient motion. Increasing the tube voltage increases the output of the X-ray tube. If the tube current and scan times are not changed, increasing the tube voltage will increase the patient dose. Changes in tube voltage also affect CT tissue attenuation values, which can change tissue contrast in a complex fashion. In practice, tube voltage is not commonly adjusted from patient to patient in chest CT examinations. It is noted that the radiation exposure delivered at a given kVp and mAs setting will vary greatly between scanners of different model and manufacturer due to differences in scanner geometry (X-ray tube-to-patient separation) and X-ray tube filtration.

Helical scans introduced a new parameter: pitch. For single-section spiral scanners pitch is defined as the table travel per 360° X-ray tube rotation divided by the beam collimation (Polacin et al. 1992). In many cases the table feed (e.g., 5 mm per 360° X-ray tube rotation) and beam collimation (e.g., 5 mm) are identical, with a resultant pitch of 1. This yields one spiral turn per section thickness and a radiation exposure equal to contiguous axial slices; however, the table can be made to feed more rapidly (e.g., 10 mm per 360° X-ray tube rotation) without changing the beam collimation (5 mm). This results in a pitch of 2. Scans with pitch values greater than 1 cover larger volumes in shorter times, providing either reduced motion artifacts or thinner slices. Scans with elevated pitch have lower image quality because of broadening of the slice profile; however, the radiation dose delivered by the scan is decreased by the value of the pitch (e.g., one-half the radiation exposure for a pitch of 2) if the kVp and mAs are kept constant. It is noted that in many multidetector-row scanners, the mAs is automatically increased to compensate for increased noise at higher pitch values, which may eliminate the radiation dose reduction. In some cases, such as spiral CT for pulmonary embolism, it has been shown that improved image contrast can be obtained with reduced radiation dose by using thinner slices at pitch values of 1.5–2 (Remy-Jardin et al. 2001).

In multidetector-row CT one manufacturer redefined pitch as the table travel divided by the detector aperture (Hu 1999) for a short time. This definition elevates the value of the pitch by the number of detector tracks. For example, the acquisition of four 1.25-mm slices at a table speed of 10 mm per second in a 0.5-s scanner results in a pitch of 1 using the standard definition; however, using the same parameters, but changing the denominator to the detector aperture, increases the value of pitch to 4. In response to the argument that this new definition of pitch did not clearly demonstrate the relationship between radiation dose and X-ray beam overlap found with the original definition this manufacturer has discontinued this definition of pitch (International Electrotechnical Commission 2002; McCollough and Zink 1999).

In the past the tube current (mA) of CT scanners was uniform at all angles around the patient; however, the chest is an elliptical object, which has higher attenuation left to right than anterior to posterior. Manufacturers have introduced programs that alter the mA, increasing radiation dose laterally and decreasing it in the thinner anteroposterior direction. This has been shown to decrease radiation dose (Greess et al. 2000; Kalender et al. 1999a, 1999b) with minimal effect on image quality. In the future we believe CT scanners will automatically adjust dose during the scanning process to compensate for the size and density of the body section being scanned, resulting in a signal-to-noise ratio that is adequate for diagnosis but not excessive.

Repeated scans of the same region (e.g., pre-contrast, contrast enhanced) increase the radiation dose in a linear fashion; therefore, if a non-contrast acquisition is routinely performed prior to administration of intravenous contrast, the radiation dose is doubled. This effect can be markedly reduced if the non-contrast scan is a high-resolution study (e.g., 1-mm collimation at 10-mm spacing), for which the radiation dose is 10% of that of a contiguous conventional CT or spiral CT with a pitch of 1.

The mA and kVp settings are usually set according to local experience and practice. Radiation dose surveys have noted wide variation in these settings between institutions (Conway et al. 1992; Nishizawa et al. 1991; Panzer et al. 1989; Shrimpton and Edyvean 1998; Shrimpton et al. 1991a, 1991b). To decrease this variation and protect the public from inadvertent overexposure, the World Health Organization and the European Community have published suggested reference values (European 2000) for many CT examinations (Table 2.3). Surveying a large number of institutions in Europe and adopting the 75th percentile as the reference dose obtained these reference dose values. These values serve as a guide to acceptable European practice.

2.6 Dose Reduction in Chest CT

The concept of reduced tube current for conventional 10-mm collimation chest CT was introduced

Table 2.3. Proposed reference dose values for routine CT examinations on the basis of absorbed dose to air. *CTDI* computed tomography dose index, *DLP* dose-length product. (From EUROPEAN 2000)

Examination	Reference dose value	
	$CTDI_w$ (mGy)	DLP (mGy cm)
Routine head[a]	60	1050
Face and sinuses[a]	35	360
Vertebral trauma[b]	70	460
Routine chest[b]	30	650
HRCT of lung[b]	35	280
Routine abdomen[b]	35	780
Liver and spleen[b]	35	900
Routine pelvis[b]	35	570
Osseous pelvis[b]	25	520

[a]Data relate to head phantom (PMMA, 16-cm diameter)
[b]Data relate to body phantom (PMMA, 32-cm diameter)

by NAIDICH et al. (1990) in 1990 with demonstration of acceptable image quality for assessment of lung parenchyma with low tube current settings (20 mAs). While these images were adequate for assessing lung parenchyma, they had a considerable increase in noise, which resulted in marked degradation of image quality on mediastinal windows. For this reason the authors noted that such low-dose techniques were most suited for assessment of children and possibly for screening patients at high risk for lung cancer. These recommendations have been implemented and further studied in lung cancer screening programs (HENSCHKE et al. 1999; ITOH et al. 2000; SWENSEN et al. 2002)

Similar dose-reduction strategies have been applied to high-resolution CT (HRCT) of the chest, where no significant difference in lung parenchymal structures was seen between low-dose (40 mAs) and high-dose (400 mAs) HRCT images (ZWIREWICH et al. 1991); however, although not statistically significant, ground-glass changes were difficult to assess on low-mA images due to increased image noise; therefore, 200 mAs was recommended for initial HRCT images, with lower doses (i.e., 40–100 mAs) used for follow-up examinations.

The radiation dose associated with HRCT has been controversial, with Di Marco quoting the high figure of 120–140 mGy (DI MARCO and BRIONES 1993), which had been reported in an early HRCT paper (MAYO et al. 1987). This dose estimate was measured using contiguous 1.5-mm sections, 510 mAs, and CTDI methodology in a head-sized (16 cm) CT quality-control phantom. The CTDI measurement was designed to facilitate dose comparisons between CT scanners and was not appropriate to describe the relative dose of HRCT. As previously noted, the effective dose is a better measure as it takes into account the significant reduction in radiation risk associated with the noncontiguous sections used in HRCT. With 10-mm intersection gaps the effective dose of HRCT is 10% that of either conventional contiguous CT sections or spiral CT with a pitch of 1. The effective dose of HRCT is reduced to approximately 5% with the use of 20-mm intersection gaps. As noted previously, low-dose HRCT can also be utilized in selected patients. It has been shown that three low-dose HRCT sections provide an effective dose comparable to that of a posteroanterior chest radiograph (0.05 mSv), with no significant loss of diagnostic accuracy in interstitial lung disease (LEE et al. 1994).

The relationship between radiation exposure and image quality on both mediastinal and lung windows has been evaluated on conventional 10-mm collimation chest CT images (MAYO et al. 1995) on a single CT scanner model. Although this study showed a consistent increase in mean image quality with higher radiation exposure, no significant difference in the detection of mediastinal or lung parenchymal abnormalities was seen from 20 to 400 mAs. The authors concluded that adequate image quality could be consistently obtained in average-sized patients on their specific CT scanner using tube currents of 100–200 mAs. This study was limited by a small number of patients (n=30), the specific CT scanner factors (geometry, filtration, tube voltage), and the experimental design, which limited low-dose sections to two levels that often were not those with clinically relevant findings. The authors noted that comparison of complete chest CT studies at a variety of radiation exposures in a large number of patients would be required to evaluate further the effect of reduced radiation dose on diagnostic accuracy in chest CT; however, they noted that such a study was not possible on patients due to the unacceptable radiation dose that would result from multiple scans at differing radiation exposures. Additionally, the variable effect of motion artifacts on repeated scans would make comparison difficult.

A practical method to evaluate the effect of reduced radiation dose on image quality is computer simulation (MAYO et al. 1997). The technique consists of obtaining a standard-dose diagnostic scan and then modifying the raw scan data by adding Gaussian distributed random noise to simulate the increased noise associated with reduced radiation exposure. The raw scan data is then reconstructed using the same field of view and reconstruction algorithm as the reference high-dose scan. In a validation trial, experienced chest radiologists were unable to distinguish simulated reduced-dose CT images from real reduced-dose images (Mayo et al. 1997). Computer simulation allows investigators to determine the effect of dose reduction on diagnostic accuracy without radiating subjects unnecessarily. In addition, the simulated images are in exact registration with the original images, eliminating artifacts due to volume averaging or motion. This technique has recently been used to evaluate the diagnostic impact of radiation dose reduction in pediatric abdominal CT examinations (Frush et al., in press).

Finally, it is noted that, although CT is a relatively high radiation dose modality, in some cases it has replaced studies with higher radiation exposures such as pulmonary angiography or bronchography (Table 2.4).

2.7 Conclusion

The introduction of helical and multidetector-row scanners has resulted in an increased number of indications and diagnostic accuracy of CT; however, the current level of radiation exposure provided by CT is high, particularly in the pediatric population. Radiation dose surveys have indicated that there is large variation in the technical factors employed, with resultant large variation in the radiation dose to patients. Reference dose values for chest CT examinations have been developed and published. Radiologic societies should be encouraged to consider the benefits that adoption of such standards would have on medical practice. Further research into the complex relationship between radiation exposure, image noise, and diagnostic accuracy should be encouraged to scientifically establish the minimum radiation doses that provide adequate diagnostic information for standard clinical questions. Once these minimum image quality levels are determined and validated, automatic exposure controls for CT scanners should be developed to ensure that all patients receive scans obtained with techniques that are as low as reasonably achievable (ALARA). Radiologists must take the lead in promoting these measures for patient protection. Because of the increased radiation sensitivity of children, initial dose-reduction efforts should be focused on the pediatric population. The Society of Pediatric Radiology has recently made recommendations in this regard (Brenner 2002; Brody 2002; Donnelly 2002; Fearon 2002; Frush 2002; Huda 2002; Nickoloff 2002; Ron 2002; Slovis 2002a, 2002b, 2002c; Toth 2002; Varchena 2002).

Finally, it is noted that the complexity of CT requires a close collaboration between radiologists and medical physicists to successfully reduce radiation dose while maintaining diagnostic accuracy.

Table 2.4. Comparison of effective doses. (From Mayo and Aldrich 1996)

Procedure	Effective dose (mSv)
Posteroanterior chest radiograph	0.05[a]
Conventional CT	7.0[b]
Spiral CT pitch 1	7.0[b]
Spiral CT pitch 2	3.5[b]
HRCT 10-mm intersection gap	0.7[b]
HRCT 20-mm intersection gap	0.35[b]
Thin-section low-dose HRCT	0.02[c]
Conventional pulmonary angiography	9.0[d]
Digital pulmonary angiography	6.0[d]
Conventional bronchography	3.0[e]
Natural background radiation	2.5[a]

[a] UNSCEAR 1993
[b] NRPB 1992
[c] Lee et al. 1994
[d] Calculated using data from NRPB (1994) report R262 assuming pulmonary angiography with 5 min of fluoroscopy and the equivalent of 30 posteroanterior and 30 lateral views
[e] Bronchography performed with the assumption of 2 min of fluoroscopy and six posteroanterior and six lateral views

References

Atherton JV, Huda W (1996) Energy imparted and effective dose in computed tomography. Med Phys 23:735–741

Beir V (1990) Health effects of exposure to low levels of ionizing radiation. National Academy Press, Washington

Berland LL, Smith JK (1998) Multidetector-array CT: once again, technology creates new opportunities. Radiology 209:327–329

Brenner DJ (2002) Estimating cancer risks from pediatric CT: going from the qualitative to the quantitative. Pediatr Radiol 32:228–231

Brenner DJ, Elliston CD, Hall EJ et al. (2001) Estimated risks of radiation-induced fatal cancer from pediatric CT. AJR 176:289–296

Brody AS (2002) CT scanner design and patient radiation exposure. Pediatr Radiol 32:268–271

Chapple C-L, Willis S, Frame J (2002) Effective dose in paediatric computed tomography. Phys Med Biol 47:107–115

Conway BJ, McCrohan JL, Antonsen RG et al. (1992) Average radiation dose in standard CT examinations of the head: results of the 1990 NEXT study. Radiology 184:135–140

Cunningham IA (1995) Computed tomography: instrumentation. In: Bronzino JE (ed) The biomedical engineering handbook. CRC Press, Boca Raton, Florida, pp 990–1002

Curry TS III, Dowdey JE, Murray RC Jr (1984) Christensen's

introduction to the physics of diagnostic radiology. Lea and Febiger, Philadelphia, p 73
Donnelly LF (2002) Lessons from history. Pediatr Radiol 32: 287–292
European C (2000) European guidelines on quality criteria for computer tomography. EUR 16262EN. Office for Official Publication of the European Communities, Luxemberg
Evans SH, Davis R, Cooke J et al. (1989) A comparison of radiation doses to the breast in computed tomographic chest examinations for two scanning protocols. Clin Radiol 40: 45–46
Fearon T (2002) CT dose parameters and their limitations. Pediatr Radiol 32:246–249
Frush DP (2002) Strategies of dose reduction. Pediatr Radiol 32:293–297
Golding SJ, Shrimpton PC (2002) Commentary. Radiation dose in CT: Are we meeting the challenge? Br J Radiol 75:1–4
Greess H, Wolf H, Baum U et al. (2000) Dose reduction in computed tomography by attenuation-based on-line modulation of tube current: evaluation of six anatomical regions. Eur Radiol 10:391–394
Haaga JR, Miraldi F, MacIntyre W et al. (1981) The effect of mAs variation upon computed tomography image quality as evaluated by in vivo and in vitro studies. Radiology 138: 449–454
Henschke CI, McCauley DI, Yankelevitz DF et al. (1999) Early Lung Cancer Action Project: overall design and findings from baseline screening. Lancet 354:99–105
Hu H (1999) Multi-slice helical CT: scan and reconstruction. Med Phys 26:1–18
Huda W (1997) Radiation dosimetry in diagnostic radiology. AJR 169:1487–1488
Huda W (2002) Effective doses to adult and pediatric patients. Pediatr Radiol 32:272–279
Huda W, Atherton JV (1995) Energy imparted in computed tomography. Med Phys 22:1263–1269
ICRP-60 (1991) Recommendations of the International Commission on Radiological Protection. Pergamon Press, Oxford
International Electrotechnical Commission I (2002) Amendment 1 to IEC 60601-2-44, 2nd edn. Medical electrical equipment, parts 2--44: Particular requirements for the safety of X-ray equipment for computed tomography – final draft international standard. International Electrotechnical Commission, Geneva, pp 1–7
Itoh H, Ikeda M, Arahata S et al. (2000) Lung cancer screening: minimum tube current reqired for helical CT. Radiology 215:175–183
Jessen KA, Shrimpton PC, Geleijns J et al. (1999) Dosimetry for optimisation of patient protection in computed tomography. Appl Radiat Isot 50:165–172
Jones AP, Mott DJ, Parkinson L (1992) Experience with a new simple method for the determination of doses in computed tomography. Radiat Prot Dosim 43:139–142
Jones DG, Shrimpton PC (1993) Normalized organ doses for X-ray CT calculated using Monte Carlo techniques NRPB-SR250. NRPB, Chilton, Oxon
Jucius RA, Kambic GX (1977) Radiation dosimetry in computed tomography. Appl Opt Instr Eng Med VI 127:286–295
Kalender WA, Polacin A (1991) Physical performance characteristics of spiral CT scanning. Med Phys 18:910–915
Kalender WA, Seissler W, Klotz E et al. (1990) Spiral volumetric CT with single-breath-hold technique, continuous transport, and continuous scanner rotation. Radiology 176:181–183
Kalender WA, Wolf H, Suess C (1999a) Dose reduction in CT by anatomically adapted tube current modulation. II. Phantom measurements. Med Phys 26:2248–2253
Kalender WA, Wolf H, Suess C et al. (1999b) Dose reduction in CT by on-line tube current control: principles and validation on phantoms and cadavers. Eur Radiol 9:323–328
Khursheed A, Hiller MC, Shrimpton PC, Wall BF (2002) Influence of patient age on normalized effective doses calculated for CT examinations. Br J Radiol 75:819–830
Lee KS, Primack SL, Staples CA et al. (1994) Chronic infiltrative lung disease: comparison of diagnostic accuracies of radiography and low- and conventional-dose thin-section CT. Radiology 191:669–673
Marco AF di, Briones B (1993) Is chest CT performed too often? Chest 103:985–986
Marco AF di, Renston JP (1994) In search of the appropriate use of chest computed tomography. Chest 106:332–333
Mayo J, Aldrich J (1996) Radiation exposure. In: Remy-Jardin M, Remy J (eds) Spiral CT of the chest. Springer, Berlin, Heidelberg New York, p 39
Mayo JR, Webb WR, Gould R et al. (1987) High-resolution CT of the lungs: an optimal approach. Radiology 163:507–510
Mayo JR, Jackson SA, Müller NL (1993) High-resolution CT of the chest: radiation dose. AJR 160:479–481
Mayo JR, Hartman TE, Lee KS et al. (1995) CT of the chest: minimal tube current required for good image quality with the least radiation dose. AJR 164:603–607
Mayo JR, Whittall KP, Leung AN et al. (1997) Simulated dose reduction in conventional chest CT: validation study. Radiology 202:453–457
McCollough CH, Schueler BA (2000) Calculation of effective dose. Med Phys 27:828–837
McCollough CH, Zink FE (1999) Performance evaluation of a multi-slice CT system. Med Phys 26:2223–2230
McGee PL, Humphreys S (1994) Radiation dose associated with spiral computed tomography. Can Assoc Radiol J 45: 124–129
Mettler FA Jr, Upton AC (1995) Medical effects of ionizing radiation. Saunders, Philadelphia
Mettler FA Jr, Wiest PW, Locken JA et al. (2000) CT scanning: patterns of use and dose. J Radiol Prot 20:353–359
Metz CE, Wagner RF, Doi K et al. (1995) Toward consensus on quantitative assessment of medical imaging systems. Med Phys 22:1057–1061
Naidich DP, Marshall CH, Gribbin C et al. (1990) Low-dose CT of the lungs: preliminary observations. Radiology 175: 729–731
Naidich DP, Pizzarello D, Garay SM et al. (1994) Is thoracic CT performed often enough? Chest 106:331–332
Nickoloff E (2002) Current adult and pediatric CT doses. Pediatr Radiol 32:250–260
Nickoloff EL, Alderson PO (2001) Radiation exposures to patients from CT: reality, public perception and policy. AJR 177:285–287
Nishizawa K, Maruyama T, Takayama M et al. (1991) Determinations of organ doses and effective dose equivalents from computed tomographic examination. B J Radiol 64:20–28
National Council on Radiation Protection and Measurements (1993) Risk estimates for radiation protection. NCRP report no. 115. Bethesda, Maryland
NRPB (1992) Documents of the NRPB National Radiological

Protection Board. III. Chilton, England: National Radiological Protection Board, 1992; 1–16
Panzer W, Scheurer C, Zankl M (1989) Dose to patients in computed tomography examinations: results and consequences from a field study in the Federal Republic of Germany. In: Moores BM, Wall BF, Eriskat H, Schibilla H (eds) Optimization of image quality and patient exposure in diagnostic radiology. British Institute of Radiology, London, report 20
Pentlow KS, Beattie JW, Laughlin JS (1977) Parameters and design considerations for tomographic transmission scanners. In: Ter-Pogossian MM, Phelps ME (eds) Reconstructive tomography in diagnostic radiology and nuclear medicine. University Park Press, Baltimore, pp 267–279
Pierce D, Shimizu Y, Preston D et al. (1996) Studies of the mortality of atomic bomb survivors. Report 12, part 1. Cancer: 1950–1990. Radiat Res 146:1–27
Polacin A, Kalender WA, Marchal G (1992) Evaluation of section sensitivity profiles and image noise in spiral CT. Radiology 185:29–35
Remy-Jardin M, Remy J, Mayo JR et al. (2001) Acquisition, injection, and reconstruction techniques. CT angiography of the chest. Lippincott Williams and Wilkins, Philadelphia, pp 1–14
Rogers L (2001a) Radiation exposure in CT: Why so high? AJR 177:277
Rogers LF (2001b) Serious business: radiation safety and radiation protection. AJR 177:1
Ron E (2002) Ionizing radiation and cancer risk: evidence from epidemiology. Pediatr Radiol 32:232–237
Rothenberg LN, Pentlow KS (1992) Radiation dose in CT. Radiographics 12:1225–1243
Shope TB, Gagne RM, Johnson GC (1981) A method for describing the doses delivered by transmission X-ray computed tomography. Med Phys 8:488–495
Shrimpton PC, Edyvean S (1998) CT scanner dosimetry. Br J Radiol 71:1–3
Shrimpton PC, Wall BF (2000) Reference doses for paediatric computed tomography. Radiat Prot Dosim 90:249–252
Shrimpton PC, Hillier MC, Wall BF et al. (1991a) Survey of CT practice in the UK. Part 1: Survey of CT practice in the UK. Chilton, Oxon, NRPB report R-248
Shrimpton PC, Jones DG, Hillier MC et al. (1991b) Survey of CT practice in the UK. Part 2: dosimetric aspects. Chilton, Oxon, NRPB report R-249
Sinclair WK (1994) The concept of effective dose. Health Phys 66:586
Slovis TL (2002a) Welcome and introduction to the ALARA Conference on the ALARA concept in pediatric CT intelligent dose reduction. Pediatr Radiol 32:222
Slovis TL (2002b) Discussion, consensus, and mandate. Pediatr Radiol 32:301–313
Slovis TL (2002c) The ALARA concept in pediatric CT: myth or reality? Radiology 223:5–6
Sprawls P Jr (1992) AAPM tutorial. CT image detail and noise. Radiographics 12:1041–1046
Sternberg S. CT scans in children linked to cancer later. USA Today 2001; Jan 22:1
Swensen SJ, Jett JR, Sloan JA et al. (2002) Screening for lung cancer with low-dose spiral computed tomography. Am J Respir Crit Care Med 165:508–513
Toth TL (2002) Dose reduction opportunities for CT scanners. Pediatr Radiol 32:261–267
Toth TL, Bromberg NB, Pan TS et al. (2000) A dose reduction X-ray beam positioning system for high-speed multislice CT scanners. Med Phys 27:2659–2668
UNSCEAR (1993) United Nations Scientific Committee on the effects of atomic radiation. Sources and effects of ionizing radiation: UNSCEAR 1993 report to the General Assembly with scientific annexes. New York, NY: United Nations 1993
Varchena V (2002) Pediatric phantoms. Pediatr Radiol 32: 280–284
Zankl M, Panzer W, Drexler G (1991) The calculation of dose from external photon exposures using reference human phantoms and Monte Carlo methods. Part VI: Organ doses from computed tomographic examinations. GSF-Forschungszentrum für Umwelt und Gesundtheit, Institut für Strahlenschutz, Neuherberg, Germany
Zankl M, Panzer W, Drexler G (1993) Tomographic anthropomorphic models. Part II: Organ doses from computed tomographic examinations in paediatric radiology. GSF-Forschungszentrum fur Umwelt und Gesundtheit, Institut fur Strahlenschutz, Neuherberg, Germany
Zwirewich CV, Mayo JR, Müller NL (1991) Low-dose high-resolution CT of lung parenchyma. Radiology 180:413–417

3 Strategies for Dose Reduction and Improved Image Quality in MSCT

M. Kachelriess, S. Schaller, W. A. Kalender

CONTENTS

3.1 Introduction

Since the introduction of the first computed tomography (CT) scanner in 1972, the importance of CT for the medical community has increased drastically. Presently, whole-body scans with isotropic sub-millimetre resolution are acquired routinely during a single breath-hold.

The decisive step towards three-dimensional isotropic data was the introduction of spiral CT in 1989 by W. A. Kalender. This scan mode is based on a continuous rotation of the gantry while simultaneously translating the patient along the axis of rotation. The scan trajectory is a spiral and allows for truly 3D data acquisition. The z-interpolation step allows one to select the longitudinal position (z-position) of the reconstructed images arbitrarily and retrospectively. The continuous axial sampling allows for high-quality 3D displays and led to a renaissance of CT (Kalender 2001). The introduction of multi-slice spiral CT (MSCT) in 1998, which allows simultaneous scanning of currently up to 16 slices, further improved the scanner's volume coverage, z-resolution and scan speed. For example, typical chest exams are carried out with collimations of 1×5 mm in 36 s with single-slice, 4×1 mm in 30 s with 4-slice and 16×0.75 mm in 10 s with 16-slice scanners (Fig. 3.1).

Recently, patient dose has become an increasingly more important issue: increasing the information density of a scan, e.g. the spatial resolution, requires to increase the photon density (absorbed photons per volume element) by at least the same factor if the signal-to-noise ratio (SNR) is to be maintained. Currently, less than 5% of all X-ray exams are performed with CT. The cumulative dose of CT, however, is of the order of 40% of all X-ray exams. Dose is especially critical in paediatric CT (Brenner et al. 2001). Practical hardware- and software-based solutions to reduce patient dose are strongly required.

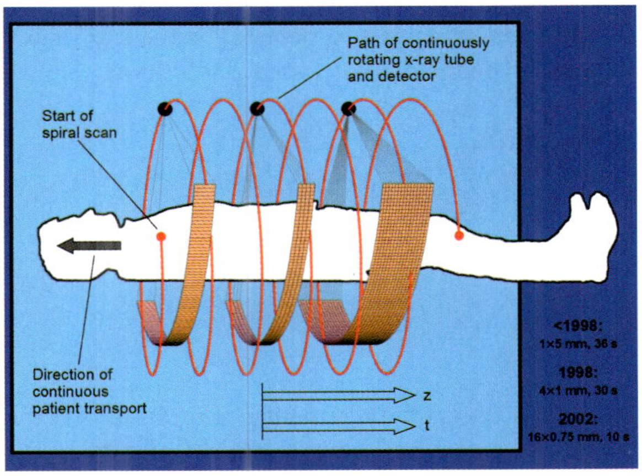

Fig. 3.1. Three generations of spiral CT scanners. The sizes of the detector elements indicate the slice thickness of single-slice, 4-slice and 16-slice scanners for typical exams. These slice dimensions (or "logical" detector dimensions) may differ from the physical dimensions since detector slices are often made up by electronically combining several detector rows

M. Kachelriess, PhD
Institute of Medical Physics, Krankenhausstrasse 12, 91054 Erlangen, Germany
W. A. Kalender, PhD
Professor, Institute of Medical Physics, Krankenhausstrasse 12, 91054 Erlangen, Germany
S. Schaller, PhD
Siemens Medical Solutions, Siemensstrasse 1, 91301 Forchheim, Germany

This paper gives an overview of CT dose issues and of strategies to reduce the patient dose or, alternatively, to improve the image quality for a given dose level. Note that in all attempts to reduce dose, image quality is crucial since the diagnostic outcome must not be jeopardized.

3.2 Dose and Image Quality

Image quality is a function of dose. We can quantify image quality in CT mainly by giving two parameters: (a) the pixel noise σ that is measured as the standard deviation of the pixel values within a homogeneous image region; and (b) the spatial resolution. Due to the circular symmetry of CT scans one usually distinguishes between the in-plane resolution Δr and the axial- or z-resolution S_{eff} (effective slice thickness). For example, an image noise of $\sigma = 30$ HU, an in-plane resolution of $\Delta r = 0.7$ mm and a z-resolution of $S_{\text{eff}} = 0.8$ mm are typical values for the present standard exams. Please note that the resolution values are not identical to the voxel size of the image data which may be chosen to be arbitrarily small during image reconstruction.

Dose is usually quantified by specifying the organ dose or the effective dose (values in mSv). For our purposes, it suffices to regard the effective tube current time product $(I{\cdot}t)_{\text{eff}}$, i.e. the "effective mAs value", as being the characteristic dose parameter since this parameter is proportional to the physical dose values. It is defined as the product of the tube current with the time under which a given z-position (slice) is exposed to X-rays; therefore, the effective mAs depends on the scan's pitch value p and on the rotation time t_{rot} as follows:

$$(I \cdot t)_{\text{eff}} = \frac{I_0 \cdot t_{\text{rot}}}{p} .$$

Recall that the pitch value is defined as

$$p = \frac{d}{M \cdot S}$$

where d is the table increment per rotation, S is the collimated (nominal) slice thickness and M is the number of simultaneously scanned slices. Its inverse p^{-1} gives the number of rotations that cover a given z-position. Consider a scan with a table increment of 6 mm and a collimation of 16×0.75 mm. This situation corresponds to a pitch of 0.5 and, consequently, each z-position is exposed to X-rays during two full rotations (twofold overlapping scan). Further assume a rotation time of 0.4 s and a tube current of 200 mA. Then, according to the definition above, the effective mAs value is 160 mAs. It is this effective mAs value, and not the tube current itself, that is directly related to the image noise σ. The present scanners make use of this fact by allowing the user to specify the effective mAs value. Internally, the scanner computes the correct tube current from the specified effective mAs value and the selected pitch. Consequently, dose and image noise and the effective mAs value do *not* depend on the spiral pitch, a fact that has often been misunderstood.

Quantitatively, the proportionality

$$\sigma^2 \propto \frac{1}{(I \cdot t)_{\text{eff}} \cdot S_{\text{eff}} \cdot \Delta r^3} \tag{1}$$

holds. The constant of proportionality depends in a complicated way on the patient size and density, on the tube voltage and on the prefiltration.

Prior to the scan, the user specifies the three parameters effective mAs value, effective slice thickness and the in-plane resolution (via the name of the reconstruction kernel) at the scanner console. He is thereby aiming at his preferred image quality. The image noise σ is the only dependent parameter since it cannot be controlled directly.

Equation has important consequences: increasing the spatial resolution requires to dramatically increase the effective mAs value and thereby the dose given that the image noise σ is to be held constant. For example, doubling spatial resolution (i.e. reducing S_{eff} and Δr to 50%) requires to increase patient dose by a factor of 16 if the pixel noise shall remain at its original level. Since such dose increases are hardly acceptable, scan protocols must carefully balance between spatial resolution and image noise; therefore, many applications are designed to either aim at good low-contrast resolution (low image noise) or to produce high spatial resolution. The first is the case in tumour detection tasks where lower spatial resolution is acceptable. In contrast, lung exams and, especially, exams of the inner ear, require to scan with the highest spatial resolution available.

3.3 Dose Reduction with Multidimensional Adaptive Filtering

To allow for even higher image quality in the future, new software- and hardware-based methods that make better use of the applied dose have been furnished.

This includes so-called adaptive filtering approaches that seek to reduce image noise either by directly manipulating the reconstructed images or by performing dedicated raw-data preprocessing prior to image reconstruction (Eklundh and Rosenfeld 1981; Lauro et al. 1990; Keselbrener et al. 1992; Hsieh 1994, 1998). Directly manipulating images turns out to be less efficient and more critical, even if the filters are applied locally (adaptively), since respective algorithms tend to smooth parts of the image; therefore, raw-data-based approaches, as they are often provided by the manufacturers, are preferred.

A highly effective method is multi-dimensional adaptive filtering (MAF) which is a raw-data-based algorithm using two detector dimensions plus the view dimension (rotation direction) to locally smooth data. The MAF allows to reduce image noise in cross sections of high eccentricity such as the pelvis, thorax or shoulder without affecting spatial resolution. In contrast to the said image-based smoothing approaches (including the selection of smooth reconstruction kernels), the raw-data-based MAF operates only on a tiny fraction of the acquired raw data. The MAF selects those attenuation values for filtering that suffer from photon starvation due to high attenuation. Typically, 5% of the data are modified; 95% of the acquired data remain unchanged (Kachelriess and Kalender 2000; Kachelriess et al. 2001b).

The MAF can be used to remove the well-known streak-like noise artefacts that are oriented along the direction of highest attenuation (typically the lateral direction). Low-contrast objects are often completely hidden by this kind of structured and correlated noise. Increasing the tube current to avoid these artefacts would be the wrong strategy since global improvements are not required. The effect of applying MAF is illustrated in Fig. 3.2. The patient exhibits severe streak artefacts in the shoulder region due to photon starvation. They are largely removed by MAF. Even more, the difference images show no patient structure. This proves that MAF does not simply smooth the image. The MAF instead man-

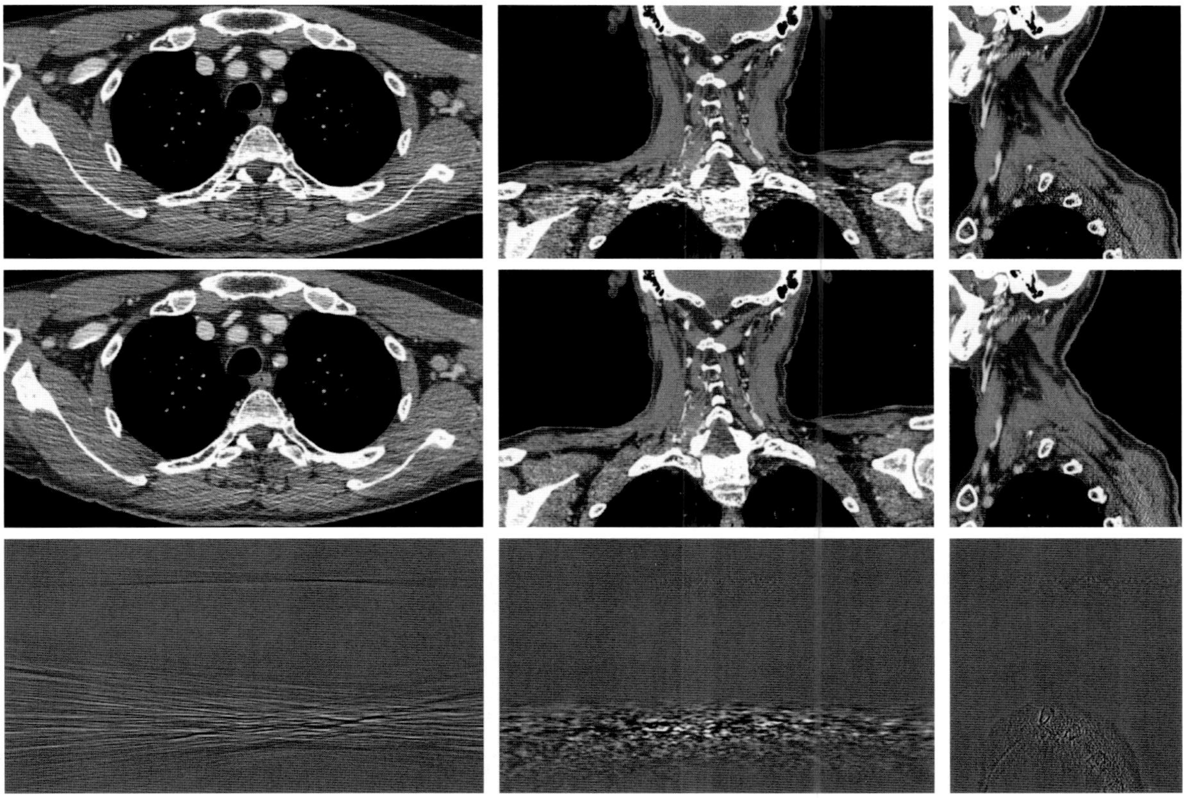

Fig. 3.2. Noise in the original data (*top row*) is reduced by up to 50% with multi-dimensional adaptive filtering (MAF; *middle row*). Since streaks are oriented laterally, the transaxial slice and the coronal MPR show great improvements, whereas there are no modifications in the anteroposterior direction and, consequently, the sagittal reformation is hardly modified. The subtraction images (*bottom row*) prove that MAF does remove noise but not structure details

ages to reduce noise and to remove the correlated noise without affecting spatial resolution; thereby, the visibility of low-contrast objects can be greatly improved (Baum et al. 2000).

3.4 Dose Reduction with Automatic Exposure Control

Similar to conventional radiography, an automatism to obtain a defined image quality is needed for CT. The present CT scanners allow to specify the spatial resolution, but it is not possible to specify the image noise. One must instead set the effective mAs product which influences image noise only indirectly. The outcome is strongly dependent on patient size, density and shape.

The dependence on patient size and its implications on dose values are best illustrated using a numerical example: a 20 cm water-equivalent object (representing an adult head) attenuates the X-rays by a factor of approximately 50 and only 2% of the photons reach the detector. For a small object of half size (representing a child head), the attenuation factor decreases to 7 and it becomes likely that too many quanta reach the detector. Due to this exponential behaviour, it is hard to manually extrapolate scan parameters from the standard adult patient to small children. This fact is one of the major causes for using too high doses in paediatric CT.

A first step towards AEC has been the introduction of the dose modulation technique. It modulates the tube current during each rotation as a function of patient anatomy to compensate for the different attenuation properties; typically, for anteroposterior projections the tube current is decreased and for lateral projections the tube current is increased (Gies et al. 1999; Kalender et al. 1999b).

It can be shown that the optimal way to modulate the tube current as a function of the rotation angle α is proportional to the square root of the attenuation $p(\alpha)$ measured at that angle (Gies et al. 1999; Harpen 1999):

$$I_0(\alpha) \propto e^{\frac{1}{2}p(\alpha)}.$$

To achieve optimal modulation, attenuation values must be known. The most effective (in terms of dose utilization) implementations use attenuation values that have been measured 180° in advance to control the tube at the current projection on-line. Figure 3.3 illustrates this principle by giving typical quantum number values. Typical mAs-reduction values that can be achieved with this on-line dose modulation technique are given in Table 3.1, taken from Kalender et al. (1999c) and Greess et al. (2000).

These mAs-reduction values have been achieved without increasing image noise. It further turns out that the noise structure of the images acquired with dose modulation is less pronounced and less correlated than the noise structure of the standard acquisition, thereby indicating improved image quality. Even more, Monte Carlo calculations of the organ dose and effective dose with and without dose modulation have shown that the mAs-reduction values underestimate the physical dose reduction (Kalender et

Table 3.1. Typical mAs-reduction values that can be achieved with on-line dose modulation technique

Region	mAs reduction (%)
Head	18
Shoulder	53
Thorax	22
Abdomen	15
Pelvis	25
Extremity	39

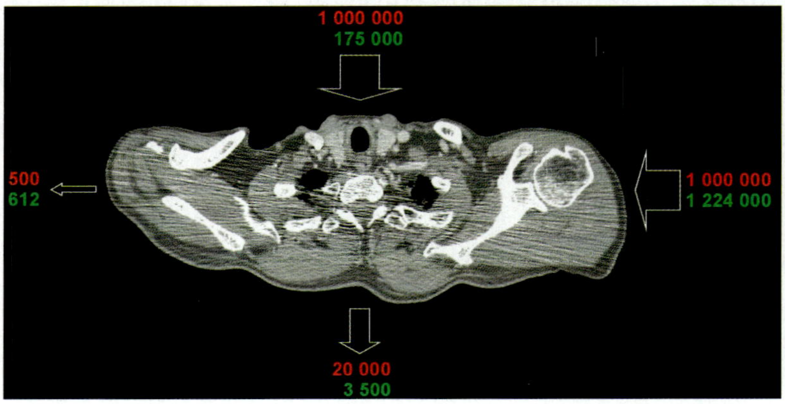

Fig. 3.3. Scans with constant tube current (red) suffer from extremely different attenuation properties within eccentric objects. Here, photon starvation occurs in the lateral direction while more than sufficiently many photons are measured anteroposteriorly. Tube current modulation (green) greatly reduces these discrepancies by modulating the tube current as a function of anatomy. In total, it reduces the mAs product (here by 30%) and, consequently, patient dose without increasing image noise

al. 1999c; SCHMIDT and KALENDER 2001, 2002): the values given in the table are only a conservative estimate of the true dose reduction achieved with tube current modulation.

Besides the on-line dose modulation techniques, other implementations make use of topogram (or scout view) data from an anteroposterior and a lateral view (KOPKA et al. 1995). Sinusoidal curves are fitted to the topogram data to predict the angle-dependent attenuation for all α; however, besides the need for two topograms, the mAs-reduction values reported are significantly lower than with the on-line method (KALENDER et al. 1999c).

All dose-modulation methods have in common that there are only local (rotation-wise) adaptations of the current. Variations of the mean attenuation properties in the longitudinal direction are not taken into account as the tube current's mean or maximum value is retained after each rotation.

The remaining step towards AEC is to combine the tube current modulation with a tube current control. The tube current control slowly varies the current's mean value according to the patient anatomy and thus is able to compensate for varying image noise along the z-direction. The AEC comprises a method to "foresee" the image noise as a function of anatomy. Then, the tube current can be controlled to achieve a given target noise. Again, there are topogram-based implementations and more sophisticated raw-data-based implementations (KACHELRIESS et al. 2001a). In the future, scanners will make use of AEC to assist the user in adapting the tube current to patient anatomy or even to replace the tube current parameter in favour of directly specifying image noise and hence image quality.

Figure 3.4 shows the tube current curve and the resulting image noise as a function of the anatomical level during a spiral 16-slice scan from neck to thorax. The red and blue graphs correspond to the conventional case: the mean level of the tube current is held constant. The noise curves (red is hidden by blue) show excellent image quality in the neck and insufficient image quality in the shoulder. Without AEC, image quality can only be increased by increasing the tube current. With AEC, in contrast, it is possible to accept more noise in the neck and to reduce noise in the thorax at the same time. Assume that the user specifies a constant noise level corresponding to the green horizontal curve. Then, AEC controls and modulates the tube current to achieve the desired level (green oscillating curve). The running mean (green slowly varying curve) gives the local mAs-reduction value as a function of the z-position.

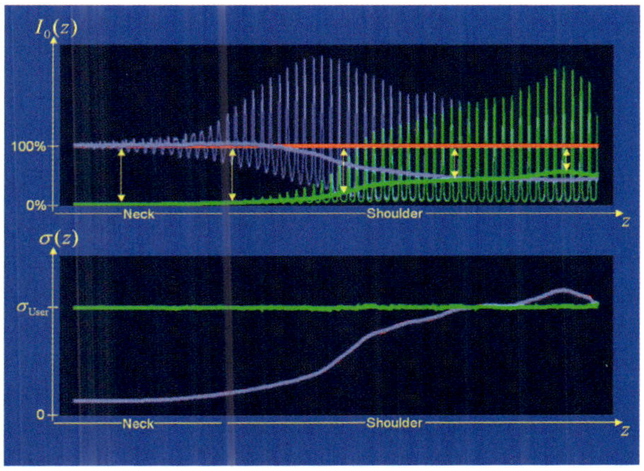

Fig. 3.4. Tube current (*top*) and resulting image noise (*bottom*) for a scan from neck to shoulder. *Red:* constant tube current (conventional scan). *Blue:* tube current modulation. *Green:* tube current control and modulation (AEC). The *thick lines in the top image* are the local averages of the modulated graphs and illustrate the dose savings as a function of the z-position. The *red graph* is hidden by the *blue graph* in the bottom image

The phantom experiment of Fig. 3.5 demonstrates the performance of AEC. The step phantom consists of three elliptical cylinders of decreasing diameter. The standard acquisition (constant tube current) suffers from varying image quality along the z-axis: high noise in the large cylinder; acceptable noise in the medium cylinder; and unnecessary low noise in the small cylinder. The three axial images further suffer from streak artefacts due to correlated noise. The AEC scan, in contrast, is as specified: constant noise for the complete scan range and reduced noise correlations in the axial images. Besides constant noise, one may also specify other noise profiles, if desired.

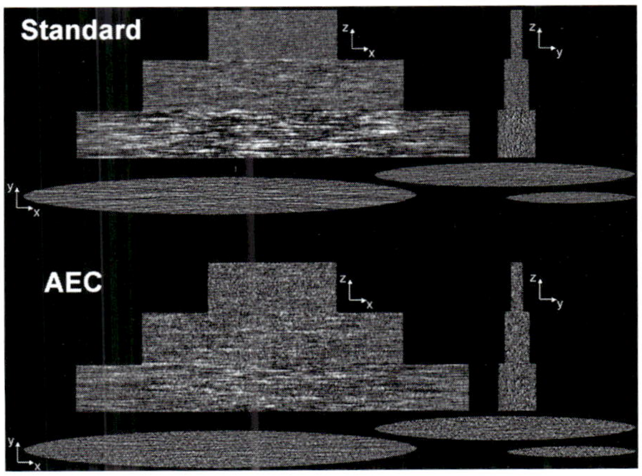

Fig. 3.5. This phantom experiment demonstrates that AEC achieves constant image noise for all z-positions and that noise structure can be significantly reduced

Even more potential for dose reduction lies in the combination of AEC and MAF (Kachelriess et al. 2002). Both methods are complementary: AEC globally influences complete projections and MAF is able to locally adjust the noise statistics of single detector readouts. The synergetic effects are illustrated in Fig. 3.6. The AEC reduces the tube current at the lung level where the attenuation is quite low. The increased noise is acceptable. In the shoulder, however, the tube current is globally increased by AEC. Here, MAF further reduces noise in the most central lateral rays.

An interesting specialization to the tube current modulation and tube current control technique has been recently introduced to reduce dose of retrospectively gated cardiac CT exams (Kachelriess and Kalender 1998): The so-called ECG pulsing technique reduces the tube current for those ECG phases that are unlikely to contribute to the reconstructed images (Jakobs et al. 2002).

3.5 Dose Reduction by User Education

When installed at a location, the CT system is usually adjusted to standard factory settings to give good image quality. This does not automatically mean the lowest possible radiation dose. Learning how to customize and optimize the scan parameters (which constitute the scan protocols) with regard to dose and image quality is therefore a promising strategy to reduce dose.

However, customizing scan protocols to optimally meet all criteria is a difficult task. This is due to the complex dependence of image noise on the patient cross section (including size, weight, etc.). Finding the optimal mAs value, for example, is an iterative process that requires profound experience and, in principle, the possibility to repeat scans with different parameters until the preferred image quality is achieved. Dose considerations, however, forbid to repeat scans on a given subject. Phantom or cadaver scans may help, but the results are often too far from reality.

Recently, industry has started to provide tools that retrospectively simulate arbitrary scan parameters (Leidecker et al. 2002). Basically, these tools consist of simulating arbitrary tube currents or, equivalently, mAs products. The resolution can be varied retrospectively by selecting different reconstruction kernels and different effective slice thicknesses.

Two classes of simulation methods are available. One approach adds random noise to reconstructed CT images. The standard deviation of the random values is a function of the voxel grey value, the source

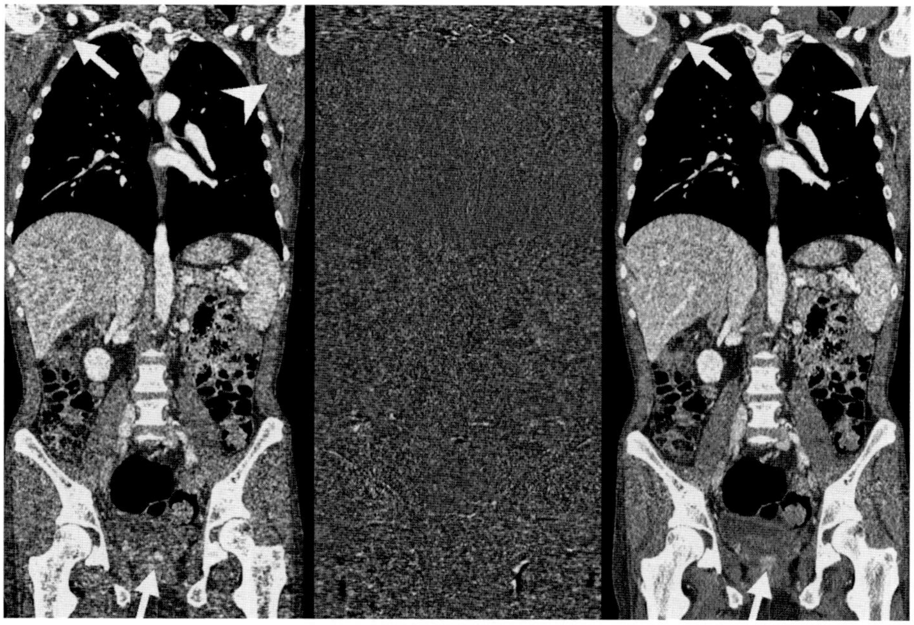

Fig. 3.6. The combination of AEC with MAF currently is the optimum dose-reduction strategy: due to its tube current modulation and control, AEC increases noise in regions of low attenuation (arrowheads) and decreases noise and noise correlation in regions of high attenuation and high eccentricity. In contrast to tube current modulation techniques that influence the photon statistics of complete projections, MAF can modify single-detector element readings and further reduce the noise in the shoulder and pelvis region (*arrows*). The difference in image indicates that no structure has been smoothed by the procedure

mAs and the desired destination mAs; however, this simple method does not correctly consider the X-ray physics which demand to add noise to the X-ray photon attenuation instead of adding noise to image pixels. Consequently, it cannot reproduce noise structure and artefacts characteristic to CT images.

The second class of algorithms correctly simulates the physics behind CT imaging. To do so, it requires CT raw data and the complete image reconstruction pipeline. Noise is added to the projection values to account for the desired destination mAs product. Figure 3.7 shows respective results using a raw-data-based tube-current simulator. As expected, image noise increases with decreased tube current and the noise structure generated is physically correct.

3.6 Tube Voltage and Filtration

As we have seen, there is much potential in optimizing the dose usage by optimizing the tube current (or, equivalently, the effective mAs value). What remains to be considered are the effects of the tube voltage U and of the prefiltration on image quality and on patient dose. It is well known that a high tube voltage yields a high-energy X-ray spectrum and that the X-ray attenuation coefficients μ decrease with increased energy. In other words: fewer photons are absorbed in the patient. The dose itself scales with both the number and the mean energy of absorbed photons. The number of photons available is proportional to the tube current but is a complicated function of U.

Although these relationships are already complex enough, we have not yet included image quality into these considerations. Since the attenuation coefficients vary with the tube voltage, the reconstructed grey values will also do so (μ is a function of U); therefore, it does not suffice to regard image noise σ alone as the indicator of image quality. Equation (1) must instead be extended to put the noise σ and the signal μ into relation:

$$(\sigma/\mu)^2 \propto \frac{e^{\mu D}}{\mu^2 (I \cdot t)_{\mathrm{eff}} \cdot S_{\mathrm{eff}} \cdot \Delta r^3}$$

Here, D is the object diameter and the numerator accounts for the total object attenuation. Low values of (σ/μ) are desired. Its inverse μ/σ is commonly known as the signal-to-noise ratio (whenever signal differences $\Delta\mu$ are of interest the SNR is given as $\Delta\mu/\sigma$). Image quality increases with increasing SNR. The complex dependence between the SNR and the tube voltage cannot be handled analytically, however. Monte Carlo simulations or phantom experiments are required to analyse the effect of tube voltage on image quality and dose.

For example, a recent study evaluated iodine contrast as a function of tube voltage to improve the scan protocol design for paediatric CT (Schaller et al. 2001). Iodine contrast $\Delta\mu = \mu_{\mathrm{I}} - \mu_{\mathrm{H_2O}}$ and image noise were measured in a thorax phantom equipped with an iodine insert for 80, 120 and 140 kV. Dose was estimated using the CT dose index (CTDI) measured in a 16 cm CTDI phantom. The CTDI is defined as the integral over the axial dose profile normalized to the nominal collimation:

$$CTDI_{100\mathrm{mm}} = \frac{1}{M \cdot S} \int_{-50\mathrm{mm}}^{50\mathrm{mm}} dz\, D(z)$$

The study resulted in the following values (Table 3.2): image quality, given by the SNR, must be normalized with the dose value: Quality=SNR^2/Dose serves as an adequate image quality measure. The Table 3.2 clearly shows the strong dependency of image quality on the tube voltage: the quality of the 80 kV scan differs from that of the 140 kV scan by a factor 2.9. This means that the SNR at 80 kV is 70% better than at 140 kV when the same dose is applied. Alternatively, one can obtain the same image quality at 80 kV with only 34% of the dose.

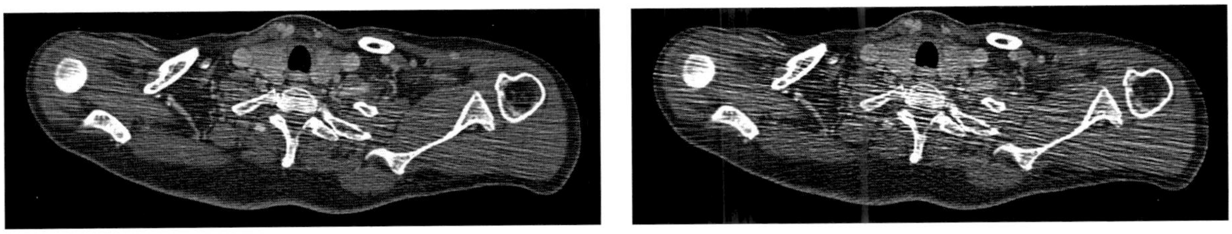

Fig. 3.7. The dose tutor helps to decrease the tube current from its original level to the desired low-dose protocol (*left:* original 160 mAs, *right:* simulated 40 mAs). Noise structure is correctly reproduced. The user can experience with realistic examples which tube current is acceptable

Table 3.2. Value results of the study

Protocol	Dose (mGy)	Iodine contrast (HU)	Image noise (HU)	Quality (mGy)
80 kV, 120 mAs	4.9	528	15.0	252
120 kV, 37 mAs	4.5	336	14.4	121
140 kV, 26 mAs	4.4	284	14.5	86

These results, however, must be taken with care and cannot be applied to the general case. They instead emphasize the potential that lies in varying the X-ray spectrum. Note that all parameters have been correctly taken into account: contrast; noise; spatial resolution; and dose. Here, comparisons were made at equal spatial resolution.

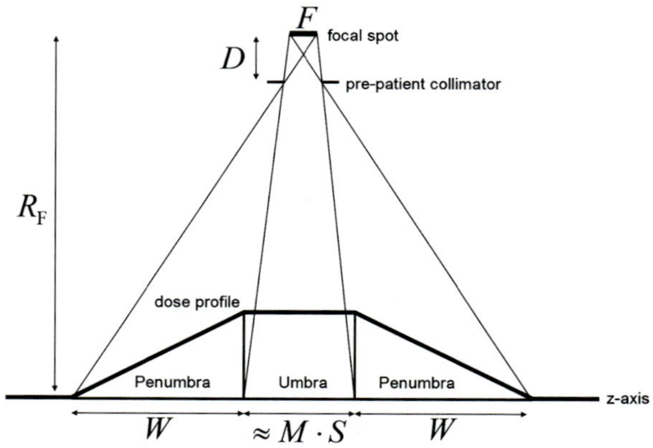

Fig. 3.8. Finite-sized focal spots yield trapezoidal primary dose profiles, whereas rectangular profiles are desired. The penumbra size W is constant, whereas the size of the umbra varies with the collimation

3.7 Penumbra Effects

In addition to the dose reduction strategies that have been mentioned, it is of great importance to know about fundamental differences between single-slice and multi-slice scanners. Theoretically, there should be no difference in dose usage if comparisons are performed at equal spatial resolution and at equal image noise. Practically, however, penumbra effects in the axial-dose profile must be taken into account.

Due to the finite size of the X-ray tube's focal spot, the desired rectangular distribution of primary X-rays in the z-direction cannot be achieved. In reality, the dose profile has to be approximated by a trapezoidal function. The shape of this function is a function of scanner-dependent geometrical parameters: the size F of the focal spot; the distance D of the pre-patient collimation to the focal spot; and the distance R_F of the focal spot to the centre of rotation (isocentre). The relations are illustrated in Fig. 3.8. The profile's triangular tails are called penumbra, its constant rectangular region is called umbra.

To make full use of the exposure to the patient it is of interest to use not only the constant umbra region, but to include also the penumbras into the measurement. This can be easily achieved with single-slice scanners by opening the post-patient collimation until the penumbra is included. For multi-slice scanners ($M > 1$), however, it is not possible to include the penumbra since the outermost slices (penumbra region) would record a different intensity than the innermost slices (umbra region) and image artefacts occur for this case; therefore, the penumbra region has to be cut off by the post-patient collimation for scanners with two or more slices (Fig. 3.9). A dose increase relative to single-slice scanners is to be expected.

A simple geometric consideration shows that the width W of the penumbra at the isocentre is related to the size F of the focal spot as

$$W = \frac{R_F - D}{D} F .$$

Inserting values typical for modern MSCT scanners (e.g. R_F=600 mm, D=200 mm, F=0.5 mm) yields a penumbra size of W=1 mm. To estimate the "geometrical" dose increase of multi-slice scanners as compared with single-slice scanners one must regard

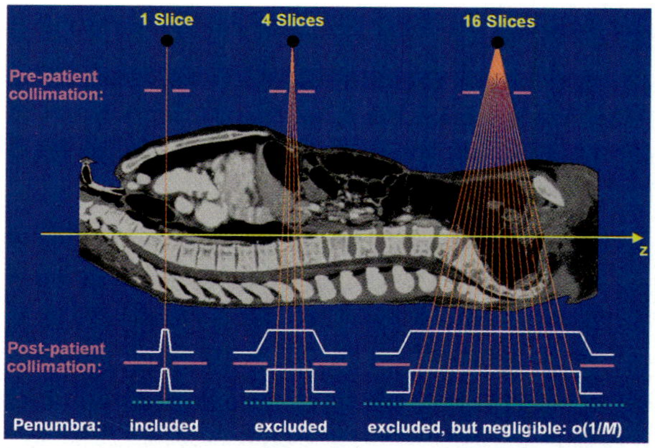

Fig. 3.9. Differences in the post-patient collimation yield a slight dose increase with multi-slice scanners due to the exclusion of the penumbra region. This increase becomes negligible with wider cone angles and a higher number of slices

the ratio of the total dose profile area (umbra plus penumbra) to the umbra area (umbra only). This ratio is given by

$$1+\frac{W}{M\cdot S}\ .$$

Consequently, the dose increase itself is given by the term $W/M{\cdot}S$ which decreases with an increasing number M of slices and with increasing slice thickness S. Table 3.3 gives examples for 4- and 16-slice scanners with typical collimations assuming W=1 mm.

Apparently, the dose increase compared with single-slice CT becomes smaller for larger collimations and will become negligible with the introduction of scanners with even larger cone angles (e.g. 32 slices or more).

3.8 Dose Information

Individual dose assessment will play a significant role in the future. For example, the European Union Directive (European Communities 1997) demands the specification of the individual patient dose for every CT examination. To directly assess scanner- and organ-specific dose values, dose calculators have become

Table 3.3. Examples for 4- and 16-slice scanners with typical collimations assuming W=1 mm

Collimation (mm)	Geometrical dose increase (%)
4×1	25
4×2.5	10
16×0.75	8
16×1.5	4

available. Based on Monte Carlo dose calculations (Schmidt and Kalender 2002), they allow to compute organ-dose and effective-dose values as a function of the scanner type and scan protocol (Fig. 3.10). The effective dose is regarded as the best indicator of stochastic risk such as induction of malignancy. It expresses the sum dose value over all organs weighted by their radiation sensitivities. The weighting factors are recommended by the International Commission on Radiation Protection (ICRP 1990).

Dose calculators should also be used to answer justified questions about dose and risk values. Here it is of advantage to know the annual effective dose caused by natural internal and external radiation sources (e.g. 2.1 mSv in Germany, between 2.0 and 7.0 mSv in Europe, and 3.0 mSv in the United States; NCRP 1988; BMU 2000). When reporting to a patient, effective dose values should be put into relation in that context. Statements such as "the exposure of this examination corresponds to two years of natural background radiation

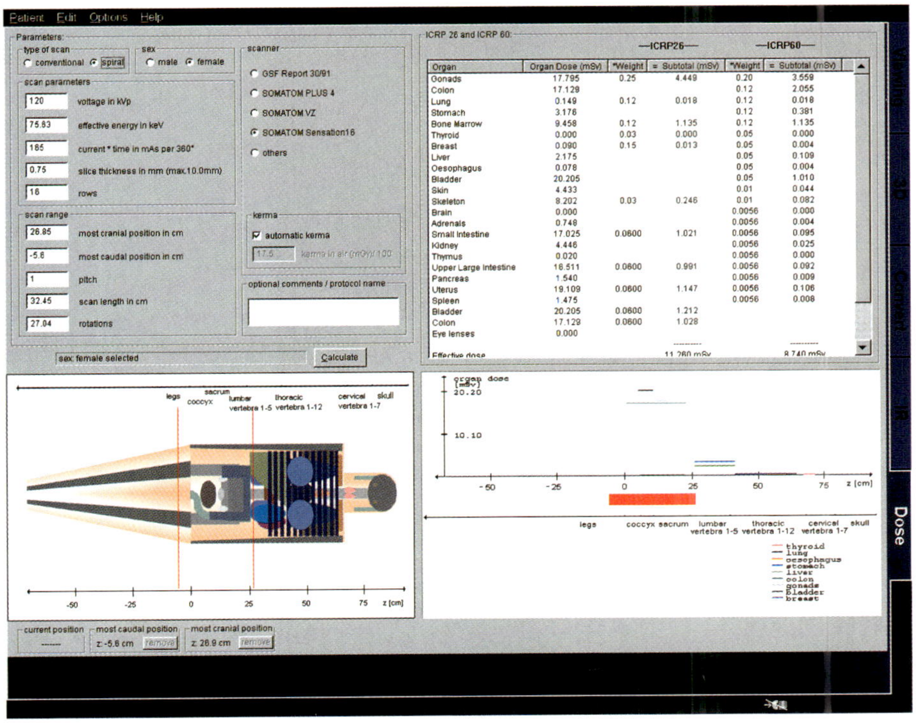

Fig. 3.10. A typical dose calculator computes organ dose values and the weighted effective dose as a function of the anatomical region and the scan parameters. It can be integrated into the scanner environment (Kalender et al. 1999a)

in the United States" are more informative than stating that the effective dose is 6.0 mSv.

3.9 Discussion

The demand for higher spatial resolution and lower image noise is limited by the increasing patient dose values according to Eq (1). Nevertheless, we have seen a number of strategies that help to compensate for the dose increase. This occurs either by making more efficient use of the available dose or by adequate training programs.

On the one hand, manufacturers' efforts will further improve dose utilization. Automatic exposure control, dose modulation, and intelligent adaptive filtering algorithms bear the highest potential for dose reduction. The design of optimized scan protocols adds to these improvements.

On the other hand, there will always be enough degrees of freedom available to the radiologist to significantly influence patient dose (in the positive or in the negative sense). The exposure to the patient should be adjusted to obtain the required diagnostic information and not to get the best image quality possible. Training tools to learn about the influence of scan parameters help to iteratively seek for the preferred image quality. Figure 3.11 shows a fully qualified image reconstruction software (VAMP GmbH, Möhrendorf, Germany). It optionally allows to artificially increase the mAs product from the original level to any value below by adding noise to the raw data and performing an image reconstruction. One may further start a multidimensional adaptive filtering algorithm and study the combined effects.

The decisive step in the near future will be the introduction of automatic exposure control which allows to directly specify the image quality (e.g. in terms of s). The mAs parameter may then vanish from the user interface to be replaced by one or more "image quality" parameters. Alternatives are the introduction of an "equivalent mAs value" corresponding to some normalized patient or the development of sophisticated user interfaces that graphically display reference images as a function of the selected parameters. These would illustrate the expected image quality before the scan is started.

Combining these strategies will help to limit the patient dose to reasonable values even if CT further goes to higher spatial resolution.

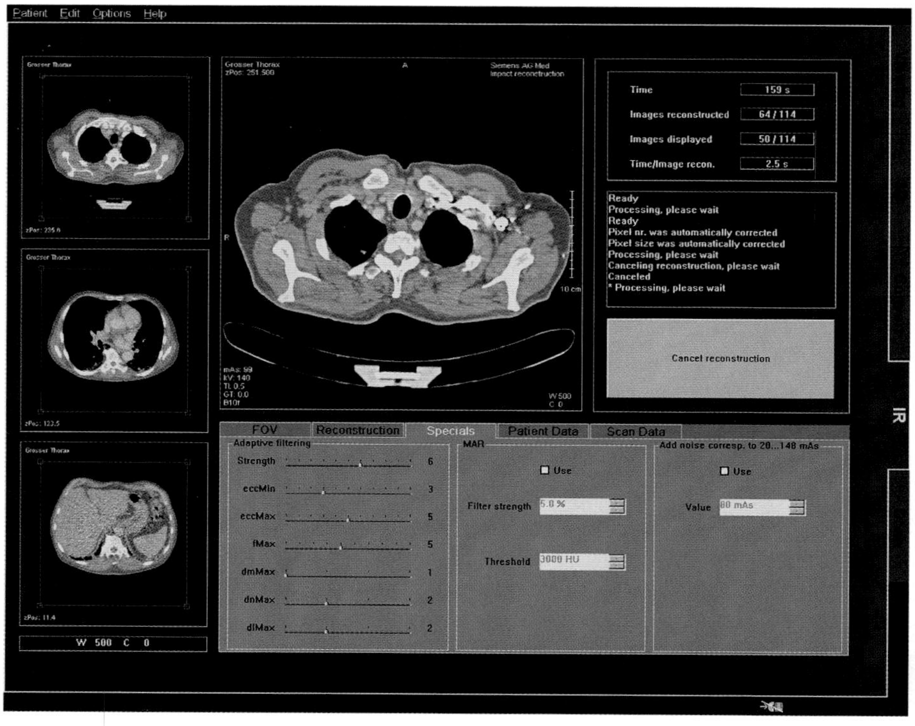

Fig. 3.11. The software-based dose-reduction algorithm MAF (*left group of the open tab*) and dose-training tools that retrospectively allow for a virtual decrease of patient dose (*right group of the open tab*) are readily available in medical applications such as the VAMP Syngo Explorer workstation

References

Baum U, Lell M, Kachelriess M, Greess H, Kalender WA, Bautz WA (2000) Rawdata-based 3D adaptive filtering for CT scans of the cervicothoracic region: Clinical evaluation. Radiology 217:413

BMU (2000) (Bundesministerium für Umwelt, Naturschutz und Reaktorsicherheit) Umweltradioaktivität und Strahlenbelastung im Jahr 2000. Unterrichtung durch die Bundesregierung

Brenner DJ, Elliston CD, Hall EJ, Berdon WE (2001) Estimated risks of radiation induced fatal cancer from pediatric CT. Am J Roentgenol 176:289–296

Eklundh JO, Rosenfeld A (1981) Imaging smoothing based on neighbor linking. IEEE Trans Pattern Anal Mach Intell 3: 679–683

European Communities (1997) Council Directive 97/43/ Euratom of 30 June 1997 on health protection of individuals against the dangers of ionising radiation in relation to medical exposure, and repealing Directive 84/466/Euratom. Official Journal of the European Communities no. L 180/22

Gies M, Kalender WA, Wolf H, Suess C, Madsen MT (1999) Dose reduction in CT by anatomically adapted tube current modulation. I. Simulation studies. Med Phys 26: 2235–2247

Greess H, Wolf H, Baum U, Lell M, Pirkl M, Kalender WA, Bautz WA (2000) Dose reduction in computed tomography by attenuation-based on-line modulation of tube current: evaluation of six anatomical regions. Eur Radiol 10:391–394

Harpen MD (1999) A simple theorem relating noise and patient dose in computed tomography. Med Phys 26:2231–2234

Hsieh J (1994) Generalized adaptive median filter and their application in computed tomography. SPIE Proc 2298: 662–672

Hsieh J (1998) Adaptive streak artifact reduction in computed tomography resulting from excessive X-ray photon noise. Med Phys 25:2139–2147

ICRP (1990) (International Commission on Radiological Protection) Publication 60. Recommendations of the International Commission on Radiological Protection. Pergamon, Oxford

Jakobs T, Becker C, Ohnesorge B, Flohr T, Schoepf UJ, Reiser M (2002) Multislice helical CT of the heart with retrospective ECG-gating: reduction of radiation exposure by ECG-controlled tube current modulation. Eur Radiol 12:1081–1086

Kachelriess M, Kalender WA (1998) Electrocardiogram-correlated image reconstruction from subsecond spiral CT scans of the heart. Med Phys 25:2417–2431

Kachelriess M, Kalender WA (2000) Computertomograph mit reduzierter Dosisbelastung bzw. reduziertem Bildpunktrauschen. Deutsches Patent- und Markenamt. Germany, Patent Specification DE 198 53 143

Kachelriess M, Leidecker C, Kalender WA (2001a) Image quality-oriented automatic exposure control (iqAEC) for spiral CT. Radiology 221:366

Kachelriess M, Watzke O, Kalender WA (2001b) Generalized multi-dimensional adaptive filtering for conventional and spiral single-slice, multi-slice, and cone-beam CT. Med Phys 28:475–490

Kachelriess M, Leidecker C, Kalender WA (2002) Patient dose reduction by combining automatic exposure control (AEC) with multidimensional adaptive filtering (MAF) for spiral CT. Eur Radiol 12 (Suppl 1):196

Kalender WA (2001) Computed tomography. Wiley, New York

Kalender WA, Schmidt B, Zankl M, Schmidt M (1999a) A PC program for estimating organ dose and effective dose values in computed tomography. Eur Radiol 9:555–562

Kalender WA, Wolf H, Suess C (1999b) Dose reduction in CT by anatomically adapted tube current modulation. II. Phantom measurements. Med Phys 26:2248–2253

Kalender WA, Wolf H, Suess C, Gies M, Greess H, Bautz WA (1999c) Dose reduction in CT by on-line tube current control: principles and validation on phantoms and cadavers. Eur Radiol 9:323–328

Keselbrener L, Shimoni Y, Akselrod S (1992) Nonlinear filters applied on computerized axial tomography. Theory and phantom images. Med Phys 19:1057–1064

Kopka L, Funke M, Breiter N, Hermann K-P, Vosshenrich R, Grabbe E (1995) Anatomisch adaptierte Variation des Röhrenstroms bei der CT. Untersuchungen zur Strahlendosisreduktion und Bildqualität. Fortschr Röntgenstr 163: 383–387

Lauro KL, Heuscher DJ, Kesavan H (1990) Bandwidth filtering of CT scans of the spine. Radiology 177:307

Leidecker C, Fuchs T, Kachelriess M, Schaller S, Kalender WA (2002) Comparison of different methods for adding virtual noise to measured rawdata in order to estimate the dose reduction potential for clinical protocols in CT. Radiology 225:592

NCRP (1988) (National Counsel on Radiation Protection and Measurement) Exposure of the population in the United States and Canada from natural background radiation. Report 94

Schaller S, Niethammer MU, Chen X, Klotz E, Wildberger TG, Flohr T (2001) Comparison of signal-to-noise and dose values at different tube voltages for protocol optimization in pediatric. Radiology 221:366

Schmidt B, Kalender WA (2001) Calculation of dose reduction by tube current modulation in pediatric CT. Radiology 221:365

Schmidt B, Kalender WA (2002) A fast voxel-based Monte Carlo method for scanner- and patient-specific dose calculations in computed tomography. Phys Med 18:43–53

4 Contrast Medium Injection Technique

D. FLEISCHMANN

CONTENTS

4.1 Introduction

The general goal of intravenous contrast medium (CM) delivery in CT is to achieve adequate enhancement of the organ or vessels within the anatomic territory of interest, synchronized with the CT acquisition. This apparently simple goal is increasingly difficult to achieve with rapidly and continuously evolving multiple detector-row CT (MDCT) technology. Given the substantially shorter acquisition times which have become possible with each new generation of MDCT scanners, correct scan timing and tailoring clinical injection protocols is ever more challenging and less forgiving; thus, a basic understanding of early CM dynamics has become a prerequisite for the rational design of current and future injection strategies. The selection of CM and its iodine concentration, considerations regarding the interrelated effects of injection flow rates, injection duration, and injection volume, new injection devices and individual patient factors all have to be integrated to match the clinical needs of a diagnostically meaningful MDCT examination.

The purpose of this chapter is to provide the reader with the basic tools for designing rational CM injection protocols for various applications of thoracic MDCT. This encompasses a review of physiologic and pharmacokinetic principles, as well as a discussion of CM properties, injection devices and tools for accurate scan timing. In addition, practical examples of injection protocols are provided.

4.2 Contrast Media for Multiple Detector-Row CT

All currently used angiographic X-ray CM are water-soluble derivates of symmetrically iodinated benzene. They are either negatively charged ionic molecules (ionic CM) or nonionic molecules (nonionic CM). The diagnostic use of X-ray CM is based on the physical ability of iodine to absorb X-rays, not on pharmacological effects, and is similar for all angiographic CM. Although small differences have been demonstrated in the rate of diffusion of different CM into organ parenchyma, the magnitude of these differences is not such as to affect the choice of CM in practice.

D. FLEISCHMANN, MD
Associate Professor of Radiology, Department of Angiography and Interventional Radiology, University of Vienna, Waehringer Guertel 18–20, 1090 Vienna, Austria; *and* Assistant Professor of Radiology, Divisions of Thoracic and Cardiovascular Imaging, Department of Radiology, Stanford University Medical Center, Stanford, California, USA

The selection of intravenous CM for MDCT is not so much governed by physicochemical properties such as osmotic pressure, viscosity and electrical charge, but primarily by safety considerations and rate of expected adverse reactions. Non-ionic CM are generally safer than ionic CM, with less adverse reactions (Katayama et al. 1990). In addition, CM delivery for MDCT requires the use of a power injector and comparably high injection rates – notably for CT angiography. Injection rates greater than 2.0–2.5 ml/s have a greater potential to cause acute nausea and vomiting, and, as a result, motion, if ionic CM are used. Furthermore, extravasation of ionic CM is less well tolerated than non-ionic CM; therefore, non-ionic CM are probably the best choice for contrast-enhanced MDCT in general (Hopper 1996).

Because of the unique anatomy of large vessels in the chest and the complexity of early CM dynamics, an increased awareness towards the iodine concentration of the contrast agent is critical in thoracic MDCT applications.

4.3 Pharmacokinetic and Physiologic Principles

From a pharmacokinetic point of view, all angiographic X-ray CM represent extracellular fluid markers. After intravenous administration, these agents are rapidly distributed between the vascular and interstitial spaces (Dawson and Blomley 1996a). The volume of distribution is approximately 0.25 l/kg body weight, which typically represents the extracellular fluid space. The main process of elimination is renal glomerular filtration. In general, kinetics were found to be linear or proportional to the dose. Because relative CT attenuation values (ΔHU, i.e., Δ Hounsfield Units), derived by subtracting background attenuation before administration of CM, are linearly related to the concentration of CM (iodine), contrast medium dynamics may be expressed in these units (Dawson and Blomley 1996a,b).

Pharmacokinetic studies on CM have typically concentrated on the phase of elimination (following CM injection), rather than on the very early phase of CM distribution (during CM administration). For the time frame relevant to contrast-enhanced thoracic MDCT, however, it is this particularly complex phase of early CM dynamics, which determines vascular enhancement, perivenous artifacts, and, to a lesser degree, parenchymal enhancement.

It is important to recognize at this stage that early vascular enhancement and subsequent tissue enhancement phases utilized in MDCT are affected by different kinetics, which will be reflected in the timing and composition of injection techniques. Early vascular enhancement is essentially determined by the relationship between iodine administration per unit of time (mg I/s) vs blood flow per unit of time (i.e., cardiac output, in l/min). Parenchymal enhancement is governed by the relationship of total iodine dose (mg I) vs total volume of distribution (i.e., body weight, in kilograms).

4.3.1 Early Contrast Medium Dynamics in the Chest

The sequence of early vascular enhancement effects in the thorax following intravenous administration of CM is particularly complex, because it differs between the great veins, the heart, and the pulmonary and systemic arteries. This is illustrated in Fig. 4.1. Figure 4.1a shows a series of non-incremental dynamic images obtained every two seconds at the level of the pulmonary artery during the injection of a small test bolus. The CM appears 4 s after the beginning of the injection, relatively undiluted and incompletely mixed, in the superior vena cava [which collects approximately one-third (~25 ml/s) of the cardiac output (~80 ml/s)]. This causes both bright enhancement and also perivenous streak artifacts. The subsequent enhancement of the pulmonary arteries and of the thoracic aorta is less strong, because it has mixed in the right atrium and ventricle with blood from the inferior vena cava and coronary sinus. The magnitude (in Hounsfield units) and the time course (in seconds) of opacification for each vascular territory is plotted in Fig. 4.1c. Note that pulmonary arterial enhancement begins immediately (2 s) after enhancement of the superior vena cava. The bolus, which is subsequently delayed and broadened in the pulmonary circulation and left heart chambers, appears in the thoracic aorta after another 10 s (14 s after initiation of the injection). Figure 4.1d integrates the relative enhancement effects (in ΔHU, above baseline) for a prolonged injection of 20 s for each vessel, respectively. Note that the enhancement events overlap in time. During a prolonged MDCT acquisition of, for example, 20 s, the enhancement is expected to be substantially greater in the superior vena cava than in the pulmonary vasculature and in the aorta (Fig. 4.1b). With respect to perivenous artifacts, it is pertinent that the time window, which shows maximum pulmonary arterial and aortic enhancement without dense opacification of the superior vena cava, is particularly narrow.

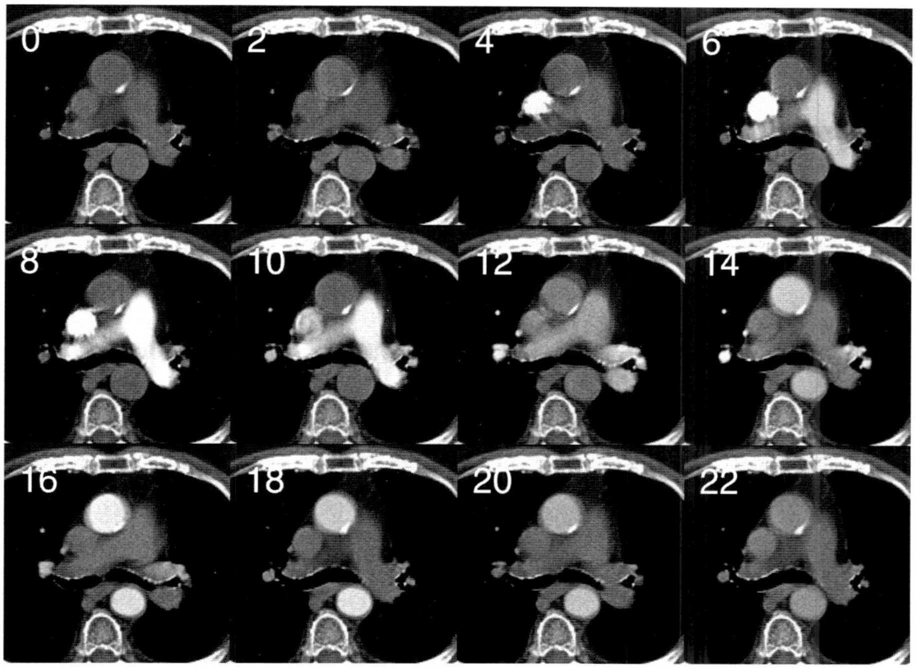

a

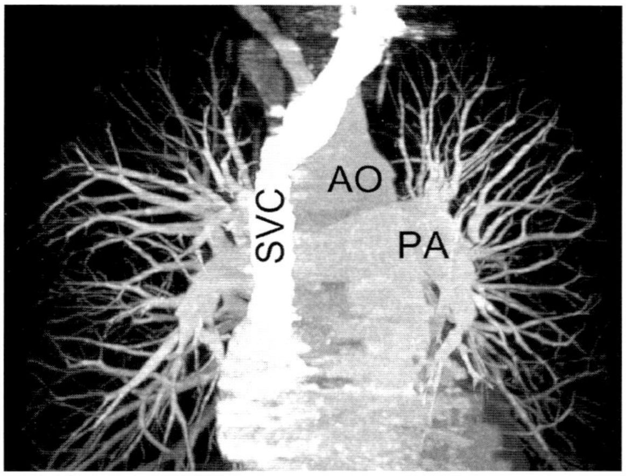

b

Fig. 4.1a–d. Early contrast medium dynamics in the chest. **a** Sequence of vascular enhancement observed in a non-incremental dynamic CT acquisition following the intravenous injection of a small test bolus are shown (see text for details). **b** Maximum intensity projection of a multiple detector-row CT (MDCT) pulmonary angiogram shows extensive opacification of the left brachiocephalic vein and superior vena cava (*SVC*). As densely opacified blood is mixed with unenhanced blood from the inferior vena cava in the right atrium and ventricle, the pulmonary arterial enhancement is substantially smaller than the enhancement in the SVC. Aortic enhancement is again slightly less than pulmonary artery (*PA*) enhancement. Analysis of the time-attenuation curves from a **c** 4-s test injection allows to predict the time attenuation curves for **d** a prolonged, 20-s injection. Note that the time window of maximum aortic enhancement without SVC enhancement is particularly narrow. *AO* thoracic aorta

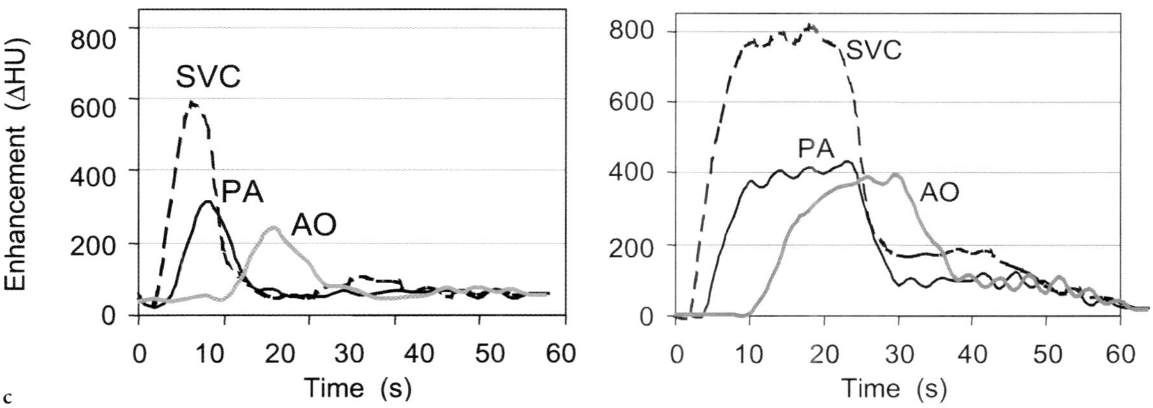

c d

4.3.2 Early Arterial Contrast Medium Dynamics

Early CM dynamics for a given vascular territory, such as the pulmonary or systemic arteries, have gained substantial interest because of their implications for CT angiography. Whereas time-attenuation responses to intravenously injected CM vary widely between vascular territories and across individuals (as discussed below), some basic principles apply to all arterial (pulmonary and systemic) vessels.

Figure 4.2 illustrates the early arterial CM dynamics as observed in the supra-celiac abdominal aorta: When a 16-ml test bolus of CM is injected intravenously, it causes an arterial enhancement response in the aorta. The time interval needed for the CM to arrive in the arterial territory of interest is referred to as the CM transit time (t_{CMT}). The first peak in the enhancement response is also referred to as the "first pass" effect. For a given individual and vascular territory, the enhancement response is proportional to the iodine injection rate.

After the CM is distributed throughout the intravascular and interstitial fluid compartments of the body, a certain proportion of CM reenters the right heart ("recirculation"). It is important to realize that within the time frame relevant to MDCT acquisition one will not only observe the first pass of contrast material but also its recirculation. As shown in Fig. 4.2, a larger (128 ml), prolonged (32 s) bolus of CM can be viewed as the sum of eight subsequent injections of small "test boluses" of 16 ml each. Each of these eight test boluses has its own effect on arterial enhancement. Under the assumption of a time-invariant linear system, the cumulative enhancement response to the entire 128 ml injection equals the sum (time integral) of each enhancement response to their respective eight test boluses (Fleischmann 2002). Note that the recirculation effects of the previous test-bolus overlap (and thus sum up) with the first-pass effects of later test boluses.

In other words, when CM is injected intravenously over a prolonged period of time (e.g., over 15–40 s), the arterial enhancement will continuously increase over time, before it decreases rapidly after the end of the injection. This well-documented effect is particularly important for CTA injection protocols, because it refutes the widely held misconception that continuous-rate prolonged injections lead to an arterial enhancement plateau. Biphasic (or multiphasic) injections with high initial and lower continuing flow rates lead to a more favorable plateau-like arterial enhancement (Fleischmann et al. 2000).

From the erroneous assumption that constant-rate injections cause a constant plateau enhancement comes another widely held misconception. One might intuitively assume that the average arterial enhancement from a 30 s CTA acquisition achieved with a 30-s CM injection is identical to the average enhancement from a 15 s CTA acquisition achieved with a 15-s injection duration. Again, it is apparent from Fig. 4.2, that if only 50% of CM was

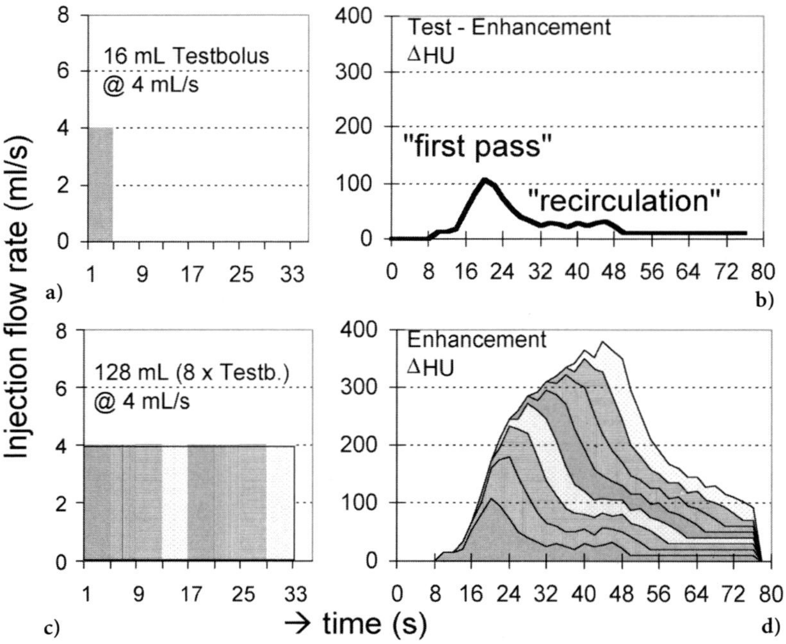

Fig. 4.2. Simple "additive model" illustrates the relationship between **a**, **c** contrast medium injection, and **b**, **d** cumulative arterial enhancement. Note that due to the asymmetric shape of the test-enhancement curve (**b**) and recirculation effects (the "tail" in the test enhancement), arterial enhancement (the "time integral of 8 test boluses") increases continuously over time (**d**). There is no enhancement plateau. (Adapted from Fleischmann 2002)

injected (corresponding to the first four of eight test boluses), the cumulative enhancement (the sum of the first four test-enhancement curves) is substantially less compared with the cumulative enhancement from the total dose (eight test boluses). It follows that if one wants to achieve the same level of enhancement with shorter injection times, the injection flow rate and/or the iodine concentration of the agent has to be increased. Alternatively, the injection delay may be increased relative to the t_{CMT}. This relative increase of the delay plus the scan time should equal the injection duration (see section 4.5).

4.3.3 Physiologic Parameters Affecting Vascular Enhancement

The vascular enhancement response to intravenously injected CM is characteristic for a given vascular territory and for a given patient. It is determined by individual physiologic parameters, and is beyond the control for the observer. The contrast material transit time (t_{CMT}) from the injection site to the vascular territory of interest depends on the anatomic distance between them, but also on the encountered physiologic flow rates between these landmarks. Except for the veins used for intravenous access, injection flow rates hardly affect the t_{CMT}. For systemic arteries, the t_{CMT} is primarily controlled by cardiac output. Cardiac output also accounts for most of the wide interindividual variability of the t_{CMT}. Low cardiac output prolongs and high cardiac output decreases the t_{CMT}. Obviously, the t_{CMT} can be substantially delayed in patients with venous obstructions downstream the injection site.

The degree of arterial enhancement following the same intravenous CM injection is also highly variable between individuals. Even in patients considered to have normal cardiac output, mid-aortic enhancement may range from 140 to 440 HU (a factor of three) between patients (Sheiman et al. 1996). Even if body weight is taken into account, the average aortic enhancement ranges from 92 to 196 HU/ml kg^{-1} (a factor of two; Hittmair and Fleischmann 2001). Adjusting the contrast medium volume (and injection rates) to body weight will therefore reduce interindividual differences of arterial enhancement, but will not completely eliminate them. The key physiologic parameters affecting individual arterial enhancement are cardiac output and the central blood volume.

Cardiac output is inversely related to the degree of arterial enhancement, particularly in first-pass dynamics (Bae et al. 1998b): If more blood is ejected per unit of time, the contrast medium injected per unit of time will be more diluted; hence, arterial enhancement is lower in patients with high cardiac output, but it is stronger in patients with low cardiac output (despite the increased t_{CMT} in the latter). This effect is illustrated in two patients with chronic thromboembolic pulmonary hypertension, in whom cardiac output was known from invasive measurements (Fig. 4.3).

Central blood volume is also inversely related to arterial enhancement, but presumably affects recirculation and tissue enhancement rather than the first-pass effect (Dawson and Blomley 1996a). Central blood volume correlates with body weight. If total contrast medium volumes are chosen relative to body weight, then 1.5–2.0 ml/kg body weight (450–600 mg I/kg) are a reasonable quantity for arterial CTA.

Other physiologic factors which affect the t_{CMT}, but also pulmonary as well as arterial enhancement, is a temporarily diminished venous return caused by a forced Valsalva maneuver of the patient in an attempt to hold his or her breath. In patients with known but also in previously undiagnosed asymptomatic individuals with a patent foramen ovale, such a maneuver may cause a temporary right-to-left shunt with early arterial enhancement.

4.3.4 Physiologic Parameters Affecting Tissue Enhancement

Parenchymal and soft tissue enhancement also diverges between different organs and tissues (Leggett and Williams 1995). Arterial blood flow, the relative proportions of intravascular to interstitial fluid compartments, and diffusion coefficients between compartments all play a role. Well-perfused tissue, such as the renal cortex, the spleen, but also hypervascular neoplasms, exhibit a similar, but somewhat delayed, enhancement course (e.g. 10- to 15-s delay relative to arterial enhancement for hypervascular liver lesions). Maximum lesion-to-background contrast between many other moderately enhancing pathologic lesions (inflammatory or neoplastic) occurs after 60 s or longer following CM administration (Foley 2002). It is again noted that such attenuation differences are generally dose dependent and less affected by the injection flow rate.

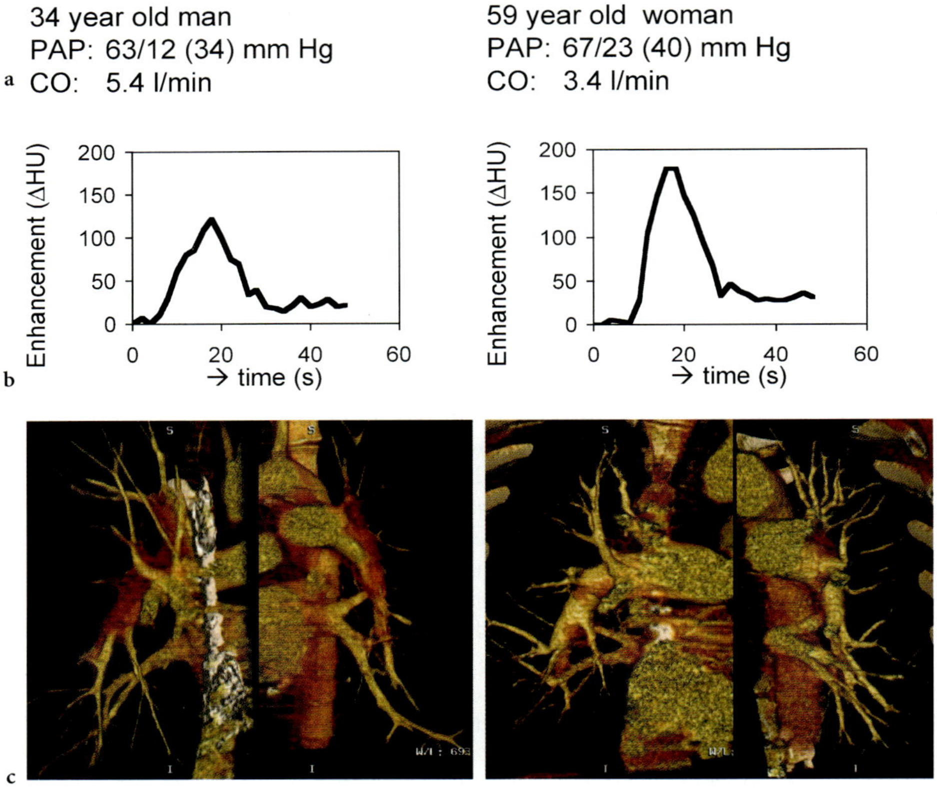

Fig. 4.3a–c. Cardiac output and pulmonary arterial enhancement. **a** Two patients with chronic thrombo-embolic pulmonary hypertension (CTEPH) are compared. *PAP* pulmonary arterial pressure [systolic/diastolic (mean)]; *CO* cardiac output. **b** Following a small test-bolus injection (16 ml at 4 ml/s), the time-attenuation response measured in the pulmonary artery is smaller in the patient with greater cardiac output. **c** Corresponding thin-slab volume-rendered images of pulmonary vessels

4.3.5 Perivenous "Streak" Artifacts

Streak artifacts arising from densely opacified brachiocephalic veins or the superior vena cava during CM administration are a well-known problem in thoracic CT. Streak artifacts may obscure neighboring structures and pathology, or lead to spurious abnormalities, such as a pseudo-intimal flap suggestive of aortic dissection. Similarly, artifacts arising from the right atrium and ventricle of the heart may obscure the right coronary artery in coronary CT angiography.

In technical terms, these artifacts are caused by beam hardening (e.g., in the vicinity of subclavian and brachiocephalic veins) or by the acquisition of inconsistent projection data (views) collected during the time window needed for the reconstruction of a given CT cross-sectional image. The latter situation occurs when densely opacified blood is incompletely mixed with unopacified blood and swirls within the superior vena cava during data acquisition.

Streak artifacts can therefore be reduced or completely avoided if the CT acquisition is performed after contrast material is already removed from the large veins. This can be accomplished by flushing the venous system with saline immediately after the CM injection (Hopper et al. 1997; Haage et al. 2000). Hand exercising during CM administration has also been reported to exhibit this effect (Nakayama et al. 2000). It is important to keep in mind, though, that the time window exhibiting strong pulmonary and systemic arterial but minimal venous enhancement is remarkably short. Artifacts can also be reduced if the attenuation difference between newly injected swirling CM and blood is minimized (Fleischmann et al. 1997). This can be accomplished by using lower injection flow rates and less concentrated CM (Rubin et al. 1996), and/or by scanning during a recirculation phase. Diminished arterial opacification is a potential trade-off when such a strategy is used.

New double-piston power injectors, which allow automated saline flushing and online variation of CM concentration, may be the most versatile tools for CM administration while minimizing streak artifacts at the same time during fast MDCT acquisitions.

4.3.6 Mathematical Modeling

Accurate prediction and controlling of time-dependent arterial enhancement is highly desirable for MDCT, particularly with faster scanners and for CTA. Ideally, one wants to predict and control the time course as well as the degree of vascular enhancement in each individual, independent of an individual's underlying physiology. Two mathematical techniques addressing this issue have been developed.

The first is a sophisticated compartmental model, which predicts vascular and parenchymal enhancement using a system of more than 100 differential equations to describe the transport of contrast medium between intravascular and interstitial fluid compartments of the body (Bae et al. 1998a). For CTA, this model suggests multiphasic injections to achieve uniform vascular enhancement. The injection flow rate is maximum at the beginning of the injection followed by a continuous, exponential decrease of the injection rate (Bae et al. 1998b).

The second black-box model approach is based on the mathematical analysis of a patient's characteristic time-attenuation response to a small test-bolus injection (Fleischmann and Hittmair 1999). Assuming a time-invariant linear system, one can mathematically extract and describe each individual's response to intravenously injected CM ("patient factor") and use this information to individually tailor biphasic injection protocols to achieve uniform, prolonged arterial enhancement at a predefined level. The principle of this technique is outlined in Fig. 4.4. The method is robust and has been successfully used in clinical practice.

Despite the advantages of mathematically derived injection protocols, both models are not widely used because they are not commercially available, because of the additional time needed for calculating individual injection protocols, and because of the need for a test-bolus injection. The greatest value of mathematical modeling comes from the gained insights into early CM dynamics for the time frame relevant for current and future CT technology, which allows a more rational design of empiric but routinely applicable injection techniques.

4.4 Instrumentation and Technique

4.4.1 Intravenous Access

Adequate intravenous CM administration for MDCT requires the use of a mechanical, programmable power injector. A large cubital or antebrachial vein is the most favorable injection site. For a given vein the largest-diameter peripheral catheter to accommodates the desired injection rate, is selected. Whereas cannula lumen diameters as small as 22 g (0.71 mm) may suffice for routine thoracic MDCT, diameters up to 17 g (1.47 mm) have been used for dedicated CTA of the thoracic aorta. If high injection flow rates are desired, a fast manual saline injection with the patient's arms in scanning position (usually above the head) before mechanical CM delivery is recommended to assure correct peripheral catheter position. Injections through a central venous catheter reduce the CM transit time (t_{CMT}), injections in a peripheral vein at the dorsum of the hand slightly prolong the t_{CMT}. In both instances, the flow rates need to be adopted in order to prevent CM extravasation or catheter rupture.

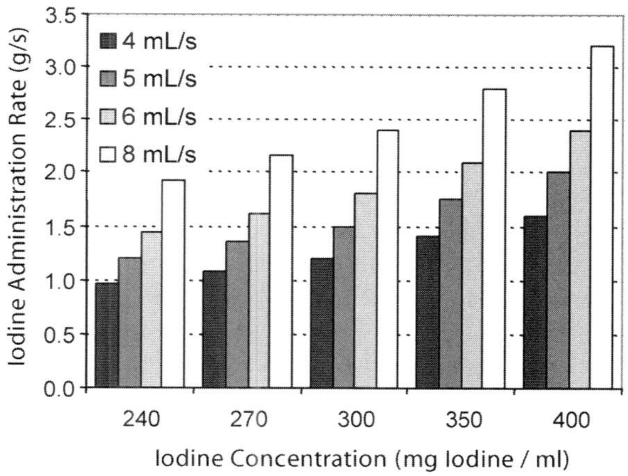

Fig. 4.4. Iodine administration rates and CM concentration. For a given CM concentration, the iodine administration rate (g/s) can be varied by selection of the injection flow rate (in ml/s). High-concentration agents permit greater iodine administration rates at the same injection rates

4.4.2 Power Injectors and Safety Issues

The use of CM in MDCT carries the same risk of idiosyncratic (non-dose-dependent) adverse reactions as in other applications. These allergy-like effects are well described (Katayama et al. 1990) and their discussion is beyond the scope of this chapter. Because MDCT requires faster injections and the use of a power injector, dose-dependent (non-idiosyncratic) adverse effects, and the risk of CM extravasation have recently regained interest.

Dose-dependent adverse reactions include nausea, vomiting, arrhythmia, pulmonary edema, and cardiovascular collapse. Based on clinical and experimental evidence for ionic CM, one might naturally assume that rapid injections would be less well tolerated than slower injections (Dawson 1998); however, at least for injection flow rates up to 4 ml/s, there seems to be no correlation between injection rate and the overall rate of adverse reactions (Jacobs et al. 1998).

The rate of CM extravasation during the intravenous administration of CM with power injectors is low, ranging from 0.2 to 0.6% (Bellin et al. 2002). Whereas this is presumably higher when compared with hand-injection and drip-infusion technique, no correlation was found between extravasation frequency and injection rates up to 4 ml/s (Jacobs et al. 1998). Most extravasations involve only small volumes and result in minimal to mild symptoms if non-ionic CM is used.

Large volumes of CM may be involved, however, in non-communicative patients such as infants and children, elderly, or unconscious patients. Monitoring of the injection site during CM administration is recommended in this group, because severe extravasation injuries have occasionally been reported, and guidelines for management of extravasation injuries should be at hand (Bellin et al. 2002). Recently, an automated CM extravasation device has been developed, which interrupts the mechanical injection when a skin-impedance change due to fluid extravasation is detected (Nelson et al. 1998). Such a device might prove useful in high-flow-rate MDCT applications (Birnbaum et al. 1999).

4.4.3 Saline Flushing of the Veins

Flushing the venous system with saline immediately after CM injection pushes the CM column from the veins into the circulation. This has two desirable effects in thoracic MDCT.

Firstly, because the CM which would otherwise remain in the arm veins after the end of the injection contributes to vascular enhancement, opacification of intrathoracic vessels is improved. This effect can also be exploited to reduce the total CM volume in routine thoracic MDCT (Hopper et al. 1997; Haage et al. 2000). Secondly, because saline flushing removes CM from the brachiocephalic veins and the superior vena cava, it reduces perivenous streak artifacts in thoracic and cardiac CT.

Saline flushing has been performed (a) manually, using a three-way valve, or (b) by layering saline above contrast in the syringe of a power injector, or (c) by using two interconnected power injectors. The former techniques, however, are impractical for routine CT, because the manual technique may expose the radiologist or technologist to radiation, and the layering technique is time consuming and poses a risk for contamination.

The most convenient technique for routine saline flushing after CM injection are new programmable double-piston power injectors (one syringe for CM, one for saline) similar to those used in MR angiography. Furthermore, these devices may allow not only to vary the injection rates, but also to vary the CM concentration during a single injection (through saline admixture). Such a strategy might allow to achieve the desired enhancement profile by initially injecting non-diluted CM, followed by a phase of diluted CM injection, with subsequent saline flushing to avoid artifacts.

4.4.4 Scanning Delay and Automated Bolus Triggering

A fixed, empiric injection-to-scan delay may be adequate for many routine thoracic and abdominal CT acquisitions, particularly if maximum vessel opacification is not of critical importance. The greatest advantage of fixed-delay protocols is obviously their ease of use. As early CM dynamics in patients without cardiocirculatory disease are within a comparable range, and as it is easier to achieve good opacification in the pulmonary arteries compared with more distant systemic arteries, fixed scanning delays have also been employed successfully for pulmonary CTA acquisitions.

For dedicated arterial or organ (liver) MDCT imaging studies a fixed scanning delay cannot be recommended, because the arterial CM transit time (t_{CMT}) is prohibitively variable between individual patients – ranging from 8 to as long as 40 s in patients with cardiovascular diseases. One might completely miss the bolus with a fast MDCT acquisition if the delay is not properly chosen.

In vascular MDCT, therefore, the delay needs to be timed relative to the contrast transit time (t_{CMT}). It is important to realize that with the possibility of very fast MDCT acquisitions the t_{CMT} itself does not necessarily serve as the scanning delay, but rather as a means of individualizing the delay relative to it. Depending on the vessels or organ of interest an additional delay relative to the t_{CMT} needs to be selected. In CTA, this additional delay may be as short as 0–2 s added to the t_{CMT} ("t_{CMT}+2 s"). For visualizing hypervascular liver lesions this additional delay may be 10–15 s ("t_{CMT}+15 s"). Transit times can be easily determined using either a test-bolus injection or an automatic bolus-triggering technique.

Test Bolus: The injection of a small test bolus (15–20 ml) while acquiring a low-dose dynamic (non-incremental) CT acquisition is a reliable means to determine the t_{CMT} from the intravenous injection site to the arterial territory of interest (van Hoe et al. 1995). The t_{CMT} equals the time-to-peak enhancement interval measured in a region of interest (ROI) placed within a reference vessel. Furthermore, time-attenuation curves obtained from one or more regions of interest can be used for individual bolus-shaping techniques using one of the previously described mathematical models. A test bolus is particularly useful to determine the t_{CMT} if unusual CM injection sites need to be used (e.g., lower extremity veins).

Bolus Triggering: Many CT scanners have this feature built into their system. A circular region of interest (ROI) is placed into the target vessel on a non-enhanced image. While CM is injected, a series of low-dose non-incremental scans are obtained, whereas the attenuation within a ROI is monitored or inspected visually. The t_{CMT} equals the time when a predefined enhancement threshold ("trigger level") is reached (e.g., 100 DHU) or observed by the person performing the scan. The minimal trigger delay to initiate the MDCT acquisition after the threshold has been reached ("trigger delay") depends on the scanner model and on the longitudinal distance between the monitoring series and the starting position of the actual MDCT series. The minimal "trigger delay" before a scan can be initiated after the trigger threshold is reached is currently between 2 and 8 s. Bolus triggering is a very robust and practical technique for routine use and has the advantage that it does not require an additional test-bolus injection.

4.4.5 Contrast Medium Concentration

Vascular enhancement (over time) is generally determined by the number of iodine molecules administered (over time). This iodine administration rate can therefore be increased either by increasing the injection flow rate, and/or by increasing the iodine concentration of the CM used (Fig. 4.4); thus, if one aims at a certain iodine administration rate (e.g., 1.2 g/s), this requires a faster (e.g., 4 ml/s) injection flow rate with standard (300 mg I/ml) compared with a slower (e.g., 3 ml/s) flow rate with high-concentration (400 mg I/ml) CM. Very high iodine administration rates, up to 2.4 g/s or more, can be safely injected with a 400-mg I/ml solution at 6 ml/s, whereas an injection flow rate of 8 ml/s would be required using standard (300 mg I/ml) solution. High iodine administration rates are useful in CTA, notably in patients with a shallow enhancement response due to underlying cardiocirculatory disease, and to avoiding high injection flow rates. Furthermore, high iodine administration rates are particularly desirable for non-vascular imaging purposes, e.g., for detecting hypervascular liver lesions, or in organ perfusion studies.

Low-concentration contrast media, on the other hand, have the advantage that they cause less perivenous artifacts at the level of the brachiocephalic veins and the superior vena cava in thoracic MDCT, particularly if no saline flushing of the veins is employed (Rubin et al. 1996).

4.5 Clinical Contrast Medium Injection Protocols

This section provides an overview of clinically applicable CM injection protocols for various thoracic MDCT applications. The suggested protocols are based on pharmacokinetic considerations, published clinical and experimental data, mathematical approximations, and practical experience. An attempt is made to provide both, a universal approach to injection strategies as well as specific examples of injection protocols.

Because of different MDCT scanner types (ranging from dual-channel to 16-channel MDCT systems, with different rotation times and selectable table increments) the protocols are tabulated according to the acquisition times. Abbreviations for temporal variables are indexed as follows: t_{SCAN}=acquisition time; and t_{INJ}=injection duration.

The actual CM injection protocols need to be adjusted to match the suggested iodine doses and administration rates. The CM doses and injection rates should also be adopted (±20%) in patients with a body weight <60 kg and >90 kg.

4.5.1 Routine Thoracic and Mediastinal MDCT

Indications: Evaluation of various systemic or thoracic diseases; staging/follow up malignancies (lymphoma, bronchogenic carcinoma).

Objectives: Opacification of thoracic vessels for better delineation of mediastinal and hilar structures.

Strategy: A small to moderate amount of iodine (20–35 g I) CM (60–120 ml of 300mgI/ml CM) delivered at a slow injection rate (1.5–3.0 ml/s) and comparably long injection duration (>30 s) results in sufficient opacification of thoracic vessels. Low-concentration agents or saline flushing are favorable to reduce perivenous artifacts. A fixed delay is adequate and should be determined so that the injection ends 5 s earlier than the MDCT acquisition (Delay=t_{INJ}+5 s-t_{SCAN}). This minimizes perivenous artifacts, particularly when a saline flush and a caudocranial scanning direction is used. Examples are shown in Table 4.1.

Table 4.1a. Routine thoracic multiple detector-row CT (MDCT)

Acquisition time (s)	Scanning delay (s)	Iodine dose (g)	Iodine administration rate (g/s)	CM volume (ml)[a]	Injection rate (ml/s)[a]	Injection duration (s)
30	25	30	0.60	100	2	50
25	30	30	0.60	100	2	50
20	25	30	0.75	100	2.5	40
15	30	30	0.75	100	2.5	40
10	28	30	0.90	100	3	33
5	33	30	0.90	100	3	33

[a] Volume and flow rate calculated for 300 mgI/ml concentration CM

Table 4.1b. Routine thoracic MDCT, high CM dose protocol

Acquisition time (s)	Scanning delay (s)	Iodine dose (g)	Iodine administration rate (g/s)	CM volume (ml)[a]	Injection rate (ml/s)[a]	Injection duration (s)
30	23	36	0.75	120	2.5	48
25	20	36	0.90	120	3	40
20	25	36	0.90	120	3	40
15	30	36	0.90	120	3	40
10	25	36	1.20	120	4	30
5	30	36	1.20	120	4	30

High CM dose protocol applicable if soft tissue enhancement (e.g., chest wall) is also desired; provides good pulmonary and systemic arterial enhancement as well. Patients with >90 kg b.w.
[a] Volume and flow rate calculated for 300 mg I/ml concentration CM

Table 4.1c. Thoracic MDCT, minimum dose protocol

Acquisition time (s)	Scanning delay (s)	Iodine dose (g)	Iodine administration rate (g/s)	CM volume (ml)[a]	Injection rate (ml/s)[a]	Injection duration (s)
30	20	18	0.75	60	1.3	46
25	20	18	0.90	60	1.5	40
20	25	18	0.90	60	1.5	40
15	30	18	0.90	60	1.5	40
10	25	18	1.20	60	2	30
5	20	18	1.20	60	2	30

Minimum dose protocol suffices for vessel delineation, if saline flush is used
[a] Volume and flow rate calculated for 300 mg I/ml concentration CM

4.5.2 Pulmonary Arteries

Indications: Acute pulmonary embolism, chronic thrombo-embolic pulmonary hypertension (CTEPH), pulmonary arteriovenous malformations (AVM), pulmonary artery aneurysms, and arteriovenous fistulas.

Objectives: Bright opacification of pulmonary arteries, in order to detect vascular abnormalities – notably filling defects or mural thrombus.

Strategy: Moderate to large amounts of iodine are required to allow a distinction between opacified blood and intraluminal abnormalities. Large amounts of iodine are necessary if an additional, delayed (approximately 2 min) acquisition of the lower extremity veins is desired. Moderate to high injection flow rates (3.0–4.0 ml/s) are required with a standard concentration agent. If a higher concentration agent is used, flow rates can be slower. Saline flushing is recommended. A fixed delay is adequate in the majority of patients, and should again be determined so that the injection ends 3 s earlier than the end of MDCT acquisition (Delay=t_{INJ}+3 s-t_{SCAN}). For patients with severely compromised cardiocirculatory distress (CTEPH), slower injection rates suffice (because diminished cardiac output leads to brighter enhancement). Image quality is more consistent if the delay is timed relative to the CM transit time. (Table 4.2)

4.5.3 Thoracic and Coronary CT Angiography

Indications: Aneurysms and dissections of the thoracic aorta and its branches, atherosclerotic or inflammatory (arteriitis) arterial stenosis or occlusions, thoracic outlet syndrome, chest trauma. Coronary CT angiography.

Objectives: Bright opacification of systemic or coronary arteries.

Strategy: For fast acquisitions (8- and 16-channel MDCT), moderate amounts of iodine at high iodine administration rates are required (i.e., high injection flow rates and/or high iodine concentration agent). For slower acquisitions, larger total CM volumes with longer injection durations and preferably biphasic injections are optimal. Individual scan timing relative to the t_{CMT} is mandatory. Saline flushing is beneficial in thoracic outlet CTA, and in coronary CTA in order to reduce artifacts in the vicinity of large veins as well as the right atrium and ventricle (Table 4.3)

Table 4.2a. Pulmonary artery CTA, fixed delay

Acquisition time (s)	Scanning delay (s)	Iodine dose (g)	Iodine administration rate (g/s)	CM volume (ml)[a]	Injection rate (ml/s)[a]	Injection duration (s)
30	13	36	0.90	120	3	40
25	18	36	0.90	120	3	40
20	23	36	0.90	120	3	40
15	18	36	1.20	120	4	30
10	23	36	1.20	120	4	30
5	28	36	1.20	120	4	30

[a] Volume and flow rate calculated for 300 mg I/ml concentration CM

Table 4.2b. Pulmonary artery CTA, with individual timing

Acquisition time (s)	Scanning delay (s)	Iodine dose (g)	Iodine administration rate (g/s)	CM volume (ml)[a]	Injection rate (ml/s)[a]	Injection duration (s)
30	t_{CMT}+5	33	0.90	110	3	37
25	t_{CMT}+5	30	0.90	100	3	33
20	t_{CMT}+8	30	0.90	100	3	33
15	t_{CMT}+10	27	1.20	90	4	30
10	t_{CMT}+15	27	1.20	90	4	30
5	t_{CMT}+20	27	1.20	90	4	30

t_{CMT}=contrast medium transit time, as established with a test-bolus or bolus-triggering technique
[a] Volume and flow rate calculated for 300 mg I/ml concentration CM

Table 4.3a. Thoracic CTA, uniphasic injection

Acquisition time (s)	Scanning delay (s)	Iodine Dose (g)	Iodine Administration rate (g/s)	300 mg I/ml CM: CM volume at injection rate (ml at ml/s)[a]	400 mg I/ml CM: CM volume at injection rate (ml at ml/s)[b]
30	t_{CMT}+8	45	1.2	150 at 3	115 at 3
25	t_{CMT}+8	42	1.2	140 at 3	105 at 3
20	t_{CMT}+8	39	1.2	130 at 3	100 at 3
15	t_{CMT}+8	36	1.5	120 at 5	90 at 3.8
10	t_{CMT}+8	33	1.8	110 at 6	85 at 4.5
5	t_{CMT}+12	27	1.8	90 at 6	70 at 4.5

t_{CMT}=contrast medium transit time, as established with a test-bolus or bolus-triggering technique
[a]Volume and flow rate calculated for 300 mg I/ml concentration CM
[b]Volume and flow rate calculated for 400 mg I/ml concentration CM

Table 4.3b. Thoracic CTA, biphasic injection

Acquisition time (s)	Scanning delay (s)	Iodine: Total dose (g)	Iodine: Biphasic administration (g at g/s)	300 mg I/ml CM: Total volume (ml)[a]	300 mg I/ml CM: Biphasic injections (ml at ml/s)[a]	400 mg I/ml CM: Total volume (ml)[b]	400 mg I/ml CM: Biphasic injections (ml at ml/s)[b]
30	t_{CMT}+8	42	9 at 1.8+33 at 1.2	140	30 at 6+110 at 4	95	23 at 4.5+82 at 3.0
25	t_{CMT}+8	36	9 at 1.8+27 at 1.2	120	30 at 6+90 at 4	90	23 at 4.5+67 at 3.0
20	t_{CMT}+8	34	9 at 1.8+25 at 1.4	115	30 at 6+85 at 4.5	90	23 at 4.5+67 at 3.4
15	t_{CMT}+8	32	9 at 1.8+23 at 1.4	105	30 at 6+75 at 4.5	80	23 at 4.5+57 at 3.4
10	t_{CMT}+8	29	9 at 1.8+20 at 1.5	95	30 at 6+65 at 5	75	23 at 4.5+52 at 3.8
5	t_{CMT}+12	24	9 at 1.8+15 at 1.5	80	30 at 6+50 at 5	65	23 at 4.5+42 at 3.8

t_{CMT}=contrast medium transit time, as established with a test-bolus or bolus-triggering technique
[a]Volume and flow rate calculated for 300 mg I/ml concentration CM
[b]Volume and flow rate calculated for 400 mg I/ml concentration CM

4.5.4 Thoracic Veins

Indications: Assessment of venous thrombosis, obstruction, or occlusion.

Objective: Delineation of venous anatomy and pathology for treatment planning

Strategy A: Intravenous CM injection into the contralateral (non-diseased) arm requires large iodine doses (e.g., 100–150 ml) at slow to moderate injection rates in order to visualize the diseased venous territory during a recirculation phase. A long delay (end of MDCT acquisition should be approximately 15 s after the end of the injection) and saline flushing is recommended. This strategy also allows assessment of systemic arteries.

Strategy B: 200 ml of diluted CM (1:10 to 1:20) injected into the diseased arm (or both arms using a Y-connector) at a slow injection rate (2–4 ml/s) is sufficient to directly opacify the thoracic veins.

4.5.5 Thoraco-Abdominal MDCT

Indications: Assessment of thoracoabdomial diseases, such as staging of lymphoma.

Objectives: Delineation of hilar and mediastinal structures, combined with adequate parenchymal enhancement of abdominal and pelvic organs.

Strategy: As mere delineation of thoracic vessels is easily achieved, CM delivery is weighted towards adequate parenchymal and soft tissue enhancement. Large iodine doses (0.5–0.6 g of iodine/kg b.w.) corresponding to approximately 100–150 ml (depending on the iodine concentration and on the patient's body weight) are required. Injection rates can be moderate to slow, and the scan delay should be long enough to allow tissue enhancement (≥60 s).

Dedicated biphasic acquisitions (with high iodine administration rates!) are also possible with MDCT, where the first acquisition includes the thorax and upper abdomen, and the second acquisition includes the abdomen and pelvis (other sequences are possible if the MDCT scanner permits). Timing is optimized for biphasic abdominal imaging, i.e., the first acquisition should include the liver in a late arterial phase (Delay=t_{CMT}+10 s, or Delay at 25 s), the second acquisition is obtained during a hepatic parenchymal phase (Delay=t_{CMT}+40 s, or Delay at 60 s).

4.6 Conclusion

A basic understanding of early CM dynamics provides the foundation for the design of current and future CM injection protocols for various clinical applications of thoracic MDCT. Further ingredients are a thorough knowledge of the technical and safety aspects of the injection equipment and CM used. With these tools at hand, CM utilization can be optimized towards the clinical necessities while exploiting the full capabilities of latest and continuously evolving MDCT technology.

References

Bae KT, Heiken JP, Brink JA (1998a) Aortic and hepatic contrast medium enhancement at CT. Part I: Prediction with a computer model. Radiology 207:647–655

Bae KT, Heiken JP, Brink JA (1998b) Aortic and hepatic contrast medium enhancement at CT. Part II: Effect of reduced cardiac output in a porcine model. Radiology 207:657–662

Bellin MF, Jakobsen JA, Tomassin I et al. (2002) Contrast medium extravasation injury: guidelines for prevention and management. Eur Radiol 12:2807–2812

Birnbaum BA, Nelson RC, Chezmar JL et al. (1999) Extravasation detection accessory: clinical evaluation in 500 patients. Radiology 212:431–438

Dawson P (1998) Does injection rate affect the tolerance? In: Dawson PH, Clauss W (eds) Contrast media in practice: questions and answers. Springer, Berlin Heidelberg New York, pp 135–136

Dawson P, Blomley MJ (1996a) Contrast agent pharmacokinetics revisited I. Reformulation. Acad Radiol 3 (Suppl 2): S261–S263

Dawson P, Blomley MJ (1996b) Contrast media as extracellular fluid space markers: adaptation of the central volume theorem. Br J Radiol 69:717–722

Fleischmann D (2002) Present and future trends in multiple detector-row CT applications: CT angiography. Eur Radiol 12:S11–S16

Fleischmann D, Hittmair K (1999) Mathematical analysis of arterial enhancement and optimization of bolus geometry for CT angiography using the discrete fourier transform. J Comput Assist Tomogr 23:474–484

Fleischmann D, Ringl H, Nowotny R et al (1997) Streak artifacts arising from the superior vena cava in contrast enhanced CT: qualitative and quantitative assessment. Eur Radiol 7:285

Fleischmann D, Rubin GD, Bankier AA et al. (2000) Improved uniformity of aortic enhancement with customized contrast medium injection protocols at CT angiography. Radiology 214:363–371

Foley WD (2002) Special focus session: multidetector CT: abdominal visceral imaging. Radiographics 22:701–719

Haage P, Schmitz-Rode T, Hubner D et al. (2000) Reduction of contrast material dose and artifacts by a saline flush using a double power injector in helical CT of the thorax. Am J Roentgenol 174:1049–1053

Hittmair K, Fleischmann D (2001) Accuracy of predicting and controlling time-dependent aortic enhancement from a test bolus injection. J Comput Assist Tomogr 25:287–294

Hopper KD (1996) With helical CT, is nonionic contrast a better choice than ionic contrast for rapid and large IV bolus injections? Am J Roentgenol 166:715

Hopper KD, Mosher TJ, Kasales CJ et al. (1997) Thoracic spiral CT: delivery of contrast material pushed with injectable saline solution in a power injector. Radiology 205:269–271

Jacobs JE, Birnbaum BA, Langlotz CP (1998) Contrast media reactions and extravasation: relationship to intravenous injection rates. Radiology 209:411–416

Katayama H, Yamaguchi K, Kozuka T et al. (1990) Adverse reactions to ionic and nonionic contrast media. A report from the Japanese Committee on the Safety of Contrast Media. Radiology 175:621–628

Leggett RW, Williams LR (1995) A proposed blood circulation model for reference man. Health Phys 69:187–201

Nakayama M, Yamashita Y, Oyama Y et al. (2000) Hand exercise during contrast medium delivery at thoracic helical CT: a simple method to minimize perivenous artifact. J Comput Assist Tomogr 24:432–436

Nelson RC, Anderson FA Jr, Birnbaum BA et al. (1998) Contrast media extravasation during dynamic CT: detection with an extravasation detection accessory. Radiology 209: 837–843

Rubin GD, Lane MJ, Bloch DA et al. (1996) Optimization of thoracic spiral CT: effects of iodinated contrast medium concentration. Radiology 201:785–791

Sheiman RG, Raptopoulos V, Caruso P et al. (1996) Comparison of tailored and empiric scan delays for CT angiography of the abdomen. Am J Roentgenol 167:725–729

Van Hoe L, Marchal G, Baert AL et al. (1995) Determination of scan delay-time in spiral CT-angiography: utility of a test bolus injection. J Comput Assist Tomogr 19:216–220

Airways / Diffuse Lung Disease

5 Multi-Detector-Row CT of the Airways

P. A. Grenier, C. Beigelman-Aubry, C. Fetita, Y. Martin-Bouyer

CONTENTS

5.1 Introduction

By combining both helical volumetric acquisition and thin slice thickness over the entire lungs during a simple breath hold, multi-detector row CT (MDCT) has the ability to acquire contiguous high-resolution CT images throughout the thorax permitting a global high-resolution assessment of the airways. This offers the advantage to provide an accurate assessment of focal or diffuse, proximal or distal airways disease. One of the greatest advantages of this new technology is the improved quality of the two-dimensional (2D) multiplanar images and three-dimensional (3D) reconstruction images, including those developed specifically for airway imaging such as CT bronchography and virtual bronchoscopy.

The clinical applications of MDCT should include the detection of bronchial lesions in patients with unexplained hemoptysis, the diagnosis and assessment of extent of tracheobronchial stenosis for planning treatment and follow-up, the assessment of complex airways abnormalities as well as congenital anomalies, bronchial fistula and dehiscence, the diagnosis and assessment of extent of bronchiectasis and small airways disease.

Improvement in image-analysis techniques and the use of spirometric control of lung volume acquisition have made possible accurate and reproducible quantitative assessment of airway wall and lumen areas and lung density. This will lead to the increasing use of CT as a research tool for better insights in physiopathology of obstructive lung disease, particularly in chronic obstructive pulmonary disease (COPD) and asthma, with an ultimate benefit in clinical practice.

P. A. Grenier, MD; C. Beigelman-Aubry, MD
Service de Radiologie, Hôpital de la Pitié–Salpêtrière, AP–HP, 47–83, boulevard de l'Hôpital, 75651 Paris cedex 13, France
C. Fetita, PhD
Department ARTEMIS, Institut National des Télécommunications, 9, rue Charles Fourier, 91011 Evry cedex, France
Y. Martin-Bouyer, MD
Service de Radiologie, Clinique du Val d'Or, 16, rue Pasteur, 92210 St. Cloud, France

5.2 Acquisition Parameters and Image Processing

5.2.1 Scanning Protocol

Fast acquisitions of approximately 10 s for the entire thorax with 1.25-mm collimation is recommended because slice thickness has the greatest impact on the quality of 2D and 3D reconstructions (Figs. 5.1, 5.2). The z-axis resolution is directly related to the effective slice thickness. The smaller the effective slice thickness, the more precise are 2D reformats or 3D reconstructions. The optimal effective slice thickness is therefore of 1.25 mm or less (0.6 or 0.75 mm when using a 16-detector rows CT scanner) rendering isotropic or near isotropic image reconstruction feasible. In all cases, overlapping transaxial images reconstruction by 50% is recommended to provide the highest morphologic detail. Because of the great natural contrast between the airways and their environment, relatively low kilovoltage (100–120 kV) and milliamperage (60–100 mA) can be used (Feretti et al. 2001). Choi et al. (2002) showed recently that image quality of surface-rendered 3D images of the central airways is preserved when the tube current decreases from 240 to 50 mA.

An advantage of MDCT is its ability to allow slice thickness to be changed retrospectively, thus enabling one to obtain high-quality reconstruction images from routine CT studies. This feature is particularly helpful in daily practice because it allows patients undergoing routine imaging to potentially benefit from the creation of 2D multiplanar and 3D reconstructions without the need for additional acquisitions (Feretti et al. 2001; Summers et al. 1998). The routine images of the airways could be reconstructed with 1.25-mm thickness and if 2D and 3D reconstructions are requested prospective reconstructions with overlap 0.6 mm is recommended. Thinner section (0.6–0.75 mm) in reconstruction is recommended if quantitative assessment of the airways is requested. It is of interest to remember that intravenous injection of contrast material is unnecessary when the examination is specifically dedicated to the airways.

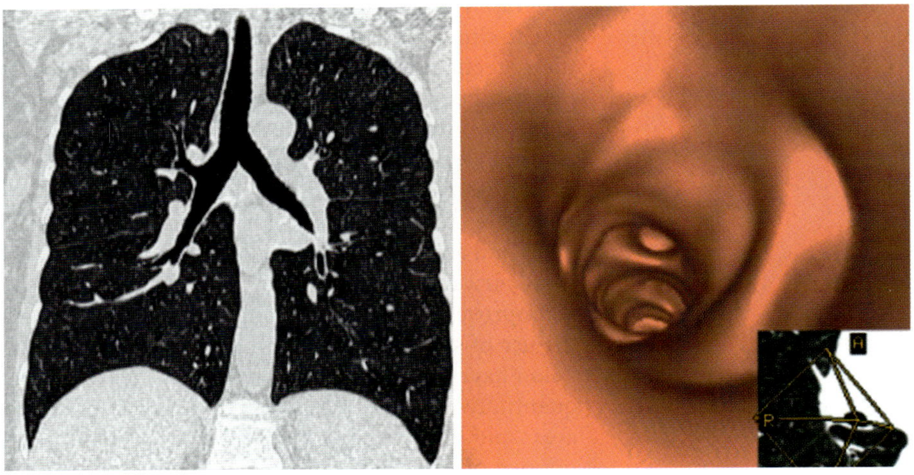

Fig. 5.1. Multi-detector row CT (MDCT) in a patient with normal airways. *Left:* Multiplanar reformation (MPR) in coronal oblique direction along the long axis of the trachea. *Right:* virtual bronchoscopy showing a descending view of the basal divisions in the right lower lobe from the intermediate bronchus

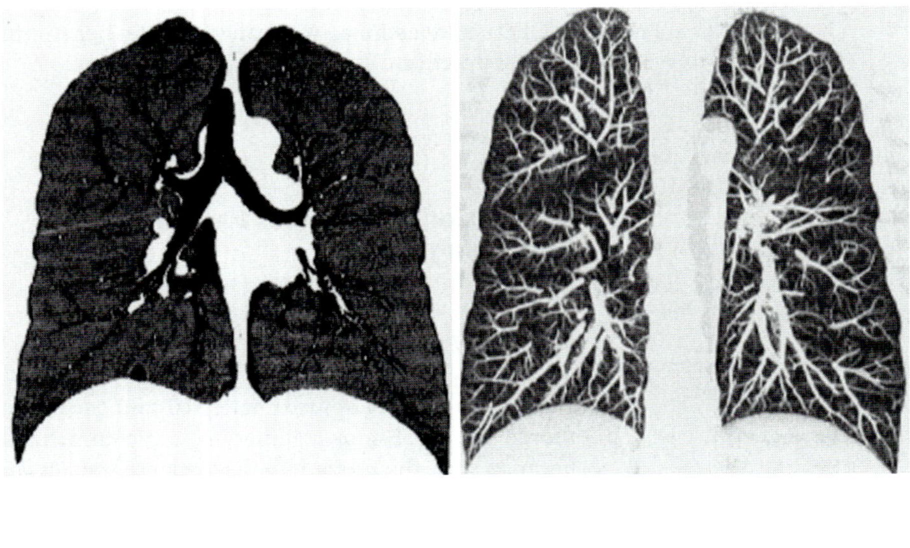

Fig. 5.2. The MDCT in a patient with normal airways. *Left:* Multiplanar volume reformation (MPVR; 5-mm-thick slab) in a coronal view with minimum intensity projection (MIP) technique. *Right:* MVPR (7.5-mm slab) in a coronal view with maximum intensity projection (MIP) technique

5.2.2
Expiratory CT

Airway imaging is routinely performed at end inspiration during a simple breath hold. Additional scanning is also required at expiration in patients with either suspected tracheobronchomalacia to assess the degree of abnormal expiratory collapse of the proximal airways at expiration, or those with suspicion of small airways disease to assess the presence and extent of expiratory air trapping (Fig. 5.3). In such cases, low-dose technique (40 mA) is recommended to decrease radiation exposure (Gotway et al. 2000).

The most commonly used technique for the assessment of air trapping at CT is based on post expiratory CT scans, obtained during suspended respiration following a forced exhalation. Dynamic CT acquisition during continuous expiration is the second technique available (Gotway et al. 2000; Lucidarme et al. 2000). Motion artifacts, which increase as temporal resolution decreases, represent the major limitations of continuous expiratory CT; however, a dynamic expiratory maneuver performed during helical CT acquisition may provide good results despite a 0.5-s scanning time per image. The use of 180° linear interpolation algorithms with a 0.5-s rotation time provides images representing scanning periods of approximately 250 ms. Moreover, motion artifacts are at maximum during the early phase of expiration and at a minimum during its late phase, which thereby allows good visualization of lobular air trapping with helical CT. Actually, a dynamic expiratory maneuver performed during helical CT acquisition, particularly during the last part of the expiratory maneuver, may provide good results without too many artifacts. This is called continuous expiratory CT (Lucidarme et al. 2000). Patients can have greater difficulty maintaining the residual volume after an exhalation than during an active exhalation when they have to continue the expiratory effort until the end of the acquisition. The air trapping extent and the relative contrast scores obtained with continuous expiratory CT have proven to be significantly higher than those obtained with suspended end expiratory CT (Lucidarme et al. 2000).

Low-dose continuous expiratory MDCT over the chest has become routine in some institutions to depict air trapping (Gotway et al. 2000). Elsewhere, it is proposed as an alternative to improve the conspicuity and the apparent extent of air trapping when patients have difficulty performing the suspended end-expiration maneuver adequately (Lucidarme et al. 2000).

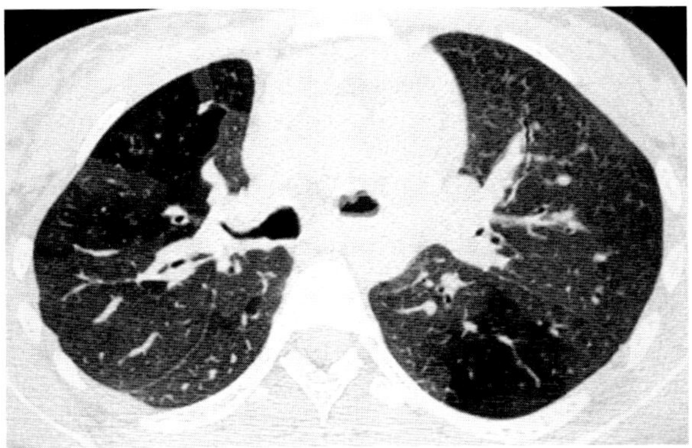

Fig. 5.3. Thin transversal slice obtained with MDCT at continuous expiration in a patient with post-infectious constrictive bronchiolitis. Areas of abnormal expiratory air trapping are depicted in the anterior segment of the right upper lobe and the superior segment of the left lower lobe. Focal bronchiectasis is also depicted in the right upper lobe

5.2.3
Cine viewing

Visualization of the overlapped thin axial images sequentially in a cine mode allows the bronchial divisions to be followed from the segmental origin to the distal bronchial lumens down to the smallest bronchi which can be identified on thin-section images. This viewing technique helps indicate the segmental and subsegmental distribution of any airway lesion and may serve as a road map for the endoscopist (Grenier et al. 2002). Moving up and down through the volume at the monitor has become an alternative to film-based review.

5.2.4
Multiplanar Reformations

Multiplanar reformations are the easiest reconstructions to generate and can be interactively performed in real time at the console or at the dedicated console or workstation. They allow to obviate the underestimation of the limits of the craniocaudal extent of a vertically oriented disease as tracheobronchial stenosis (Fig. 5.4; Quint et al. 1995). They are of particular value for better detection and evaluation of mild focal stenosis. Whereas the thickness of the displayed planar image is 0.6–0.8 mm, depending on the dimension of the field of view, multiplanar volume reconstruction (MPVR) consists of a slab with a thickness of several pixels and in a less noisy reformation (Fig. 5.4). Because underestimation of a stenosis may occur if the reformation plane is not adequately chosen, simultaneous reading of the native cross-sectional images and a selection of reformation plane from the 3D reconstructed image of the airways are recommended. Multiplanar volume reformation may be associated with the use of the intensity projection techniques (Fig. 5.5; Rémy-Jardin et al. 1996).

5.2.5 Minimum (m) and Maximum (M) Intensity Projection (IP)

The minimum intensity projection (mIP) technique projects the tracheobronchial air column into a viewing plane. Pixels encode the minimum voxel value encountered by each ray. It is usually applied to a selected volume of the thorax containing the airway under evaluation (MPVR–mIP technique; Fig. 5.5; Rubin 1996). Airways are visualized because air contained within the tracheobronchial tree is lower in attenuation than surrounding pulmonary parenchyma, with a small density difference between pulmonary parenchyma and airways between 50 and 150 HU (Rubin 1996). Numerous drawbacks have limited indications of mIP in assessing airway disease. The size of asymmetrical stenoses may be artificially decreased (Kauczor et al. 1996). The technique is very vulnerable to varying width of volume of interest and to partial-volume effects. Even minor partial-volume

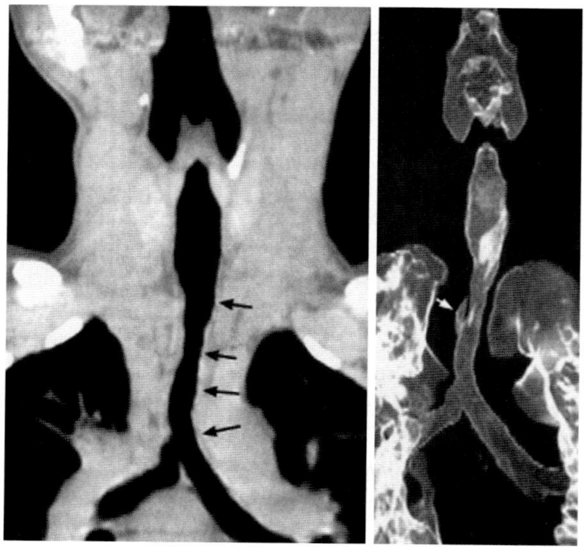

Fig. 5.4. Tracheal stenosis occurring after longstanding tracheal intubation. Assessment of the lesion before surgical treatment. *Left:* Coronal oblique volume reformation along the long axis of the trachea assessing accurately the extent and degree of the stenosis (*arrows*). *Right:* Three-dimensional volume-rendering technique displaying the tracheal stenosis. Note the visibility of small amount of intra-esophageal air reconstructed by the 3D reconstruction procedure (*arrow*)

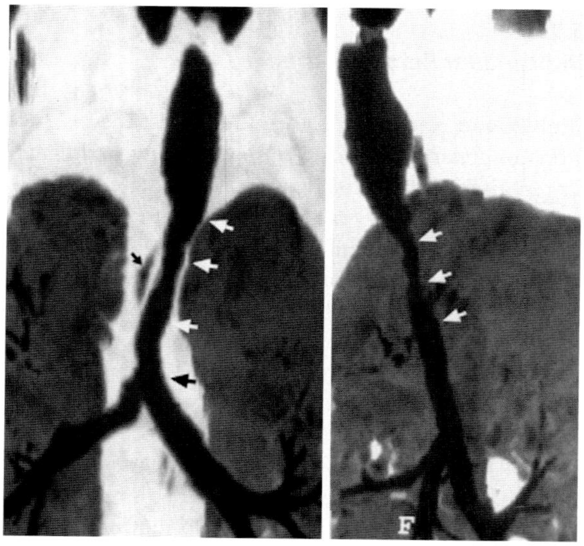

Fig. 5.5. Same patient as in Fig. 4. Coronal oblique (*left*) and sagittal (*right*) views obtained with MVPR–mIP technique, which assess the extent and morphology of the tracheal stenosis (*large arrows*). The *small arrow* shows air into the esophagus

averaging leads to underestimation of the airway caliber. This effect grows with increasing effective slice thickness, decreasing bronchial diameter, and horizontal course of a bronchus. Sometimes, high-grade stenoses can be imaged as pseudo-occlusions. The intraluminal growth of eccentric tumors is generally underestimated and may even be completely missed. Intraluminal structures of higher density (e.g., stents) are not displayed. Other air-containing structures, such as esophagus, may simulate tracheal fistulas if careful analysis of all angles of view is not performed (Fig. 5.5A). Despite these limitations, MPVR–mIP technique may be used in the detection of air bronchogram in focal areas of air-space consolidation, ground-glass opacification, or cavitation (Fig. 5.6). The recognition of the involved airways may help the endoscopist select the segmental or subsegmental bronchi for aspiration, bronchoalveolar lavage or transbronchial biopsy. The MPVR–mIP technique may also increase the depiction and visualization of any bronchial fistula or dehiscence (Fig. 5.4). By increasing the contrast between areas of normal lung attenuation and areas of lung hypoattenuation, it may facilitate the depiction of mosaic perfusion pattern in small airways disease. Its application on expiratory CT scans can be appreciated to facilitate the assessment of presence and extent of expiratory air trapping (Fig. 5.7; Fotheringham et al. 1999).

In maximum intensity projection (MIP) technique, pixels encode the maximum voxel value

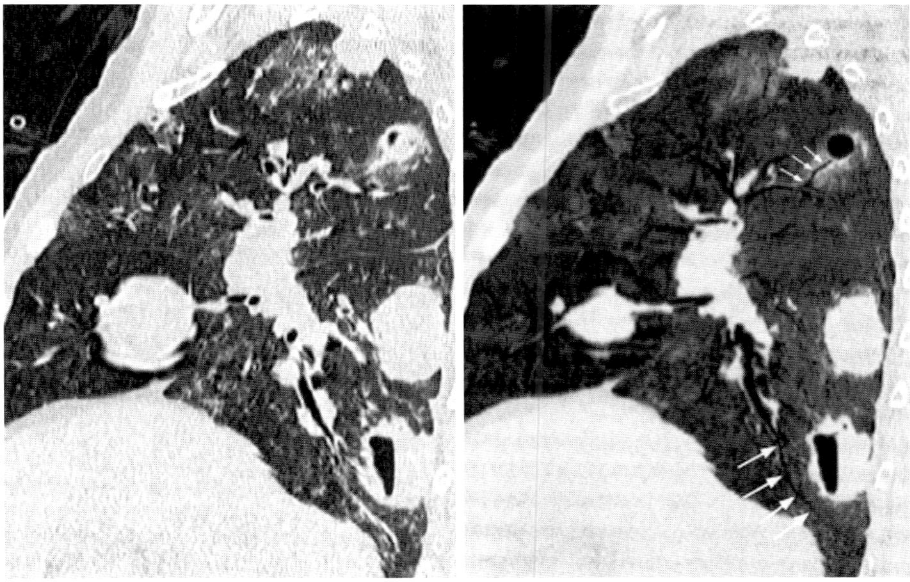

Fig. 5.6. The MDCT in a patient with multiple infected metastases. *Left:* Sagittal reformation showing multiple cavitated lung masses in the peripheral part of the right upper and lower lobes. *Right:* Sagittal volume reformation (5-mm-thick slab) with mIP. The relationships between subsegmental bronchi and cavitated masses are well depicted (*arrows*). A direct communication between a peripheral bronchus and a cavitated nodule in the posterior segment of the right upper lobe is visible

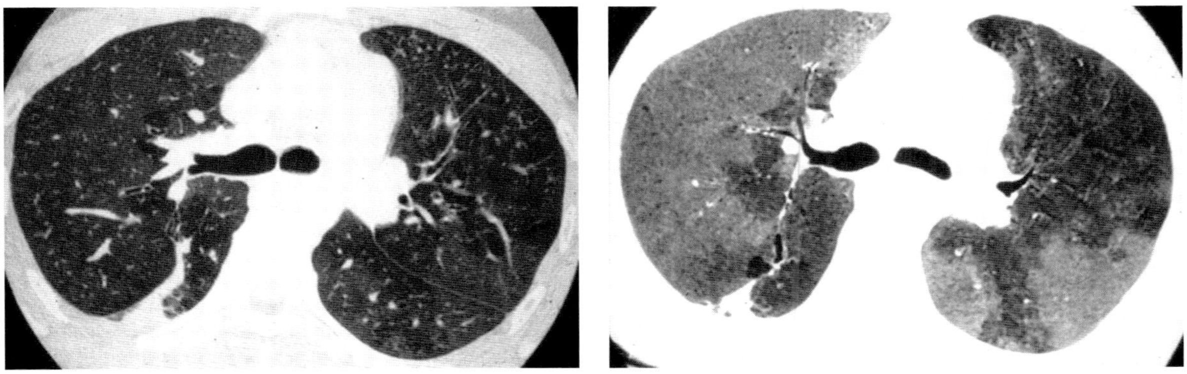

a b

Fig. 5.7a, b. Expiratory air trapping in a patient with post-tuberculous constrictive bronchiolitis. **a** Thin transverse scan at expiration showing patchy areas of air trapping. **b** A 7-mm-thick transverse slab with MPVR–mIP technique increases the contrast in attenuation between areas of air trapping (decreased lung attenuation) and normal areas encountered by each ray. The thickness of the slab is selected interactively at the console or workstation (MPVR–MIP technique; Rémy et al. 1998). This benefits in the display of the mucoid impactions seen in dilated bronchi (Fig. 5.8), or the display of the small centrilobular nodular and/or linear opacities (tree-in-bud appearance) expressing infectious or inflammatory bronchiolitis (Fig. 5.9).

5.2.6 3D Surface- and Volume-Rendering Techniques

The surface of the volume of air contained in the airways is isolated from the initial volume data by thresholding segmentation. Volume-rendering techniques are preferable to shaded-surface display to image the airways (Fig. 5.4b). The technique allows for a better understanding of the longitudinal extent of airway stenoses than axial CT images (Rémy-Jardin et al. 1996; Kauczor et al. 1996; Boiselle et al. 2002). The 3D images offer an overview of the pathology, particularly appreciated in complex airway anatomy, and may be used to select the best orientation for multiplanar reformations. The major limits of this technique are related to thresholding range. The results of reconstructions are sensitive to partial-volume artifacts and motion-related artifacts.

5.2.7 CT Bronchography

Computed tomographic bronchography is a new functionality consisting in a segmentation of the lumen–wall interface of the airways. Rémy-Jardin et al. (1998a) used a continuous rim of peripheral voxels and the volume-rendering algorithm. This technique has proven to be of particular interest in diagnosing mild changes in airway caliber and understanding complex tracheobronchial abnormalities (Rémy-Jardin et al. 1998b). Using the same concept, we developed a fully automatic method for 3D bronchial tree reconstruction based on bronchial lumen detection within the thoracic volume data set

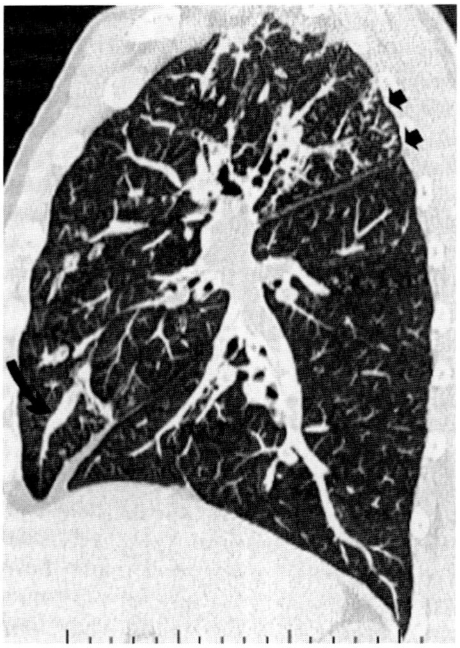

Fig. 5.8. Patient with cystic fibrosis. Sagittal 7-mm-thick slab with MIP technique showing mucoid impactions in dilated bronchi in the right middle lobe (*curved arrow*) and foci of tree-in-bud sign in the posterior segment of the left upper lobe (*straight arrows*)

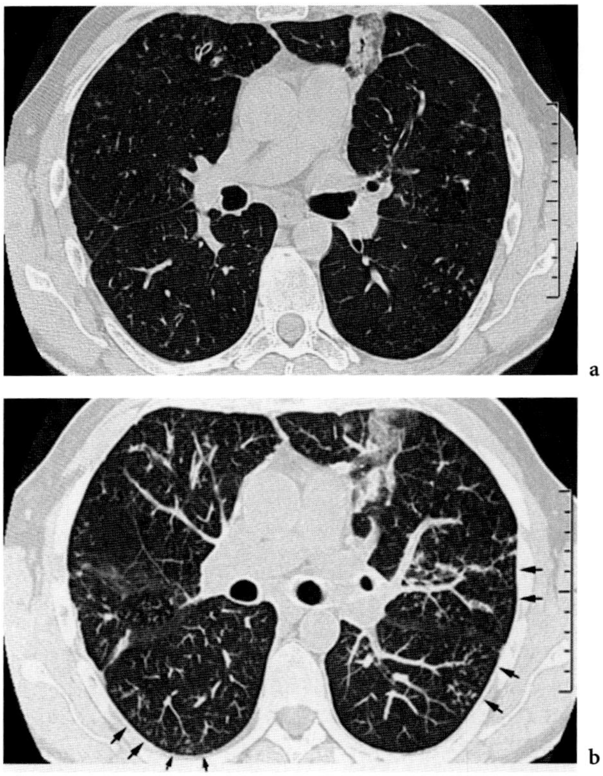

Fig. 5.9a, b. Infectious bronchiolitis in a patient with bronchiectasis. **a** Thin transverse slice and **b** 5-mm-thick slab in MPVR–MIP technique. Several foci of small centrilobular, nodular and branching linear opacities (tree-in-bud sign) are only depicted (*arrows*) on MPVR–MIP image. Note the presence of a focal area of air-space consolidation and ground-glass attenuation within the anterior segment of the left upper lobe due to bronchopneumonia

obtained from thin multidetector CT acquisition and thin collimation during breath hold (Grenier et al. 2002). It provides a specific visualization modality relying on an energy-based 3D reconstruction of the bronchial tree up to the sixth- to seventh-order subdivisions with a semi-transparent volume-rendering technique (Fig. 5.10). In addition, automatic delimitation and indexation of anatomical segments makes possible local and reproducible analysis at a given level of the bronchial tree, and an automatic extraction of the central axis of the bronchial tree which simplifies the interactivity during the navigation within CT bronchography or virtual endoscopy modes. These tools can also be used for quantitative assessment of the wall and lumens of the airways on cross-sectional images of the bronchi reconstructed perpendicular to their central axis.

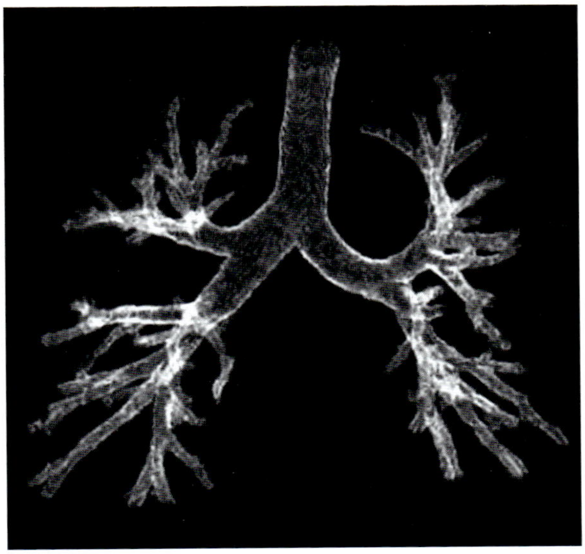

Fig. 5.10. A CT bronchography after MDCT. Coronal view of the 3D reconstructed bronchial tree with a semi-transparent volume-rendering technique in a normal individual

5.2.8 Virtual Bronchoscopy

Virtual bronchoscopy provides an internal rendering of the tracheobronchial walls and lumen. Owing to a perspective rendering algorithm, this simulates an endoscopist's view of the internal surface of the airways (Fig. 5.1). The observer may interactively move through the airways. This technique may be obtained from both 3D surface-rendering and volume-rendering techniques (Fig. 5.11; Rémy-Jardin et al. 1996; Remy et al. 1998). Volume-rendering technique is less sensitive to partial-volume effects than surface rendering. Powerful computers permit real-time rendering (15–25 images/s) making flying within the airways in a virtual manner possible. The technique allows accurate reproduction of major endoluminal abnormalities with an excellent correlation with fiberoptic bronchoscopy results regarding the location, severity, and shape of airway narrowing (McAdams et al. 1998). Virtual bronchoscopy is also able to visualize the bronchial tree beyond an obstructive lesion and thus to perform a retroscopy when looking back toward the distal part of the stenosis. Despite these

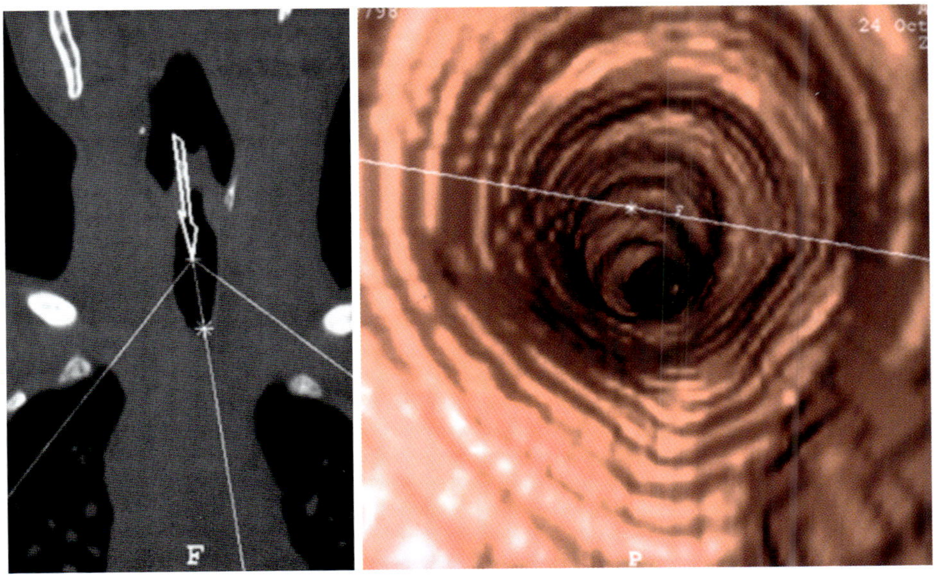

Fig. 5.11. Tracheal stenosis (same patient as in Figs. 4 and 5). Virtual bronchoscopy. Descending view from the origin of the trachea with a perspective internal volume-rendering technique, showing the progressive and regular narrowing of the tracheal lumen

appreciable abilities, virtual bronchoscopy remains very sensitive to the partial-volume averaging effect and motion artifacts. In addition, this technique is unable to identify the causes of bronchial obstruction; mild stenosis, submucosal infiltration, and superficial spreading tumors are not identified (Rémy-Jardin et al. 1996).

5.2.9 Quantitative Assessment of the Airways

Airway lumen and airway wall areas may be quantitatively assessed on CT images by using specific techniques that must be reproducible as well as accurate in order to compare the airways pre- and post-intervention (bronchoprovocation, bronchodilatation, therapeutic response) and to carry out longitudinal studies of airway remodeling. Airway lumen and wall areas measured on axial images depend on the lung volume, and angle between the airway central axis and the plane of section. Volumetric acquisition at controlled lung volume is required in order to precisely match the airways of an individual on repeated studies. The control of lung volume at CT is obtained by spirometric triggering (Grenier et al. 2002). Measurements of airway lumen and wall area have to be restricted to airways that appear to have been cut in cross section (King et al. 2000). With MDCT, it becomes possible to acquire a volume of lung with 0.6- to 0.75-mm slice thickness leading to CT voxels having cubic dimensions (isotropic voxels) (Wood et al. 1995). The segmentation of bronchial lumens and reconstruction of the airways in 3D allow determining of the central axis of the airways and reconstruct the airway cross section in a plane perpendicular to this axis (Fig. 5.12; Grenier et al. 2002). Although they have been used almost exclusively for research purposes, these techniques with continued refinements will eventually be of benefit in the clinical practice of radiology (King et al. 2000). They will also contribute to better insights in physiopathology of obstructive lung disease, particularly in COPD and asthma.

Extent of air trapping can also be measured using a semi-quantitative scoring system which estimates the presence of lung that appears abnormal on each expiratory scan (Ng et al. 1999). An automatic and more reproducible technique has also been proposed. It is based on thresholding at –900 HU on expiratory scan. All the pixels included in areas of air trapping may be highlighted and automatically counted (Newman et al. 1994). Using MDCT over the lungs at full expiration, an exhaustive assessment of the volume of air trapping and a 3D display of distribution of air trapping can be obtained.

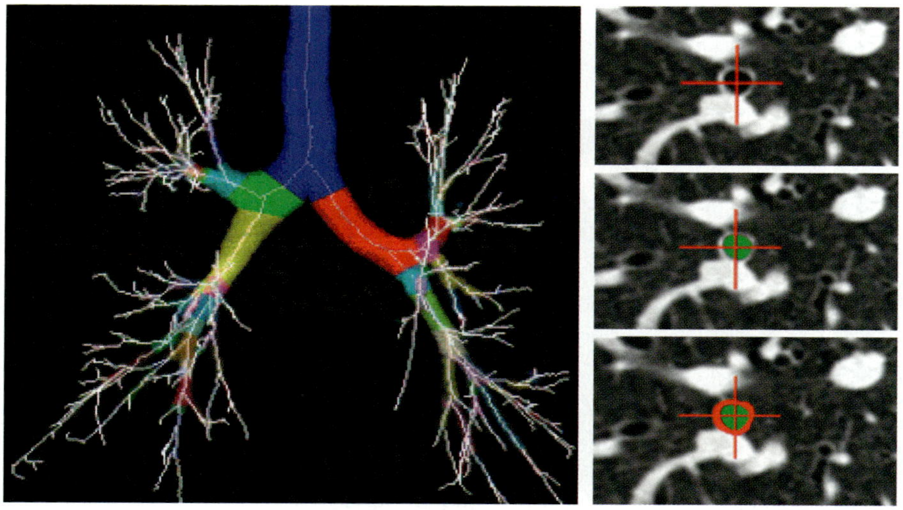

Fig. 5.12. Quantitative assessment of the airways. *Left:* A 3D reconstruction of the bronchial tree after MDCT and automatic indexation of the trachea, main and lobar bronchi (color-coded) and 3D representation of the central axis of the tracheobronchial tree. *Right:* Cross section (*top*) of the posterobasal segmental bronchus of the right lower lobe strictly perpendicular to the scanning plane. Automatic detection of the inner contour of the bronchial wall and segmentation of the bronchial lumen area (*middle*; *green*). *Bottom:* the automatic detection of the outer contour of the bronchial wall permitting the segmentation and quantitative assessment of the bronchial wall cross-section area (*red*)

5.3 Clinical Applications

5.3.1 Tracheobronchial Stenoses

Multiplanar volume reformations, CT bronchography, and virtual bronchoscopy may prove valuable in patients with tracheal or bronchial stenosis from central tumors as well as from inflammatory diseases or fibrosis after surgery or interventional endoscopic or radiologic treatment (Figs. 5.4, 5.5, 5.11). Imaging may contribute to image guidance of endobronchial treatment modalities such as endobrachytherapy, laser treatment planning, or endoprosthesis (Boiselle et al. 2002; Grenier et al. 1996). Imaging is also helpful in the follow-up after such treatment to search for complications such as recurrence of stenosis, stent misplacement, or displacement. It provides information that allows more precise direction of a real bronchoscopy, including demonstration of the length of a stricture and depiction of additional areas of strictures beyond an area of narrowing that is not traversable by the bronchoscope. This capacity is particularly important in patients who are prone to multiple strictures. It may also be easier to measure the degree of stenosis at CT compared with the view obtained at bronchoscopy. Whereas the extraluminal extent of an abnormality is not visible at bronchoscopy, it can generally be demonstrated at CT (Fig. 5.13). In addition, imaging may help to precisely visualize the attachment site of a benign bronchial tumor which can strongly influence the surgical decision making (Rémy et al. 1998).

Analysis of the shape, content, density, and anatomic relationships of the lesion on CT images can contribute to determining the precise etiology of a bronchial stenosis. Focal or diffuse fat infiltration visible within an endoluminal bronchial mass is characteristic of hamartoma. The association with central or "popcorn" calcification reinforces this diagnosis. Broncholithiasis, a condition in which peribronchial calcified nodal disease erodes into or distorts an adjacent bronchus, is recognized at CT by the presence of a calcified endobronchial or peribronchial lymph node, associated with bronchopulmonary complications due to obstruction (including atelectasis, pneumonia, bronchiectasis, and air trapping), in the absence of an associated soft tissue mass (Conces et al. 1991). Focal

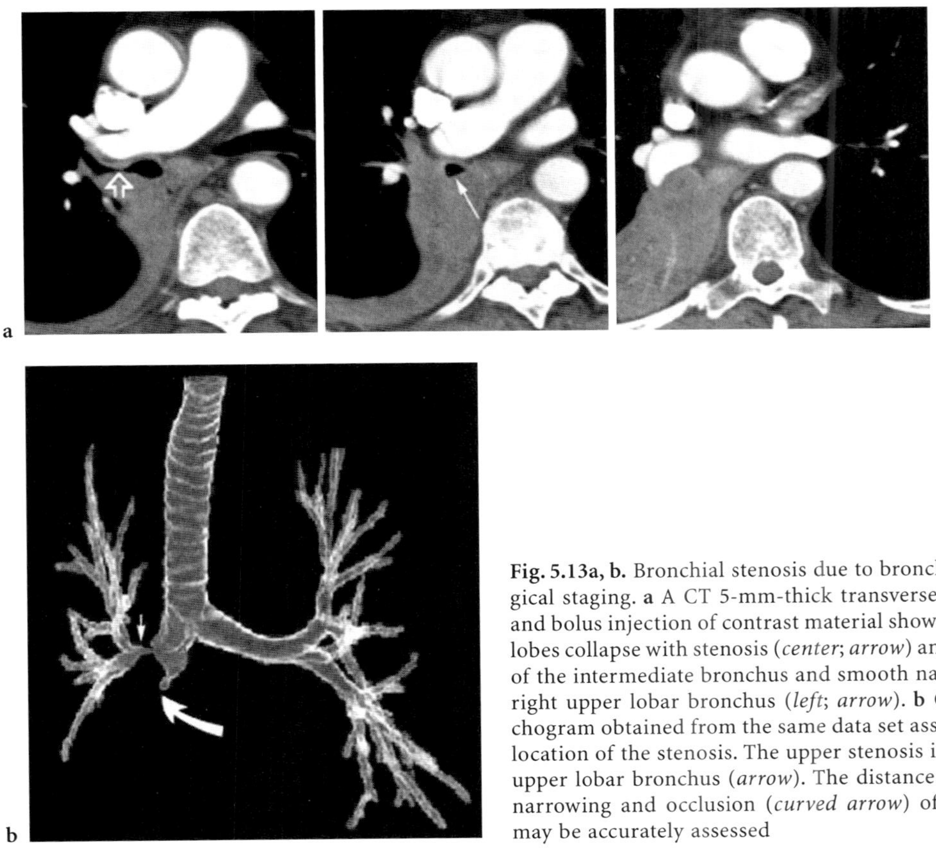

a

b

Fig. 5.13a, b. Bronchial stenosis due to bronchogenic carcinoma. Pre-surgical staging. **a** A CT 5-mm-thick transverse scan after MDCT scanning and bolus injection of contrast material showing a right middle and lower lobes collapse with stenosis (*center*; *arrow*) and complete occlusion (*right*) of the intermediate bronchus and smooth narrowing of the lumen of the right upper lobar bronchus (*left*; *arrow*). **b** Coronal view of a CT bronchogram obtained from the same data set assessing the shape, extent, and location of the stenosis. The upper stenosis is located at the origin of the upper lobar bronchus (*arrow*). The distance between the carina and the narrowing and occlusion (*curved arrow*) of the intermediate bronchus may be accurately assessed or diffuse bronchial stenosis can be observed in several inflammatory diseases, such as sarcoidosis, Wegener's granulomatosis, amyloidosis, and relapsing polychondritis. Computed tomography can demonstrate regular or irregular narrowing of the airways, thickening of the bronchial wall, sometimes with dense calcium deposits, or extrinsic airway compression by enlarged nodes (GRENIER et al. 1996).

When bronchopulmonary tumors are not visible at endoscopy, CT can be useful to guide the taking of bronchial or transbronchial biopsy by showing the relationships between the bronchial tree and peripheral carcinomatous lesions. The ability to make a definite diagnosis after bronchial forceps biopsy and bronchial brushing has proven to be better for lesions characterized by a bronchus cutoff or bronchus contained within a tumor (GAETA et al. 1993). Transbronchial needle aspiration has proven to be best able to provide a diagnosis in patients with a bronchus compressed by the tumor or with a thickening and narrowing of the bronchus leading to the tumor. The MDCT fluoroscopy now provides real-time guidance of any transbronchial needle procedures of tumor or lymph nodes (BOISELLE et al. 2002).

5.3.2 Airway Fistula and Dehiscence

The MDCT with thin collimation is the most accurate technique to identify peripheral bronchopleural fistulas that are most commonly caused by necrotizing pneumonia or secondary to traumatic lesions (Fig. 5.14; WESTCOTT and VOLPE 1995). Nodobronchial and nodobronchoesophageal fistulas that are most commonly caused by Mycobacterium Tuberculosis infection are depicted by the presence of gas in cavitated hila or mediastinal lymphadenopathy adja-

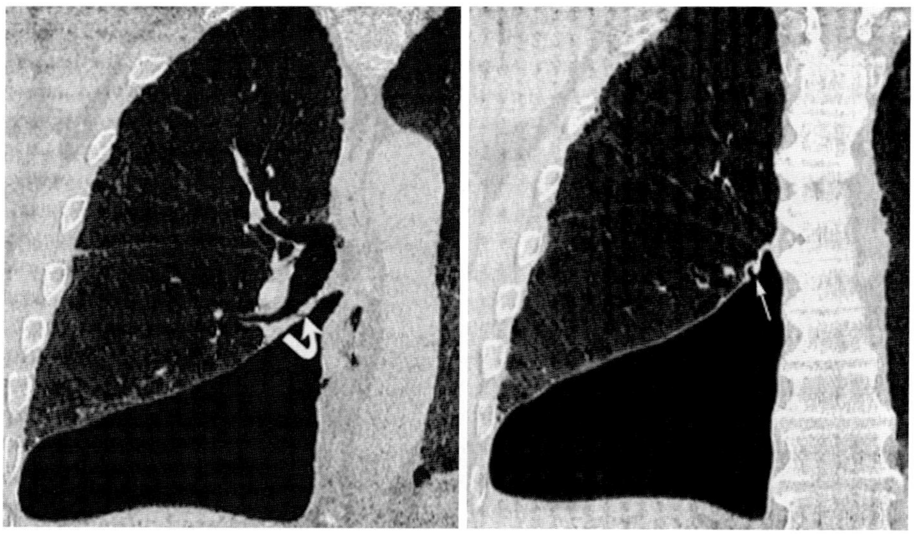

a

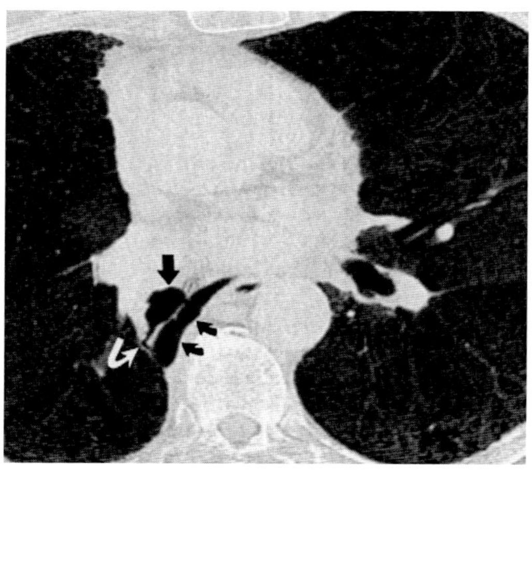

b

Fig. 5.14a, b. Bronchopleural fistula in a patient suffering from an idiopathic non-specific interstitial pneumonia who underwent lobectomy of the right lower lobe for primary lung adenocarcinoma (stage IA). The patient was referred for the assessment of a persistent air collection within the lobectomy space. **a** Coronal reformation with MPVR–mIP technique showing a small tubular connection between the intermediate bronchus (*curved arrow*) and the pleural air collection (*arrow*). **b** Transverse MPVR (7 mm thick)–mIP image confirming the presence of the postoperative bronchopleural fistula (*curved white arrow*). *Large black arrow* shows the intermediate bronchus and the small *curved black arrows* show the upper part of the pleural air-space collection cent to the airways. Direct visualization of the sinus tract between the bronchial lumen and the hypertrophied cavitated lymph node and/or the esophagus can be helpful in planning therapy. Tracheal diverticula and tracheo-broncho-esophageal fistula may also be diagnosed even in adults (GRENIER et al. 2002). Computed tomography has a high degree of sensitivity and specificity for depicting bronchial dehiscence occurring after lung transplantation and seen as bronchial wall defect associated with extraluminal air collections (SEMENKOVICH et al. 1995).

5.3.3 Congenital Abnormalities of the Airways

The MDCT easily detects as an asymptomatic incidental finding congenital anomalies of the bronchial branching pattern such as ectopic bronchi, supernumerary anomalous bronchus, bronchial atresia, and lobar hypoplasia. A focal mucoid impaction projecting into a hyperinflated and oligemic segment or lobe is highly suggestive of the diagnosis of bronchial atresia. Segmental or lobar hyperinflation distal to the atretic bronchus with develops early in life as a result of collateral ventilation is easily identified on CT scans, whereas bronchoscopy is usually interpreted as being normal (RÉMY-JARDIN et al. 1989). Multiplanar reformation enables the visualization of the linear opacity connecting the bronchocele and the bronchial tree corresponding to the atretic bronchial segment (BEIGELMAN et al. 1998).

Hemoptysis or recurrent infection may occur as secretions can be retained with resultant inflammation, and hypervascularity, and reveal an ectopic bronchus, particularly the tracheal bronchus or accessory cardiac bronchus. These abnormalities are easily analyzed by CT using cine viewing, multiplanar reformation, and 3D techniques (BEIGELMAN et al. 1998).

5.3.4 Bronchiectasis

Despite its decreased prevalence in developed countries, bronchiectasis remains an important cause of hemoptysis and chronic sputum production. It is now generally accepted that thin-section CT is the imaging modality of choice to establish the presence of bronchiectasis and to determine its precise extent (FRASER et al. 2000).

5.3.4.1 CT Characteristics

The characteristic CT findings of bronchiectasis include the following (MCGUINESS et al. 1993; KIM et al. 1997): (a) an internal bronchial diameter greater than that of the adjacent pulmonary artery; (b) lack of bronchial tapering, defined as a bronchus that has the same diameter as its parent bronchi for a distance of more than 2 cm; (c) visualization of bronchi abutting the mediastinal pleura; and (d) visualization of bronchi within 1 cm of the costal pleura. A bronchial wall thickening is also often present but this abnormality is a non-specific finding that may also be seen in other conditions, particularly asthma, and in asymptomatic smokers.

The thin-section CT appearance of dilated bronchi varies depending on the type of bronchiectasis and the orientation of the airways relative to the

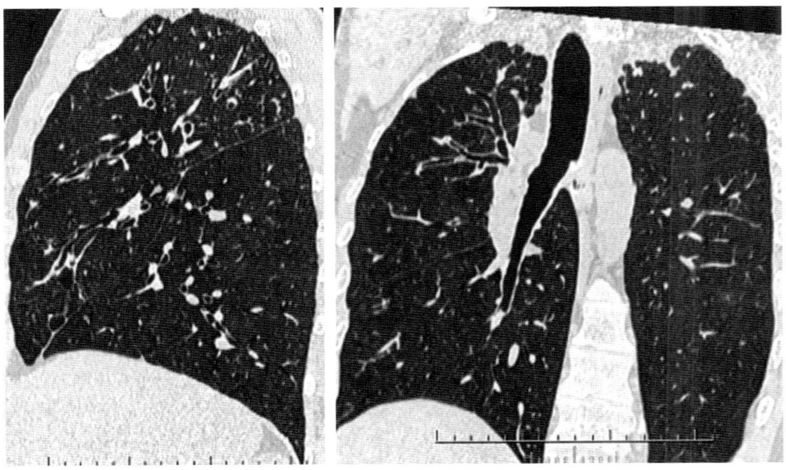

Fig. 5.15. Patient with post tuberculosis; bilateral cylindrical bronchiectasis. *Left:* Sagittal reformation after MDCT showing cylindrical bronchiectasis in the right upper and middle lobes. *Right:* Coronal oblique reformation depicting cylindrical bronchiectasis in the superior and posterior segments of the right upper lobe (lack of distal tapering of the bronchial lumens)

plane of the thin-section CT scan. In cylindrical bronchiectasis, bronchi coursing parallel and in the plane of section are visualized as parallel lines (Fig. 5.15), whereas bronchi coursing perpendicular to the plane of scanning appear as circular lucencies larger than the diameter of the adjacent pulmonary artery, resulting in a signet ring appearance. Varicose bronchiectasis is characterized by the presence of non uniform bronchial dilatation (Fig. 5.16), whereas cystic bronchiectasis results in a cluster of cystic spaces sometimes containing air–fluid levels.

Secretion accumulation within bronchiectatic airways is generally easily recognizable as lobulated glove-finger, lobulated V- or, lobulated Y-shaped densities. When oriented perpendicular to the scanning plane the filled dilated bronchi are visualized as nodular opacities and recognized by the observation of the homologous pulmonary arteries whose diameters are smaller than those of the dilated filled bronchi.

The size of the ectatic bronchi decreases on end expiratory as compared with inspiratory thin-section CT scans. Occasionally, they collapse completely because of their increased compliance.

In addition to bronchiectasis itself, a number of other abnormalities are seen with increased frequency in patients who have the disease, including areas of decreased lung attenuation and perfusion, expiratory air trapping, tracheomegaly and mediastinal lymph node enlargement.

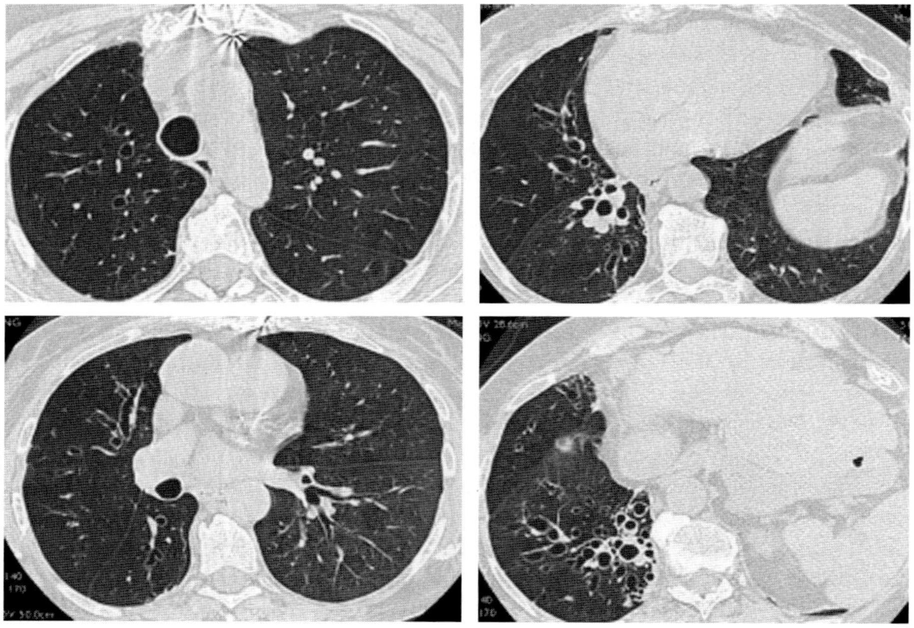

a

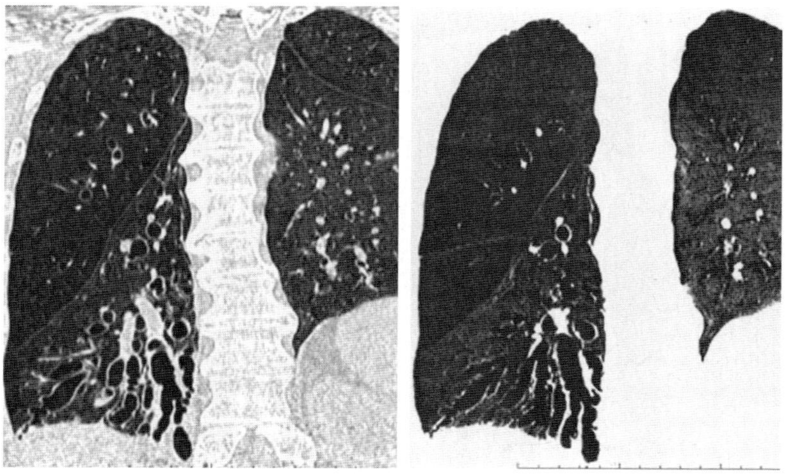

b

Fig. 5.16a, b. Bronchiectasis associated with constrictive bronchiolitis occurring after right lung transplantation (chronic rejection). **a** Transverse thin slice after MDCT showing thin-walled varicose and cystic bronchiectasis within the three lobes of the right lung. Oligemia and decreased lung attenuation are present in the right lung due to constrictive bronchiolitis. **b** Coronal reformation with MPVR (*left*) and MPVR-mIP (*right*) images displaying the distribution and extent of bronchiectasis in the right lower lobe and the increased volume of the right lung

5.3.4.2
CT Accuracy

Thin-section CT has been proven to be a reliable and non-invasive method for the assessment of bronchiectasis and has largely eliminated the need for bronchography (GRENIER et al. 1986). Thin-section CT is not, however, 100% sensitive and specific, and several limitations of the technique need to be recognized (KANG et al. 1995). These limitations include: (a) artifacts resulting from both respiratory and cardiac motion; (b) overlooking of areas of focal bronchiectasis located exclusively in skipped areas; and (c) difficulty of perceiving the slight dilatation of mild cylindrical bronchiectasis.

Motion degradation of bronchial images can be reduced by using a 180° interpolation algorithm to reconstruct axial images after helical scanning. The ECG gating may be used to reduce cardiac motion artifacts that may mimic disease (SCHOEPF et al. 1999). In addition, volumetric helical acquisition during breath holding eliminates the potential risk of missing small subtle bronchiectasis in areas skipped by the interspacing between thin-section CT scans (LUCIDARME et al. 1996). Because of many factors that can cause transient or permanent changes in diameter of the relatively compliant pulmonary arteries, invalidating the finding of cylindrical bronchiectasis based on the bronchoarterial diameter ratio >1, the lack of tapering of bronchial lumen has proven to be the most reliable sign of cylindrical bronchiectasis (KANG et al. 1995); however, this finding is difficult to perceive on successively spaced thin-section CT scans and its assessment is significantly improved by using helical CT with thin collimation and viewing the contiguous scans in a cine mode. As mucoid impaction filling bronchiectatic bronchi can simulate pulmonary nodules or masses on a single thin-section CT scan and pulmonary arteries are not recognized because of intense vasoconstriction in hypoventilated areas, MDCT with thin collimation provides a multiplanar display of the radiopaque tubular structures converging toward the hilum in a segmental or subsegmental distribution, corresponding to filled dilated bronchi (Fig. 5.8).

By comparing helical CT with 3-mm collimation and thin-section CT scans with 10-mm intervals in a series of 50 patients with suspicion of bronchiectasis, LUCIDARME et al. (1996) showed that the number of patients, segments, and bronchi affected with bronchiectasis was higher on helical CT than on thin-section CT scans. In addition, the interobserver agreement was significantly better with helical CT than with thin-section CT scans for the presence or absence of bronchiectasis on a per-segment basis, and also for assessing the extent of bronchiectasis in a given lobe and the distribution of disease in a given segment (LUCIDARME et al. 1996). A such accurate assessment of extent of disease is particularly required before surgery for focal bronchiectasis. Indeed, the surgeon must identify with certainty which segments are diseased, since surgical techniques frequently permit preservation of one or more normal pulmonary segments from a lobe in which bronchiectasis is present. For all these reasons, MDCT with thin-slice thickness using low dose should become the recommended routine protocol for the diagnosis and assessment of bronchiectasis (Figs. 5.15, 5.16). In addition, CT bronchography reconstructed after MDCT acquisition with thin-slice thickness should permit to increase the confidence level of diagnosis of mild cylindrical bronchiectasis or to improve the visual assessment of the extent of disease (Fig. 5.17; GRENIER et al. 2002).

5.3.5
Small Airways Disease

Thin-section CT scan is currently the best imaging technique for assessment of diseases of the small airways (MULLER and MILLER 1995). The MDCT may contribute in improving the visualization of the characteristic findings. The use of MPVR–MIP technique has been proven to increase the number of bronchiolar changes compared with single thin-section CT scans (Fig. 5.18; RÉMY-JARDIN et al. 1996).

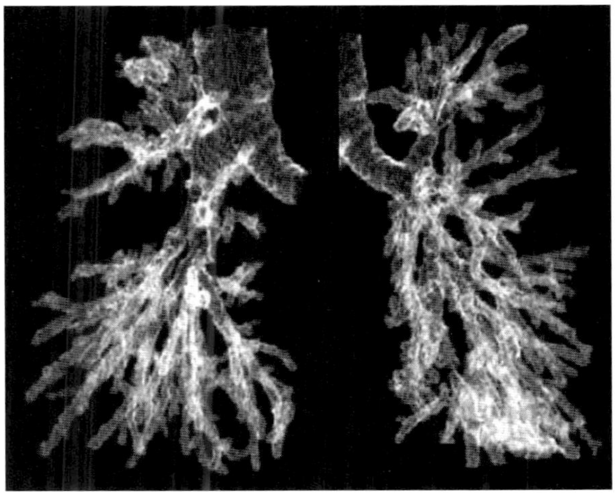

Fig. 5.17. A CT bronchogram after MDCT in a patient with chronic obstructive pulmonary disease (COPD) and diffuse cylindrical bronchiectasis. *Left:* Right bronchogram in a right posterior oblique view. *Right:* Left bronchogram in a left posterior oblique view

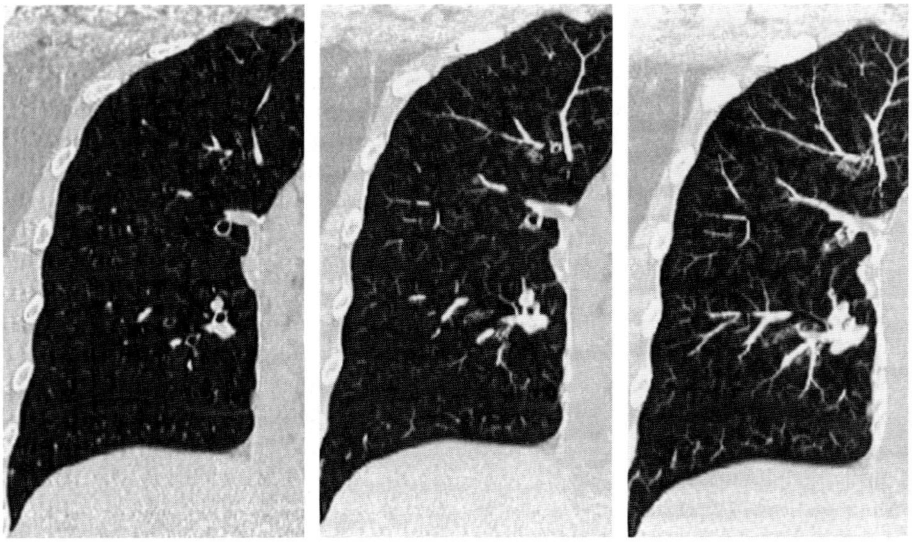

Fig. 5.18. Respiratory bronchiolitis in an asymptomatic smoker. Coronal reformations after MDCT. Increasing the thickness of the slab from 0.6 mm (*left*) to 3.3 mm (*center*) and 7.7 mm (*right*) increases the profusion and visibility of multiple small ill-defined and hazy dense centrilobular nodules

In cellular bronchiolitis, CT findings consist of small centrilobular nodular and/or branching linear opacities. The association of both nodular and linear branching opacities gives the tree-in-bud appearance, characteristic of infection. These abnormalities represent enlarged bronchioles filled with mucous or pus coursing perpendicular and parallel to the CT plane of section (Figs. 5.8, 5.9).

The CT findings of constrictive bronchiolitis express the airway obstruction due to bronchiolar fibrosis which leads to decreased ventilation and reflex vasoconstriction. They consist of areas of decreased lung attenuation and perfusion and air trapping. Redistribution of blood flow to areas of normal lung leads to a pattern of mosaic attenuation and perfusion (Worthy et al. 1997). The air trapping is best seen on expiratory scans (Fig. 5.3, 5.7). The abnormalities have often a patchy bilateral distribution. In case of more global involvement of the small airways, the lack of regional homogeneity of the lung density is difficult to perceive on inspiratory scans (Hansell et al. 1997). Mosaic perfusion becomes only visible on expiratory scans. In patients with particularly severe and widespread involvement of the small airways, inspiratory scans appear with an apparent uniformity of decreased attenuation in the lungs and scans taken at end expiration may appear unremarkable. In these patients, the most striking features are paucity of pulmonary vessels and lack of change of the cross-sectional areas of the lung at comparable levels on inspiratory and expiratory scans.

The extent of air trapping rather than the lung attenuation better predicts pulmonary function tests findings of obstruction. Although abnormal expiratory air trapping may be depicted in patients with normal pulmonary function tests, significant correlations have been shown between extent of air trapping at expiratory CT and indices of airflow obstruction at pulmonary function tests in patients with various types of small airway disease (Hansell et al. 1996, 1997; Lucidarme et al. 1998; Padley et al. 1993; Roberts et al. 2000). The CT features of small airway diseases are common findings in patients with bronchiectasis and the extent of CT evidence of small airway disease (decreased lung attenuation and expiratory air trapping) has been proven to be the major determinant of airflow obstruction (Roberts et al. 2000). In contrast, the obstructive defect found at pulmonary function tests was not related to the degree of collapse of large airways on expiratory CT or the extent of mucus plugging of the airways.

5.3.6 Chronic Obstructive Pulmonary Disease

Involvement of proximal airways in patients with COPD includes bronchial wall thickening, saber-sheath trachea, and expiratory airway collapse due to abnormal flaccidity. Bronchial wall thickening

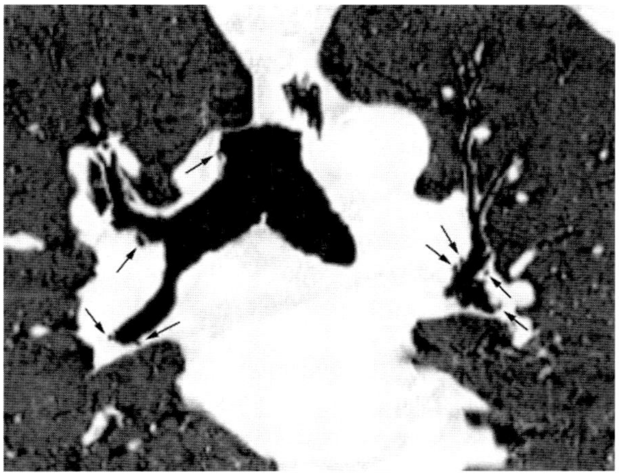

Fig. 5.19. Bronchial diverticula in a COPD patient. Coronal MPVR-mIP image showing the presence of small outpouchings of the bronchial lumen visible along the trachea as well as the upper and lower lobar bronchi (*arrows*)

is commonly present on thin-section CT scans of patients with COPD (Tagasuki and Godwin 1998). This abnormality, however, has been assessed only subjectively. The increase in size of tracheobronchial glands in patients with COPD is sometimes apparent on MDCT scans as small depression or diverticula on the airway lumen surface (Fig. 5.19)

5.3.6.1 Expiratory Bronchial Collapse and Tracheobronchomalacia

The quantity of bronchial cartilage has been found to be decreased in patients who have COPD in some investigations (Tandon and Campbell 1969; Thurlbeck et al. 1974; Maisel et al. 1968). The most severe deficiency has been seen in the segmental and subsegmental bronchi, generally being more apparent in the lower than the upper lobes. Because cartilage provides an important contribution to the relative incompressibility of these airways, its deficiency may be expected to result in more prominent collapse. Expiratory bronchial collapse in patients who have COPD may be apparent using CT (Fig. 5.20). Tracheobronchomalacia is a variant of expiratory airway collapse due to abnormal flaccidity involving the trachea and main bronchi. The increase in compliance is due to the loss of integrity of the wall's structural components and is particularly associated with damaged or destroyed cartilages. The coronal diameter of the trachea becomes significantly larger than sagittal one, producing a lunate configuration to the trachea. The flaccidity of the trachea or bronchi is usually most apparent during coughing or forced expiration. In patients with COPD with high downstream resistance particularly high dynamic pressure gradients can be generated across the tracheal wall, and it is likely that caliber changes of more than 50% can occur at expiration with normal tracheal compliance. As a result, only

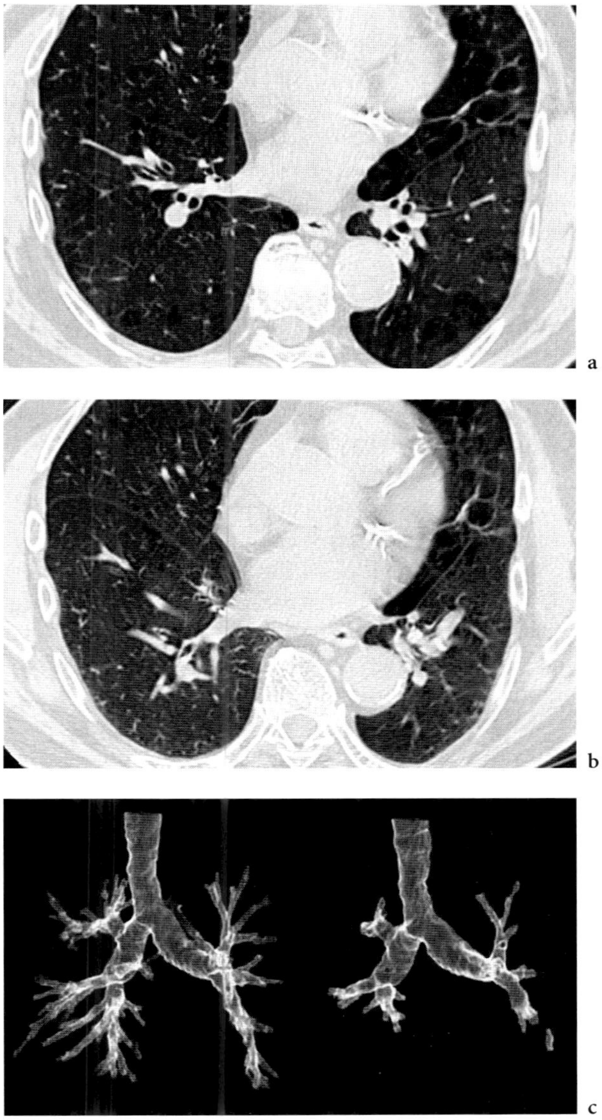

Fig. 5.20a–c. Expiratory bronchial collapse in a COPD patient. Transverse thin slices at **a** full inspiration and **b** expiration after MDCT, and **c** CT bronchograms obtained from the same data (*left:* inspiration; *right:* expiration). Expiratory bronchial collapse is seen in the segmental and subsegmental bronchi within the lower lobes (**b**, **c**)

a decrease in cross-sectional area of the tracheal lumen greater than 70% at expiration indicates tracheomalacia (Stern et al. 1993). Dynamic expiratory multislice CT may offer a feasible alternative to bronchoscopy in patients with suspected tracheobronchomalacia. Dynamic expiratory CT may show complete collapse or collapse of greater than 75% of airway lumen. Involvement of the central tracheobronchial tree may be diffuse or focal. The reduction of airway may have an oval or crescentic shape. The crescentic form is due to the bowing of posterior membranous trachea (Gilkeson et al. 2001).

5.3.6.2 *Saber-Sheath Trachea*

Saber-Sheath Trachea is a deformity defined as excessive coronal narrowing of the intrathoracic trachea in tandem with widening of the sagittal tracheal diameter. Concurrently, the cross-sectional diameter of the trachea decreases to less than 60% of normal (Stark and Norbash 1998). This deformity is highly characteristic of COPD. It affects primarily the intrathoracic trachea and the main bronchi and usually spares the cervical trachea, which retains normal dimensions and a normal configuration. The tracheal wall is slightly thickened, rigid, smooth, or slightly corrugated with occasional ossification or calcification of the cartilaginous elements.

5.3.6.3 *Involvement of Distal Airways*

It is commonly present in patients with COPD. Small centrilobular nodules or linear branching opacities may represent mucous plugging of bronchioles and small bronchi more or less associated with inflammatory bronchiolitis. These abnormalities could be the precursors of small airway obstruction and of centrilobular emphysema, but they can disappear if the patient stops smoking.

As with other airway diseases, COPD may result in expiratory air trapping. At CT scans performed 10% of vital capacity, patients with chronic bronchitis have lower attenuation than that of normal individuals (Lamers et al. 1994). This lower attenuation at expiration is considered as a finding of bronchiolar lumen obstruction. When emphysema is present, air trapping can be due to either airway obstruction caused by a loss of alveolar attachment to the airways directly related to emphysema, or to intrinsic bronchial or bronchiolar abnormalities associated with cigarette smoking.

5.3.7 Asthma

The most common abnormalities seen on thin section CT are bronchial wall thickening, narrowing of the bronchial lumen, bronchial dilatation, patchy areas of decreased lung attenuation and vascularity, and air trapping (Lynch 1998; Grenier et al. 1996; Lynch et al. 1993; Paganin et al. 1992; Park et al. 1997). The distribution of bronchial abnormalities is often heterogeneous; some airways have normal thickness and diameters, whereas others have thick walls and are narrowed or dilated. The prevalence of high-resolution CT abnormalities increases with increased severity of symptoms (Grenier et al. 1996; Paganin et al. 1996). Considerable variations exist, however, in the reported frequency of abnormalities. This variation is related to differences in diagnostic criteria and patient selection (Lynch 1998; Grenier et al. 1996; Lynch et al. 1993; Paganin et al. 1992; Park et al. 1997).

Park et al. (1997) demonstrated that only three findings were significantly more frequent in asthmatic patients than in normal individuals: bronchial wall thickening; bronchial dilatation; and expiratory air trapping.

The real current challenge for CT in asthma is to visualize and quantify the lumen and wall of airways and lung attenuation to assess the extent of airway obstruction, and to evaluate airway wall remodeling. This will become crucial in the monitoring of current and future therapy. The CT scanning of the airways has allowed to demonstrate in patients with mild intermittent asthma, the presence of basal bronchoconstriction that is reversible after salbutamol inhalation (Beigelman-Aubry et al. 2002). Abnormal expiratory air trapping is depicted in approximately 50% of asthmatic patients (Park et al. 1997); it may be induced by methacholine challenge and is partly reversible after salbutamol inhalation (Beigelman-Aubry et al. 2002). Bronchial wall thickening, frequently observed in patients with persistent asthma, reflects airway wall remodeling due to structural changes in the airways with smooth muscle hypertrophy and hyperplasia, responsible for the faster and higher decrease related to age of forced expiratory volume per second (FEV1) in asthmatics than in controls (Lange et al. 1998). Bronchial wall thickness measured at CT has been proven to be prominent in patients with more severe asthma. This is correlated with the duration and severity of the disease and the degree of air-flow obstruction (Niimi et al. 2000). This observation supports the concept that quantitative assessment of bronchial wall area at CT could be used to assess airway wall remodeling in asthmatic patients for longitudinal studies to evaluate the effects of new therapies.

References

Beigelman C, Howarth NR, Chartrand-Lefebvre C et al. (1998) Congenital anomalies of tracheobronchial branching patterns: spiral CT aspects in adults. Eur Radiol 8:79–85

Beigelman-Aubry C, Capderou A, Grenier PA et al. (2002) Mild intermittent asthma: CT assessment of bronchial cross-section area and lung attenuation at controlled lung volume. Radiology 223:181–187

Boiselle PM, Reynolds KF, Ernst A (2002) Multiplanar and three-dimensional imaging of the central airways with multidetector CT. Am J Roentgenol 179:301–308

Choi YW, McAdams HP, Jeon SC et al. (2002) Low-dose spiral CT: application to surface-rendered three-dimensional imaging of central airways. J Comput Assist Tomogr 26: 335–341

Conces DJ, Tarver RD, Vix VA (1991) Broncholithiasis: CT features in 15 patients. Am J Roentgenol 157:249–254

Ferretti GR, Bricault I, Coulomb M (2001) Virtual tools for imaging of the thorax. Eur Respir J 18:381–392

Fotheringham T, Chabat F, Hansell DM et al. (1999) A comparison of methods for enhancing the detection of areas of decreased attenuation on CT caused by airways disease. J Comput Assist Tomogr 23:385–389

Fraser RS, Muller NL, Coman N et al. (2000) Diagnosis of disease of the chest, vol 3, 4th edn. Saunders, Philadelphia, pp 2274–2277

Gaeta M, Barone M, Russi EG, Volta S, Casablanca G, Romeo P, La Spada F, Minutoli A (1993) Carcinomatous solitary pulmonary nodules: evaluation of the tumor-bronchi relationship with thin-section CT. Radiology 187:535–539

Gilkeson RC, Ciancibello LM, Hejal RB et al. (2001) Tracheobronchomalacia: dynamic airway evaluation with multidetector CT. Am J Roentgenol 176:205–210

Gotway MB, Lee ES, Reddy GP et al. (2000) Low-dose, dynamic, expiratory thin-section CT of the lungs using a spiral CT scanner. J Thorac Imaging 15:168–172

Grenier P, Maurice F, Musset D et al. (1986) Bronchiectasis: assessment by thin section CT. Radiology 161:95–99

Grenier P, Mourey-Gerosa I, Benali K et al. (1996) Abnormalities of the airways and lung parenchyma in asthmatics: CT observations in 50 patients and inter- and intraobserver variability. Eur Radiol 6:199–206

Grenier PA, Beigelman-Aubry C, Fétita C et al. (2002) New frontiers in CT imaging of airway disease. Eur Radiol 12: 1022–1044

Hansell DM, Rubens MB, Padley SP et al. (1997) Obliterative bronchiolitis: individual CT signs of small airway disease and functional correlation. Radiology 203:721–726

Hansell DM, Wells AU, Padley SP et al. (1996) Hypersensitivity pneumonitis: correlation of individual CT patterns with functional abnormalities. Radiology 199:123–128

Kang EY, Miller RR, Muller NL (1995) Bronchiectasis: comparison of preoperative thin-section CT and pathologic findings in resected specimens. Radiology 195:649–654

Kauczor HU, Wolcke B, Fischer B et al. (1996) Three-dimensional helical CT of the tracheobronchial tree: evaluation of imaging protocols and assessment of suspected stenoses with bronchoscopic correlation. Am J Roentgenol 167: 419–424

Kim JS, Muller NL, Park CS et al. (1997) Cylindrical bronchiectasis: diagnostic findings on thin-section CT. Am J Roentgenol 168:751–754

King GG, Muller NL, Whittall KP et al. (2000) An analysis algorithm for measuring airway lumen and wall areas from high-resolution computed tomographic data. Am J Respir Crit Care Med 161:574–580

Lamers RJ, Thelissen GR, Kessels AG et al. (1994) Chronic obstructive pulmonary disease: evaluation with spirometrically controlled CT lung densitometry. Radiology 193:109–113

Lange P, Parner J, Vestbo J et al. (1998) A 15-year follow-up study of ventilatory function in adults with asthma. N Engl J Med 339:1194–1200

Lucidarme O, Grenier PA, Coche E et al (1996) Bronchiectasis: comparative assessment with thin-section CT and helical CT. Radiology 200:673–679

Lucidarme O, Coche E, Cluzel P et al. (1998) Expiratory CT scans for chronic airway disease: correlation with pulmonary function test results. Am J Roentgenol 170:301–307

Lucidarme O, Grenier PA, Cadi M et al. (2000) Evaluation of air trapping at CT: comparison of continuous versus suspended expiration CT techniques. Radiology 216:768–772

Lynch DA (1998) Imaging of asthma and allergic bronchopulmonary mycosis. Radiol Clin North Am 36:129–142

Lynch DA, Newell JD, Tschomper BA et al. (1993) Uncomplicated asthma in adults: comparison of CT appearance of the lungs in asthmatic and healthy subjects. Radiology 188:829–833

Maisel JC, Silvers GW, Mitchell RS et al. (1968) Bronchial atrophy and dynamic expiratory collapse. Am Rev Respir Dis 98:988–997

McAdams HP, Palmer SM, Erasmus JJ et al. (1998) Bronchial anastomotic complications in lung transplant recipients: virtual bronchoscopy for noninvasive assessment. Radiology 209:689–695

McGuinness G, Naidich DP, Leitman BS et al. (1993) Bronchiectasis: CT evaluation. Am J Roentgenol 160:253–259

Muller NL, Miller RR (1995) Diseases of the bronchioles: CT and histopathologic findings. Radiology 196:3–12

Newman KB, Lynch DA, Newman LS, Ellegood D, Newell JD Jr (1994) Quantitative computed tomography detects air trapping due to asthma. Chest 106:105–109

Ng CS, Desai SR, Rubens MB et al. (1999) Visual quantitation and observer variation of signs of small airways disease at inspiratory and expiratory CT. J Thorac Imaging 14:279–285

Niimi A, Matsumoto H, Amitani R et al. (2000) Airway wall thickness in asthma assessed by computed tomography. Relation to clinical indices. Am J Respir Crit Care Med 162:1518–1523

Padley SPG, Adler BD, Hansell DM et al. (1993) Bronchiolitis obliterans: high-resolution CT findings and correlation with pulmonary function tests. Clin Radiol 47:236–240

Paganin F, Trussard V, Seneterre E et al. (1992) Chest radiography and high resolution computed tomography of the lungs in asthma. Am Rev Respir Dis 146:1084–1087

Paganin F, Seneterre E, Chanel P et al. (1996) Computed tomography of the lungs in asthma: influence of disease severity and etiology. Am J Respir Crit Care Med 153: 110–114

Park CS, Muller NL, Worthy SA et al. (1997) Airway obstruction in asthmatic and healthy individuals: inspiratory and expiratory thin-section CT findings. Radiology 203: 361–367

Quint LE, Whyte RI, Kazerooni EA et al. (1995) Stenosis of the central airways: evaluation by using helical CT with multiplanar reconstructions. Radiology 194:871–877

Rémy J, Rémy-Jardin M, Artaud D et al. (1998) Multiplanar and three-dimensional reconstruction techniques in CT: impact on chest diseases. Eur Radiol 8:335–351

Rémy-Jardin M, Rémy J, Ribet M, Gosselin B (1989) Bronchial atresia: diagnostic criteria and embryologic considerations. Diagn Intervent Radiol 1:45–51

Rémy-Jardin M, Rémy J, Deschildre F et al. (1996) Obstructive lesions of the central airways: evaluation by using spiral CT with multiplanar and three-dimensional reformations. Eur Radiol 6:807–816

Rémy-Jardin M, Rémy J, Artaud D et al. (1998a) Tracheobronchial tree: assessment with volume rendering-technical aspects. Radiology 208:393–398

Rémy-Jardin M, Rémy J, Artaud D et al. (1998b) Volume rendering of the tracheobronchial tree: clinical evaluation of bronchographic images. Radiology 208:761–770

Roberts HR, Wells AU, Milne DG et al. (2000) Airflow obstruction in bronchiectasis: correlation between computed tomography features and pulmonary function tests. Thorax 55:198–204

Rubin GD (1996) Techniques of reconstruction. In: Rémy-Jardin M, Rémy J (eds) Medical radiology spiral CT of the chest. Springer, Berlin Heidelberg New York, pp 101–127

Schoepf UJ, Becker CR, Bruening RD et al. (1999) Electrocardiographically gated thin-section CT of the lung. Radiology 212:649–654

Semenkovich JW, Glazer HS, Anderson DC et al. (1995) Bronchial dehiscence in lung transplantation: CT evaluation. Radiology 194:205–208

Stark P, Norbash A (1998) Imaging of the trachea and upper airways in patients with chronic obstructive airway disease. Radiol Clin North Am 36:91–105

Stern EJ, Graham CM, Webb WR et al. (1993) Normal trachea during forced expiration: dynamic CT measurements. Radiology 187:27–31

Summers RM, Shaw DJ, Shelhamer JH (1998) CT virtual bronchoscopy of simulated endobronchial lesions: effect of scanning, reconstruction, and display settings and potential pitfalls. Am J Roentgenol 170:947–950

Tagasuki JE, Godwin D (1998) Radiology of chronic obstructive pulmonary disease. Radiol Clin North Am 36:39–55

Tandon MK, Campbell AH (1969) Bronchial cartilage in chronic bronchitis. Thorax 24:607–612

Thurlbeck WM, Pun R, Toth J et al. (1974) Bronchial cartilage in chronic obstructive lung disease. Am Rev Respir Dis 109:73–80

Westcott JL, Volpe JP (1995) Peripheral bronchopleural fistula: CT evaluation in 20 patients with pneumonia, empyema, or postoperative air leak. Radiology 196:175–181

Wood SA, Zerhouni EA, Hoford JD et al. (1995) Measurement of three-dimensional lung tree structures by using computed tomography. J Appl Physiol 79:1687–1697

Worthy SA, Muller NL, Hartman TE, Swensen SJ, Padley SPG, Hansell DM (1997) Mosaic attenuation pattern on thin-section CT scans of the lung: differentiation among infiltrative lung, airway, and vascular diseases as a cause. Radiology 205:465–470

6 MDCT in Diffuse Lung Disease

H.-U. Kauczor

CONTENTS

6.1 Introduction

Computed tomography is generally accepted as the most powerful tool for the assessment of the lung parenchyma in patients known to have or suspected of having diffuse lung disease (Kazerooni 2001). Diffuse lung disease in this context comprises parenchymal diseases with an increase or a decrease of lung tissue, such as fibrosis and emphysema. Chest radiography, usually the initial imaging modality in these patients, has limited sensitivity and specificity for detection, characterization, and quantification. A significant number of disease will appear absolutely non-specific or remain completely occult (Grenier et al. 1991; Mathieson et al. 1989).

The inherent properties of CT as a cross-sectional imaging modality provide transversal images of the lung with high spatial resolution and without superimposition. In addition, the augmented contrast resolution of CT improves the detection of pathological processes within the body. The large attenuation difference between air-filled alveolar space and tissue makes the lung a high-contrast organ and allows for the detection of very subtle changes within the parenchyma. It is well known that the sensitivity of CT is much higher than for projection radiography; thus, CT may show clinically suspected disease which is not apparent on a chest radiograph or even non-suspected lung disease. The higher sensitivity of CT also results in early detection of parenchymal disease, e.g., in a comparative study CT was able to detect infiltrates approximately 5 days earlier than the chest radiograph (Heussel et al. 1999). Specificity and accuracy of CT are significantly higher than for chest radiographs which is an important advan-

H.-U. Kauczor, MD
Professor, Department of Radiology, Deutsches Krebsforschungszentrum Heidelberg, Im Neuenheimer Feld 280, 69120 Heidelberg, Germany

tage in the differential diagnosis of diffuse lung disease (Lee et al. 1994). At the same time CT has an unmatched negative predictive value for the exclusion of parenchymal abnormalities. For the tailored investigation of the lung parenchyma high-resolution CT (HRCT) has been proposed by many groups as most accurate (Mayo et al. 1987; Müller 1991). It has been widely accepted as the imaging gold standard for the lung parenchyma. Although optimal use and interpretation of HRCT requires clinical correlation, it is accepted that in particular clinical settings typical patterns from HRCT may be sufficient to come up with a presumptive diagnosis (Grenier et al. 1994). This information might be sufficient to start treatment even without histological verification.

6.2 High-Resolution Computed Tomography

The remarkable ability of HRCT to provide sufficient morphological detail of normal and abnormal lung parenchyma is based on high-quality examinations. With optimal scan technique the spatial resolution is as low as 0.5 mm. Due to the high contrast within the lung parenchyma, even structures as small as 0.2 mm may be visualized (Murata et al. 1989). Before the future role of multidetector-row CT (MDCT) in diffuse lung disease is discussed the technical characteristics of HRCT are reviewed.

Optimal visualization of the lung parenchyma is achieved by enhanced spatial resolution. The two most important factors in increasing spatial resolution were the use of thin collimation and reconstruction of the scan data with a high-spatial frequency algorithm. These two factors are essential for the definition of HRCT of the lung (Mayo et al. 1987; Müller 1991). Additional techniques, such as an increase of matrix size, reduction of the field of view, and alterations of voltage and tube current, were regarded as less contributory. Although they may be used additionally, they are not part of the definition of HRCT; however, they may gain increased recognition while using MDCT for volumetric high-resolution CT.

6.2.1 Collimation

To optimize image resolution a very thin collimation is indispensable. Usually, it is 1 mm. Such narrow collimation improves spatial resolution (Mayo et al. 1987). With optimal scanning technique, such as limitation of the field of view to the parenchyma of both lungs, the spatial resolution is between 0.5 and 0.3 mm. Depending on orientation, position and contrast within the lung parenchyma structures as small as 0.2 mm are occasionally identified (Murata et al. 1989); thus, pulmonary artery branches down to the 16th and bronchi down to the 8th generation will be depicted. They can even be characterized due to a significant reduction of partial-volume effects from adjacent structures by the thin collimation. Since the volume averaging effects of the margins of such small structures are minimized, HRCT provides a more accurate image of their true size. With respect to thick collimation CT, more small airways can be perceived and variations in lung attenuation are much more apparent with HRCT (Fig. 6.1). The reduction of partial-volume effects and volume averaging brings about some drawbacks. The identification of pulmonary arteries, veins and septa may appear more complicated since we are only looking at a single thin cut through these structures (Fig. 6.1). Their typical course within the parenchyma is much more difficult to follow, especially when it is oblique with respect to the transversal orientation of scanning. In this regard, despite high spatial resolution, HRCT leads to interpretive challenges because familiar landmarks in the lung parenchyma may be harder to recognize. This holds especially true since HRCT slices are not contiguous and obtained at 10- or 20-mm intervals.

6.2.2 High-Frequency Algorithm

The HRCT improves spatial resolution also by the application of a high spatial frequency reconstruction algorithm (Mayo et al. 1987). In comparison with standard algorithms which are regarded necessary for the assessment of soft tissues, high-resolution algorithms do not perform the smoothing used to decrease the perception of image noise. Anatomic margins and tissue interfaces, such as the fissure, pleura or septa, appear sharper. Increased spatial resolution, however, goes along with increased image noise and decreased contrast resolution. These factors are of limited impact in lung imaging which benefits significantly from the high intrinsic contrast between air-filled alveolar space and the higher density of the soft tissue components.

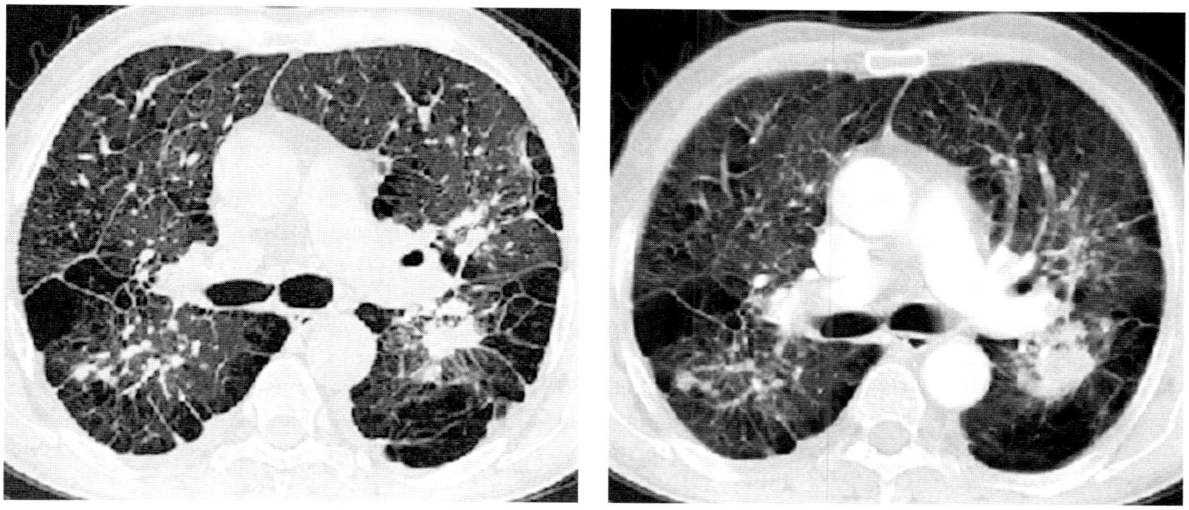

a b

Fig. 6.1a, b. A 67-year-old man with silicosis, progressive massive fibrosis and concomitant paracicatricial emphysema. **a** 1-mm thin slice shows irregular nodules, a septal pattern, architectural distortion, and widespread concomitant paracicatricial emphysema. Note that peripheral airways can be perceived and variations in lung attenuation are much more apparent than on the 5-mm-thick slice at the same position (**b**) due to reduction of partial-volume effects and volume averaging

6.2.3 Field of View

The field of view should be adjusted to the size of the lungs. For any given matrix size, this reduces the anatomic dimensions of the voxels and thus increases spatial resolution. Volume averaging and partial-volume effects are also reduced which can either be regarded as an advantage providing higher spatial resolution or as a disadvantage because the identification of small structures by their typical orientation of course within the lung parenchyma is more difficult. To ensure that the field of view does not cut off any part of the lung, it should be limited by the diameter of the external cortex of the ribs. To increase spatial resolution even further, targeting of the field of view onto a single lung or particular lobes or regions can be performed. Such an approach must be regarded as an additional reconstruction for the minute evaluation of the parenchyma or peripheral bronchi beyond the regular evaluation of images demonstrating both lungs (Remy-Jardin et al. 2002).

6.2.4 HRCT Protocols

Most HRCT protocols obtain images at 10- or 20-mm intervals between the single slices which makes it particularly difficult to depict the characteristic branching and distribution pattern of arteries, veins, bronchi and septa. At the same time, 90% of the lung parenchyma is not scanned if HRCT is performed as a stand-alone procedure. The HRCT for diffuse lung disease is based on the understanding that representative areas of lung disease will be present and are depicted for analysis; thus, it only requires the acquisition of some images at selected levels. Since many diffuse lung diseases are not uniform in distribution throughout the lung random sampling is generally performed; however, as only approximately 10% of the lung parenchyma is scanned, characteristic foci of disease may be missed. Some centers even obtain fewer HRCT slices for the assessment of diffuse lung disease in addition to a contiguous thick collimation coverage of the whole lung. This approach makes clear that HRCT alone should only be used in widespread diffuse or generalized lung disease.

6.3 Multidetector-Row Computed Tomography

6.3.1 Volumetric High-Resolution Computed Tomography

Multidetector-row CT represents an enormous achievement in the field of cross-sectional imaging. The combination of continuous rotation of the X-ray tube, continuous table feed, and multiple detector rows allows for acquisition of real volumetric data sets. The introduction of volumetric MDCT scan protocols has the advantage of great lung coverage, more complete assessment of the lung, and almost isotropic data sets. In diffuse lung disease, MDCT is performed with a collimation of 1 mm. To mimic traditional HRCT 1-mm thin slices can be reconstructed every 10 mm with the high-frequency algorithm; however, MDCT can provide much more information. To benefit from its huge potential, reconstruction of the whole data set with 1-mm thin slices and a high-frequency algorithm is recommended. This procedure generates volumetric high-resolution CT with almost isotropic resolution which provides contiguous visualization of the lung parenchyma. Obviously, hard-copy reading is inappropriate since not all images are to be filmed. Soft-copy reading on a workstation is mandatory to cope with the huge amount of images generated. Stack-mode viewing facilitates the depiction of parenchymal lung disease and the perception of image patterns which is extremely important in diffuse disease. This alone already requires a change in the protocols to be used and the workflow for patients with diffuse lung disease. From the volumetric high-resolution MDCT data sets with almost isotropic voxels high-quality images in different, non-axial planes can be reconstructed (Honda et al. 2001); thus, reading of chest CT will go far beyond the standard assessment of the transaxial slices since multiplanar reformations (MPR) and three-dimensional volume reconstructions are easily performed. Radiologists must be familiar with the huge potential of this technology and the necessity for a paradigm shift in the reading strategy (Rubin et al. 1996).

6.3.2 Performance of Volumetric High-Resolution Computed Tomography

Several studies have already looked into the performance of volumetric high-resolution MDCT and demonstrated that MDCT is approximately equivalent to HRCT in some respect, but offers a huge amount of additional information which will make the assessment of diffuse lung disease much easier. The use of volumetric MDCT is also particularly useful for the evaluation of nodular disease. Abnormalities are more easily identified to be related to the underlying vascular, bronchial, and lobular anatomy.

Studies comparing MDCT (1- and 5-mm slice thickness reconstructed from 1-mm collimation) with HRCT (1-mm slices) complemented by spiral CT (5-mm slices) have shown significant advantages for MDCT; these were apparent when the 5-mm slices at spiral CT were compared with the fused 5-mm slices at MDCT, which were based on 1-mm collimation. Regarding the assessment of the parenchyma with high resolution, both techniques were equivalent for the 1-mm slices (Schoepf et al. 1999; Honda et al. 2001). A different study looked at image quality and findings of high-resolution imaging more closely. The 1-mm slices from MDCT and HRCT were equivalent in terms of image quality, noise, as well as visualization of the central vessels, bronchi, and their related pathologies. Traditional HRCT was advantageous with regard to spatial resolution, which allowed better visualization of peripheral vessels and bronchi (Mehnert et al. 2000). This difference was attributed to the broader slice sensitivity profile in MDCT which causes a more blurred appearance of the very small intrapulmonary structures (Schorn et al. 1999). At the same time, however, MDCT was superior to traditional HRCT in demonstrating interlobar septa. Even more important will be the advantages of MDCT over HRCT with regard to motion, since respiratory or pulsation artifacts were more or less absent on MDCT images. Diagnostic relevant differences between volumetric high-resolution MDCT and traditional HRCT were only noted in 2.2% of cases (Mehnert et al. 2000).

On a single 1-mm HRCT slice a small, round subcentimeter structure will be better visualized than on MDCT; however, the interpretation is more difficult since this structure may represent an end-on vessel or a nodule. On a thicker section this differentiation would be an easy call. The MDCT with reconstruction of thin (1 mm) and thicker (5 mm) slices from the same data set is capable to provide visualization with both high resolution and with volume averaging to facilitate depiction and interpretation. Similarly, small irregularly marginated nodules on a single HRCT scan will represent impacted bronchioles. The typical tree-in-bud pattern of the same disease, however, will not be appreciated on a single thin collimation slice. Again, the use of a volumetric high-resolution acquisition will facilitate pattern detection of both, centrilobular nodules and tree-in-bud, significantly. Besides the assessment of thin and thick collimation slices reconstructed from the same data set, they can be summed up (fused) and viewed with a maximum intensity projection (MIP; Eibel et al. 2001a), or even a minimum intensity projection (MinIP). Multiplanar reformations (MPRs) in coronal plane should be reconstructed routinely, whereas MPRs in additional planes are optional.

6.3.3 Maximum Intensity Projection

Several studies have used MIP to demonstrate that the identification of pulmonary nodules can be improved. In one study 103 patients with suspicion or evidence of pulmonary nodules were enrolled and underwent MDCT with a collimation of 1 mm. The MIP and MPR were reconstructed in all three planes. The MIP were superior in the depiction of pulmonary nodules at a statistically significant level. Additional lesions were identified with MIP that were missed with transaxial slices and MPR. The improvement by MIP was based on the identification of nodules smaller than 5 mm in diameter. The improvement by MIP also led to an increase in diagnostic confidence (Eibel et al. 2001a). In a different study, MIP led to the detection of additional findings in 27% of patients with nodular disease (Gavelli et al. 1998). The advantage was particularly obvious within the central parts of the lung due to better distinction between nodules and vessels (Vernhet et al. 1999). In very extensive disease, MIP will show the nodules as a blurred, irregular pattern due to superimposition of nodular opacities. This might pose a potential problem in some patients.

6.3.4 Minimum Intensity Projection

Although minimum intensity projections (MinIP) are not widely used, they improve the assessment of lung disease associated with a decrease in attenuation. Single HRCT slices are not well suited for this type of postprocessing; however, it could be demonstrated that MinIP enhances the changes of small airway disease resulting in increased observer confidence and agreement as compared with HRCT alone (Fotheringham et al. 1999). Volumetric high-resolution MDCT provides a much better database than HRCT for the application of MinIP in low attenuation lung disease or ground-glass opacities. When using spiral CT for volumetric high resolution acquisitions MinIP revealed additional findings in 8% of patients with emphysema and in 25% of cases with ground-glass opacities (Gavelli et al. 1998). These results have been confirmed by a different study where MinIP improved the detection of pulmonary cysts and their differentiation from honeycomb cysts as well as the detection of ground-glass opacities not visible on HRCT (Vernhet et al. 1999). It has to be noted that MinIP was particularly prone to motion artifacts; thus, the image quality of MinIP derived from MDCT will be far superior to that obtained from traditional spiral CT as the source data set.

6.3.5 Multiplanar Reformations

Thin slices throughout the entire lung as provided by volumetric MDCT are best suited for high-quality multiplanar reformations (MPR). In diffuse lung disease, coronal or sagittal MPRs can be regarded as the primary plane for reading. A slice thickness of 5 mm for MPR yielded best results. Coronal reformations are superior to the transaxial slices because they better display the topology of the lungs and offer improved anatomic orientation (Eibel et al. 2001b). The detection of radiological patterns is facilitated, and the diagnostic yield is improved significantly (Figs. 6.2–6.9). Only the lung parenchyma directly adjacent to the heart and the great vessels might be visualized with limited quality due to cardiac pulsation artifacts. Coronal MPRs in particular are also more easily appreciated by our clinical partners because they are used to coronal projections from chest radiography and MRI of the chest. Advantages of sagittal MPR include the sharper delineation of interlobar fissures and thus improved anatomic localization of a lesion when compared with transaxial slices and coronal MPR (Eibel et al. 2001b). The usefulness of coronal MPRs from MDCT on work-flow related issues was demonstrated in a recent study in 50 patients with suspected or confirmed interstitial lung disease. This study showed that the number of images to be interpreted could be reduced by 40% without affecting diagnostic accuracy if a coronal plane was reconstructed rather than the routine transaxial plane. The actual number of images to read will be almost as low as with traditional transaxial HRCT. There is a high level of concordance between reading coronal and transaxial slices regarding the identification of nodules or fibrosis. Distribution of abnormalities and patterns are more easily and precisely observed on coronal MPR images. For the dedicated evaluation of the relationship between nodules and airways even the application of curved MPR is useful (Raman et al. 2002).

6.3.6 Patient Position

In the normal lung with the patient supine, there is a gradual increase in attenuation and vessel size from the more ventral to the more dorsal lung regions. This attenuation gradient is caused by the effect of gravity on blood flow and gas volume as well as some non-gravity-dependent effects. The density gradient is accentuated on expiration (Verschakelen et al. 1998). Hypoventilation and atelectasis in the dependent lung will cause areas of dependent density or subpleural lines; thus, in some cases it may be necessary to obtain prone images to differentiate actual disease from physiologically dependent density or atelectasis. This is particularly true in patients with suspected diffuse lung disease, when the detection of ground-glass opacities or curvilinear subpleural lines are of diagnostic importance. Prone scanning is useful in almost 20% of patients. The proportion is even higher in patients with a normal or near-normal chest radiograph (Volpe et al. 1997). The MDCT allows for very fast acquisition and complete coverage of the lung in a single breath hold. Since planning and data acquisition are so fast, the development of atelectasis formation due to supine posture and regional hypoventilation is less likely than at HRCT which requires more time and repeated breath holds. Nevertheless, routine MDCT in supine position should be complemented by a scan acquired in prone position if early diffuse lung disease is suspected in a dependent lung region.

6.3.7 Patient Respiration

Motion artifacts due to non-suspended respiration are common. Manifestations of respiratory motion include blurring of normal detail, ground-glass opacities, and linear streaks or star artifacts from the edges of vessels and other high-density structures (Fig. 6.2). Motion of linear structures, such as fissures, vessels, and bronchial walls, may result in artifactual parallel opacities which are also called double images or ghosting. On lung window setting respiratory motion artifacts are normally easily recognized. Respiratory motion artifacts not identified on a single scan are easily appreciated by stack mode viewing, where they are even more obvious. The cyclic appearance of the artifacts is characteristic for respiratory motion (Fig. 6.2). Since gross motion artifact is usually easily recognized, it degrades image quality, but it will not interfere with image interpretation. Subtle motion-related ground-glass opacities may mimic an infiltrative process, and doubling of vascular structures can mimic thickened interlobular septa or the walls of a dilated bronchus. If they are not recognized as respiratory motion artifacts, they will represent a false-positive finding of interstitial lung disease or bronchiectasis. In general, there are fewer respiratory motion artifacts at MDCT than at HRCT. The single, short breath-hold period at MDCT is normally better tolerated than the multiple consecutive breath holds at HRCT. If cluster scanning is used for HRCT, progressive respiratory motion artifacts are sometimes observed from one image to the next within a cluster of acquisitions (Engeler 1994). A single breath hold also provides a constant respiratory depth throughout the lung, whereas HRCT can be impaired by different depths of inspiration from one scan or cluster to another.

a 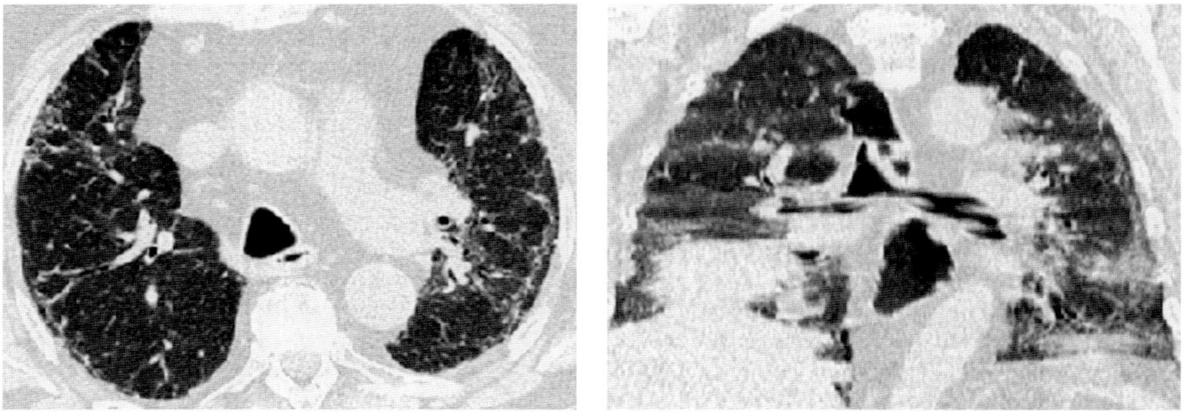 b

Fig. 6.2a, b. A 61-year-old woman with collagen vascular disease and fibrosis. **a** 1-mm thin slice shows a reticular pattern with predominance in the peripheral and subpleural lung zones. This slice was reconstructed for a given time when the patient held her breath in inspiratory position. **b** Coronal MPR shows severe cyclic artifacts caused by breathing. They are more pronounced in the lower and middle lung zones. The assessment of the extent of fibrosis is markedly impaired.

6.3.8 Inspiratory and Expiratory Scans

Scans are routinely obtained at full inspiratory position with the lungs fully expanded; thus, the contrast between low-attenuation aerated air space and high-attenuation lung structure is maximized. At the same time, full inspiration minimizes the frequency of confounding densities due to subsegmental and mostly gravity-dependent atelectasis. Sometimes a geographic pattern of heterogeneous lung attenuation is appreciated on scans obtained at full inspiratory position. This pattern fulfills the definition of ground-glass opacities (see below); however, it has a distinctive distribution pattern. It is usually caused by regional variations of pulmonary perfusion, and that is why it is called mosaic perfusion. It can reflect primary vascular disease, such as in chronic thromboembolic pulmonary hypertension, or hypoxic vasoconstriction secondary to primary airway disease, such as in bronchiectasis (Fig. 6.3). In primary vascular disease the density pattern is almost identical on scans obtained at full expiratory position. On the contrary, the pattern is very much accentuated at expiration in primary airway disease having led to fixed hypoxic vasoconstriction. Scans at full expiratory position, however, should also be obtained in a wide variety of different diffuse lung diseases in order to detect air trapping and make the diagnosis of bronchiolitis (Fig. 6.4; Kauczor et al. 2000). The visual assessment of severity and extent of air trapping, which is much more common on expiratory scans (Ng et al. 1999), can be complicated. A fine visual grading system has shown unacceptable observer variation, whereas a coarse grading system provides much more reliable results (Ng et al. 1999). Visual assessment of scans from an unselected patient population alone, however, does not allow for confident estimation of functional compromise due to obstructive lung disease (Kauczor et al. 2000). In

a

b

c

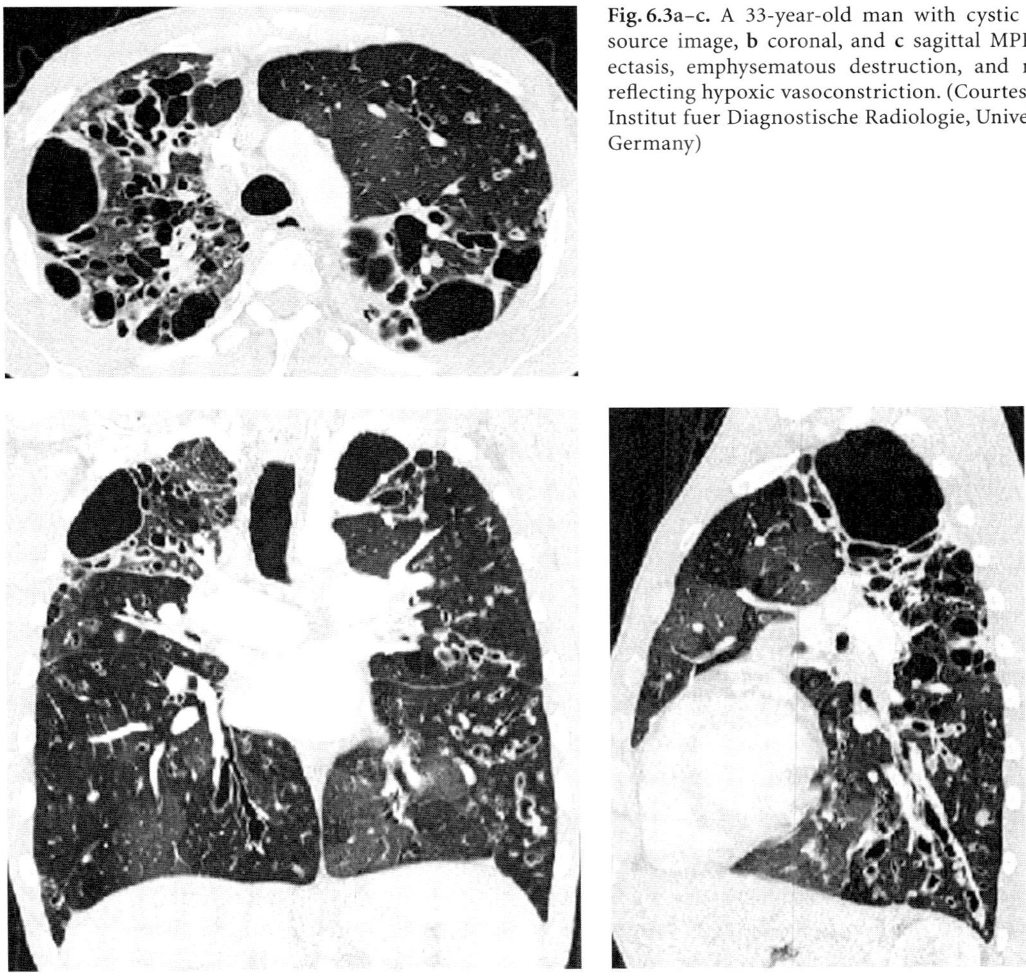

Fig. 6.3a–c. A 33-year-old man with cystic fibrosis. **a** Axial source image, **b** coronal, and **c** sagittal MPR show bronchiectasis, emphysematous destruction, and mosaic oligemia reflecting hypoxic vasoconstriction. (Courtesy of A. Noemayr, Institut fuer Diagnostische Radiologie, Universitaet Erlangen, Germany)

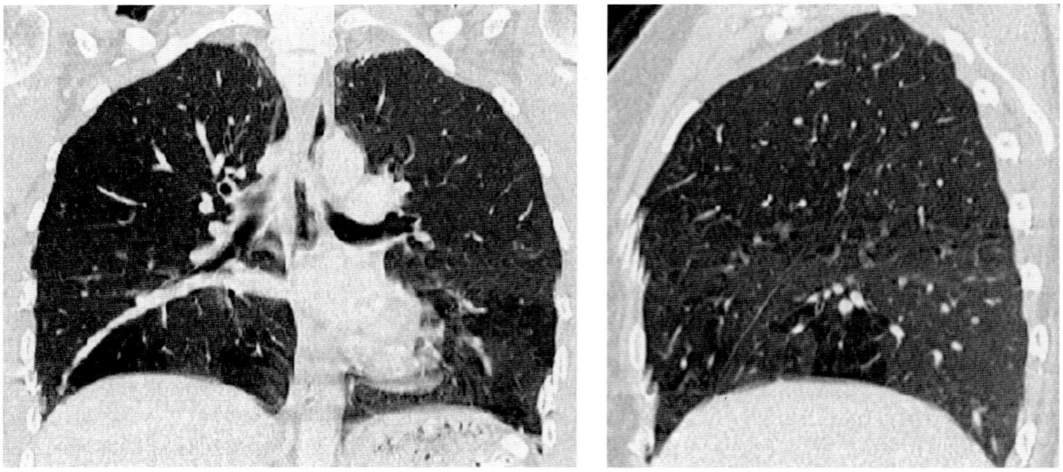

Fig. 6.4a, b. A 32-year-old woman with bronchiolitis obliterans after chemotherapy for non-Hodgkin's lymphoma. **a** Coronal MPR in expiration shows areas of focal air trapping in both lower lobes. **b** Sagittal MPR in expiration delineates an area of focal air trapping in the right lower lobe. (Courtesy of A. Noemayr, Institut fuer Diagnostische Radiologie, Universitaet Erlangen, Germany)

well-characterized patients, such as in bronchiectasis, the extent of air trapping on expiratory CT scans correlated with the severity of air-flow obstruction measured by FEV1 (r=0.55; Roberts et al. 2000).

6.3.9 Cardiac Pulsation Artifacts and Cardiac Gating

Cardiac pulsation artifacts typically affect the paracardiac regions of the lingula and the right middle lobe (Figs. 6.4, 6.5). Aortic pulsation most likely affects lung areas adjacent to the aortic arch or the descending thoracic aorta being segments 6 and 10 of the left lower lobe. These pulsation artifacts can be misleading and cause positive findings. Cardiac gating is especially helpful for the visualization of the lobes adjacent to the heart, in particular the left ventricle, as well as the thoracic aorta during its whole course. Image quality can be significantly improved in the affected areas, especially the lingula, when ECG triggering is used (Schoepf et al. 1999). Prospective ECG triggering leads to a significant prolongation of measurement time, which interferes with the breath-hold capabilities of many patients (Becker et al. 2000); thus, retrospective cardiac gating should be regarded as the method of choice to get rid of disturbing pulsation artifacts in the lingula, if present; both will also reduce the amount of pulsation artifacts within the ascending aorta mimicking a plane of dissection and within the lung regions adjacent to the thoracic aorta. Besides ECG triggering, another factor which reduces the number of artifacts significantly is the faster rotation time which can be used on MDCT scanner. It is 0.5 s instead of 1 s on older spiral CT scanners or as an option on MDCT scanners (Montaudon et al. 2001). Rotation time also has a significant positive effect on reduction of cardiac pulsation artifacts, which might even be more important than ECG triggering.

6.3.10 Window Setting

There is no single ideal window setting for evaluating the lung parenchyma. Window settings have to be optimized with regard to the settings of scanners, monitors, and laser imagers. For the assessment of parenchymal disease a relatively wide window width (1400–1800 HU) together with a high window level (–700 to –500 HU) is recommended. Wider window settings are generally better for the evaluation of high-contrast interfaces, especially pleural interfaces; thus, wide windows are especially advised for the assessment of asbestosis. Narrower window settings are better suited for the detection of emphysema or air trapping, since they allow for detection of subtle attenuation differences. The use of individual modifications for particular tasks is strongly encouraged. They should be performed on the monitor to emphasize subtle attenuation differences, such as those seen in lungs with emphysema or air trapping, as well as pleural pathologies such as in asbestosis.

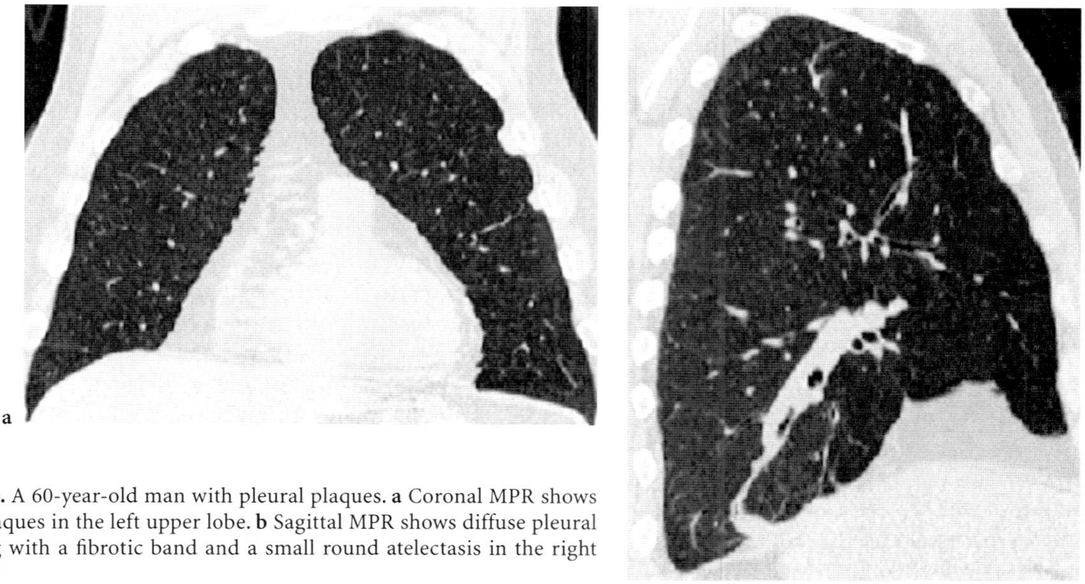

Fig. 6.5a, b. A 60-year-old man with pleural plaques. **a** Coronal MPR shows pleural plaques in the left upper lobe. **b** Sagittal MPR shows diffuse pleural thickening with a fibrotic band and a small round atelectasis in the right lower lobe

The window setting has a substantial effect on the accuracy of size measurements. This is particularly important for the assessment of bronchial lumen diameter and bronchial wall thickness. It has been demonstrated that an intermediate window width between –1000 and –1400 HU together with a window level between –250 and –700 HU best reflects the real size of the bronchi and especially the thickness of the bronchial wall (Bankier et al. 1996). Although studied with HRCT, these results are also valid for MDCT; thus, it is not unlikely that different window settings have to be used for the identification of pathological changes of the parenchyma or the pleura and the for the measurement of bronchial diameter and wall thickness. In the future, dedicated software will allow to measure the cross-sectional area of the bronchial lumen and the wall thickness automatically with a high degree of accuracy (Beigelman-Aubry et al. 2002). Under these circumstances the window setting on the screen does not affect the measurements anymore.

6.4 CT Patterns in Diffuse Lung Disease

6.4.1 Introduction

Many acute and chronic lung diseases are characterized by diffuse infiltrations of the lung parenchyma. The differential diagnosis is based on patterns and distribution of findings. Diffuse lung diseases can be divided into diseases with decreased and increased lung attenuation. Diseases with decreased attenuation comprise the emphysemas and all the different varieties of a cystic pattern, so-called holes in the lung. The patterns of diffuse lung diseases with increased density are multiple. They include septal, reticular, and nodular patterns as well as ground-glass opacities and consolidations.

A pattern or sign in CT refers to a radiological finding or a combination of findings which suggest the diagnosis of a specific disease process. Identification of a CT sign or pattern requires the understanding of the meaning of it. For communication with clinicians it is important to use a cohesive terminology of signs and patterns describing the findings so that they will know how a certain differential diagnosis has come up and what the confidence level of this diagnosis is. Quite a number of interstitial lung diseases are associated with characteristic signs and patterns on CT scanning. They will substantially support a certain specific diagnosis, such as Langerhans cell histiocytosis, lymphangioleiomyomatosis, or end-stage lung disease as a sequel of usual interstitial pneumonia (UIP). In these cases, a reticular and cystic pattern with predominance in the costophrenic angles is present. The signs of fibrosing alveolitis are observed additionally. A number of combinations of findings as mentioned below allow formulation of quite specific differential diagnoses.

The different patterns of lung disease have all been described on the basis of HRCT. This knowledge has now to be transferred to high-resolution MDCT.

Obviously, the different CT patterns are still valid, but MDCT now offers the third dimension by providing a volumetric data set. Instead of looking at single two-dimensional HRCT slices, we have to get used to perceiving them in a three-dimensional volume. Once accomplished detection of the different patterns will be easier than in the past. At the same time it will also be easier to recognize the predominant distribution pattern, which is another important hint in differential diagnosis.

6.4.2 Normal Anatomy

To describe the localization of parenchymal abnormalities, well-known anatomic terms, such as lobes and segments, are used in volumetric HRCT. They are easily identified while using CT because the normal interlobar fissures are seen as smooth, linear opacities measuring less than 1 mm in thickness. The mere categorization in lung fields or levels is very easy to handle but is very difficult to be transferred for further invasive diagnostic or therapeutic procedures, such as bronchoscopy; therefore, the accurate localization of abnormal findings to certain segments is essential to guide bronchoscopy, video-assisted thoracoscopy, or open surgery. Regarding pulmonary physiology the categorization of the pulmonary core (medulla) and rind (cortex) is also useful.

The smallest anatomic unit of the pulmonary parenchyma visible at CT is the secondary lobule which is associated with a secondary bronchiole and is enclosed by connective tissue septa. Secondary lobules consist of 3–24 acini which are distal to the terminal bronchioles depending on location. The terminal bronchioles are the last generation of purely air-conducting, non-gas-exchanging airways. The distal acinus is the largest unit entirely involved in gas exchange. In general, the secondary lobules measure between 1 and 2.5 cm in diameter. They are bigger and rectangular in the periphery, whereas they are smaller and hexa- or polygonal in the center. The regular structure of the secondary lobule shows a central axial compartment with the centrilobular structures. They consist of a pulmonary artery branch, the secondary bronchiole, lymphatics, and some connective tissue. It is important to note that under normal conditions only the pulmonary artery branch is visible on the CT scan. Together they form the "bronchovascular bundle." More distally in the parenchymal compartment terminal and respiratory bronchioles, acini, alveolar ducts, and alveoli are present; however, since all of them are very small, they cannot be visualized by CT under normal conditions. Interlobular and perilobular septa represent the outer margin of the secondary lobule. They contain lung veins and lymphatics. The identification of the structures of the secondary lobule and their appearance when they are affected by disease is important. The knowledge of particular patterns of spread of disease is of great support for the differential diagnosis of pathological abnormalities. The patterns are mainly related to a leading finding, such as an increase or decrease in lung attenuation together with a certain shape, e.g., nodular, or size, e.g., less than 1 cm in diameter, and localization, such as in the central axial compartment. They mostly involve a substantial lung area with some kind of regional predominance which will be much easier depicted on volumetric high-resolution CT.

6.4.3 Septal Pattern

The normal interlobular septa marginate parts of the secondary lobule. Also, as mentioned previously, they contain venous and lymphatic structures. They measure approximately 0.1 mm in thickness, and are only occasionally or partially seen on CT scans under normal conditions. Thickening of interlobular septa will make these septa a striking finding. A regular network becomes apparent, and the centrilobular artery is easily identified as a small dot in the center of a hexa- or polygon. Thickening of the interlobular septa may be caused by interstitial fluid, such as in pulmonary congestion, by cellular infiltration, such as in lymphangitic carcinomatosis, or by tissue, such as in fibrosis or storage diseases (Stein et al. 1987; Munk et al. 1988; Meziane et al. 1988). Septa are most prominent in the lung periphery where they can be seen as 1- to 2-cm-long lines. They course perpendicularly to the pleural surface which they usually reach. Although the margins of the secondary lobules are outlined in part or completely, the normal architecture of the lung parenchyma is not distorted. The thickening of the interlobular septa can be smooth, nodular, or irregular (Kang et al. 1996). Clearly marginated regular thickened septa are a non-specific finding. It is apparent in all processes which have a component of pulmonary edema or hemorrhage; thus, smooth thickening of the septa is associated with a predominant perilobular distribution since veins and lymphatics are equally affected. The septal pattern with its perilobular distribution will also be associated with ground-glass opacity which can also be caused by fluid overload and congestion (see below). The septal pattern can develop very quickly in acute pulmonary congestion, but it may also resolve very fast. Nodular or beaded thickening of the septa is a typical finding in lymphangitic spread of carcinoma or lymphoma (Munk et al. 1988). Less frequent differential diagnoses of nodular thickening of the septa are sarcoidosis, silicosis (Fig. 6.1), lymphocytic interstitial pneumonia, amyloidosis, and Kaposi sarcoma. All of these go along with focal clusters of immunocompetent cells, such as lymphocytes or macrophages, or focal deposition of inflammatory or proteinaceous material, such as granulomas or amyloid. Since the pathological process takes place within the lymphatic pathways not only the perilobular septa are affected. There is additional disease in the lymphatics which course in the central compartment of the secondary lobule; thus, nodular thickening will also be present along the bronchovascular bundles, which is an especially typical finding in sarcoidosis. The distribution is also referred to as perilymphatic pattern. Irregular thickening of the septa is seen in interstitial fibrosis (Nishimura et al. 1992). There is a predominance of the subpleural and basal lung zones. The septal pattern can be a precursor of architectural distortion and formation of a reticular pattern (see below). The distribution of reticulation and associated findings often enables refinement of the differential diagnosis.

6.4.4 Reticular Pattern

A reticular pattern consists of linear shadows which do not respect the normal architecture of the lung parenchyma. They are referred to as trans- or intralobular lines or septa. They result in irregular linear opacities which appear as an irregular mesh or network (Figs. 6.2, 6.6, 6.7). The lines exhibit irregular margins and lead to distortions of secondary lobules and bronchi. They result in traction bronchiectasis and bronchiolectasis as well as displacement of fissures. The reticular pattern with sharply marginated translobular septa is typical for fibrosing alveolitis, pulmonary manifestations in connective tissue disease, or asbestosis. The reticular pattern is frequently associated with a septal pattern (see above). Together they represent the typical fibrotic appearance with parenchymal destruction in end-stage lung disease. These changes mostly have a peripheral and caudal predominance. In advanced disease, reticular patterns are also associated with a cystic pattern, in particular the formation of honeycomb cysts (see below).

The reticular pattern is associated with a heterogeneous group of interstitial lung diseases. These include idiopathic pneumonias [usual interstitial pneumonia (UIP), desquamative interstitial pneumonia (DIP), acute interstitial pneumonia (AIP) and non-specific interstitial pneumonia (NSIP)], idiopathic pulmonary fibrosis (IPF), collagen vascular disease, drug-induced lung disease, radiation pneumonitis, and asbestosis. The idiopathic interstitial pneumonias have no well-defined cause.

The UIP is the most common type. It has a typical subpleural and lower lung zone predominance (Figs. 6.2, 6.6). It is characterized histologically by a patchy heterogeneous pattern with foci of normal lung, interstitial inflammation, fibroblastic proliferation, interstitial fibrosis, and honeycombing. In early disease, CT will show ground-glass opacification (see below). It represents active alveolitis which will progress to overt fibrosis; thus, in general, the reticular pattern is the leading feature of UIP. It is frequently associated with the development of traction bronchiectasis and honeycombing. Ground-glass opacity and consolidation are also seen but are not dominant features. The accuracy of a confident diagnosis of UIP made on CT by a trained observer is consistently 90% or higher (Lynch et al. 1995; Mathieson et al. 1989). Temporal heterogeneity is an important histological feature. It allows to distinguish UIP from DIP. The UIP can result from dust exposure, drugs radiation, or collagen vascular disease (Fig. 6.2). If no cause is found, it is classified as an idiopathic interstitial pneumonia and considered synonymous with IPF (Fig. 6.6). Patients with IPF have a substantially increased risk of lung cancer, estimated to be between 10 and 17% (Lee et al. 1996). Fibrosis-related lung cancer is more often located peripherally in the lower lobes. Volumetric high-resolution MDCT with coverage of the entire lung has a significant advantage over simple HRCT for the detection or follow-up of nodules in IPF.

The presence of a predominantly ground-glass opacity pattern should suggest the possibility of an alternative diagnosis, such as desquamative interstitial pneumonia (DIP), acute interstitial pneumonia (AIP) or non-specific interstitial pneumonitis (NSIP).

Desquamative interstitial pneumonia (DIP) is characterized histologically by a relatively uniform pattern of macrophages within the alveoli. Most patients are smokers, and it is likely that DIP represents a reaction to cigarette smoke. The features are similar to those encountered in respiratory bronchiolitis interstitial lung disease (RBILD), although the distribution is dif-

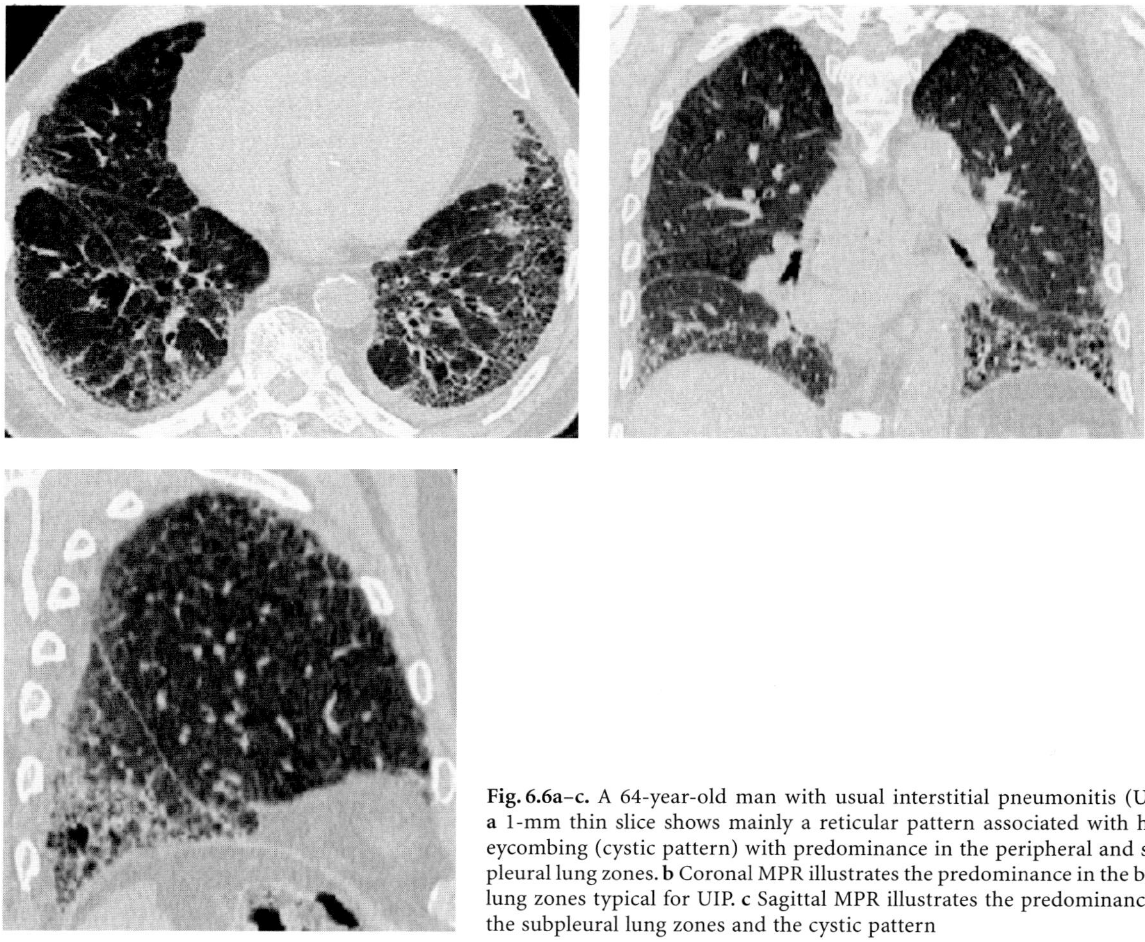

a b c

Fig. 6.6a–c. A 64-year-old man with usual interstitial pneumonitis (UIP). **a** 1-mm thin slice shows mainly a reticular pattern associated with honeycombing (cystic pattern) with predominance in the peripheral and subpleural lung zones. **b** Coronal MPR illustrates the predominance in the basal lung zones typical for UIP. **c** Sagittal MPR illustrates the predominance in the subpleural lung zones and the cystic pattern

fuse in DIP and bronchiolocentric in RBILD. The typical CT feature of DIP is diffuse ground-glass opacity, and reticulation is uncommon.

Acute interstitial pneumonia (AIP) is characterized histologically by hyaline membranes within the alveoli and diffuse, active interstitial fibrosis. Patients with AIP often present with respiratory failure developing over days or weeks. No etiologic agent is identified. Typical CT features are ground-glass opacity and consolidation with a geographic distribution. In later stages honeycombing and reticulation develop.

Nonspecific interstitial pneumonia (NSIP) is characterized histologically by interstitial inflammation and fibrosis without any specific features indicative for UIP, DIP, or AIP. It is a diagnosis of exclusion. The typical CT feature is ground-glass opacity, and although reticulation and consolidation are common, honeycombing is uncommon (Kim et al. 1998). The ground-glass opacity is usually bilateral and symmetric, and less commonly it is peribronchovascular. It has a peripheral and basal predominance.

The subpleural and lower zone predominance of the reticular pattern known from UIP also occurs in asbestosis. Common findings in asbestosis are subpleural curvilinear lines which run parallel to the pleural surface and parenchymal bands which are several millimeters thick and 2–5 cm long with contact to the pleura. Although subpleural curvilinear lines are not pathognomonic for pulmonary asbestosis, it is important to check for any potential exposure to asbestos in the past. Sometimes these subpleural curvilinear lines are caused by posture and gravity effects. In such cases, additional prone scanning is helpful to confirm the presence of these lines as fixed fibrotic changes instead of mere sign of hypoventilation in the dependent lung region. Pulmonary asbestosis is frequently associated with pleural plaques and diffuse pleural thickening. Their presence will be just another important indicator of check for any potential exposure to asbestos in the past.

In sarcoidosis, fibrosis occurs in the late stages of the disease. It typically affects the central lung regions in the middle and upper lung zone. It can be observed as nodular thickening of the bronchi and pulmonary vessels, interlobular septa, and interlobar fissure. This results in central clustering of ectatic and distorted bronchi, called traction bronchiectasis. Associated nodular disease with a perilymphatic distribution pattern reflecting multiple granulomas is common and allows to diagnose sarcoidosis as the underlying disease causing lung fibrosis.

In hypersensitivity pneumonitis reticulation and honeycombing representing fibrosis is seen predominantly in the mid- and lower lung regions. The relative sparing of the posterior costophrenic recesses and the presence of centrilobular nodules allows its distinction from UIP in most cases (Fig. 6.7).

6.4.5 Nodular Pattern

Nodular opacities or pulmonary nodules are spherical or ovoid. They are categorized according to size, attenuation, margination, and localization. The association between these findings and dignity of a particular etiology is limited. A general categorization of size in micronodules (<5 mm), nodules (5–20 mm), and masses (>20 mm) is helpful. Measurements of attenuation are problematic. Values higher than 150 HU are typical for calcifications and indicate benign, postinflammatory granuloma (Siegelman et al. 1986). Faint and nodular increases of density with a centrilobular localization are also regarded as a nodular pattern and not as ground-glass opacities (see below). Ill-defined peribronchial nodules measuring less than 10 mm are highly specific for acute bronchial infections. A surrounding area with a small increase in density is called "halo." By definition, it represents an area of ground-glass opacity, although it is just the interface between the nodule and the normal lung parenchyma. The halo sign is said to indicate acute inflammation or hemorrhage.

According to localization five distribution categories of nodules should be differentiated.

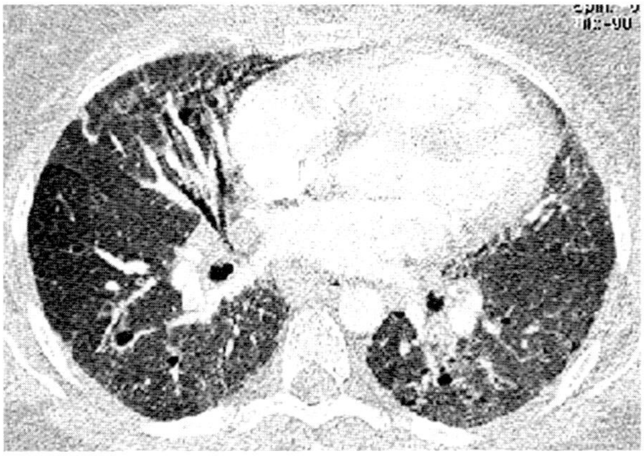
a

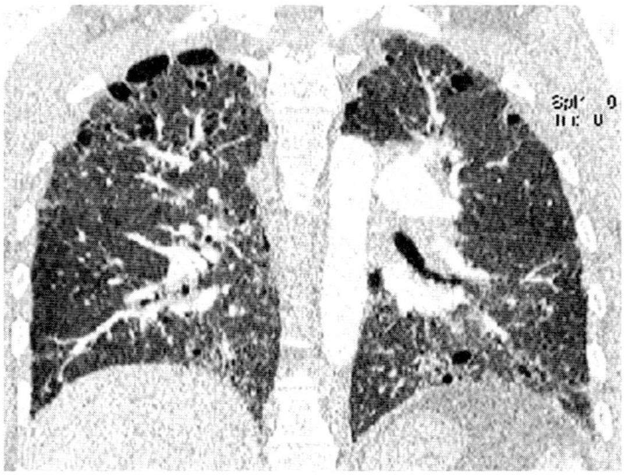
b

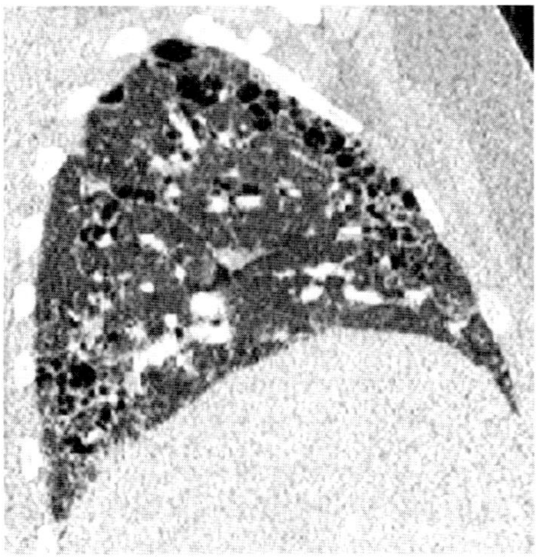
c

Fig. 6.7a–c. A 41-year-old woman with hypersensitivity pneumonitis. **a** Axial source image, **b** coronal, and **c** sagittal MPR show mainly a cystic pattern (honeycombing) associated with a reticular pattern and traction bronchiectasis. There is no obvious predominance of the findings in the upper, mid, or lower lung zones, which together with the relative sparing of the posterior costophrenic recesses allows for distinction of hypersensitivity pneumonitis from usual interstitial pneumonia (UIP). (Courtesy of A. Noemayr, Institut fuer Diagnostische Radiologie, Universitaet Erlangen, Germany)

Peribronchovascular Distribution. These nodules originate from the wall of a bronchus or pulmonary artery. They are well defined and often have a beaded appearance. They measure less than 5 mm. Computed tomography is not capable of differentiating nodules which originate from the bronchus from those originating from the pulmonary artery wall. Typically, these nodules are granulomas, e.g., as they may be encountered in vasculitis (Seo et al. 2000).

Centrilobular Distribution. These nodules are also referred to as parenchymal nodules. They originate from the terminal and respiratory bronchioles, which are normally invisible. They can also originate from the peripheral pulmonary artery branches. They have a distance of 3–10 mm from interlobular septa, fissure, or pleura. Enlargement of centrilobular structures, and lack of definition or the depiction of dilated, branching bronchioles are features of centrilobular nodules. They often present as focal, ill-defined, centrilobular ground-glass opacities. They indicate alveolitis, bronchiolitis, or even small foci of bronchopneumonia as they occur in acute exacerbations of chronic obstructive lung disease. In silicosis, nodules frequently have a centrilobular or subpleural distribution pattern with a predominance in the posterior aspect of the upper lobe. Typically, they are smoothly marginated. The nodules range between 2 and 5 mm in diameter, and can be calcified. Concomitant nodular thickening of the interlobular septa is uncommon.

Perilobular Distribution. Perilobular nodules are localized along the interlobular septa and the pleura surfaces. They are infrequently encountered as a single distribution pattern for nodules.

Perilymphatic Distribution. Much more frequent is a perilymphatic distribution pattern of nodules. It relates to the presence of nodules along the different lymphatic pathways within the lung, such as along the bronchovascular bundles, the interlobar fissures, the interlobular septa, and the subpleural regions. It is a typical distribution pattern for granuloma in sarcoidosis. Here the nodules measure less than 5 mm and have irregular margins. They have a predominance for the perihilar regions and the upper lobes which is particularly well depicted on coronal reformations. Confluence of granuloma may result in large nodules, ground-glass opacities, or consolidation (Nishimura et al. 1993). The nodular pattern in lymphangitic carcinomatosis can also show a perilymphatic distribution; however, for reasons unknown, lymphangitic carcinomatosis has a predominance for the perilobular distribution pattern.

A nodular pattern with a random distribution with respect to the leading structures of the secondary lobule is indicative for a disease process with hematogenous spread as it occurs in malignant disease and hematogenous metastases, miliary tuberculosis, miliary histoplasmosis, cytomegaly, or herpes virus infections.

6.4.6 Cystic Pattern

A cystic pattern results from a heterogeneous group of diseases, all having in common the presence of focal, multifocal, or diffuse parenchymal lucencies and lung destruction. The cystic pattern is also referred to as "holes in the lung." Some "holes" are part of well-known and frequent diseases such as bullae in emphysema, centrilobular lucencies, honeycombing in fibrosis, and end-stage lung disease or cavitations in inflammatory disease. Other "holes" present with specific cystic patterns such as in Langerhans cell histiocytosis, lymphangioleiomyomatosis, sarcoidosis, lymphocytic interstitial pneumonitis, or *Pneumocystis carinii* pneumonia.

6.4.6.1 Cysts

The term "cyst" itself is non-specific and refers to a thin-walled (usually less than 3 mm thick), well-defined and circumscribed air- or fluid-filled lesion. Only air-filled cysts appear as a cystic pattern on a CT scan and are discussed here. Cysts with a liquid, semi-solid, or solid contents appear as a nodule. The nature of the contents can sometimes be differentiated by the use of CT. Air-filled cysts typically measure 1 cm or more in diameter and have a fibrous or epithelial wall (Klein et al. 1992). The presence of a definable wall demonstrated at CT differentiates cysts from emphysema. Cysts are usually multiple, have different sizes, and are sharply marginated with respect to the surrounding parenchyma. Intrapulmonary air-filled cysts can occur spontaneously without being associated with any other disease. Besides the cyst itself there is no architectural distortion. Cysts can also be the leading pattern of specific lung diseases, such as Langerhans cell histiocytosis and lymphangioleiomyomatosis, where they result in destruction of the normal lung parenchyma.

6.4.6.2
Langerhans Cell Histiocytosis and Lymphangioleiomyomatosis

In case of Langerhans cell histiocytosis, the cysts have a mid and upper lung zone predominance with sparing of the lung bases (Brauner et al. 1997; Kazerooni 2001) which is better depicted on coronal reformations than on cross-sectional images. In the early phase, Langerhans cell histiocytosis have a typical nodular pattern with multiple, <10-mm small centrilobular nodules with irregular margins. Later these nodules increase in size and have a tendency to cavitate and to develop into cystic lesions with a diameter of up to 2 cm. The cysts are usually thin walled, often confluent, and have bizarre or lobulated shapes. Since the thin walls of the cysts are prone to rupture, there is an increased risk of pneumothoraces. Concomitant nodules are usually irregular, measure 1–5 mm, and often have a centrilobular distribution. The interspersed pulmonary parenchyma is typically normal, without evidence of fibrosis or septal thickening.

In lymphangioleiomyomatosis, the cysts are distributed diffusely throughout the lung (Akkermann and Eberhardt 1992; Haubold-Reuter et al. 1995). They are thin walled, round, and measure 0.2–5 cm. Their wall is thin, ranging from and barely seen to 4 mm in thickness (Lenoir et al. 1990). Since the thin walls of the cysts are prone to rupture there is an increased risk of pneumothoraces. The surrounding parenchyma is typically normal. Nodules are uncommon. Sometimes it may be difficult to distinguish lymphangioleiomyomatosis and Langerhans cell histiocytosis from emphysema. There is a helpful finding as the cystic spaces in lymphangioleiomyomatosis and Langerhans cell histiocytosis do not have any central nodular opacities, whereas the cystic spaces seen with centrilobular emphysema contain a small central nodular opacity representing the centrilobular artery.

6.4.6.3
Honeycomb Cysts

Honeycomb cysts constitute the irreversible final stage of parenchymal destruction in lung fibrosis (end-stage lung), mainly due to UIP, collagen vascular disease, asbestosis, hypersensitivity pneumonitis, or drug-related fibrosis (Figs. 6.2, 6.6, 6.7). They usually are round or ovoid and measure between 0.3 and 1 cm in diameter, although they can range from several millimeters to several centimeters in size. In an individual, however, they are uniform. They have clearly definable walls which are 1–3 mm thick (Webb et al. 1988). The walls consist of fibrous tissue with or without signs of chronic inflammation. In general, they are lined by bronchiolar epithelium. Honeycomb cysts seem to develop from massively dilated terminal and respiratory bronchioles. Honeycombing is associated with other findings of lung fibrosis such as septal and reticular pattern, architectural distortion, and traction bronchiectasis. The combination of honeycomb cysts and a large-mashed reticular pattern presents as a joint honeycomb pattern. It consists of multiple irregular cystic spaces (honeycombs) which are separated from each other by irregular thick walls and the intralobular septa and lines. Even CT is not capable of separating the walls of the honeycomb cysts from the thickened intralobular fibrous bands. According to the predominance of the underlying disease, honeycombing is typically subpleural and worse at the lung base or apices. Honeycomb cysts occur in botryoidal groups. Their distribution within the lung reaches from a single location to an almost complete involvement of both lungs. Frequently, there is a patchy distribution. The differential diagnosis of honeycomb cysts is important, but not extensive. Due to superimposition of multiple localized changes of lung attenuation, it is sometimes difficult to decide whether the increase or decrease in lung attenuation represents the real lesion; thus, the differentiation between a honeycomb pattern in fibrosis and multiple nodules in an interstitial granulomatous disease might be difficult. In contrast, the differentiation between honeycomb cysts and different air-filled cysts is easy. Size, wall thickness, as well as the variability between the individual cysts together with the surrounding structures are valuable hints; thus, honeycomb cysts are usually readily differentiated from the cysts seen in Langerhans cell histiocytosis and lymphangioleiomyomatosis.

6.4.6.4
Bullae

Bullae can be solitary or multiple. They are usually associated with any type of emphysema. They are supposed to take their origin from confluent emphysematous secondary lobules and result in architectural distortion and destruction (Fig. 6.3); thus, bullae are substantially larger than normal secondary lobules and measure more than 1 cm in diameter. They only partially participate in ventilation. The wall surrounding bullae is usually very thin (less than 1 mm) (Klein et al. 1992). This thin wall is even difficult to depict at CT. The bulla is detected because of their low attenuation in comparison with the surrounding lung parenchyma (Schurawitzki 1992). Since the wall is so thin, there is a substantial risk for the development of a pneumothorax.

6.4.6.5
Cavities

Cavities are mostly caused by necrotic inflammatory processes with cavitation such as in tuberculosis or aspergillosis. Alternatively, they can be caused by necrotic tumors. Cavities usually present with clearly visible walls which are thicker than 3 mm. These walls typically have irregular outer and inner margins. Cavities per se do not cause widespread destruction of the parenchyma. Cavities regularly have a connection of the bronchial tree which can be demonstrated with the use of MDCT. Cavities frequently contain some fluid or debris, which can be caused by mucus hypersecretion, cavitating tumors, hemorrhage, hydatid disease, and mycetoma. Mycetomas are a sequel of the bronchogenic secondary colonization of the cavity with micro-organisms, especially *Aspergillus* species. The contents of the cavity creates a visible air-fluid level or a so-called air-crescent sign. Air–fluid levels are gravity dependent. Additional prone scanning proves the air–fluid level and the amount of fluid. It also demonstrates the exact localization of the fluid collection, whether it is intrapulmonary or intrapleural. The air crescent separates the round or irregular contents of the cavity from the inner wall (Austin et al. 1996). The air-crescent sign is typical for cavitating inflammations, which gain contact with the bronchial tree. It frequently occurs at an intermediate stage of an *Aspergillus* infection (Blum et al. 1994). In mycetoma, the air crescent delineates a fungus ball. Again, prone scanning demonstrates rolling of the fungus ball and prove the diagnosis.

6.4.7
Consolidation

Consolidation of lung is caused by the complete replacement of alveolar air by fluid, cells, tissue, or other substances thus leading to an extensive, homogeneous increase in lung attenuation. Consolidations are frequently related to hemorrhage, infections, or inflammations (Fig. 6.8). The finding is non-specific and should not be applied for differential diagnosis. The underlying vascular structures are obscured by definition (Remy-Jardin et al. 1993a). Positive air bronchograms are observed frequently (Fig. 6.8). Consolidations are focal processes in most cases, and the normal pulmonary parenchyma itself is not affected. Larger consolidations are frequently symptomatic and lead to lung function impairment because there is no gas exchange within the consolidated area (Aberle 1993; Kohno et al. 1993).

In the setting of chronic diffuse infiltrative lung disease, consolidation is seen in chronic eosinophilic pneumonia (CEP), bronchiolitis obliterans organizing pneumonia (BOOP) or cryptogenic organizing pneumonia (COP), bronchioloalveolar carcinoma, lipoid pneumonia, sarcoidosis, and lymphoma. Acute consolidations are commonly caused by pulmonary edema, hemorrhage, extrinsic allergic alveolitis, radiation pneumonitis, infarction, or infectious pneumonia. Alveolar proteinosis can also present as acute or recurrent pulmonary consolidation.

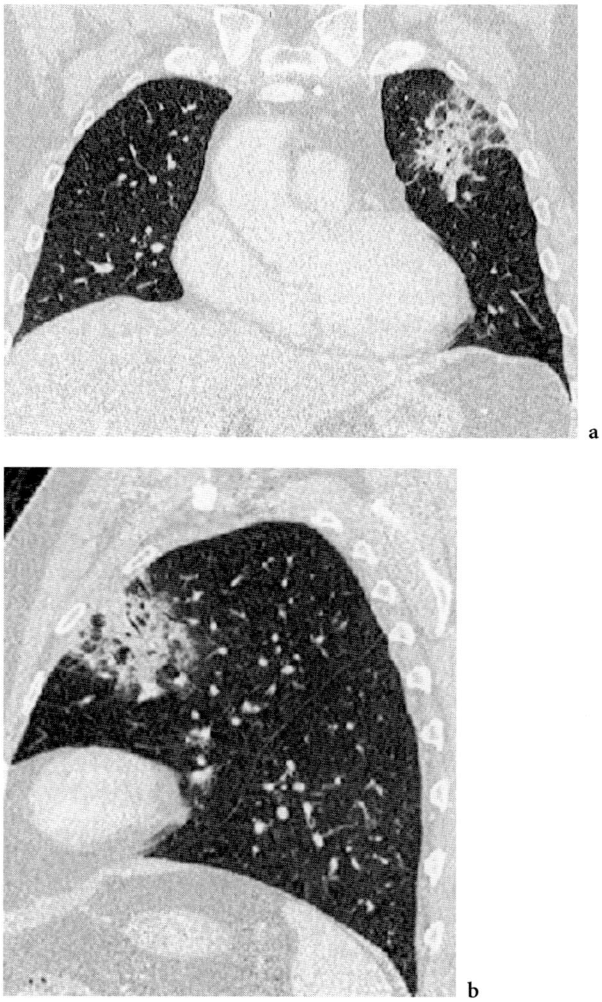

Fig. 6.8a, b. A 53-year-old man with pneumonia (tuberculosis) in the left upper lobe. **a** Coronal MPR shows ground-glass opacification and consolidation. **b** Sagittal MPR shows positive bronchograms within the consolidation. (Courtesy of A. Noemayr, Institut fuer Diagnostische Radiologie, Universitaet Erlangen, Germany)

Chronic eosinophilic pneumonia (CEP) and bronchiolitis obliterans organizing pneumonia (BOOP) or cryptogenic organizing pneumonia (COP), typically result in subpleural consolidations. The BOOP/COP is characterized by the presence of unilateral or more commonly bilateral areas of consolidation. They often have a predominant subpleural or peribronchial distribution. Poorly defined centrilobular or peribronchial nodules or masses may also be present. The patterns of BOOP/COP and CEP are frequently indistinguishable; however, although CEP usually has an upper lobe predominance, BOOP/COP typically involves predominantly the middle and lower lung zones. Patients with CEP and BOOP/COP can rapidly respond to steroid therapy. In the resolution phase linear opacities may be seen paralleling the pleural surface.

Sarcoidosis can also manifest as peripheral areas of consolidation on CT, although this is not the most common appearance of the disease. Alveolar proteinosis typically manifests as patchy or diffuse consolidation and ground-glass opacity with geographic margins and septal thickening. Unilateral or bilateral patchy airspace consolidation may also be a presenting feature of bronchioloalveolar carcinoma. It must be considered when consolidations progress over several months or are associated with lung nodules.

Consolidations which are caused by aerogenic infections show a typical relationship to the bronchus involved. Their extension then surrounds a bronchus; less frequently, when localized in the lung periphery, the consolidations in aerogenic infections are wedge shaped. In parallel, consolidations with hematogenous causes, such as infarction, have a spatial relationship to a pulmonary artery branch; thus, infarctions are characterized by one or more wedge-shaped areas of consolidation along the pleural surface. Multiple or extensive pulmonary infarcts can easily mimic other peripheral lung diseases. Consolidations with a relationship to a pulmonary artery branch are also called "infarct-like lesions," and diseases with infiltration of the pulmonary artery, such as invasive pulmonary aspergillosis, will have an unambiguous spatial relationship between a pulmonary artery branch and the concomitant wedge-shaped consolidation; thus, the infarct-type distribution pattern is also called angiotropic.

Consolidations often present with large caliber vessels which are easily seen after the administration of a contrast agent. The obvious contrast between the vessel and the consolidation has been named "CT angiogram sign." The pulmonary artery branch is a strongly enhancing, branching structure clearly delineated within the consolidation which has a low density due to mucus and debris. The "CT angiogram sign" was first described as fairly typical for bronchioloalveolar tumors; however, it can also be observed in different types of pneumonias, pulmonary edema, obstruction atelectasis, round atelectasis, lymphoma manifestation, and metastases of gastrointestinal tumors (Maldonado 1999).

6.4.8 Ground-Glass Opacities

Ground-glass opacity is defined as an extensive increase in lung attenuation without obscuration of the vascular markings (Engeler et al. 1993), which is the decisive difference with regard to "consolidation" (Figs. 6.2–6.4, 6.6, 6.7). Thin collimation is often necessary to detect subtle forms of ground-glass opacity, whereas volume averaging can obscure ground-glass opacities on thick collimation scans (Remy-Jardin et al. 1993a). Ground-glass opacities can be generalized or limited to particular secondary lobules, segments, or lobes. The underlying parenchyma is not affected. A mild degree of ground-glass opacities corresponds to an increase in density of 100–200 HU, a moderate degree to an increase of 200–400 HU, and a severe degree to an increase on more than 400 HU. Multiple pathogenetic processes can lead to ground-glass opacities, which are caused by an increase of fluid, cells, or tissue within the axial interstitium and the alveoli. This pattern is highly sensitive with respect to physiological and pathological changes within the interstitium and the alveoli; however, it is highly non-specific, and not helpful to support a particular diagnosis. Comparative studies with histology demonstrated that ground-glass opacities are caused by pure interstitial changes in 45%, by pure alveolar infiltrations in 10%, and by a combination of both in 45% of cases (Remy-Jardin et al. 1993b). The spatial resolution of CT is not sufficient to separate the interstitial and the alveolar component. Approximately two-thirds of ground-glass opacities corresponded to inflammatory and one-third to fibrotic changes. Additional criteria, such as the presence of traction bronchiectasis, are helpful indicators for fibrosis which might not be eligible for certain therapies.

In chronic interstitial lung diseases, ground-glass opacities are mostly related to inflammatory, potentially reversible infiltrations. They occur in subacute hypersensitivity pneumonitis, NSIP, DIP, and RBILD. In subacute hypersensitivity pneumonitis, areas of ground-glass opacity are usually bilateral and involve mainly the mid- and lower lung zones. It is frequently associated with poorly defined centrilobular nodules and lobular areas of reduced attenuation due to air trapping (see below).

Non-specific interstitial pneumonitis (NSIP) is a histological entity characterized by homogeneous interstitial inflammation and fibrosis mainly involving the alveolar walls without specific features. It can be idiopathic or associated with collagen vascular disease or drug reaction. The most common finding of NSIP is bilateral ground-glass opacity with or without consolidation. The abnormalities mainly involve the mid- and lower lung zones and often have a subpleural predominance. A fine reticular pattern and traction bronchiectasis are often evident within the areas of ground-glass opacity, reflecting the presence of fibrosis. Honeycombing is usually not a prominent feature.

Desquamative interstitial pneumonia and RBILD form part of the spectrum of cigarette-smoking-related disease characterized by pigmented macrophage infiltration of the alveolar space. In RBILD the abnormalities mainly involve the peribronchovascular regions, whereas in DIP they are diffuse. The radiologic appearance of DIP substantially differs from that of UIP and IPF. The predominant feature in DIP is the presence of patchy areas of ground-glass opacification often with a subpleural and basal predominance (Hartman et al. 1993). The RBILD is typically characterized by the presence of patchy ground-glass opacities and poorly defined centrilobular nodules. The abnormalities are bilateral and symmetric and can involve mainly the upper and lower lung zones.

Lymphocytic interstitial pneumonia is characterized histologically by a diffuse interstitial mononuclear cell infiltrate. Bilateral areas of ground-glass opacities together with centrilobular nodules are the predominant finding. Subpleural nodules, thickening of the peribronchovascular interstitium, and thin-walled cystic airspaces are also frequently seen.

In some diseases ground-glass opacities indicate potentially reversible disease (Leung et al. 1993), and the finding can be used to initiate anti-inflammatory treatment (Müller et al. 1987). In other diseases, such as sarcoidosis, the extent of ground-glass opacities did not correlate with the clinical development and the results of pulmonary function tests (Remy-Jardin et al. 1994). An additional reason for ground-glass opacities is the increase of blood volume within the peripheral capillaries. In arterial hyperperfusion, e.g., in pulmonary arterial hypertension, bronchiectasis, or emphysema, a typical irregular subsegmental pattern of ground-glass opacity is observed, which is called mosaic perfusion (see below). In pulmonary venous congestion, however, there is a clear predominance of the dependent lung zones dorsally and caudally. Further causes and differential diagnoses of ground-glass opacities are: shallow breathing; (alveolar hypoventilation or respiratory artifacts); artifacts due to contractions of the left ventricle (lingula); and supine position (posterior lung zones). On scans obtained in full expiratory position, there is a physiological, gravity-dependent homogeneous increase of lung attenuation in the posterior lung zones. Bronchial or bronchiolar diseases often present with marked differences within the expiratory increase in lung density, such as hyperinflated areas (lobular, acinar), due to impeded expiration resulting in air trapping.

A lot of acute lung diseases are characteristically associated with ground-glass opacities. They include extrinsic allergic alveolitis, pulmonary edema, hemorrhage, and pneumonia. In immunocompromised patients, focal or diffuse ground-glass opacities are highly suggestive for *Pneumocystis carinii* pneumonia or viral infections such as cytomegaly virus pneumonia.

The simultaneous appearance of an area of ground-glass opacity together with an overlying septal pattern due to thickening of the interlobular septa creates a "crazy paving" pattern (Johkoh et al. 1999). The network of branching linear densities generates geometric structures with polygonal, triangular, or quadratic shape reflecting the margins of the secondary lobules. Ground-glass opacity is caused by partial filling of the alveolar space, whereas the thickened appearance of the septa is caused by proteins and cells. "Crazy paving" was first described as a typical finding of alveolar proteinosis (Collins and Stern 1997), where ground-glass opacities are frequent and usually have a patchy or geographic distribution. It is noted that in alveolar proteinosis, thickening of the septa is mimicked by accumulation of intra-alveolar proteinaceous material along the septa, which should not be confused with fibrotic thickening of the septa. "Crazy paving" has also been described in acute respiratory distress syndrome, idiopathic pulmonary fibrosis, lipoid pneumonia, drug-induced pneumonitis, and bronchioloalveolar carcinoma (Johkoh et al. 1999).

6.4.8.1 Mosaic Pattern

Heterogeneous lung attenuation on inspiratory scans is called a mosaic pattern. It is usually caused by inhomogeneous pulmonary perfusion leading to ground-glass opacities with an irregular subsegmental distribution pattern. The mosaic perfusion pattern can be observed in vascular obstruction (pulmonary hypertension, chronic pulmonary thromboembolism), airway obstruction with subsequent hypoxic vasoconstriction (bronchiectasis, emphysema, bronchiolitis) (Fig. 6.3), or from infiltrative processes. Vascular obstruction, such as in chronic thromboembolic pulmonary hypertension, results in decreased perfusion in some areas with compensatory hyperperfusion in other areas. This results in the same mosaic pattern which is then also called mosaic oligemia (Martin et al. 1986). Areas distal to vascular obstruction have small-caliber vessels resulting in decreased perfusion and lower attenuation due to oligemia. On the contrary, areas without vascular obstruction have large caliber vessels providing hyperperfusion which causes higher attenuation.

In advanced primary airway disease, such as bronchiectasis, poor ventilation and air trapping of some lung regions are a typical manifestation. Insufficient ventilation makes gas exchange in this lung region ineffective. To reduce the amount of blood flowing through the lungs without taking part in gas exchange (shunt perfusion), the pulmonary artery branches are constricted. This mechanism is called reflex hypoxic vasoconstriction. The subsequent hypoperfusion of the poorly ventilated area induces a further decrease in lung attenuation. Again, compensatory increased perfusion in other areas results in an increase of lung attenuation similar to ground-glass opacity. Assessment of vessel size and expiratory CT are helpful in elucidating whether the cause is primarily vascular or bronchogenic. Scans performed in full expiratory position are most helpful for the differentiation between vascular and bronchial diseases (Stern and Frank 1994). In patients with a mosaic pattern resulting from airway disease, attenuation differences are accentuated on expiration. In patients with vascular diseases or infiltrative processes, expiratory CT shows a proportional increase in attenuation in areas of both increased and decreased density. Air trapping is not a dominant feature of vascular or infiltrative disease.

6.4.9 Emphysema

Emphysema is defined histologically as a constant, irreversible, abnormal enlargement of the alveoli distal to the terminal bronchioles (Snider et al. 1985). It is associated with destruction of the intralobular interstitium and the perilobular septa without an increase of the soft tissue structures. The increased air content and the loss of lung structure together cause a decrease in lung attenuation (Figs. 6.1, 6.9). Areas with decreased attenuation are easily detected if they are inhomogeneous providing contrast with respect to the surrounding non-emphysematous lung areas, such as in centrilobular emphysema. The emphysematous areas with decreased attenuation do not show any visible margin or wall. The decrease in lung attenuation can also be generalized, i.e., in panlobular emphysema. Visual assessment is complicated by the lack of contrast. Measurements of lung attenuation, however, prove the presence of emphysema. Such measurements can be performed on a local basis using a region of interest (ROI) or after segmentation of the entire lung. In HRCT studies with pathological–anatomical correlation and correlation with pulmonary function tests different density ranges have been investigated to show which range best represents emphysematous and destroyed lung parenchyma. Different upper thresholds have been proposed: −900 HU, −910 HU (Archer et al. 1993; Müller et al. 1988; Kinsella et al. 1990), and also −950 HU (Gevenois et al. 1992). The lower threshold was always −1024 HU. It is unclear which threshold values can be easily transferred to MDCT for the assessment of emphysema. It is of great interest whether the quantitative evaluation of emphysema could be done on coronal reformats from MDCT data sets. The thus defined density range (density mask) can be applied to determine the area of emphysema with respect to the entire lung area or volume (emphysema index). Although different thresholds have been used, CT has shown a very high level of concordance with pathological–anatomical investigations. The CT is far superior to the chest radiograph in the verification of subtle emphysematous changes, because the chest radiograph shows mainly indirect signs in advanced disease, such as hyperinflation (Klein et al. 1992). At the same time we have to be aware of the fact that histologically discernible emphysematous changes can be missed at CT, if they are smaller than the spatial resolution of CT (Miller et al. 1989). The CT also visualizes the consequences of emphysema formation onto the vascular system. In mild emphysema the architecture of the pulmonary vasculature remains normal. In advanced disease vascular pruning occurs predominantly in the lung periphery. This can be detected at CT (Spouge et al. 1993) together with alteration of the course of the pulmonary vessels due to local destruction or bullae. These findings are easily appreciated on coronal reformats from MDCT data sets. In contrast to the chest radiograph, CT is capable of differentiating macroscopic and microscopic types of emphysema. Again, volumetric MDCT allows for an assessment of emphysema in three dimensions facilitating the categorization of emphysema.

6.4.9.1 Centrilobular Emphysema

Chronic destructive bronchiolitis leads to destruction and dilatation of the respiratory bronchioles in the proximal acinus. The enlargement of these air spaces is defined as centrilobular emphysema. It is typically associated with smoking and chronic obstructive pulmonary disease. The CT shows centrilobular emphysema as an area of decreased attenuation within the central parts of the secondary lobules. Emphysematous areas are interspersed within the normal parenchyma. Interfaces or wall structures are absent. The architecture of the normal lung parenchyma is maintained. Comparisons of CT obtained in vivo and in vitro with histology of lung specimens have demonstrated that CT shows centrilobular emphysema with a high level of accuracy (significant correlations in vitro, r=0.91; Foster et al. 1986, 1993; Hruban et al. 1987). During the course of the centrilobular emphysema there is central to peripheral progression of the initially partial, later complete, destruction of the air spaces. Finally, the appearance meets the criteria of advanced emphysematous lung destruction. Centrilobular emphysema is typically predominant in the upper lobes and is associated with obstructive lung function impairment. It has been shown that patients whose emphysema involves mainly the upper lobes have a better response to lung volume reduction surgery than patients with diffuse emphysema or with disease involving mainly the lower lobes. The craniocaudal distribution of emphysema is easier to visualize on coronal reconstructions than on single cross-sectional images. Since up to 5% of patients undergoing lung volume reduction surgery have lung cancer (Kazerooni et al. 1995), volumetric high-resolution CT in these patients is preferable to limited sampling while using traditional HRCT.

6.4.9.2 Panlobular Emphysema

Panlobular emphysema equally affects all parts of the secondary lobule. It has a typical basal predominance and a mild obstructive component which appears late during the course of the disease (Fig. 6.9). Obvious cases of panlobular emphysema can be observed in senile emphysema and emphysema in alpha-1-antitrypsin deficiency (Guest and Hansell 1992). In panlobular emphysema CT shows a homogeneous decrease in attenuation throughout the entire secondary lobule, sometimes even entire segments or lobes. Since panlobular emphysema is so homogeneous, it can be easily overlooked during visual assessment (Spouge et al. 1993). Density measurements with values less than –900 or –950 HU and vascular pruning prove the presence of emphysema. Density measurements should also be used during follow-up of the disease with or without treatment.

6.4.9.3 Paraseptal Emphysema

Paraseptal emphysema is a special type of panlobular emphysema. Peripheral secondary lobules adjacent to the visceral pleura or the interlobular septa are involved. Other lung areas are normal. Since paraseptal emphysema only has a subpleural manifestation, it does not result in hyperinflation of the entire lung. The CT demonstrates the secondary lobules involved with low attenuation because they represent a hard contrast with respect to the surrounding parenchyma. The secondary lobules with decreased attenuation are predominantly found in the subpleural regions of the anterior and posterior upper lobes as well as the posterior lower lobe. Paraseptal emphysema respects the borders of the normal secondary lobules, and the normal interlobular septa are outlined. There is no further destruction of the pulmonary architecture. The MDCT and coronal reformats clearly demonstrate the typical distribution pattern and the extent of paraseptal emphysema.

6.4.9.4 Paracicatricial Emphysema

Paracicatricial emphysema is caused by intrapulmonary scars which are residual findings of inflammation (pneumonia), fibrosis, or pneumoconiosis (Fig. 6.1). They are responsible for a focal lucency similar to the process in compensatory hyperinflation. By definition, scars are associated with architectural distortion or destruction. The secondary lobules adjacent to the scar are fixed and induce a focal decrease of pulmonary compliance. Decreasing compliance is an important cause for impaired expiration resulting in air trapping which leads to constant hyperinflation of the secondary lobules involved. Progressing focal destruction of the

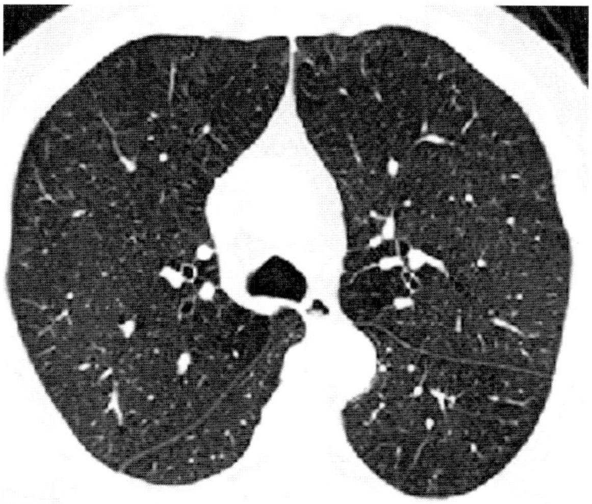
a

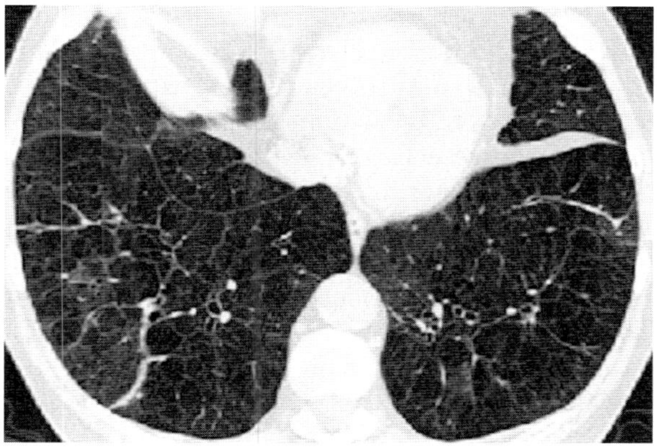
b

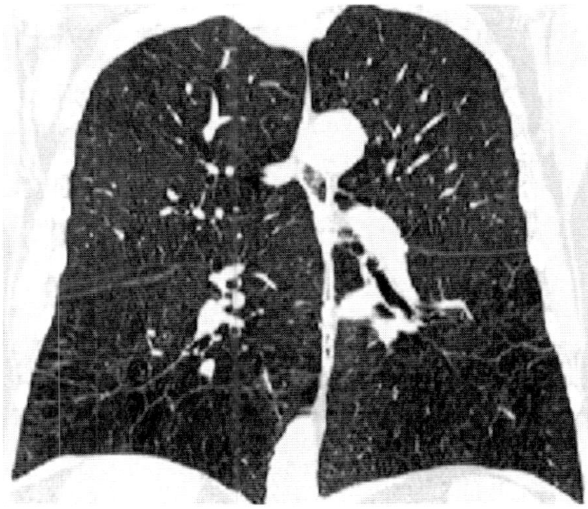
c

Fig. 6.9a–c. A 61-year-old man with alpha-1 antitrypsin deficiency and panlobular emphysema. **a** 1-mm thin slice in the upper lung zones shows mild panlobular emphysema with a slight decrease in overall attenuation. **b** 1-mm thin slice in the lower lung zones shows severe panlobular emphysema with architectural distortion and vascular pruning. **c** Coronal MPR illustrates predominance of panlobular emphysema in the basal segments of the lower lungs with significantly smaller arteries than in the upper lobes

otherwise normal parenchyma finally causes paracicatricial emphysema. At CT, it is detected as an area with decreased attenuation, which is surrounded or septated by fibrotic band-like scars. An extensive paracicatricial emphysema such as in progressive massive fibrosis in silicosis can already be detected on the chest radiograph. The CT allows for a much better visualization of these changes. It is also capable to depict small scars with concomitant surrounding emphysematous areas as an incidental finding.

6.4.9.5
Expiratory Hyperinflation–Air Trapping

In normal lungs attenuation increases significantly during expiration. In the presence of airway obstruction lung remains lucent on expiration and shows little change in cross-sectional area. This finding is called air trapping. Areas of air trapping are seen with relatively low attenuation on expiratory scans where the involved areas are in obvious contrast with the adjacent or contralateral areas which exhibit a physiological increase in attenuation (Fig. 6.4). Air trapping can be patchy and geographical in distribution, it can also correspond to individual secondary lobules, segments, lobes or even the whole lung. Air trapping is usually observed in diseases which involve the small airways, such extrinsic allergic alveolitis and sarcoidosis. Air trapping in a lobe is usually associated with large airway or generalized small airway abnormalities, whereas lobular or segmental air trapping is associated with focal small airway disease. Pulmonary vessels within the low attenuation areas of air trapping often appear relatively smaller than in the denser regions of the lung.

6.4.10
Role of Volumetric High-Resolution Multidetector-Row CT in Diffuse Interstitial Lung Disease

The different patterns of lung disease have all been described on the basis of HRCT. This knowledge has now to be transferred to volumetric high-resolution

MDCT. Obviously, the different CT patterns are still valid, but MDCT now offers the third dimension by providing an almost isotropic volume data set. Instead of looking at single two-dimensional HRCT slices, we have to get used to perceiving them as a three-dimensional volume. Once accomplished, detection of the different patterns will be easier than in the past (Johkoh et al. 2002). At the same time, it will also be easier to recognize the predominant distribution pattern, which is another important hint in differential diagnosis.

6.4.10.1 Volumetry

The MDCT with acquisition of a volume data set is a perfect database for three-dimensional reconstruction of the lung volume. From data obtained in full inspiratory position total lung capacity can be estimated (Kauczor et al. 1998). Introduction of correction factors for patient posture will improve the results for absolute quantification even further (Kauczor et al. 2001). Data obtained at full expiratory position can be used to calculate functional residual capacity (Kauczor et al. 1998). The reduction of these two volumes is a hallmark of restrictive lung function impairment caused by lung fibrosis, whereas an increase of these volumes indicates hyperinflation such as in emphysema. The MDCT will most likely provide more accurate results than spiral-CT approaches in the past. The determination of lung volumes might be an attractive by-product of a diagnostic MDCT scan of the chest. Automatic or semi-automatic tracing of the lung contours is already reality. From here calculation of lung volumes is an easy next step. The big advantage of CT with respect to pulmonary function tests is the potential to calculate the volume of the right and left lungs separately, so-called split-lung volumes (Mergo et al. 1998). This can be complemented by the determination of the volume of the central tracheobronchial tree which provides a measure for anatomical dead space (Brown et al. 2000). By the use of different density ranges it will even be possible to estimate the amount of emphysema within the lung as well as the relative volume of well-ventilated lung (Markstaller et al. 1999). All these volumes are helpful in the follow-up of patients with diffuse interstitial lung disease as well as in planning lung surgery.

6.4.10.2 Computer-Assisted Diagnosis

As the huge number of images in volumetric high-resolution MDCT is a challenge for reporting the scans, there is the general need for intelligent postprocessing tools which might support the radiologist. Since the lung is a high-contrast organ, threshold-based systems are a well-suited basis for postprocessing. Besides mere statistical approaches, more and more artificial intelligence tools, such as fuzzy-logic and neural networks, are entering the field of radiological image postprocessing. Neural networks frequently consist of three levels with input, hidden, and output levels. Before training the individual neurons, these levels are randomly connected. During training, they learn to project typical inputs onto a certain output. After training, the network is capable of evaluating unknown input data and of delivering reliable output results.

In the assessment of emphysema threshold-based evaluation tools, such as density masks, are widely accepted (Riga et al. 2000); however, they only provide a rough measure of the extent of emphysema and are not capable of characterizing the type of emphysema. More sophisticated postprocessing tools apply texture based methods and Bayesian classifiers. They combine thresholding and region growing and make use of statistical and fractal properties of the lung parenchyma (Uppaluri et al. 1997). Such tools significantly improve sensitivity and specificity of emphysema detection. Another method aims at the quantitation of emphysema prior to lung volume reduction surgery (Gierada et al. 2000). Different indices for global extent of emphysema, regional heterogeneity of emphysema, and an indicator of reserve lung parenchyma are used. The indication of lung volume reduction surgery was predicted correctly in 87% of patients as compared with the traditional work-up based on nuclear medicine and pulmonary function tests. Categorization of the type of emphysema has been rarely tried. The detection of different size clusters of bullous emphysematous destruction and their individual contribution to the total emphysematous area might be a successful way towards morphological categorization of different types of emphysema (Blechschmidt et al. 2001).

Intelligent postprocessing tools can also be applied to detect and quantify lung disease which is associated with an increase in lung attenuation. An approach based on thresholding, texture-based pattern recognition as the most important part of the program, and multivariate discrimination analysis is capable of differentiating between vessels and bronchi, emphysema and fibrosis with a sensitivity ranging between 69 and 81% (Delorme et al. 1997). Multiple neural networks complemented by an expert rule are capable of automatically detecting ground-glass opacities and of quantifying their extent (Heitmann et al. 1997). Such a postprocessing tool might prove very helpful in grading the disease activity in lung fibrosis and in detection and follow-up of pneumonic infiltrates in high-risk patients (Heussel et al. 2003). Multiple neural networks performed significantly better than a traditional density mask. When compared with an expert radiologist, the neural networks reached a sensitivity of 99% and a specificity of 83%. Typical errors were cardiac motion artifacts and partial-volume effects (Heitmann et al. 1997).

References

Aberle DR (1993) HRCT in acute diffuse lung disease. J Thorac Imaging 8:200–212

Akkermann DM, Eberhardt K (1992) Lymphangioleiomyomatose. Aktuel Radiol 2:370–372

Archer DC, Coblentz CL, deKemp RA et al. (1993) Automated in vivo quantification of emphysema. Radiology 188:835–838

Austin JHM, Müller NL, Friedman PJ et al. (1996) Glossary of terms for CT of the lungs: recommendations of the nomenclature committee of the Fleischner Society. Radiology 200:327–331

Bankier A, Fleischmann D, Mallek R et al. (1996) Bronchial wall thickness: appropriate window settings for thin-section CT and radiologic-anatomic correlation. Radiology 199:831–836

Becker C, Ohnesorge B, Schoepf U et al. (2000) Current development of cardiac imaging with multidetector-row CT. Eur J Radiol 36:97–103

Beigelman-Aubry C, Capderou A, Grenier P et al. (2002) Mild intermittent asthma: CT assessment of bronchial cross-sectional area and lung attenuation at controlled lung volume. Radiology 223:181–187

Blechschmidt R, Werthschutzky R, Lorcher U (2001) Automated CT image evaluation of the lung: a morphology-based concept. IEEE Trans Med Imaging 20:434–442

Blum U, Windfuhr M, Buitrago-Tellez C et al. (1994) Radiologische Differentialdiagnose des entzündlichen pulmonalen Rundinfiltrates bei immungeschwächten Patienten. Fortschr Röntgenstr 161:292–299

Brauner M, Grenier P, Tijani K et al. (1997) Pulmonary Langerhans cell histiocytosis: evaluation of lesions on CT scans. Radiology 204:497–502

Brown M, Goldin J, McNitt-Gray M et al. (2000) Knowledge-based segmentation of thoracic computed tomography images for assessment of split lung function. Med Phys 27:592–598

Collins J, Stern E (1997) Ground-glass opacity at CT: the ABCs. AJR 169:355–367

Delorme S, Keller-Reichenbecher M, Zuna I et al. (1997) Usual interstitial pneumonia: quantitative assessment of high-resolution computed tomography findings by computer-aided texture-based image analysis. Invest Radiol 32:566–574

Eibel R, Turk T, Kulinna C et al. (2001a) Multidetector-row CT of the lungs: multiplanar reconstructions and maximum intensity projections for the detection of pulmonary nodules. Fortschr Roentgenstr 173:815–821

Eibel R, Turk T, Kulinna C et al. (2001b) Value of multiplanar reformations (MPR) in multi-slice spiral CT of the lung. Fortschr Roentgenstr 173:57–64

Engeler C (1994) When should spiral scanning be used rather than axial cluster scanning? Am J Roentgenol 163:469

Engeler CE, Tashjian JH, Trenkner SW et al. (1993) Ground-glass opacity of the lung parenchyma: a guide to analysis with high-resolution CT. AJR 160:249–251

Foster WL Jr, Pratt PC, Roggli VL et al. (1986) Centrilobular emphysema: CT-pathologic correlation. Radiology 159:27–32

Foster WL Jr, Gimenez EI, Roubidoux MA et al. (1993) The emphysemas: radiologic–pathologic correlations. Radiographics 13:311–328

Fotheringham T, Chabet F, Hansell D et al. (1999) A comparison of methods for enhancing the detection of areas of decreased attenuation on CT caused by airway disease. J Comput Assist Tomogr 23:385–389

Gavelli G, Giampalma E, Cenni M et al. (1998) High resolution columetric computerized tomography of the lung: optimization of technique and image quality as a function of its clinical-diagnostic use and dose to the patient. Radiol Med (Torino) 95:322–328

Gevenois PA, Vuyst PD, Littani M et al. (1992) CT quantification of pulmonary emphysema – correlation with pulmonary function tests: preliminary results on 15 patients. In: Felix R, Langer M (eds) Advances in CT II. Springer, Berlin Heidelberg New York, pp 3–7

Gierada D, Yusen R, Villanueva I et al. (2000) Patient selection for lung volume reduction surgery: an objective model based on prior clinical decisions and quantitative CT analysis. Chest 117:991–998

Grenier P, Valeyre D, Cluzel P et al. (1991) Chronic diffuse interstitial lung disease: diagnostic value of chest radiography and high-resolution CT. Radiology 179:123–132

Grenier P, Chevret S, Beigelman C et al. (1994) Chronic diffuse infiltrative lung disease: determination of the diagnostic value of clinical data, chest radiography, and CT and Bayesian analysis. Radiology 191:383–390

Guest PJ, Hansell DM (1992) High resolution computed tomography (HRCT) in emphysema associated with alpha-1-antitrypsin deficiency. Clin Radiol 45:260–266

Hartman T, Primack S, Swensen S et al. (1993) Desquamative interstitial pneumonia: thin-section CT findings in 22 patients. Radiology 187:787–790

Haubold-Reuter B, Lübbering J, Schmidt (1995) High-Resolution-CT bei Früh- und Spätform einer Lymphangioleiomyomatose. Aktuel Radiol 5:59–62

Heitmann KR, Kauczor H-U, Mildenberger P et al. (1997) Automatic detection of ground glass opacities on lung HRCT using multiple neural networks. Eur Radiol 7:1463–1472

Heussel C, Kauczor H-U, Heussel G et al. (1999) Pneumonia in febrile neutropenic patients, bone-marrow and blood stem-cell recipients: use of high-resolution CT. J Clin Oncol 17:796–805

Heussel C, Kauczor H-U, Ullmann A (2003) Pneumonia in neutropenic patients. Eur Radiol. DoI 10.1007/s 00330-003-1985-6

Honda O, Johkoh T, Tomiyama N et al. (2001) High-resolution CT using multidetector CT equipment: evaluation of image quality in 11 cadaveric lungs and a phantom. Am J Roentgenol 177:875–879

Hruban RH, Meziane MA, Zerhouni EA et al. (1987) High resolution computed tomography of inflation-fixed lungs: pathologic–radiologic correlation of centrilobular emphysema. Am Rev Respir Dis 136:935–940

Johkoh T, Itoh H, Müller N et al. (1999) Crazy-paving appearance at thin-section CT: spectrum of disease and pathologic findings. Radiology 211:155–160

Johkoh T, Mueller N, Nakamura H (2002) Multidetector spiral high-resolution computed tomography of the lungs: distribution of findings on coronal image reconstructions. J Thorac Imaging 17:291–305

Kang E-Y, Grenier P, Laurent F et al. (1996) Interlobular septal thickening: patterns at high-resolution computed tomography. J Thorac Imaging 11:260–264

Kauczor H-U, Klamm R, Heussel C et al. (1998) Assessment of lung volumes using spiral CT in inspiration and expiration: comparison with pulmonary function tests. AJR 171: 1091–1095

Kauczor H-U, Hast J, Heussel C et al. (2000) Focal airtrapping at expiratory high-resolution CT: comparison with pulmonary function tests. Eur Radiol 10:1539–1546

Kauczor H-U, Markstaller K, Puderbach M et al. (2001) Volumetry of ventilated airspaces using 3He MRI: preliminary results. Invest Radiol 36:110–114

Kazerooni E (2001) High-resolution CT of the lungs. Am J Roentgenol 177:501–519

Kazerooni E, Chow L, Whyte R et al. (1995) Preoperative examination of lung transplant candidates: value of chest CT compared with chest radiography. Am J Roentgenol 165:1343–1348

Kim T, Lee K, Chung M et al. (1998) Nonspecific interstitial pneumonia with fibrosis: high resolution CT and pathologic findings. Am J Roentgenol 171:1645–1650

Kinsella M, Müller NL, Abboud RT et al. (1990) Quantification of emphysema by computed tomography using a density mask program and correlation with pulmonary function tests. Chest 97:315–321

Klein JS, Gamsu G, Webb WR et al. (1992) High-resolution CT diagnosis of emphysema in symptomatic patients with normal chest radiographs and isolated low diffusing capacity. Radiology 182:817–821

Kohno N, Ikezoe J, Johkoh T et al. (1993) Focal organizing pneumonia: CT appearance. Radiology 189:119–123

Lee H, Im J, Ahn J et al. (1996) Lung cancer in patients with idiopathic pulmonary fibrosis: CT findings. J Comput Assist Tomogr 20:979–982

Lee K, Primack S, Staples C et al. (1994) Chronic infiltrative lung disease: comparison of diagnostic accuracies of radiography and low- and conventional-dose thin-section CT. Radiology 191:669–673

Lenoir S, Grenier P, Brauner M et al. (1990) Pulmonary lymphangiomyomatosis and tuberous sclerosis: comparison of radiographic and thin-section CT findings. Radiology 175: 329–334

Leung A, Miller R, Mueller N (1993) Parenchymal opacification in chronic infiltrative lung diseases: CT-pathologic correlation. Radiology 188:209–214

Lynch DA, Newell JD, Logan P et al. (1995) Can CT distinguish hypersensitivity pneumonitis from idiopathic pulmonary fibrosis? AJR 165:807–811

Maldonado R (1999) THe CT angiogram sign. Radiology 210: 323–324

Markstaller K, Kauczor H-U, Eberle B et al. (1999) Multi-rotation CT during continuous ventilation: comparison of different density areas in healthy lungs and in the ARDS lavage model. Fortschr Roentgenstr 170:575–580

Martin KM, Sagel SS, Siegel BA (1986) Mosaic oligemia simulating pulmonary infiltrates on CT. AJR 147:670–673

Mathieson JR, Mayo JR, Staples CA et al. (1989) Chronic diffuse infiltrative lung disease: comparison of diagnostic accuracy of CT and chest radiography. Radiology 171:111–116

Mayo JR, Webb WR, Gould R et al. (1987) High-resolution CT of the lungs: an optimal approach. Radiology 163:507–510

Mehnert F, Pereira P, Dammann F et al. (2000) High resolution multislice CT of the lung: comparison with sequential HRCT slices. Fortschr Roentgenstr 172:972–977

Mergo PJ, Willliams WF, Gonzalez-Rothi R et al. (1998) Three-dimensional volumetric assessment of abnormally low attenuation of the lung from routine helical CT: inspiratory and expiratory quantification. AJR 170:1355–1366

Meziane M, Hruban R, Zerhouni E et al. (1988) High-resolution CT of the lung parenchyma with pathologic correlation. Radiographics 8:27–54

Miller RR, Müller NL, Vedal S et al. (1989) Limitations of computed tomography in the assessment of emphysema. Am Rev Respir Dis 139:980–983

Montaudon M, Berger P, Blachere H et al. (2001) Thin-section CT of the lung: influence of 0.5-s gantry rotation and ECG triggering on image quality. Eur Radiol 11:1681–1687

Müller NL (1991) Clinical value of high-resolution CT in chronic diffuse lung disease. AJR 157:1163–1170

Müller NL, Staples CA, Miller RR et al. (1987) Disease activity in idiopathic pulmonary fibrosis: CT and pathologic correlation. Radiology 165:731–734

Müller NL, Staples CA, Miller RR et al. (1988) "Density mask": an objective method to quantitate emphysema using computed tomography. Chest 94:782–787

Munk PL, Müller NL, Miller RR et al. (1988) Pulmonary lymphangitic carcinomatosis: CT and pathologic findings. Radiology 166:705–709

Murata K, Khan A, Herman PG (1989) Pulmonary parenchymal disease: evaluation with high-resolution CT. Radiology 170:629–635

Ng C, Desai S, Rubens M et al. (1999) Visual quantitation and observer variation of signs of small airways disease at inspiratory and expiratory CT. J Thorac Imaging 14:279–285

Nishimura K, Kitaichi M, Izumi T et al. (1992) Usual interstitial pneumonia: histologic correlation with high-resolution CT. Radiology 182:337–342

Nishimura K, Itoh H, Kitaichi M et al. (1993) Pulmonary sarcoidosis: correlation of CT and histopathologic findings. Radiology 189:105–109

Raman R, Napel S, Beaulieu C et al. (2002) Automated generation of curved planar reformations from volume data: method and evaluation. Radiology 223:275–280

Remy-Jardin M, Remy J, Giraud F et al. (1993a) Computed tomography assessment of ground glass opacity: semiology and significance. J Thorac Imaging 8:249–264

Remy-Jardin M, Giraud F, Remy J et al. (1993b) Importance of ground-glass attenuation in chronic diffuse infiltrative lung disease: pathologic-CT correlation. Radiology 189: 693–698

Remy-Jardin M, Giraud F, Remy J et al. (1994) Pulmonary sarcoidosis: role of CT in the evaluation of disease activity and functional impairment and in prognosis assessment. Radiology 191:675–680

Remy-Jardin M, Edme J-L, Boulenguez C et al. (2002) Longitudinal follow-up study of smoker's lung with thin-section CT in correlation with pulmonary function tests. Radiology 222:261–270

Riga B, Andres A, Stramare R (2000) Density-mask spiral computed tomography in patients who are candidates for a lung-volume-reduction intervention: a preliminary study. Radiol Med 99:150–155

Roberts H, Wells A, Milne D et al. (2000) Airflow obstruction in bronchiectasis: correlation between computed tomography features and pulmonary function tests. Thorax 55: 198–204

Rubin GD, Napel S, Leung AN (1996) Volumetric analysis of volumetric data: achieving a paradigm shift. Radiology 200:312–317

Schoepf U, Bruening R, Becker C et al. (1999) Multislice spiral CT imaging of the chest. Radiologe 39:943–951

Schorn C, Obenauer S, Funke M et al. (1999) Schichtempfindlichkeitsprofile und Bildpunktrauschen einer Mehrschicht Spiral-CT im Vergleich zu einer Einzelschicht Spiral CT. Fortschr Roentgenstr 171:219–225

Schurawitzki H (1992) Hochauflösende Computertomographie (HR-CT) der Lunge vor Transplantation. Fortschr Roentgenstr 157:21–25

Seo J, Im J, Chung J et al. (2000) Pulmonary vasculitis: the spectrum of radiological findings. Br J Radiol 73:1224–1231

Siegelman SS, Khouri NF, Leo FP et al. (1986) Solitary pulmonary nodules: CT assessment. Radiology 160:307–312

Spouge D, Mayo JR, Cardoso W et al. (1993) Panacinar emphysema: CT and pathologic findings. J Comput Assist Tomogr 17:710–713

Snider GL, Kleinemann J, Thurlbeck WA et al. (1985) The definition of emphysema. Am Rev Respir Dis 132:182–185

Stein MG, Mayo J, Müller NL et al. (1987) Pulmonary lymphangitic spread of carcinoma: appearance on CT scans. Radiology 175:535–539

Stern EJ, Frank MS (1994) Small airway diseases of the lung: findings at expiratory CT. AJR 163:37–41

Uppaluri R, Mitsa T, Sonka M et al. (1997) Quantification of pulmonary emphysema from lung computed tomography images. Am J Respir Crit Care 156:248–254

Vernhet H, Bousquet C, Vergnes C et al. (1999) Contribution of high resolution computed tomography (HRCT) for the exploration of diffuse pulmonary infiltrates. Rev Mal Respir 16:188–197

Verschakelen JA, Scheinbaum K, Bogaert J et al. (1998) Expiratory CT in cigarette smokers: correlation between areas of decreased lung attenuation, pulmonary function tests and smoking history. Eur Radiol 8:1391–1399

Volpe J, Storto M, Lee K et al. (1997) High-resolution CT of the lung: determination of usefulness of CT scans obtained with the patient prone based on plain radiographic findings. Am J Roentgenol 169:369–374

Webb WR, Stein MG, Finkbeiner WE et al. (1988) Normal and diseased isolated lungs: High-resolution CT. Radiology 166:81–87

7 Pulmonary Infections: Imaging with MDCT

B. L. Partik, A. N. Leung, C. J. Herold

CONTENTS

7.1 Introduction

Pneumonia is one of the major infectious diseases responsible for significant morbidity and mortality throughout the world. It is the most prevalent community-acquired infection and the second most common nosocomial infectious disorder. Despite the availability of antimicrobial agents, pneumonias constitute the sixth most common cause of death and are the number one cause of death from infections (Fraser et al. 1994; Moine et al. 1994; Lynch 2001; Levy et al. 1988). Pneumonias may develop into a life-threatening condition especially in immunocompromised patients, in children, and in the elderly population.

Imaging plays a crucial role in the detection and management of patients with pneumonia. Chest radiography is the imaging technique of choice in evaluating patients with suspected pneumonia because of its low radiation dose, low cost, and wide accessibility. In daily practice, radiographs are used to confirm the clinical diagnosis of pneumonia, characterize the extent and severity of disease, search for complications, monitor the response to therapy, and examine for possible alternative or additional diagnoses (Katz and Leung 1999); however, an increasing number of patients undergo thin-section CT of the chest, when there is a high clinical suspicion for pneumonia in the presence of abnormal or questionable radiographic findings (Schaefer-Prokop et al. 2000). The introduction of multi-detector row CT (MDCT) scanners in 1998 incrementally improved the capability of CT to acquire volumetric data of the lungs with unprecedented spatial resolution. Recently introduced 16-row MDCT scanners are able to acquire an isotropic volumetric data set of the entire chest during a single breathhold, thereby allowing high-quality reconstructed images in any desired plane. In the following chapters the impact of MDCT imaging for the diagnosis of infectious lung diseases will be evaluated.

Franquet and colleagues (2001) have shown that a combination of radiologic pattern recognition with knowledge of the clinical setting is the best approach to the pulmonary infectious processes; thus, the differentiation between community-acquired pneumonia, nosocomial pneumonia, and pneumonia in the immunocompromised patient is of practical interest. Although the spectrum of offending organisms (Table 7.1) differ between these disorders, considerable overlap exists between their radiologic features.

7.2 Spread of Infection and Patterns of Imaging

By far the most common route of infection occurs via the tracheobronchial tree by aspiration or inhalation of microorganisms. Traditionally, pneumonia

B. L. Partik, MD
Department of Radiology, University of Vienna Medical School, Waehringer Guertel 18–20, 1090 Vienna, Austria
A. N. Leung, MD
Department of Radiology, Stanford University Medical Center, 300 Pasteur Drive, Room S072, Stanford, CA 94305, USA
C. J. Herold, MD
Department of Radiology, University of Vienna Medical School, Waehringer Guertel 18–20, 1090 Vienna, Austria

Table 7.1. Overview of organisms potentially causing infectious lung diseases

Bacteria
Aerobic bacteria: gram positive
Streptococcus pneumoniae
Staphylococcus aureus
Bacillus anthracis
Aerobic bacteria: gram negative
Klebsiella, Enterobacter, Serratia species
Escherichia coli
Haemophilus influenzae
Pseudomonas aeruginosa
Legionellaceae
Anaerobic bacteria
Mycobacteria
Actinomycosis
Mycoplasma pneumoniae
Chlamydia pneumonia, C. psittaci
Rickettsiae
Fungi
Histoplasmosis
Coccidiomycosis
Blastomycosis
Cryptococcosis
Aspergillosis
Mucormycosis
Nocardiosis
Viruses
Respiratory syncytial virus
Adenovirus
Varicella zoster virus
Protozoa
Pneumocystis carinii
Helminths
Strongyloides stercoralis

acquired that way has been divided into air-space (lobar) pneumonia, bronchopneumonia, and interstitial pneumonia (Fraser et al. 1994). Infection by the way of the pulmonary vasculature often occurs in conjunction with extrapulmonary infection; particularly in tuberculous or fungal disease, the primary focus of infection is the lung itself. Because of preferential gravity-related blood flow to the dependent portions of the lung, hematogenously spread infection tends to show considerable basal predominance. A nodular appearance of the individual foci of infection is typical.

Direct spread across the chest wall or diaphragm or from the mediastinum may occur in association with penetrating thoracic wounds or by extension of infection from an extrapulmonary source, such as a subphrenic abscess. In these cases, pulmonary disease usually is localized to an area contiguous with the extrapulmonary source of infection and often takes the form of an abscess (Fraser et al. 1994).

7.2.1 Localized Air-Space Disease

Lobar pneumonia is characterized by homogeneous consolidation of lung parenchyma with well-defined borders, and does not typically respect segmental borders. Air bronchograms are present, and usually the lung volume is normal with the exception of gram-negative pneumonias where volume loss is frequently seen. The typical features may be altered in the presence of underlying disease. For example, the inflammatory exudate may not fill emphysematous spaces, resulting in a sponge-like appearance of the consolidated lung. Frequently, lobar pneumonias are related to bacterial organisms such as *Streptococcus pneumoniae* (Fig. 7.1), most gram-negative bacilli, and *Legionella pneumophila*. Cavitation is rare in pneumococcal infections but typical in gram-negative pneumonias (Gharib and Stern 2001).

Bronchopneumonia (Lobular pneumonia) is characterized by the absence of air bronchograms, a patchy, segmental distribution, since the infection usually occurs at multiple foci at the same time, and volume loss. Typically, lobular boundaries are respected resulting in involvement of secondary pulmonary lobules while sparing adjacent lobules. Bronchopneumonia is exemplified by infection by *Staphylococcus aureus*, many gram-negative bacteria (e.g., *Haemophilus influenzae*), *Mycoplasma pneumoniae*, and fungi (Reittner et al. 2003). In *Pseu-*

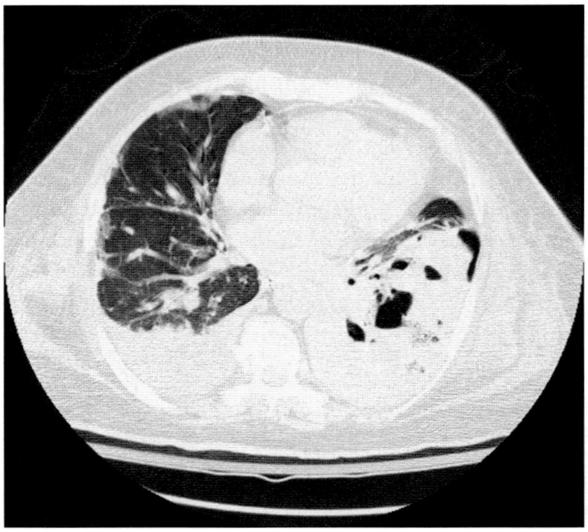

Fig. 7.1. Streptococcal pneumonia in a 61-year-old woman. Chest CT scan (collimation 4×1.25 mm) shows consolidation of left lower lobe with associated areas of cavitation

domonas aeruginosa pneumonia, bilateral disease, lower lobe predominance, and abscess formation are also common. Resolution of the infiltrates may take several weeks, particularly in *Staphylococcus aureus* infections and *Mycoplasma pneumoniae*.

In addition, rounded pneumonia represents an infection process that does not have a lobar pattern but rather presents as a rounded density that does not follow anatomic landmarks. Rounded or nodular forms of pneumonia are usually due to pneumococcal, *Legionella*, or fungal infections. This pattern is more common in children (Slone et al. 1999).

The term "atypical pneumonia" was originally applied to pneumonias with atypical clinical, laboratory, and/or radiographic features. It was primarily used to describe atypical bacterial infections. Besides numerous viruses, the main bacterial pathogens causing atypical pneumonias are *Mycoplasma pneumoniae*, two chlamydial species, *Chlamydia pneumoniae* and *Chlamydia psittaci* (Fig. 7.2), one rickettsia, *Coxiella burnetti*, and several *Legionella* species (Saikku 1997). In the group of "atypical" bacterial pneumonias, *Legionella pneumophila*, but also *Mycoplasma pneumoniae* and *Chlamydia* infections, demonstrate a radiographic pattern of air-space disease indistinguishable from that of other typical bacterial infections. It is important to know that unilateral or bilateral air-space disease may be caused by a so-called atypical organism.

Localized air-space disease may be seen as a manifestation of *Mycobacterium tuberculosis*. The typical radiographic features of postprimary disease in the adult consist of patchy areas of ill-defined opacities in the upper lobes, with or without cavitation (Fig. 7.3). In primary tuberculosis, parenchymal consolidation, with or without hilar and/or mediastinal lymphadenopathy, may be present and can overlap to some degree. In some cases, differentiation of primary and post-primary disease may be difficult. The tree-in-bud pattern has become a popular descriptive term for various diseases of the peripheral airways in which mucous plugging, bronchial dilatation, and wall thickening are present. It has primarily been used as a descriptive term for abnormalities found on CT scans of the lung in patients with endobronchial

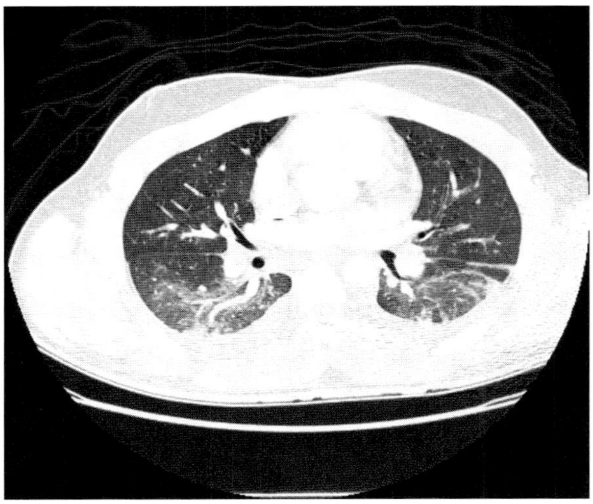

Fig. 7.2. Psittacosis in a 19-year-old man. Chest CT scan (collimation 8×1.25 mm) shows diffuse, bilateral ground-glass opacities predominating in lower lobes and associated with small pleural effusions

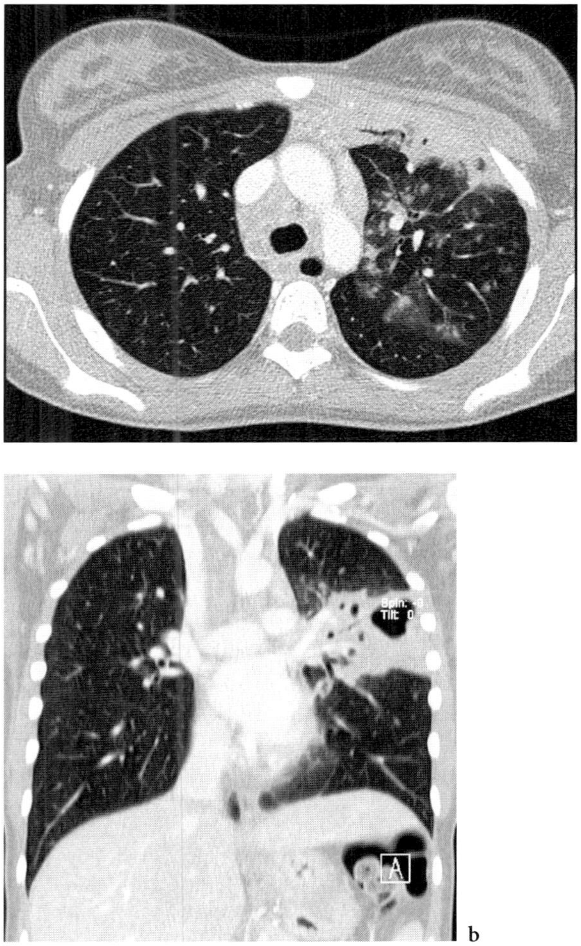

a

b

Fig. 7.3a, b. Tuberculosis in a 14-year-old girl. **a** Chest CT scan (collimation 12×0.75 mm) shows areas of consolidation in left upper lobe associated with centrilobular nodules in the lung periphery (*arrows*). Mediastinal lymphadenopathy in the right paratracheal and aortopulmonary window stations is also present. **b** Coronal reformatted image shows consolidation and associated cavitation spread of *Mycobacterium tuberculosis*; however, any infectious organism, including bacterial, mycobacterial, viral, parasitic, and fungal agents, can involve the small airways and cause a tree-in-bud pattern (Eisenhuber 2002).

Invasive pulmonary aspergillosis (IPA) and mucormycosis are fungal pneumonias seen almost exclusively in immunocompromised patients. Arising from a nodular or patchy infiltrate. They progress to homogeneous peripheral wedge-shaped (sub)segmental or lobar consolidation, which represents infarction due to infiltration of pulmonary arteries by the fungus. Finally, air-space disease may be seen in viral and protozoal infections. In patients with CAP, one should be aware that the influenza virus may cause segmental air-space disease which may simulate bacterial infections. In patients with mild immunosuppression, segmental alveolar infiltrates may be caused by *Pneumocystis carinii* pneumonia.

7.2.2 Interstitial Pneumonia

Interstitial pneumonia reveals two imaging patterns. Firstly, the inflammatory process can be localized in airway walls and alveolar septa without any air-space disease. Secondly, in a more acute setting the inflammatory reaction may progress to air-space disease due to alveolar damage and proteinaceous exudate within air-spaces leading to diffuse areas of air-space opacification; thus, although primarily an interstitial process, disease of this variety typically evolves to affect adjacent air-spaces (Fraser et al. 1994). Typically, interstitial pneumonias are caused by viruses but may also be seen with organisms such as *Pneumocystis carinii* and *Mycoplasma pneumoniae.*

Diffuse bilateral lung disease is rarely seen in bacterial pneumonias. Diffuse lung disease is also rare in patients with CAP; however, if identified in otherwise healthy people, it is most commonly caused by viral pneumonias such as the respiratory syncytial virus (RSV; Fig. 7.4). In *Herpes varicellae* (*Varicella zoster*) pneumonia, diffusely distributed and well-defined patchy or nodular densities are the characteristic features. In immunocompromised patients, particularly in organ-transplant recipients, a symmetric, diffuse bilateral linear, or nodular pattern, potentially combined with patchy alveolar densities, is most commonly caused by cytomegalovirus (CMV) infection. *Pneumocystis carinii* pneumonia may resemble CMV pneumonia and begin with a discrete increase in pulmonary parenchymal density, which progresses to a reticular or mixed reticular-alveolar pattern, and finally to diffuse air-space consolidation. A diffuse interstitial nodular pattern, with nodules ranging from 3 to 5 mm in size, is typically seen in pneumonia caused by *Candida.* Diffusely distributed micronodules (miliary disease) indicate the hematogenous spread of a mycobacterial or fungal organism.

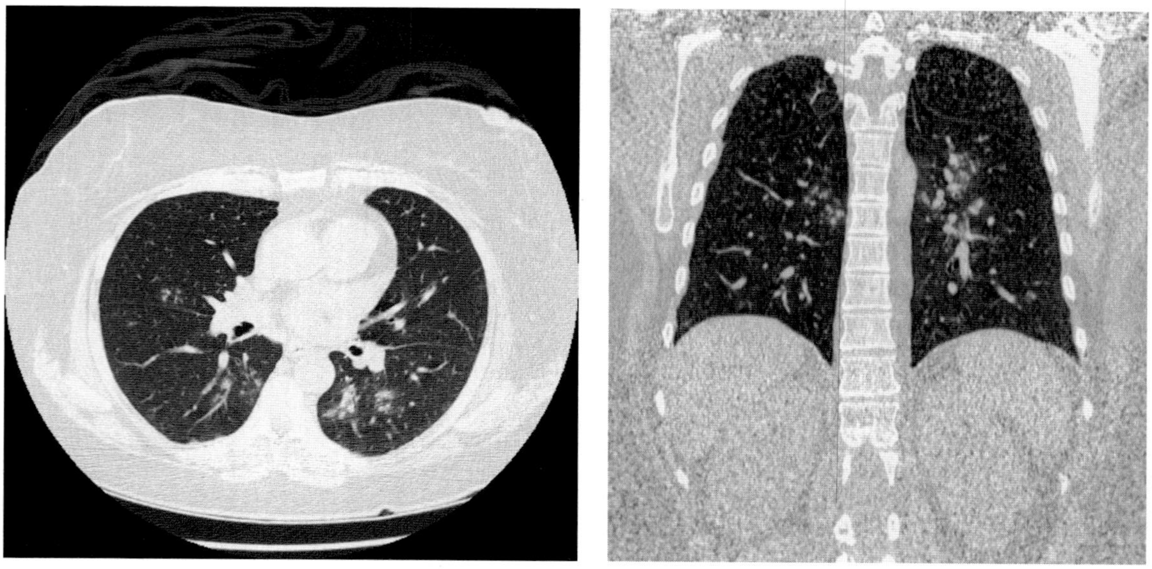

a b

Fig. 7.4a, b. Respiratory syncytial virus (RSV) infection in a 56-year-old woman after bone marrow transplantation. **a** Chest CT scan (collimation 16×1.25 mm) shows multiple centrilobular nodules located predominantly in both lower lobes. **b** Coronal reformatted image depicts craniocaudal distribution of centrilobular nodules

7.2.3
Nodular Lesions

Nodular lesions attributed to pulmonary infections are most often seen in nosocomial pneumonias and in immunocompromised patients. They may be caused by bacteria such as *Nocardia asteroides* (Fig. 7.5) and *Mycobacterium tuberculosis,* septic emboli, and fungi. *Nocardia asteroides* causes single or nodular infiltrates with or without cavitation. Invasive pulmonary aspergillosis, *Mucor,* and *Cryptococcus neoformans* may present with single or multiple nodular infiltrates, which often progress to wedge-shaped areas of consolidation. Cavitation (the "air-crescent sign") is common later in the course of the disease. In the appropriate clinical setting MDCT may aid in the diagnosis of IPA by demonstrating the so-called halo sign.

7.3
Clinical Setting of Patients

The immune status of the individual determines the type, severity, and susceptibility to infection; thus, it is useful to consider cases of pulmonary infections in three clinical and environmental groups: community acquired, nosocomial, and in the immunocompromised patient, since they differ not only in the types of offending organisms but also in their potentially different etiology, clinical features, diagnostic approaches, and therapeutic strategies.

7.3.1
Community-Acquired Pneumonia

Community-acquired pneumonia (CAP) is a major health care and economic problem. Hospital admission rates of CAP episodes vary from 22 to 51% (Niedermans et al. 1998). The spectrum of causative organisms includes gram-positive bacteria such as *Streptococcus pneumoniae (Pneumococcus), Haemophilus influenzae,* and *Staphylococcus aureus,* atypical organisms such as *Mycoplasma pneumoniae, Chlamydia pneumoniae,* or *Legionella pneumophila,* and viral agents such as the influenza A virus and the RSV. It appears from the literature that the spectrum of organisms varies according to a patient's health and socioeconomic status as well as to the affected individual's temporal, geographic, and diagnostic factors (Fraser et al. 1994). Healthy individuals are most likely to contract *Mycoplasma pneumonia* or a mild form of *Pneumococcus pneumonia.* Debilitated patients, alcoholics, and chronically ill persons, however, more often present with severe pneumococcal pneumonia, or infections caused by *Staphylococcus aureus, Haemophilus influenzae,* or other gram-negative bacilli. *Legionella pneumophila* and *Chlamydia* infections are more common in patients with some forms of mild immunologic compromise. In

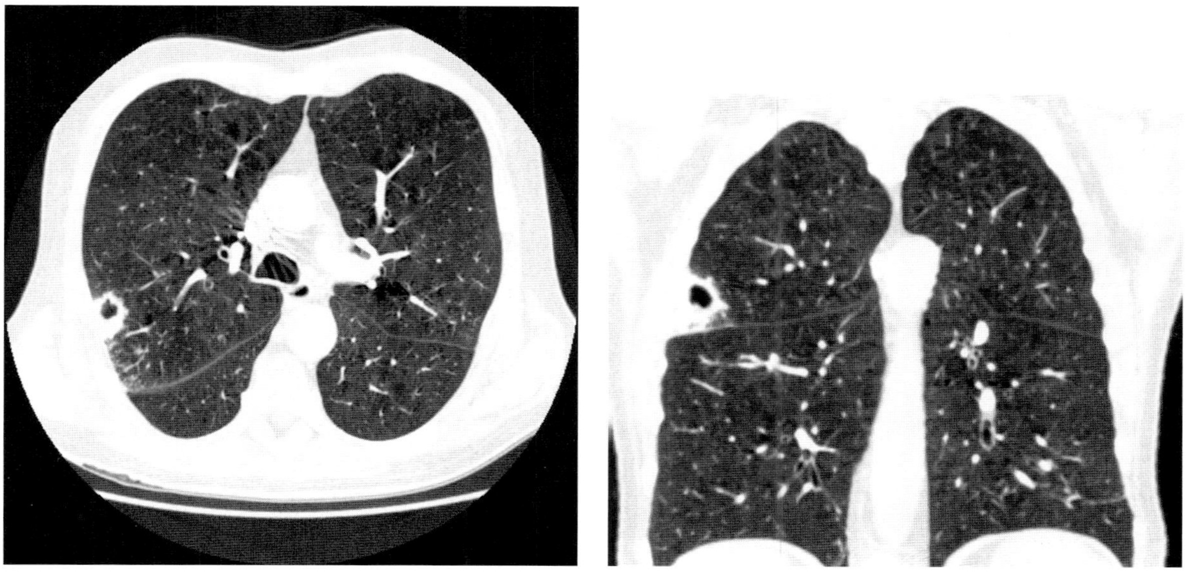

a b

Fig. 7.5a, b. *Nocardia* infection in a 67-year-old man. **a** Chest CT scan (collimation 4×1.25 mm) shows a cavitary nodule in right upper lobe which extends to the costal pleural surface. **b** Coronal reformatted image shows relationship of nodule to adjacent major fissure these patients, *Mycobacterium tuberculosis* infections are more prevalent in comparison with healthy persons without risk factors. Patients with poor oral hygiene and occasional loss of consciousness (epilepsy, alcoholism) may suffer from anaerobic pulmonary infections resulting from aspiration.

The spectrum of causative organisms of lobar pneumonia includes gram-positive bacteria such as *Streptococcus pneumoniae*, the most common cause of complete lobar consolidation, as well as *Klebsiella pneumoniae* and other gram-negative bacilli as *Legionella pneumophila, Haemophilus influenzae*, and occasionally *Mycoplasma pneumoniae*. Bronchopneumonia, characterized by peribronchial alveolar opacities leading to segmental consolidation, which may also cavitate, is typically caused by *Staphylococcus aureus* and *Haemophilus influenzae*. Bacterial infections in CAP may also produce multiple rounded pulmonary nodules or masses, with or without cavitation, occurring from infection with *Nocardia, Aspergillus, Legionella*, Q fever, and *Mycobacterium tuberculosis* (American Thoracic Society 1996; Tanaka et al. 1996). *Mycoplasma pneumoniae* is typically a disease of children and young adults. The MDCT findings consist mainly of centrilobar nodules often in a lobar distribution and thickening of the peribronchovascular and interlobar septal interstitium. These findings are often difficult to identify on chest radiographs but can usually be recognized on CT scans (Reittner et al. 2000).

When an out-patient presents with symptoms such as fever, cough, and purulent tracheobronchial secretions, he or she may or may not suffer from pneumonia; thus, the diagnosis of pneumonia is based on the detection of a pulmonary infiltrate on the chest X-ray. This practice relies on the pathophysiologic events that lead to the development of a visible pulmonary infiltrate. Although some variation exists regarding the time frame between the onset of clinical symptoms and the development of a radiographically visible pulmonary infiltrate, it has been stated that the vast majority of infiltrates appears within the time period of 12 h from development of symptoms (Spencer 1985). This time frame allows detection or exclusion in most cases of CAP as patients are generally seen by the radiologist within a few days following initial clinical presentation.

Although MDCT has no role in the primary diagnosis of CAP, recurrent pneumonias can indicate the presence of an underlying problem such as congenital or acquired immunologic disorder; airway abnormalities such as chronic bronchitis, bronchiectasis, and bronchogenic carcinoma; cardiac problems (congestive heart failure); or systemic diseases such as diabetes, chronic alcoholism, and intravenous drug abuse. In these patients, MDCT should be used to exclude the presence of a predisposing morphologic abnormality. Moreover, MDCT is indicated for the assessment of complications, or investigation of persistent infiltrates. In complicated childhood pneumonia, CT is far superior to conventional chest radiographs in revealing pleural and parenchymal complications, which may require early surgical intervention (Fig. 7.6; Tan Kendrick et al. 2002).

Moreover, some diseases may mimic infectious lung diseases and require cross-sectional imaging.

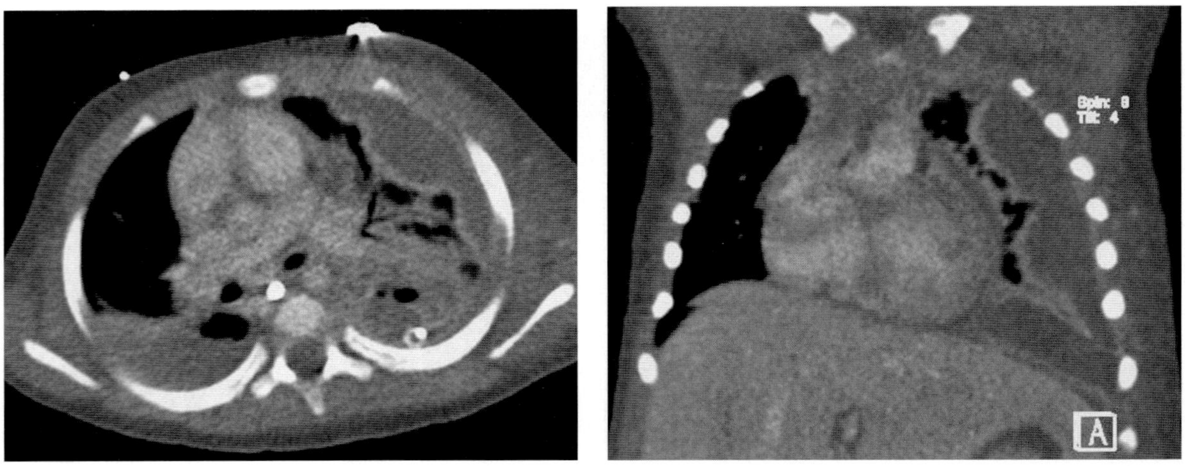

a b

Fig. 7.6a, b. Empyema (*Enterobacter* infection) following streptococcal pneumonia in a 2-year-old child. **a** Contrast-enhanced chest CT scan (collimation 12×0.75 mm) shows loculated fluid collection with enhancing pleural margins in left hemithorax. Note consolidation in adjacent left lower lobe and small right pleural effusion. **b** Coronal reformatted image shows craniocaudal extent of empyema

Extrinsic allergic alveolitis (EAA) is an immunologically mediated lung disease caused by inhalation of antigens contained in a variety of organic dusts. Heavy exposure to the inciting antigen may lead to the acute form of EAA characterized by dyspnea and fever developing within 4–6 h after exposure. Thin-section CT has been shown to be particularly helpful in the assessment of patients with subacute EAA. Characteristic features include bilateral areas of ground-glass attenuation and poorly defined centrilobular nodules. The centrilobular nodules measure less than 5 mm in diameter and are most numerous in the middle and lower lung zones (Remy-Jardin et al. 1993).

In acute interstitial pneumonia (AIP), previously healthy persons develop rapidly increasing dyspnea with fever over a few days, often following a short influenza-like prodrome (Armstrong et al. 2000). On thin-section CT, ground-glass opacity is a universal finding. It is commonly diffuse and patchy, sometimes with a geographic pattern. If related airways are of normal caliber, the histologic correlate of ground-glass opacity is exudative diffuse alveolar damage, but if airways are dilated, the histo-pathology shows proliferative or fibrotic diffuse alveolar damage. The second commonest CT finding, in two-thirds of patients, is consolidation which may have a subpleural predominance (Ichikado et al. 1997).

7.3.2 Nosocomial (Hospital-Acquired) Pneumonia

Nosocomial pulmonary infections that develop in hospital environment and were neither present nor incubating at the time of admission frequently occur in up to 5% of inpatients and are particularly common in mechanically ventilated patients in intensive care units (Eickhoff 1982). Mortality rates reported for NP have ranged from 20% in multihospital studies to 50% or higher in single referral centers and university hospitals. Mortality is related to the causative agent such that the prognosis associated with aerobic gram-negative pneumonias is considerably worse than that with gram-positive or viral agents. Typically, gram-negative bacteria have the tendency to colonize the oropharynx and gastrointestinal tract and are infrequent commensals in healthy persons, the carrier rate being estimated to range from 2–10%; however, in hospitalized patients who are not critically ill, the carrier rate has been found to approximate 30–40%, and in chronically or severely incapacitated in-hospital patients is as high as 60–75% (Fraser et al. 1994). Colonization is the result largely of contact spread from contaminated hospital personnel or equipment (e.g., inserted tubes, lines, and catheters). The persons at greatest risk are the elderly with underlying disease and patients who are malnourished or who have been inappropriately treated with broad-spectrum antibiotics. The spectrum of infectious agents has changed over the past decades. Enterobacteriaceae, *Pseudomonas aeruginosa*, and *Staphylococcus aureus* became important problems; however, multiple infecting organisms (Fig. 7.7) may be identified in 20–40% of cases (A'Court and Garrard 1992).

The NP can be difficult to diagnose, since the classical findings for pneumonia, such as new fever, new pulmonary infiltrate, cough, sputum production, and elevated leukocyte count may not be present in the hospitalized patient with NP. If present, these symptoms may not necessarily be caused by pneumonia. Microbiologic evaluation of the patient with suspected NP (sputum, bronchoalveolar lavage) may or may not be helpful because of the difficulties in differentiating contamination from true infection. In addition, pulmonary disease in a hospital environment may be produced by more than one agent; therefore, the identification of a pulmonary infection, the use of various methods to obtain a specimen, and the value of isolation of potential pathogens are matters of constant discussion in the clinical diagnosis of NP.

Radiologically, the identification of the pulmonary infiltrate may be hampered by preexisting disorders or concomitant lung disease such as fibrosing alveolitis, lupus pneumonitis, hemorrhage or contusion, tumor, atelectasis, and embolic infarcts. The most

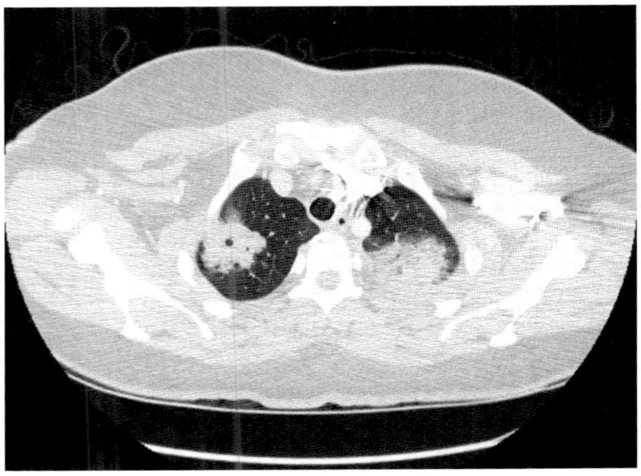

Fig. 7.7. Polymicrobial bacterial pneumonia in a 33-year-old woman. Chest CT scan (collimation 16×1.25 mm) shows bilateral nodules in upper lobes. Note small area of necrosis in right upper lobe lesion

common sources of septic emboli (Fig. 7.8) are infected venous catheters and tricuspid valve endocarditis (a major source in intravenous drug abusers; Julander 1983). The MDCT shows multiple lesions either round in shape or with the shape of a pulmonary infarct, namely a wedge-shaped density based on the pleura and pointing to the hilum. The lesions may be any size and frequently cavitate. A relatively common finding of both bland and infected infarcts, which may be helpful in differential diagnosis, is the "feeding vessel sign," a distinct vessel leading to the apex of a peripheral area of consolidation (Armstrong et al. 2000).

All of the above-mentioned disorders may obscure or alter the otherwise characteristic radiographic appearance of an infiltrate and also render the etiologic approach using pattern recognition difficult. Particularly in patients with adult respiratory distress syndrome (ARDS), the identification of ventilator-associated pneumonia is still a problem. Diagnostic accuracy for pneumonia was found to be fair (69%) owing to 70% true-negative ratings vs 59% true-positive ratings. No single CT sign was significantly different for pneumonia, but dependent atelectasis was more common in patients with early ARDS without pneumonia (Winer-Murham et al. 1998).

However, MDCT is used more often when an NP is suspected than in patients with CAP to detect early morphologic signs of infection (e.g., ground-glass opacities). The MDCT can also identify detect complications, and guide invasive diagnostic procedures such as bronchoscopy or percutaneous biopsy.

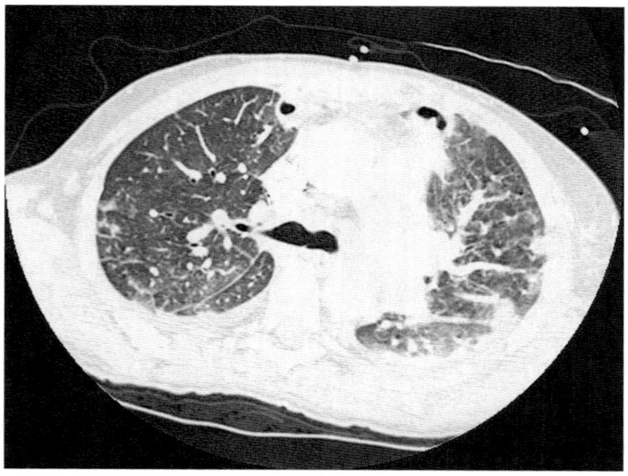

Fig. 7.8. Septic emboli in a 43-year-old woman with endocarditis. Chest CT scan (collimation 16×1.25 mm) shows multiple pleural-based nodules. Note vessel-feeding sign in left lower lobe and cavitary nodules adjacent to heart

7.3.3 Pneumonia in the Immunocompromised Patient

There has been a dramatic increase in the number of immunocompromised patients over the past two decades. The most common causes of immunosuppression are the acquired immunodeficiency syndrome (AIDS), hematologic malignancy such as leukemia or lymphoma, chemotherapy of tumors, and organ transplantation with consecutive medical immunosuppression (Naidich et al. 1998). Most notably, milder forms of immunosuppression may be seen in elderly individuals, pregnant women, alcoholics, and patients with severe malnutrition.

As the lung is particularly susceptible to infection in a compromised host, opportunistic pulmonary infections are an important cause of morbidity and mortality in the immunocompromised population. For example, pneumonia develops in up to 80% of patients with acute leukemia and is seen in up to 50% of organ transplant recipients. The mortality associated with pulmonary infection in the immunocompromised host may approach 50% (McLoud and Naidich 1992).

Pneumonia in the immunocompromised patient may represent a difficult diagnostic problem for the clinician. The spectrum of potentially causative organisms is exceedingly broad. Moreover, sputum and BAL cultures are frequently negative or contain more than one potential pathogen; thus, differentiation between contaminative, colonized, or pathogenic organisms is generally difficult. Further diagnostic invasive procedures in immunocompromised patients with thrombocytopenia or coagulopathy are problematic and are therefore frequently avoided by the clinicians. In order to make a meaningful contribution to the management of these patients, background information, such as the cause of immunodeficiency, current immunosuppressive therapy, white blood cell count (particularly the CD4 + count in AIDS patients), and overall medical status should be gathered, since these will serve as important diagnostic guides. When this information is available it is possible to extend the traditional role of a radiologist from one limited to detection and monitoring of pulmonary abnormalities.

Many of the bacteria causing CAP in the healthy community are also responsible for complicated infections in this high-risk group. In AIDS patients major causative agents for pneumonia include *Pneumocystis carinii* pneumonia (PCP; Fig. 7.9), *Mycobacterium tuberculosis*, and the *Mycobacterium avium* complex (Fig. 7.10; Chaisson and Pa 1995).

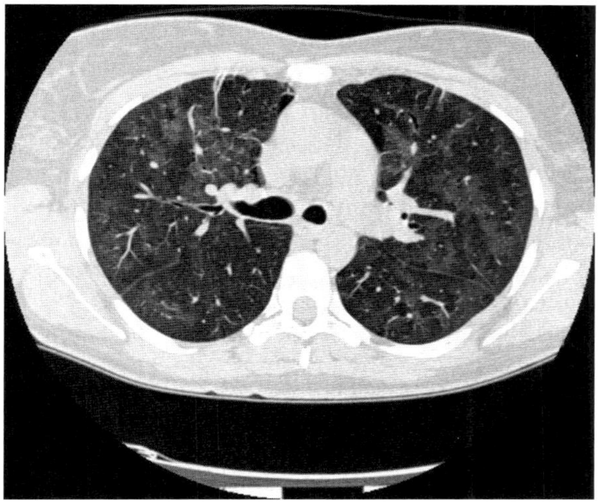

Fig. 7.9. *Pneumocystis carinii* pneumonia in a 36-year-old HIV-positive woman. Chest CT scan (collimation 12×0.75 mm) shows extensive, bilateral areas of ground-glass opacity which are found in a geographic distribution

Manifestation of opportunistic infections depends on the CD4+ cell count. Patients with CD4+cell counts of >200 cells/mm^3 are predisposed to bronchial infections and bacterial pneumonia, whereas patients with CD4+ counts of <200 cells/mm^3 are mainly predisposed to opportunistic infections such as PCP (Shah et al. 1997). The classic thin-section CT finding in PCP consists of extensive ground-glass opacities, corresponding to intraalveolar fluid exudation, often patchy or geographically distributed, with a predilection for the perihilar regions (Kuhlmann 1996). Recent literature describes the changing face of PCP as the classic radiographic presentation is being encountered less frequently (Boiselle et al. 1999): The most prevalent trend has been an increased frequency of diffuse cystic lung disease with description of cysts of different shapes, sizes, and varying degrees of wall thickness predisposing to spontaneous pneumothoraces. Upper lobe predominance of parenchymal opacities has been recognized in patients undergoing aerosolized pentamidine inhalation therapy and was initially explained by the insufficient agent distribution into the upper lobes when inhaling in an upright position. Other reports have also documented upper lobe predominance in patients without pentamidine prophylaxis. Atypical radiological features include parenchymal abnormalities as lung nodules and masses (varying in size from 2 mm to 1 cm in diameter), lobar consolidation, and interstitial fibrosis with septal thickening, bronchiectasis, and honeycombing. Nodules may also undergo calcification and rarely cavitation. Other described features are mediastinal and hilar lymph node enlargement and pleural effusion (Gruden et al. 1997).

Although *Candida* is the most common opportunistic mycosis, it rarely causes pneumonia in the absence of disseminated disease. End-stage AIDS patients and patients with severe neutropenia are more often affected by *Aspergillus fumigatus* (Fig. 7.11), causing bronchial invasive aspergillosis with clinical manifestation of acute tracheobronchitis, bronchiolitis, and bronchopneumonia. Typical thin-section CT features of angioinvasive aspergillosis are characterized by the presence of centrilobular nodules with patchy distribution and branching linear or nodular opacities giving an appearance resembling a "tree-in-bud" (Aquino et al. 1994). Conolly et al. (1999) summarized several forms of aspergillosis. Invasive pulmonary aspergillosis in patients with severe immunodeficiency is characterized on radiographs by multiple ill-defined 1- to 3-mm peripheral nodules, gradually coalescing into masses or areas of consolidation. An additional findings on CT scans are a rim of surrounding ground-glass attenuation surrounding the nodules (CT-halo sign) and the well-known air-crescent sign, indicating central cavitation. Chronic necrotizing or semiinvasive aspergillosis typically occurs in patients with mild immunodeficiency. It manifests with slowly progressive cavitary consolidation, which usually affects the upper lobes. Two forms of tracheo-

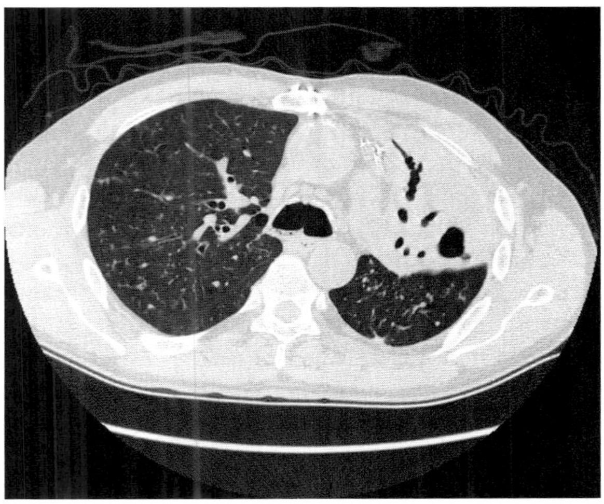

Fig. 7.10. *Mycobacterium avium* infection in a 59-year-old man. Chest CT scan (collimation 8×1.25 mm) shows left upper lobe consolidation with central necrosis and multiple centrilobular nodules in the superior segment of the left lower lobe as well as right upper lobe

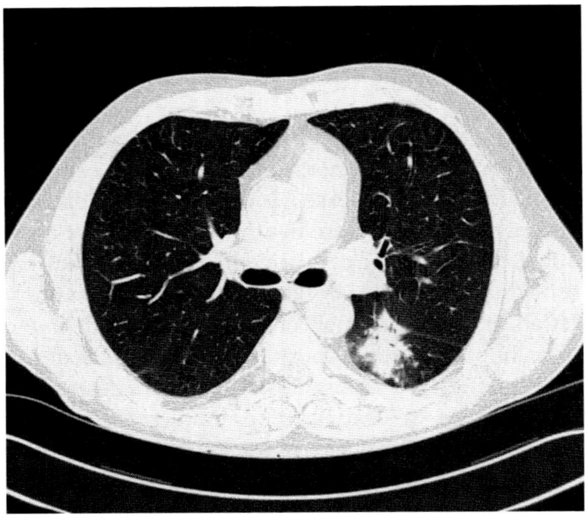

Fig. 7.11. Invasive aspergillosis in a 55-year-old man with acute myeloid leukemia. Chest CT scan (collimation 12×0.75 mm) shows nodule with surrounding ground-glass attenuation ("CT halo sign") in the superior segment of the left lower lobe

bronchial aspergillosis are described: invasive tracheobronchial and obstructing bronchopulmonary aspergillosis. Invasive tracheobronchial aspergillosis is commonly reported in patients after bone marrow or lung transplantation and is characterized by radiographic and CT findings of bronchial wall thickening, multiple poorly defined nodular opacities, atelectasis, and consolidation. Obstructing bronchopulmonary aspergillosis, typically seen in end-stage AIDS patients, is caused by an overgrowth of fungus within the tracheobronchial system without airway wall infiltration, and radiologically manifests as large mucoid impactions ("finger-in-glove sign") predominantly in the upper lobes (Conolly et al. 1999).

Occasionally, helminths, such as *Strongyloides stercoralis* (Fig. 7.12), cause pulmonary infections; however, in recent years severe disease (so-called hyperinfection) has been recognized in the immunocompromised AIDS population and in patients with asthma or chronic obstructive pulmonary disease receiving corticosteroid therapy (Fraser et al. 1994). Although reports are few, small nodules superimposed on diffuse interstitial infiltrates have been described (Makris et al. 1993). Other authors have described migratory pulmonary consolidations without recognizable segmental distribution most likely due to an allergic reaction in the lung parenchyma. Blood and sputum eosinophilia were often present, and the entity was therefore included as one of the causes of acute pulmonary infiltrates with eosinophilia (Löffler's syndrome; Armstrong et al. 2000).

Impaired host immunity is a predisposing factor for development of postprimary tuberculosis. Ikezoe and associates evaluated the CT features of pulmonary tuberculosis in immunocompromised patients compared with other patients without underlying disease and found that immunocompromised patients, who demonstrated a high prevalence of nonsegmental distribution of infiltrates and multiple small cavities within any given lesion, had a somewhat different presentation compared to patients without underlying disease who had a more segmental distribution of lesions in a single cavity within a given lesion (Ikezoe et al. 1992).

In bone marrow transplant (BMT) recipients, pulmonary infections occur in up to 50% of patients and the onset of new infiltrates on chest radiographs should prompt an early definitive diagnosis. The CMV is the most significant viral infection that occurs in BMT patients with a described prevalence of 50–70% of allogenic BMT recipients within a typical onset time of 1–4 months after transplantation. One-third of patients develop CMV pneumonia approximately 50–60 days after bone marrow transplantation (Cunningham 1992). Radiological findings of pulmonary CMV are nonspecific and may consist of lobar consolidation, diffuse and focal parenchymal haziness, and multiple small nodules with associated perifocal ground-glass attenuation ("halo"; McGuiness et al. 1994).

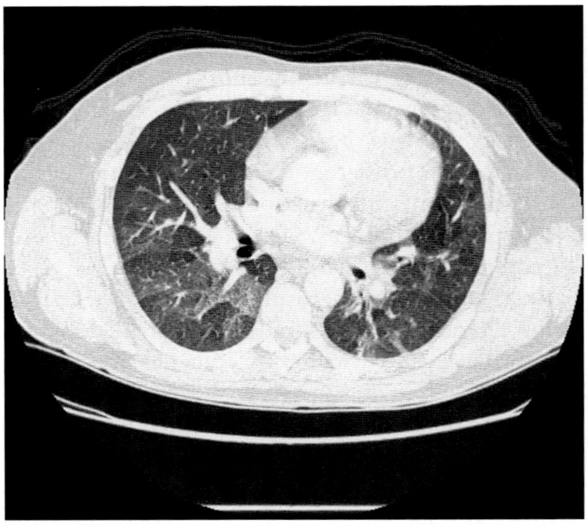

Fig. 7.12. *Strongyloides* in a 36-year-old man. Chest CT scan (collimation 16×1.25 mm) shows nonspecific bilateral areas of ground-glass opacity

Similar to patients after solid organ transplantation, the timeline of infections that occur in BMT recipients can be divided into three distinct periods differentiated on the basis of neutrophil count and degree of medical immunosuppression: 0–30 days post-, 30–120 days post-, and >120 days post-transplantation. In the early neutropenic phase, immediately after marrow ablative chemo- and radiation therapy, opportunistic fungi, such as *Aspergillus*, account for the majority of infections. While bacteremias are common, bacterial pneumonias are rare due to the widespread use of empiric broad-spectrum antibiotics for febrile episodes. In the second phase, after marrow engraftment and recovery of neutrophils, persistent deficits in cellular and humoral immunity predispose to infections with viruses, and more specifically CMV, which accounts for the majority of infections during this period. In the late post-transplantation period (>120 days), autologous recipients and allogeneic recipients without graft vs host disease (GVHD) experience relatively few late infections. Most infections occur in the setting of chronic GVHD which predisposes allogeneic recipients to infections with bacteria and opportunistic fungi (Leung et al. 1999).

Typical radiographic pattern for herpes simplex virus (HSV) pneumonia as a representative for viral pulmonary infection is diffuse and multifocal parenchymal disease with a patchy, predominantly ground-glass pattern with scattered, less dominant areas of consolidation (Aquino et al. 1998). Especially in immunocompromised patients, CT findings were described as helpful in narrowing the differential diagnoses of *Varicella zoster* pneumonia. In addition to multiple diffuse bilateral 5- to 10-mm ill-defined partially confluent intrapulmonary nodules seen on chest radiographs, CT scans also demonstrated nodules with surrounding ground-glass attenuation, patchy ground-glass opacities, and coalescence of lesions (Kim et al. 1999).

7.4 Combined Analysis of Radiologic Pattern and Clinical Setting

Many of the previously described imaging patterns are common knowledge from conventional chest X-rays. The knowledge of these signs and the distribution of abnormalities may be helpful for interpretation of MDCT images since coronal reformatted images closely resemble conventional chest films in the posterior anterior projection. In chest imaging, the value of multiplanar reformatted (MPR) images has been previously demonstrated for limited regions of interest (e.g., airway lesions, pulmonary vessels; Quint et al. 1995; Remy-Jardin et al. 1995; Storto et al. 1998); however, the value of coronal MPRs of the whole chest is still under evaluation for assessment of inflammatory lung diseases. To date, only casuistic descriptions are available regarding the value of MPR images (Johkoh et al. 2002). Multiplanar reconstructions may allow better depiction of the pattern and distribution of findings, thus improving recognition of abnormalities and narrowing the differential diagnosis.

Generally, MDCT findings of pneumonia are nonspecific and diagnosis of a specific microbial organism is frequently not possible. Ground-glass opacities, air-space consolidations, cavitations, defined linear opacities, and especially poorly defined nodules, are early indicators for pulmonary infections (Siegelmann et al. 1986; Kauczor et al. 1996; Aberle 1993). As a general rule of thumb, localized segmental or lobar alveolar densities can be attributed to typical or atypical bacterial infections. In CAP, the main feature differentiating the two groups is the presence of centrilobular nodules which are much more frequently found in atypical bacterial pneumonia (*Mycoplasma pneumonia*: 89%), viral (77%), and fungal pneumonia (65%), as compared with typical bacterial pneumonia (17%; Reittner et al. 2003).

Diffuse bilateral interstitial and/or interstitial alveolar infiltrates most commonly are caused by viruses, atypical bacteria, and protozoa. A predominantly nodular pattern of pneumonia is seen with a variety of infections. Fungal pneumonia characteristically manifests as multiple, ill-defined nodules that may gradually coalesce to form a mass or an area of air-space consolidation (Conolly et al. 1999; Kuhlmann et al. 1988). In viral pneumonia, nodules are typically associated with a background of diffuse ground-glass attenuation and/or reticulation (Conolly et al. 1999; McGuiness et al. 1994). In *Mycoplasma pneumoniae* and bacterial pneumonias caused by *Nocardia*, *Staphylococcus aureus*, and *Pseudomonas aeruginosa*, nodules may extend to involve the entire secondary pulmonary lobule (Reittner et al. 2000; Worthy et al. 1995).

In HIV-infected patients having one or more pulmonary nodules on chest CT scan, opportunistic infections are the most common cause. Specific clinical and radiographic features can suggest particular opportunistic infections. Fever, cough, and size of nodules less than 1 cm on chest CT were identified as independent predictors of having an opportunistic infection. Furthermore, a history of bacterial pneumonia, symptoms for 1–7 days, and size of nodules less than 1 cm on CT independently predicts a diagnosis of bacterial pneumonia. A history of homelessness, weight loss, and lymphadenopathy on CT independently predicted a diagnosis of tuberculosis (Jasmer et al. 2000).

The significance of ground-glass attenuation depends on the immune status of the patients. In immunocompromised patients, the presence of extensive, diffuse, bilateral ground-glass attenuation is highly suggestive for *Pneumocystis carinii* pneumonia (Gruden et al. 1997). This pattern was demonstrated to be present in up to 94% of AIDS patients with PCP (Hartmann et al. 1994). In immunocompromised patients who do not have AIDS and in immunocompetent patients with pneumonia, areas of ground-glass attenuation are a common but non-specific finding. Although viral pneumonia may produce extensive areas of ground-glass attenuation, viral infections are commonly associated with nodules and focal or diffuse areas of air-space consolidation (McGuiness et al. 1994; Kang et al. 1996). In *Mycoplasma pneumoniae* pneumonia, focal areas of ground-glass attenuation in association with centrilobular nodules are frequently present. These focal areas of ground-glass attenuation often have a lobar distribution (Reittner et al. 2000). In bacterial and fungal pneumonias areas of ground-glass attenuation tend to be minor findings adjacent to areas of air-space consolidation and nodules (Conolly et al 1999). Reticulation is a non-specific feature in all groups of pneumonias and may be associated with air-space consolidation, ground-glass attenuation, and nodules (Reittner et al. 2003). Micronodular disease is most often caused by miliary TB ("miliary pattern"), candidiasis, and histoplasmosis (small nodules), or viruses such as herpes or varicella zoster virus (diffuse nodules with hazy borders). Large, nodular lesions may represent bacterial abscesses, and in immunocompromised patients, may be caused by invasive aspergillosis and *Nocardia*.

Chest radiography is still the mainstay and primary imaging method in patients with suspected CAP. Diagnosis and disease management most frequently rely on chest radiography and do not require the use of further diagnostic tests. In these patients, MDCT scanning and invasive diagnostic procedures are reserved only for cases in which treatment failure or complications, such as abscess formation, influence the course of the disease. Conversely, in nosocomial or opportunistic infections, cross-sectional imaging techniques and invasive procedures, such as needle or bronchoscopically guided biopsies, are more often required, underlined by the fact that in most large series of pneumonia a causative organisms cannot be identified in 25–45% of patients even when extensive noninvasive diagnostic tests are performed. The NP are associated with a high mortality rate, ranging from 20 to 50%; thus, identification of the causative organism is more intensively pursued, with the use of fiberoptic bronchoscopic lavage, brushing, and/or biopsy. In many institutions, imaging methods, such as CT scans, are used for the guidance of invasive methods into areas of most severe involvement. The MDCT images (e.g., MPRs, virtual bronchoscopy) may also serve as a "road map" to direct fiberoptic bronchoscopy towards the lesion.

The use of transthoracic CT aspiration needle biopsy in the diagnosis of pulmonary infection is controversial. Nevertheless, when noninvasive techniques used to identify the underlying organism, such as sputum examination and cultures, are nondiagnostic, a choice must be made between empiric therapy and an invasive diagnostic test. While the majority of patients are treated empirically, the nature and course of pneumonias in nosocomial infections and in immunosuppressed individuals frequently dictates a more aggressive approach. In such cases, transthoracic needle biopsy may help to identify the causative organism (Sanchez-Nieto et al. 1998). Sanchez-Nieto et al. (1998) reviewed a series of 441 transthoracic needle aspiration biopsies to evaluate the use of the procedure in the diagnosis of pulmonary infections. In 67 patients in whom pulmonary infection was suspected, a specific diagnosis was made with needle biopsy in 45 cases. In 46 cases in which infection was ultimately found to be present, aspiration biopsy identified the organism in 35 cases. Overall, clinically useful information was obtained in 81% of aspiration biopsies performed for pulmonary infection. Since other authors have reported similar results, needle biopsy should be considered an important component of the radiologist's armamentarium in diagnosing and managing pulmonary infections.

It has been shown that even a small number of thin-section CT images provides adequate assessment of diffuse lung diseases (Kazerooni et al. 1997); thus, volumetric imaging throughout the chest is not likely to provide a significant advantage in the assessment of these patients. Furthermore, the potential benefits from volumetric imaging in these patients may be outweighed by the potential risks of the increased radiation exposure (Honda et al. 2002).

Overall, the role of MDCT in suspected or proven pneumonia can be summarized as follows: firstly, MDCT is a valuable tool in early diagnosis of pneumonia, especially in patient groups in which such an early diagnosis is important (immunocompromised patients and critically ill patients). Secondly, MDCT can aid in the characterization and localization of pulmonary infections and may suggest an etiologic diagnosis. Thirdly, MDCT is an excellent tool in assessing complications such as bronchopleural fistula. Fourthly, MDCT is required in the investigation of patients with persistent and recurrent pulmonary infiltrates.

References

Aberle DR (1993) HRCT in acute lung disease. J Thorac Imaging 8:200–212

A'Court C, Garrard CS (1992) Nosocomial pneumonia in the intensive care unit: mechanisms and significance. Thorax 47:465–473

American Thoracic Society (1996) Hospital-acquired pneumonia in adults: diagnosis, assessment of severity, initial antimicrobial therapy and preventive strategies. Am J Respir Crit Care Med 153:1711–1725

Armstrong P, Wilson EG, Paul D et al. (2000) Imaging of diseases of the chest, 3rd edn. Mosby, London

Aquino SL, Kee ST, Warnock ML et al. (1994) Pulmonary aspergillosis: imaging findings with pathologic correlation. Am J Roentgenol 163:811–815

Aquino SL, Dunagan DP, Chiles C et al. (1998) Herpes simplex virus I pneumonia: pattern on CT scans and conventional chest radiographs. J Comput Assist Tomogr 22:795–800

Boiselle PM, Crans CA, Kaplan MA (1999) The changing face of *Pneumocystis carinii* pneumonia in AIDS patients. Am J Roentgenol 172:1301–1309

Chaisson RE, Pa V (1995) Clinical manifestations of HIV infection. In: Mandell GL, Benett JE, Dolin R (eds) Principles and practice of infectious disease, 4th edn. Churchill Livingstone, New York, pp 1231–1236

Conolly JE, McAdams HP, Erasmus JJ et al. (1999) Opportunistic fungal infections. J Thorac Imaging 14:51–62

Cunningham I (1992) Pulmonary infections after bone marrow transplant. Semin Resp Infect 7:132–138

Eickhoff TC (1982) Nosocomial infections. N Engl J Med 306: 1545

Eisenhuber E (2002) The tree-in-bud sign. Radiology 222: 771–772

Franquet T (2001) Imaging of pneumonia: trends and algorithms. Eur Respir J 18:196–208

Fraser RS, Paré PJA, Fraser RG et al. (1994) Synopsis of diseases of the chest, 2nd edn. Saunders, Philadelphia, pp 287–395

Gharib AM, Stern EJ (2001) Radiology of pneumonia. Med Clin North Am 85:1461–1491

Gruden J, Huang L, Turner J et al. (1997) High-resolution CT in the evaluation of clinically suspected *Pneumocystis carinii* pneumonia in AIDS patients with normal, equivocal, or nonspecific radiographic findings. Am J Roentgenol 169: 967–975

Hartmann T, Primack S, Müller NL et al. (1994) Diagnosis of thoracic complications in AIDS: accuracy on CT. Am J Roentgenol 162:547–553

Honda O, Johkoh T, Yamamoto S et al. (2002) Comparison of quality of multiplanar reconstructions and direct coronal multidetector CT scans of the lung. Am J Roentgenol 179: 875–879

Ichikado K, Johkoh T, Ikeoe J et al. (1997) Acute interstitial pneumonia: radiographic and CT findings correlated with pathology. Am J Roentgenol 168:333–338

Ikezoe J, Takeuchi N, Johkoh T et al. (1992) CT appearance of pulmonary tuberculosis in diabetic and immunocompromised patients: comparison with patients who had no underlying disease. Am J Roentgenol 159:1175–1179

Jasmer RM, Edinburgh KJ, Thompson A et al. (2000) Clinical and radiographic predictors of the etiology of pulmonary nodules in HIV-infected patients. Chest 117:1023–1030

Johkoh T, Müller NL, Nakamura H (2002) Multidetector spiral high-resolution computed tomography of the lungs: distribution of findings on coronal image reconstructions. J Thorac Imaging 17:291–305

Julander I (1983) Staphylococcal septicaemia and endocarditis in 80 drug addicts. Scand J Infect Dis 41:S49–S54

Kang EJ, Patz E, Müller NL (1996) Cytomegalovirus pneumonia in transplant patients: CT findings. J Comput Assist Tomogr 20:295–299

Katz DS, Leung AN (1999) Radiology of pneumonia. Clin Chest Med 20:549–562

Kauczor HU, Heussel CP, Mildenberger P et al. (1996) How is it called? Scheme glossary for reporting and understanding HRCT of the lung. Fortschr Röntgenstr 165:428–437

Kazerooni EA, Martinez EF, Flint A et al. (1997) Thin-section CT obtained at 10 mm increments versus limited three-level thin-section CT for idiopathic pulmonary fibrosis: correlation with pathologic scoring. Am J Roentgenol 169:977–983

Kim JS, Ryu CW, Lee SI et al. (1999) High resolution CT findings of *Varicella zoster* pneumonia. Am J Roentgenol 172: 113–116

Kuhlmann JE (1996) Pneumocystis infections: the radiologist's perspective. Radiology 198:623–635

Kuhlmann J, Fishman EK, Burch PA et al. (1988) CT of invasive pulmonary aspergillosis. Am J Roentgenol 150:1015–1020

Leung AN, Gosselin MV, Napper CH et al. (1999) Pulmonary infections after bone marrow transplantation: clinical and radiographic findings. Radiology 210:699–710

Levy M, Dromer F, Biron N et al. (1988) Community acquired pneumonia. Importance of initial noninvasive bacteriologic and radiographic investigations. Chest 92:43–48

Lynch JP (2001) Hospital-acquired pneumonia: risk factors, microbiology, and treatment. Chest 119:373S–384S

Makris AN, Sher S, Bertoli C et al. (1993) Pulmonary strongyloidiasis: an unusual opportunistic pneumonia in a patient with AIDS. Am J Roentgenol 161:545–547

38. McGuiness G, Scholes JV, Garay SM et al. (1994) Cytomegalovirus pneumonitis: spectrum of parenchymal CT findings with pathologic correlation in 21 AIDS patients. Radiology 192:451–459

McLoud TC, Naidich DP (1992) Thoracic disease in the immuno-compromised patient. Radiol Clin North Am 30: 552–554

Moine P, Vercken JB, Chevret S et al. (1994) Severe community-acquired pneumonia; etiology, epidemiology, and prognosis factors. Chest 105:487–495

Naidich DP, Müller NL, Zerhouni EA et al. (1998) Computed tomography and magnetic resonance of the thorax, 3rd edn. Lippincott-Raven, New York, p 447

Niedermans MS, McCombs JS, Unger AN et al. (1998) The cost of treating community acquired pneumonia. Clin Ther 20: 820–837

Quint LE, Whyte RI, Kazerooni et al. (1995) Stenosis of the central airways: evaluation by using helical CT with multiplanar reconstructions. Radiology 194:871–877

Reittner P, Müller NL, Heyneman L et al. (2000) *Mycoplasma pneumoniae* pneumonia: radiographic and high-resolution CT features in 28 patients. Am J Roentgenol 174:37–41

Reittner P, Ward S, Heyneman L et al. (2003) Pneumonia: high-resolution CT findings in 114 patients. Eur Radiol 13:515–521

Remy-Jardin M, Remy J, Wallaert B et al. (1993) Subacute and chronic bird breed hypersensitivity pneumonitis: sequential evaluation with CT and correlation with lung function tests and bronchoalveolar lavage. Radiology 198: 111–118

Remy-Jardin M, Remy J, Cauvain O et al. (1995) Diagnosis of central pulmonary embolism with helical CT: role of two-dimensional multiplanar reformations. Am J Roentgenol 165:1131–1138

Saikku P (1997) Atypical respiratory pathogens. Clin Microbiol Infect 3:599–604

Sanchez-Nieto JM, Torres A, Garcia-Corboda F et al. (1998) Impact of invasive and noninvasive quantitative culture sampling on outcome of ventilator associated pneumonia. Am J Respir Crit Care Med 157:371–376

Schaefer-Prokop C, Prokop M, Fleischmann D et al. (2000) High resolution CT of diffuse interstitial lung disease: key findings in common disorders. Eur Radiol 11:373–392

Shah RM, Kaji AV, Ostrum BJ et al. (1997) Interpretation of chest radiographs in AIDS patients: usefulness of CD4 lymphocyte counts. Radiographics 17:47–58

Siegelmann SS, Khuori NF, Leo FB et al. (1986) Solitary pulmonary nodules: CT assessment. Radiology 160:307–312

Slone M, Gutierrez F, AJ F (1999) Thoracic imaging, 1st edn. A practical approach. McGraw-Hill, New York, pp 75–86

Spencer H (1985) Pathology of the lung, 4th edn. Pergamon Press, Oxford

Storto ML, Ciccotosto C, Guidotti A et al. (1998) Neoplastic extension across pulmonary fissures: value of spiral computed tomography and multiplanar reformations. J Thorac Imaging 1998:204–210

Tan Kendrick AP, Ling H, Subramaniam R et al. (2002) The value of early CT in complicated childhood pneumonia. Pediatr Radiol 32:16–21

Tanaka N, Masumoto T, Kuramitsu T et al. (1996) High resolution CT findings in community-acquired pneumonia. J Comput Assist Tomogr 20:600–608

Winer-Murham HT, Steiner RM, Gurney JW et al. (1998) Ventilator-associated pneumonia in patients with adult respiratory distress syndrome: CT evaluation. Radiology 208:193–199

Worthy S, Kang E, Müller NL (1995) Acute lung disease in the immunocompromised host: differential diagnosis on high-resolution CT. Semin Ultrasound CT MRI 16:353–360

8 Multidetector CT Evaluation of Acute Respiratory Distress Syndrome

L. R. Goodman and L. Gattinoni

CONTENTS

8.1 Introduction

In 1967, Ashbaugh et al. reported on 12 patients who developed acute dyspnea, tachypnea, refractory hypoxia, and diffuse bilateral infiltrates on the chest radiograph. In each patient, symptoms had developed after a major systemic insult. They coined the term "adult respiratory distress syndrome" [subsequently termed acute respiratory distress syndrome] (ARDS), a syndrome distinct from Respiratory Distress of the Newborn. Over the next three decades, these terms have been applied loosely and often imprecisely to many forms of respiratory failure in the adult and in children beyond the neonatal period.

In response to the uncertain criteria and uncertain clinical definitions of ARDS, the American-European Consensus Conference (AECC) more rigorously defined the condition so that research and clinical studies could proceed using more uniform criteria (Bernard et al. 1994). The AECC subdivided respiratory failure into two groups: "Acute Lung Injury" (ALI) and the more severe form, "Acute Respiratory Distress Syndrome" (ARDS). The term "Adult" was dropped in recognition of the occurrence of these conditions in children, as well. Although these changes are a significant move forward in defining ARDS, they are still a somewhat general definition and do not distinguish between the varied etiologies of ALI/ARDS, and they do not explain the varied responses to treatment. According to the AECC classification, a major systemic insult causing respiratory insufficiency is described as Acute Lung Injury (ALI), and its more severe form is termed Acute Respiratory Distress Syndrome (ARDS). The syndrome requires the following for diagnosis: acute onset of respiratory insufficiency, pulmonary artery wedge pressure of <18 mmHg (no CHF) and bilateral infiltrates on the chest X-ray. In ALI, the PaO_2/FiO_2 is >300 mmHg and in ARDS, it is >200 mmHg.

Prior to the use of CT to study ALI/ARDS, the basic *in vivo* morphologic understanding was derived from the portable radiograph, an imperfect tool under the best of circumstances. Emphasis was placed on radiographic appearance, correlation with clinical parameters, and temporal progression. To paraphrase Putman's 1983 description (Putman and Ravin 1983):

1) The X-ray is usually normal at the onset of symptoms.
2) At 24 hours, there is perihilar haze and radiating linear densities consistent with interstitial edema.
3) Over the next 24 hours, the densities coalesce and resemble edema or pneumonitis.
4) Once established, the radiograph is often stable for days.

Not overtly stated, but implied by most descriptions of "diffuse infiltrate," was the assumption that the lungs are relatively uniformly involved. Physiologically, the lungs were thought to be "stiff" (low compliance). Since these humble beginnings, a better definition of ARDS has been established and CT has provided valuable morphologic and physiologic insights, markedly changing our understanding of this often fatal condition.

L. R. Goodman, MD, FACR
Director, Thoracic Imaging, Medical College of Wisconsin, 9200 West Wisconsin Avenue, Milwaukee, WI 53226-3596 USA
L. Gattinoni, MD, FRCP
Professor of Anesthesiology, Istituto di Anestesia e Rianimazione, Università degli Studi di Milano, Ospedale Maggiore di Milano Italy I.R.C.C.S.

When body CT was first introduced in the 1970 s, there was little interest in studying ARDS. The time per axial image was long (8 to 18 seconds per image) and scanners were not readily available for this type of application. Furthermore, the lungs were thought to be homogeneously involved, and therefore CT was thought to offer little additional diagnostic or physiologic information. Pioneering articles by Maunder et al. (1986) and Gattinoni et al. (1986) showed that ARDS was surprisingly heterogeneous, *not* homogeneous, and scanning was now rapid enough to study the lung in different phases of respiration. Helical CT, and now multidetector CT, provide very rapid volumetric acquisition, or repeated imaging at a given anatomic level in different phases of respiration. They have and will play an increasing role in the understanding of both lung morphology and physiology in ALI/ARDS. Better temporal and spatial resolution will provide better regional, as well as global, real time imaging and the potential of measuring perfusion changes, as well. What follows is a description of the CT morphology of ARDS and then a description of the functional data derived from CT. A recently published article by Gattinoni et al. (2001a) summarizes many of these topics.

8.2 Morphologic Changes

The radiographic and CT appearance of ALI/ARDS is difficult to characterized succinctly, because the morphologic (i.e., pathologic) lung changes progress rapidly during the first few days, the lung appearance is altered by coexistent or superimposed lung disease, and mechanical ventilation and other interventions change the morphologic appearance of the lung. Therapy may also lead to its own set of unique complications. Nonetheless, some basic patterns have emerged (Goodman 1996; Gattinoni et al. 2001a; Tagliabue et al. 1994; Desai 2002; Pesenti et al. 2001).

8.2.1 Acute Phase

From the beginning, CT refuted the concept that ARDS is homogeneous. It is, in fact, usually heterogeneous and has a somewhat predictable distribution. CT usually reveals areas of apparently normal lung, areas of ground glass opacification, and areas of dense consolidation. Although the radiographic description "ground glass opacification" has many etiologies, in the setting of ALI/ARDS, it is probably due to a combination of interstitial edema, alveolar wall thickening, partial filling of alveoli with edema fluid and cell debris, and diminished aeration due to atelectasis. Areas of alveolar consolidation are more problematic. They may represent collapsed, airless lung, which are potentially re-expandable (recruitable), or they represent areas of complete alveolar filling (edema, pus, or blood), which are not easily expandable. Frequently, both are present.

These varied parenchymal patterns do not occur at random. In ALI/ARDS, the "normal" lung is usually ventral (anterior in the supine patient), the alveolar consolidation is usually dorsal, and the ground glass opacification most often in between (Fig. 8.1) (Gattinoni et al. 1988). In addition to the ventral/dorsal gradient, the density of the lung increases along a craniocaudal axis (Puybasset 1998).

For years, it was assumed that all ALI/ARDS lung injuries were similar, and that similar supportive treatment was appropriate regardless of etiology. Recent work indicates that the etiology of the respiratory insufficiency may influence morphology, pathophysiology, and response to intervention (Goodman et al. 1999; Gattinoni et al. 1998). ALI/ARDS may be due to *direct injury* to the lung from diseases such as pneumonia, aspiration, toxic inhalation, etc. In these instances of direct or *primary* lung injury ($ARDS_P$), the imaging reflects the local lung damage (often air space consolidation), the resulting generalized capillary leak edema (often ground glass opacification), and the subsequent atelectasis from prolonged supine positioning (usually gravity-dependent) (Figs. 8.2, 8.3). Conversely, when the lung injury is secondary to a systemic or *extrapulmonary* insult ($ARDS_{exp}$), such as sepsis, hypotension, or pancreatitis, the CT should show the results of the diffuse capillary leak edema and the dependent atelectasis (Figs. 8.1, 8.4).

Two recent studies indicate that the above morphologic dichotomy is often, but not universally, the case. In a CT study of 22 patients with ARDS due to pulmonary disease ($ARDS_P$) and 11 patients with ARDS due to extra pulmonary disease ($ARDS_{exp}$), we found that approximately 20% of the lung was normal in both $ARDS_p$ and $ARDS_{exp}$. (Goodman et al. 1999) In patients with $ARDS_p$, the volume of ground glass opacification and consolidation were approximately equal, whereas in $ARDS_{exp}$ ground glass opacification was the dominant pattern (Figs. 8.2, 8.3). In $ARDS_{exp}$, airspace consolidation tended to be in gravity-dependent caudal locations (Figs. 8.1, 8.4). Asymmetric and non-grav-

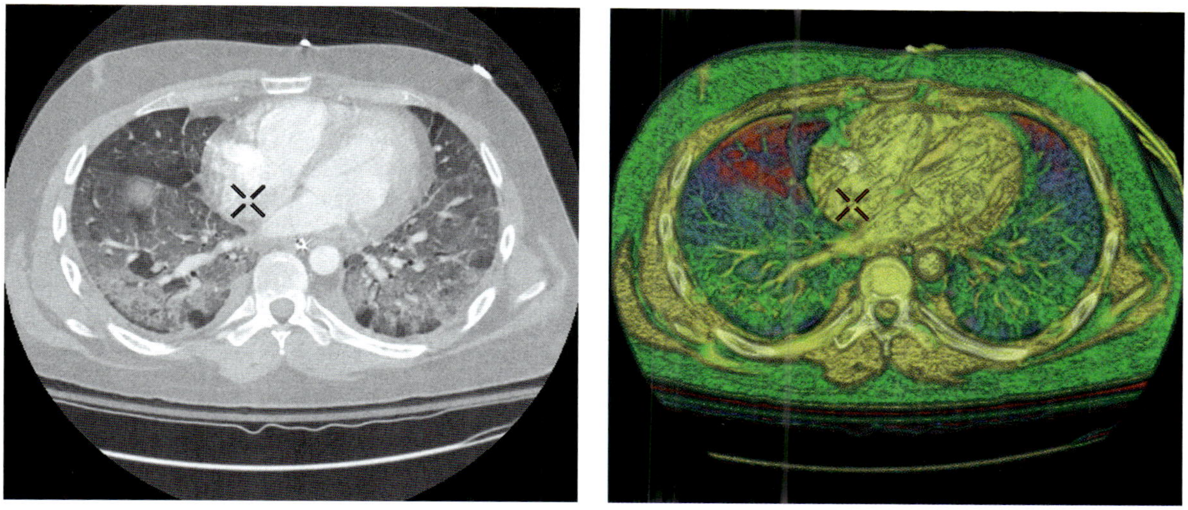

a b

Fig. 8.1. ARDS density gradient. **a** Scan through the lung base shows progressive increased density from ventral to dorsal. **b** Color coded CT shows normally aerated lung in red, ground glass areas in blue, and gravity dependent atelectasis in green

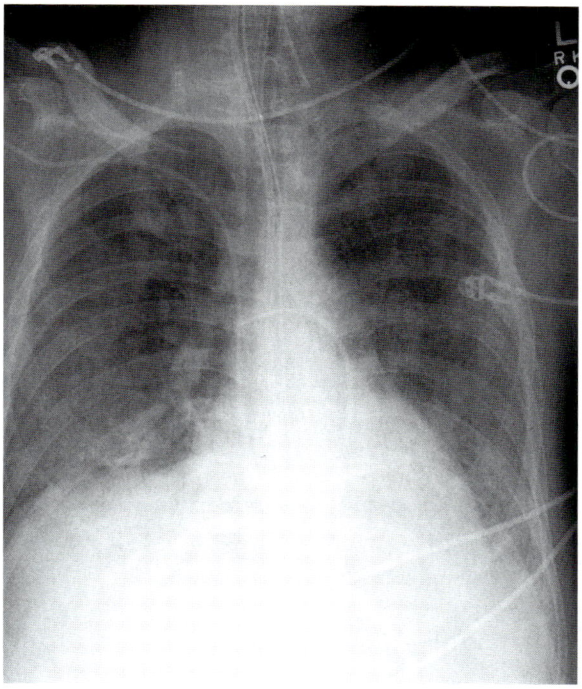

a

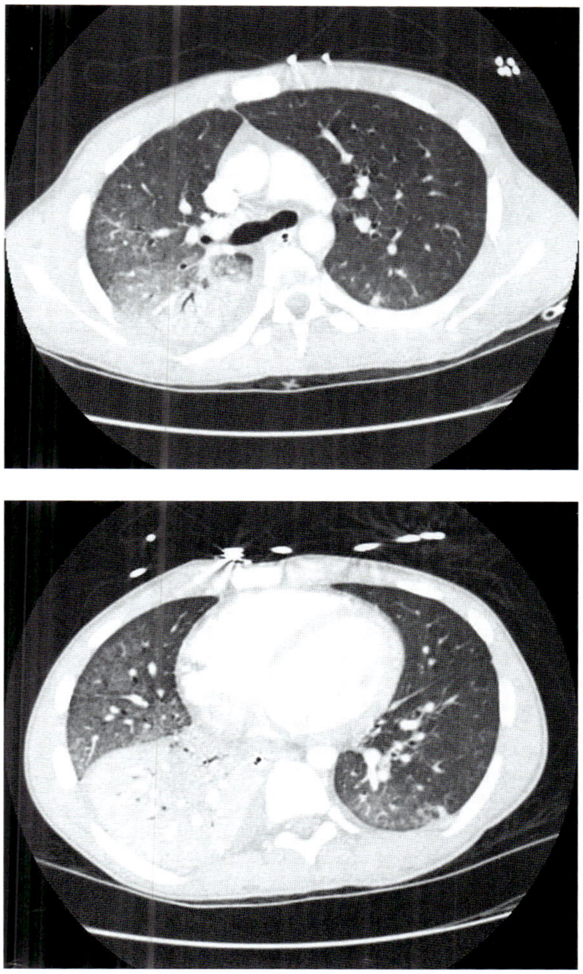

b c

Fig. 8.2. ARDS due to community acquired pneumonia (ARDS$_p$). **a** Chest X-ray shows RLL consolidation and diffuse ground glass opacification. **b** CT through carina shows diffuse ground glass opacification, sparing the ventral lung. There is consolidation of the superior segment of the RLL. **c** CT through the lung base shows right lower lobe dense consolidation due to pneumonia and diffuse ground glass opacification due to ARDS

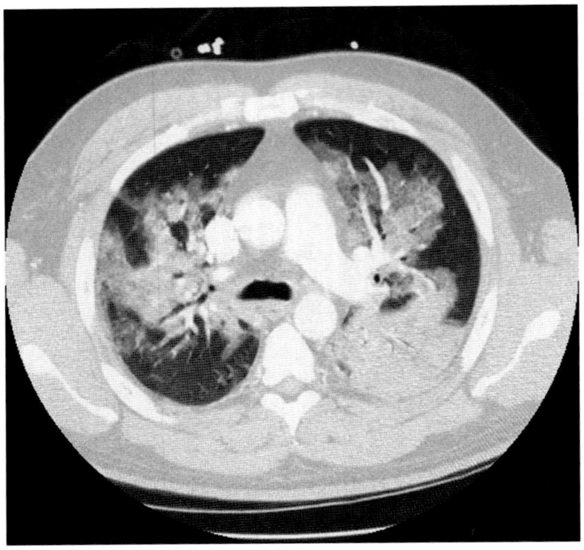

Fig. 8.3. ARDS$_p$. Dense consolidation and a small amount of ground glass opacification characterizes a patient with a hospital acquired bacterial pneumonia and ARDS

ity dependent consolidation was more prominent in ARDS$_p$, usually the primary lung process. DESAI et al. (2001) found similar differences between ARDS$_p$ and ARDS$_{exp}$, but did not find the differences great enough to distinguish between the two pathologic pathways in individual patients. They termed ARDS$_{exp}$, the pattern of ground glass opacification and gravity-dependent atelectasis, "typical" ARDS. This typical pattern was present in 72% of ARDS$_{exp}$ but **also** in 31% of ARDS$_p$ patients. This undoubtedly reflects the complexity of the problem and the multiplicity of processes in the same badly damaged lung.

Conventional radiography seldom demonstrates pleural effusions in ALI/ARDS, but CT scans show small to moderate effusions in approximately half of the patients (GOODMAN et al. 1999). Bronchial dilatation is present in about two-thirds of the lobes of patients with ALI/ARDS. Air bronchograms are present in over 90% of patients. They tend to be more frequent in ARDS$_p$. In our study, more than four segmental air bronchograms were present in 86%

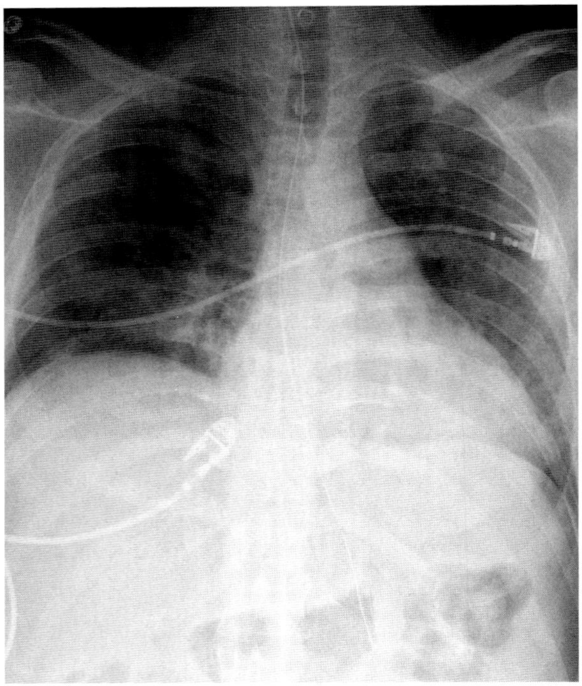

a

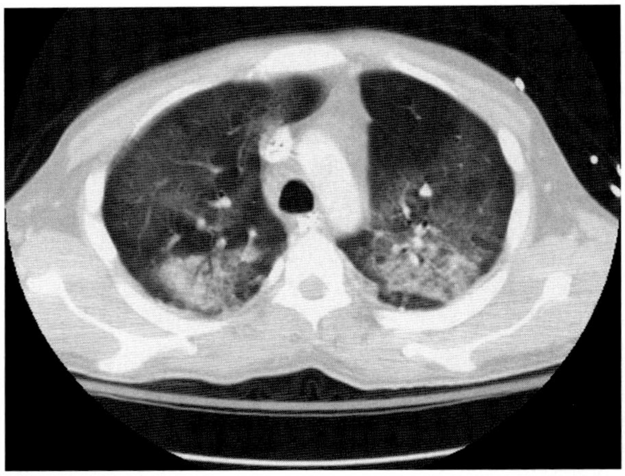

b

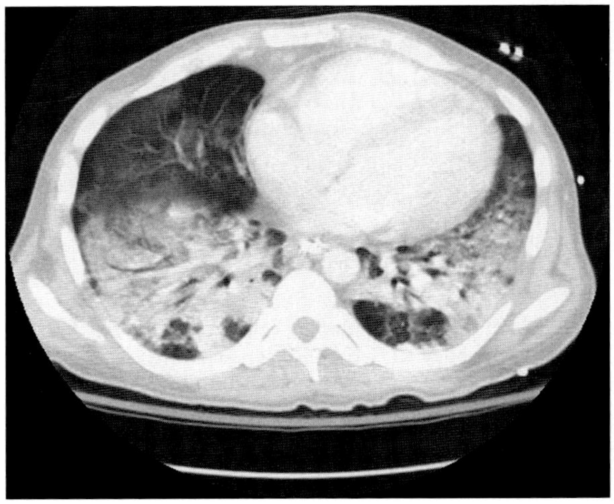

c

Fig. 8.4. ARDS due to extrapulmonary causes (ARDS$_{exp}$). Young male with abdominal sepsis and increasing dyspnea. **a** Chest X-ray after three days of increasing respiratory insufficiency, just prior to intubation. There is diffuse symmetrical ground glass opacification. The lung volumes are low. **b, c** CT scans through the upper and lower thorax show diffuse ground glass opacification, sparing the ventral lung. The dorsal and caudal lung shows more consolidation, at least in part due to atelectasis of $ARDS_p$ patients and in 54% of $ARDS_{exp}$ patients. When high resolution CT is used to study ARDS, septal lines are seen in approximately 80% of patients and lung cysts in approximately 35% of patients (Desai 2001).

Although Kerley lines are seen in many ARDS patients on HRCT, one should be able to distinguish ARDS from CHF. In ARDS, the pulmonary vessels remain normal in size, whereas in CHF, they increase. The arteries are larger than the adjacent bronchi. Peribronchial cuffing and left heart enlargement also indicate CHF. Pleural effusion is seen frequently in both (Goodman 1996).

8.2.2 Subacute Phase

After the early changes of ALI/ARDS are established, progression and resolution are variable. By the second week, overall lung density decreases, the ground glass densities become more heterogeneous, and the interstitium thickens. After several weeks, most of the ground glass opacification resolves and irregular reticulation remains (Desai et al. 1999; Gattinoni et al. 1994, 2001a). Fibrosis causes interstitial distortion and thickening of the bronchovascular markings (Fig. 8.5). The bronchi may dilate further. Beyond the first week or two, emphysematous cysts or pneumatoceles appear. These vary from a few millimeters to several centimeters and are usually associated with prolonged mechanical ventilation (Tagliabue et al. 1994). The cystic structures may be due to cavitation from abscess formation but are usually due to "volutrauma or barotrauma". Abscesses should follow the distribution of the parenchymal infection. Ventilator induced cysts have several proposed etiologies. If found in the nondependent lung, they may be due to alveolar overdistension of the relatively normal low resistance lung. If found in the mid-lung, they may be due to the shearing forces caused by opening and closing of the air spaces in the lung that is recruited by PEEP during inspiration but collapses on expiration because the residual PEEP is insufficient to keep the alveoli open. Pneumatoceles may rupture, giving rise to interstitial emphysema, pneumomediastinum, or pneumothorax.

8.2.3 Late Phase

Within six months, the majority of patients regain normal or near normal respiratory function and a relatively normal chest X-ray. However, CT scanning shows that the majority of patients have residual parenchymal abnormalities. These abnormalities tend to be in the ventral portion of the lung. Distorted reticular densities are most frequently seen (Fig. 8.5). These are often associated with areas of traction bronchiectasis. These scarred areas correspond to the areas of relatively normal lung during the acute phase, rather than the areas of consolidated lung. The degree of fibrosis correlates with the length of mechanical ventilation and with the use of inverse ratio ventilation. It is thought that the ventral lung, which is distensible with mechanical ventilation, is injured by the mechanical overdistension and collapse. Conversely, the densely opacified lung may remain collapsed during the ventilatory cycle and

a

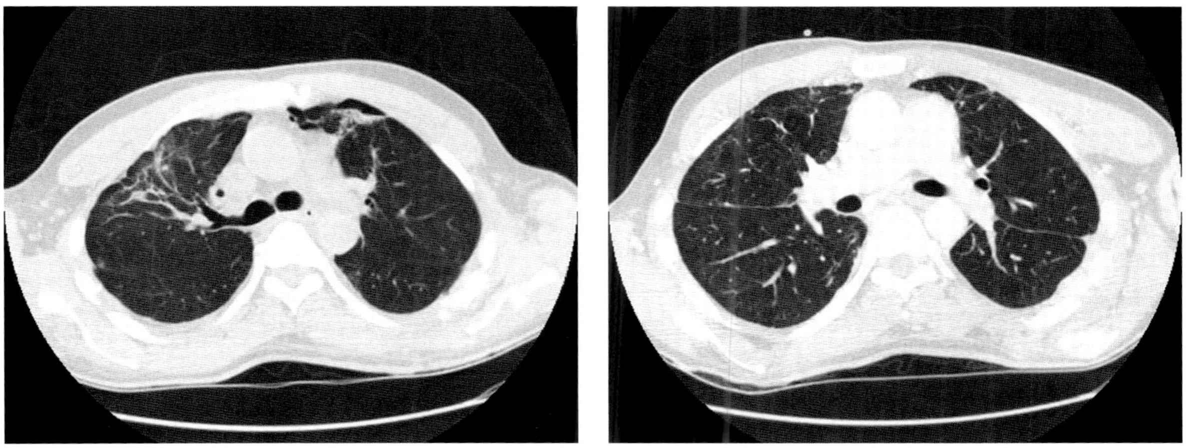

b

Fig. 8.5. Subacute phase. **a** There is residual reticular infiltrate and lung distortion in the ventral portions of the upper lobes, six weeks into $ARDS_{exp}$. **b** Four weeks later, there is improvement consequently not exposed to the trauma of mechanical ventilation or the high FiO_2. It is therefore likely that the residual CT changes are, in part, the iatrogenic sequelae of mechanical ventilation (Desai et al. 1999; Gattinoni et al. 2001a; Nobauer-Huhmann et al. 2001). Clearly, areas of lung abscess, pneumonia, laceration, etc., may cause local scarring.

8.3 Physiologic Changes

Over the last 15 years, numerous investigators have used CT to better understand the physiology of the lung in ALI/ARDS. Initial studies utilized 10 mm axial images, with images limited to 1 to 3 predetermined levels. The lung was studied at these levels under different therapeutic conditions (mechanical ventilation, prone positioning, etc.) (Gattinoni et al. 2001a). The scanning parameters were a compromise between maintaining acceptable radiation levels and achieving an adequate representation of the lung. Currently, helical CT and electron beam CT (improved temporal resolution at the cost of spacial resolution) provide rapid information about the entire lung but at an increased radiation dose. Multidetector CT provides even better spatial and temporal resolution. With the 16-slice multidetector, and very high resolution images (.6 mm), the entire thorax can be scanned in less than 5 seconds. For many applications, a low mA (40 to 80) provides adequate information while minimizing dosage. Stationary subsecond scans can be respiratory or cardiac gated to study temporal changes in ventilation and first pass perfusion. What follows is a very brief review of the morphologic/physiologic correlates elucidated by CT over the last 15 years and a look at some of the newer applications of fast CT and electron beam CT scanning. The results of multidetector studies are just starting to appear as this book goes to press.

Understanding the distribution of gas in the normal lung and the diseased lung, as well as the effects of mechanical ventilation and other maneuvers, rests on the measurement of lung density (Gattinoni et al. 1987, 1988, 2001a). If one assumes that pure air is −1000 Hounsfield units and water (tissue) is 0 Hounsfield units, a voxel of −500 Hounsfield units is 50% air and 50% water (tissue). At functional residual capacity, the lung measures approximately-700 Hounsfield units (70% air and 30% water). In ALI/ARDS, the average lung density is −300 Hu (30% air and 70% water) (Fig. 8.6). Knowing the amount of water and the lung volume, one can calculate the weight of the lung. Unfortunately, the change in density of a voxel does not indicate whether it is due to a change in the amount of air per measured volume or to a change in the amount of tissue per measured volume.

We can compute, for any lung region in which the total volume is known, the volume of gas, the volume of tissue, and the gas to tissue ratio. The later becomes important in understanding lung recruitment during mechanical ventilation. With mechanical ventilation, an increasing gas to tissue ratio, or an increasing number of voxels in the "aerated" range, indicates recruitment of underinflated areas or overinflation of already inflated areas (Figs. 8.7, 8.8). This type of analysis has led to the important reevaluation of the belief that the lung is rigid (noncompliant) in ALI/ARDS. Studying lung mechanics with pressure/volume curves, Gattinoni et al. (1987, 1995) showed that most of the aeration occurs in the relatively normal lungs located ventrally in the supine patient and the amount of aerated lung is strictly correlated with compliance. The consolidated lung changes little. Therefore, the lung is not really "stiff," but the lung is small relative to the tidal volume applied.

As stated earlier, in the supine ALI/ARDS patient, there is a gradient from normal, to ground glass, to consolidation, as one goes ventral to dorsal (Pelosi et al. 1994). Recruitment follows this same gradient. The level of PEEP needed for recruitment of the lung can

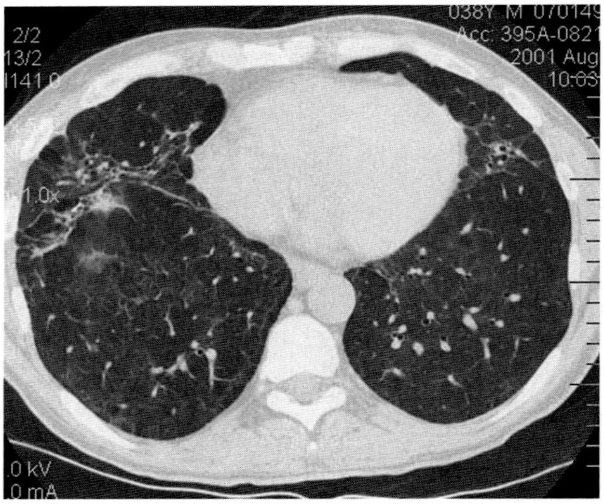

Fig. 8.6. Residual scarring, 11 years after ARDS from pancreatitis. There is marked scarring anteriorly. The remainder of the lung show areas of mosaic attenuation and slight distortion of the interstitial markings. At the time of the ARDS, the patient was 32 years old and was not known to have preexisting lung disease

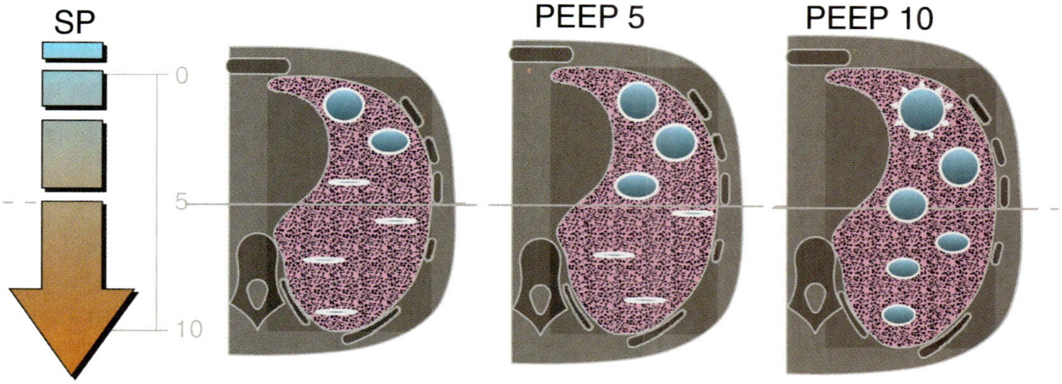

Fig. 8.7. The lungs in three states of inflation. The first depicts the lung at functional residual capacity (zero end expiratory pressure). It demonstrates the diminishing aeration of the alveoli from ventral to dorsal due to increasing superimposed pressure (SP). The next two images indicate the effects of 5 and 10 cm of PEEP on lung inflation. Five mm of PEEP expand the mid-lung zone, where the PEEP exceeds the standing pressure of the lung. Ten mm of PEEP overdistends the ventral lung, completely expands the central lung, and partially overcomes the effects of standing pressure on the dorsal lung

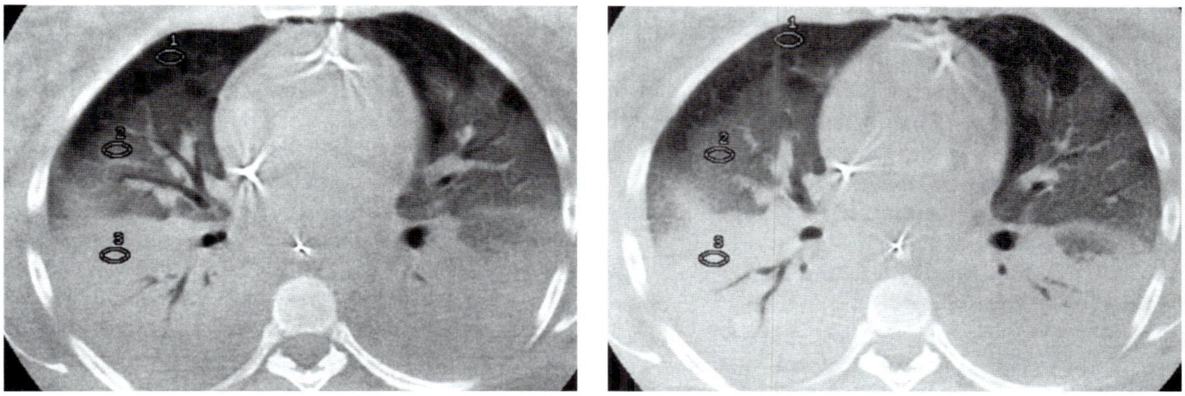

Fig. 8.8. Fig. 8 PEEP effects ¯ $ARDS_{exp}$. A Baseline expiratory CT. B During 10 cc H_2O PEEP, 700 ml tidal volume. Increased aeration most pronounced ventrally. *Zone 1,* diminished 124 Hu. *Zone 2,* diminished 66 Hu. *Zone 3,* diminished 15 Hu (Goodman 1996, with permission)

also be estimated using CT. In the supine patient, the anterior lung weighs on the posterior lung, causing atelectasis (Gattinoni et al. 1998). The lung weight increases when there is increased lung water (edema, pus, etc.). This ventral dorsal gradient is a major cause of gravity dependent atelectasis in both the ICU and in general anesthesia. Moreover, the heart weight may play a role in producing compression atelectasis in the supine patient (Malbouisson et al. 2000). CT has confirmed that the level of PEEP required to recruit nonaerated lung is proportional to the changes along the ventral/dorsal gradient (Fig. 8.7). CT has also confirmed that higher PEEP levels are needed to keep recruited lung "open". The lung in $ARDS_{exp}$ appears to be more easily recruited than the lung in $ARDS_p$ (Gattinoni et al. 1998). As one increases PEEP to recruit the areas of dense consolidation, one overdistends the already recruited areas, sometimes leading to barotrauma with subsequent air leaks or tissue damage (Gattinoni et al. 2001a).

Although three lung images are helpful in understanding the distribution of ventilation and recruitment in the lung, they do not provide the whole story. Puybassat et al. (1998) looked at helical *whole lung* scanning in healthy volunteers and patients with ALI to determine the effects of PEEP induced alveolar recruitment. The entire lung was scanned at functional residual capacity and 15 cm of PEEP. They found that the AP and transverse dimensions of the lungs were similar in patients and normal controls, but in the ALI/SRDS group, craniocaudal dimension was reduced by more than 15% and total lung volume was reduced by 27%. Upper lobe volume differed little from controls but the lower lobes were only 48% of the predicted value. Nonaerated lung was predominantly juxtadiaphragmatic. Recruitment followed a ventral/dorsal and craniocaudal gradient (Fig. 8.4).

The same group (The CT Scan ARDS Study Group – Malbouisson et al. 2001) has also used the helical scanner to take a more detailed look at lung recruitment. They measured improved aeration of *both* areas of ground glass opacification and consolidation, rather than just consolidation alone. They showed alveolar recruitment of approximately 500 ml and alveolar distension or overdistension of approximately 400 ml between expiration and 15 cm of PEEP. They found an excellent correlation (r = .76) between CT measured alveolar recruitment and the increase in PaO_2.

They also revisited how lung morphology interacts with physiologic parameters and prognosis (Rouby et al. 2000). They defined three CT patterns of lung consolidation. The first group (23%) showed diffuse bilateral increased density. Most had primary ARDS, markedly abnormal respiratory mechanics, and an overall mortality rate of 75%. The second group (41%) showed patchy consolidation with increased attenuation throughout. These patients had predominantly primary ARDS, and markedly altered mechanics, but a mortality of only 41%. The third group (36%) showed predominantly lower lobe disease. They were more likely to have extrapulmonary ALI/ARDS, less mechanical derangement, and a mortality rate of 42%. The authors developed an ARDS Severity Score, based on CT features, the degree of hypoxia, the calculated lower inflection point of recruitment, and the slope of the pressure volume curve (see Rouby et al. 2000).

The increased speed of the multidetector scanner provides a more accurate assessment of moment to moment lung inflation and deflation. A recent study of 11 ALI/ARDS patients studied changes continuously throughout the respiratory cycle. It showed that various portions of the lung inflate or deflate at different rates. For the majority of the lung, the time constant of inflation was approximately one second, but as much as 7 seconds for the rest (Yamaguchi et al. 2001).

If the patient is placed in the prone position, the lung weight gradient reverses, dorsal to ventral. In addition, the lung dorsal to the heart is no longer compressed (Albert and Hubmayr 2000). CT demonstrates that atelectasis develops ventrally and atelectasis diminishes dorsally (Langer et al. 1988). Oxygenation improves in most patients. The effects of periodic prone positioning on morbidity and mortality during mechanical ventilation, however, appear to be limited (Gattinoni et al. 2001b; Chatte et al. 1997). It is also likely that patients with ALI/$ARDS_{exp}$ have more atelectasis and are more likely to show gravity dependent shifts in the prone position. Unfortunately, Papazian et al. (2002) found no morphologic CT features that would predict response to prone positioning.

Ultimately, gas exchange is the balance between ventilation and perfusion. CT has done well at analyzing global and regional aeration but not perfusion. It is clear that hypoxia is related to poor oxygenation of consolidated lung, but it is not totally clear how much gas exchange and perfusion occurs in the partially aerated (ground glass) lung.

Multidetector CT and electron beam CT now provide tools for assessing perfusion in local areas throughout the lung. This perfusion can then be matched with ventilation maps. For example, how does perfusion change in the prone and supine patient? How does that relate to the ventilatory changes documented by CT? Jones et al. (2001) have confirmed, using contrast enhanced first pass rapid CT, the already known fact that perfusion in normal subjects is greater in the dorsal lung in the supine patient. When a normal person is placed prone, the gradient reverses. Using multiple small regions of interest, they demonstrated heterogeneous perfusion throughout the lung in both positions but less so in the prone position. This type of approach may provide the regional mapping of perfusion needed to better understand local ventilation/perfusion relationships.

CT can also be used to assess regional flow and perhaps distinguish between permeability edema and hydrostatic edema (Ullrich et al. 2002). Hydrostatic edema was induced in five piglets and oleic acid permeability edema was induced in seven piglets. CT scanning was performed 90 minutes after induction of edema. Regions of interest in normal, ground glass, and consolidated lung were measured. Intravenous contrast agent was then injected and lung enhancement was measured in both groups during the first pass and then over time. The density of ground glass areas increased continuously in both groups for the first 80 seconds. Beyond 80 seconds, lung density increased in the permeability group only. No enhancement was observed immediately, or with time, in either the normal or the consolidated lung in either group. This suggests that much of the perfusion is occurring in the ground glass areas, and capillary leak in ALI/ARDS is predominantly in the ground glass areas in early ALI/ARDS.

Schoepf et al. (2000) have used electron beam CT to study pulmonary blood flow and perfusion in patients suspected of having a pulmonary embolism. They studied a 7 cm volume of lung during the infusion of intravenous contrast. First pass measurements showed that blood flow in normal lung areas was approximately four times that of embolized areas and returned to normal after anticoagulation (Fig. 8.9). Such techniques are potentially applicable to ALI/ARDS.

In the future, multidetector and electron beam CTs will provide increasing temporal and spatial resolution. Recent technical developments suggest that four-dimensional scanning will be achievable in the near future. This will provide rapid, sequential three-dimensional images, providing a fourth dimension (time) and the next level of understanding in both ventilation and perfusion. Although global information about the lung and ALI/ARDS is important, the marked heterogeneity of the lung disease requires local analysis of both ventilation and perfusion.

Other imaging modalities will also contribute to our understanding. CT/PET scanning, available in a single unit will provide more precise anatomic correlation between structure and function (Schuster 1998). Similarly, MRI can be used to assess interparenchymal water, capillary permeability, and blood flow. MRI may also be able to analyze gas distribution using hyperpolarized helium (Eberle et al. 1999). Sophisticated computer modeling will provide three-dimensional spatial and fourth-dimensional temporal resolution (Sandiford 1995; Uematsu et al. 2001).

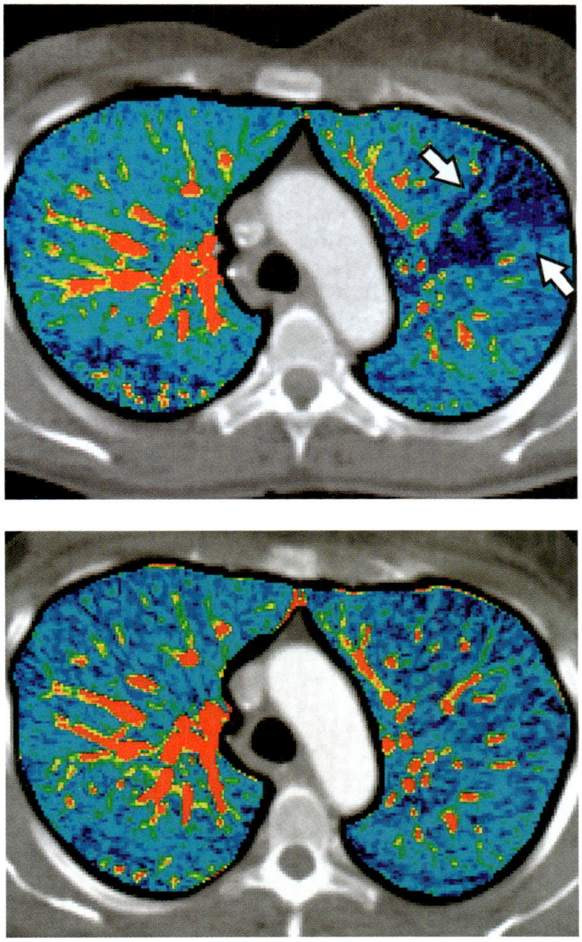

a

b

Fig. 8.9. Color coded perfusion map obtained with dynamic electron beam CT. A Perfusion defect due to pulmonary embolism (arrows) in left upper lobe. B Follow-up after heparin therapy (Schoepf et al. 2000, with permission)

8.4 Conclusion

Both ventilation and perfusion in ALI/ARDS are dynamic processes that occur inhomogeneously throughout the lung. Multidetector scanners and the next generation of four-dimensional scanners will further refine the insights provided by conventional and helical CT over the last 15 years.

References

Albert RK, Hubmayr RD (2000) The prone position eliminates compression of the lungs by the heart. Am J Respir Crit Care Med 161:1660–1665

Ashbaugh DG, Bigelow DB, Petty TL et al (1967) Acute respiratory distress in adults. Lancet 2:319–323

Bernard GR, Artigas A, Brigham KL et al (1994) The American-European consensus conference on ARDS: definitions, mechanisms, relevant outcomes, and clinical trial coordination. Am J Respir Crit Care Med 149:818–824

Chatte G, Sab JM, Dubois JM et al (1997) Prone position in mechanically ventilated patients with severe acute respiratory failure. Am J Respir Crit Care Med 155:473–478

Desai SR (2002) Acute respiratory distress syndrome: imaging of the injured lung. Clin Radiol 57:8–17

Desai SR, Wells AU, Rubens MB et al (1999) Acute respiratory distress syndrome: computed tomographic abnormalities at long-term follow up. Radiology 210:29–35

Desai SR, Wells AU, Suntharalingam G et al (2001) Acute respiratory distress syndrome caused by pulmonary and extrapulmonary injury: a comparative computed tomographic study. Radiology 218:689–693

Eberle B, Weiler N, Markstaller K et al (1999) Analysis of intrapulmonary O(2) concentration by MR imaging of inhaled hyperpolarized helium-3. J Appl Physiol 87:2043–2052

Gattinoni L, Mascheroni D, Torresin A et al (1986) Morphological response to positive end expiratory pressure in acute respiratory failure. Computerized tomography study. Intensive Care Med 12:137–142

Gattinoni L, Pesenti A, Avalli L et al (1987) Pressure-volume curve of total respiratory system in acute respiratory failure. Computed tomographic scan study. Am Rev Respir Dis 136:730–736

Gattinoni L, Pesenti A, Bombino M et al (1988) Relationships between lung computed tomographic density, gas exchange, and PEEP in acute respiratory failure. Anesthesiology 69:824–832

Gattinoni L, Bombino M, Pelosi P et al (1994) Lung structure and function in different stages of severe adult respiratory distress syndrome. JAMA 271:1772–1779

Gattinoni L, Pelosi P, Crotti S et al (1995) Effects of positive end-expiratory pressure on regional distribution of tidal volume and recruitment in adult respiratory distress syndrome. Am J Respir Crit Care Med 151:1807–1814

Gattinoni L, Pelosi P, Suter PM et al (1998) Acute respiratory distress syndrome caused by pulmonary and extrapulmonary disease. Am J Respir Crit Care Med 158:3–11

Gattinoni L, Caironi P, Pelosi P et al (2001a) What has computed tomography taught us about the acute respiratory distress syndrome? Am J Respir Crit Care Med 164:1701–1711

Gattinoni L, Tognoni G, Pesenti A et al (2001b) Effect of prone positioning on the survival of patients with acute respiratory failure. N Engl J Med 345:568–573

Goodman LR (1996) Congestive heart failure and adult respiratory distress syndrome: new insights using computed tomography. Radiol Clin North Am 34:33–46

Goodman LR, Fumagalli R, Tagliabue P et al (1999) Adult respiratory distress syndrome due to pulmonary and extrapulmonary causes: computed tomographic, clinical and functional correlations. Radiology 213:545–552

Jones AT, Hansell DM, Evans TW (2001) Pulmonary perfusion in supine and prone positions: an electron-beam computed tomography study. J Appl Physiol 90:1342–1348

Langer M, Mascheroni D, Marcolin R et al (1988) The prone position in ARDS patients: a clinical study. Chest 94:103–107

Malbouisson LM, Cornelius JB, Puybasset L et al (2000) Role of the heart in the loss of aeration characterizing lower lobes in acute respiratory distress syndrome. Am J Respir Crit Care Med 161:2005–2012

Malbouisson LM, Muller JC, Constantin JM et al (2001) CT Scan ARDS Study Group. Computed tomography assessment of positive end-expiratory pressure-induced alveolar recruitment in patients with acute respiratory distress syndrome. Am J Respir Crit Care Med 163:1444–1450

Maunder RJ, Schuman WP, McHugh JW et al (1986) Preservation of normal lung regions in the adult respiratory distress syndrome: analysis by computed tomography. JAMA 255:2463–2465

Nobauer-Huhmann IM, Eibenberger K, Scheafer-Prokop C et al (2001) Changes in lung parenchyma after acute respiratory distress syndrome (ARDS): assessment with high-resolution computed tomography. Eur Radiol 11:2436–2443

Papazian L, Paladini MH, Bregeon F et al (2002) Can the tomographic aspect characteristics of patients presenting with acute respiratory diestress syndrome predict improvement in oxygenation-related response to the prone position? Anesthesiology 97:599–607

Pesenti A, Tagliabue P, Patroniti N et al (2001) Computerised tomography scan imaging in acute respiratory distress syndrome. Ontensive Care Med 27:631–639

Pelosi P, D'Andrea L, Vitale G et al (1994) Vertical gradient of regional lung inflation in adult respiratory distress syndrome. Am Rev Respir Crit Care Med 149:8–13

Putman CE, Ravin CE (1983) Adult respiratory distress syndrome. In: Goodman LR, Putman CR (eds) Intensive care radiology: imaging of the critically ill. Saunders, Philadelphia, pp 114–123

Puybasset L, Cluzel P, Chao N et al (1998) The CT Scan ARDS Study Group. A computed tomography scan assessment of regional lung volume in acute lung injury. Am J Respir Crit Care Med 158:1644–1655

Rouby JJ, Puybasset L, Cluzel P et al (2000) CT Scan ARDS Study Group. Regional distribution of gas and tissue in acute respiratory distress syndrome. II. Physiological correlations and definition of an ARDS Severity Score. Intensive Care Med 26:1046–1056

Sandiford P, Province MA, Schuster DP (1995). Distribution of regional density and vascular permeability in the adulte respiratory distress syndrome. American Journal of Respiratory & Critical Care Med 151(3 Pt 1):737–742

Schoepf UJ, Bruening R, Konschitzky H et al (2000) Pulmonary embolism: comprehensive diagnosis by using electron-beam CT for detection of emboli and assessment of pulmonary blood flow. Radiology 217:693–700

Schuster DP (1998) The evaluation of lung function with PET. Semin Nucl Med 28:341–351

Tagliabue M, Casella TC, Zincone GE et al (1994) CT and chest radiography in the evaluation of adult respiratory syndrome. Acta Radiol 35:230–234

Uematsu H, Levin DL, Hatabu H (2001) Quantification of pulmonary perfusion with MR imaging: recent advances. Eur J Radiol 37:155–163

Ullrich R, Wassermann E, Zimpfer M et al (2002) Dynamic CT measurement of late pulmonary enhancement for differentiation of hydrostatic versus high vascular permeability edema in a piglet model. European Society of Thoracic Imaging, Brugge, Belgium, May 2002

Yamaguchi K, Soejima K, Koda E et al (2001) Inhaling gas with different CT densities allows detection of abnormalities in the lung periphery of patients with smoking-induced COPD. Chest 120:1907–1916

Focal Lung Disease / Lung Cancer

9 CT Screening for Lung Cancer

C. I. Henschke, D. F. Yankelevitz, W. Kostis

CONTENTS

9.1 Screening for Lung Cancer

Considerable screening with chest radiography has continued in the United States (Epler 1990) despite the official recommendations against it (Eddy 1989; U.S. Preventive Services Task Force 1989; American Cancer Society 1980; National Cancer Institute 2000). In Japan, on the other hand, screening for lung cancer has been offered as a matter of public-health policy for quite some time, initially with chest radiography (Sobue et al. 1992; Sobue 2000) and now with CT (Kaneko et al. 1996; Sone et al. 1998).

C. I. Henschke, PhD, MD
Department of Radiology, New York Presbyterian Hospital, Weill Cornell Medical Center, 525 East 68th Street, New York, NY 10021, USA
D. F. Yankelevitz, MD
Department of Radiology, New York Presbyterian Hospital, Weill Cornell Medical Center, 525 East 68th Street, New York, NY 10021, USA
W. Kostis, PhD
Department of Radiology, New York Presbyterian Hospital, Weill Cornell Medical Center, 525 East 68th Street, New York, NY 10021, USA

Recently, the Early Lung Cancer Action Project (ELCAP) a prospective trial, demonstrated that earlier diagnosis of lung cancer with CT can be achieved (Henschke et al. 1999; Henschke et al.), and these results have led to considerable demand for CT screening. The ELCAP results confirmed that, relative to traditional chest radiography, CT-based screening markedly enhances the detection of lung cancer at earlier and more curable stages relative to what is known to prevail in the absence of screening. It was confirmed, as expected, that the experience with annual repeat screening was quite different from that with baseline screening, notably with respect to the number of false-positive results of the initial test; positive results on annual repeat were much less common than on baseline (3 vs 23%). The nodule-associated malignancies on annual repeat screening were, as was also anticipated, typically of stage IA. While over 80% of the malignancies were of stage IA on baseline and annual repeat examinations, the median size was considerably smaller on annual repeat. The ELCAP recommendations also succeeded in minimizing biopsies of benign nodules.

Translation of the diagnostic distribution of the malignancies found on the annual repeat screening to its estimated corresponding overall rate of curability under screening requires information on the stage- and size-specific rates of curability by relevant subtypes of lung cancer (Henschke et al. 2002, 2003). In the future, ELCAP and its subsequent projects will provide detailed information as to the consequent decrease in deaths due to lung cancer by early diagnosis and early treatment. A lower bound for the curability of CT screen-diagnosed lung cancer, however, was obtained from the data on the curability of lung cancers diagnosed by chest radiographic screening. These tumors averaged approximately 20 mm in diameter (Henschke et al. 2003). Using the data from Flehinger et al. (1992), which showed that the 5-year lung cancer fatality rates in the absence and presence of treatment (resection) were 90 and 30% respectively, we found that the curability rate was (90–30)/90 or 67% – much higher than that in the context of symptom-prompted diagnosis (Henschke et al. 2003). It was only that, despite the high frequency of repeat screening with chest radiography and sputum cytology, stage-I diagnosis was achieved in only 29% of the diagnosed cases (Fontana et al. 1996), whereas it was achieved in over 80% of the cases with annual CT screening (Sone et al. 1998; Henschke et al.).

The ELCAP and its sister projects, the NY-ELCAP and I-ELCAP, have already screened more than 20,000 people using a common protocol which prescribes the screening regimen (I-ELCAP). This protocol minimizes the frequency of overdiagnosed cases of lung cancer as the screening regimen properly requires documentation of growth of the smallest nodules before proceeding to obtain pathologic evidence by requiring demonstration of in vivo growth. The pathology protocol (Vazquez et al. 2002a; Vazquez et al. 2002b) details careful pathologic evaluation to identify whether there is evidence of invasion. Those who choose not to have resection are followed to learn about the natural history. Finally, if a category of cancers that might qualify for "overdiagnosed" cancers can be identified, a randomized trial of these lesions to immediate resection and no resection might be possible to answer the question of overdiagnosis directly (International Conferences on Screening for Lung Cancer).

9.2 Basis of Current Recommendations Against Screening for Lung Cancer

Had prior studies on chest radiography screening for lung cancer shown the benefit of screening, the ELCAP data would be sufficient to recommended CT screening as it clearly demonstrated the marked improvement of CT over chest radiography. For example, the recommendations for colonoscopy screening for colon cancer are based on a similar study showing the improved detection of colon carcinoma with colonoscopy as compared with guaiac positive stools (Mandel et al. 1993), as previously guaiac positive stools had been shown to be useful (Newcomb et al. 1992).

The recommendations against screening for lung cancer were essentially based on the results of the Mayo Lung Project (MLP), published in 1986 (Fontana et al. 1986). The long-term follow-up results published in 2000 attempted to reinforce these recommendations (Marcus et al. 2000). In the MLP, over 10,000 men each had two diagnostic tests, chest radiography and sputum cytology, to identify those with lung cancer on this first, baseline screening. Those men who had no evidence of lung cancer on the baseline screening were then randomized, half to an "intervention" cohort in which men were screened with chest radiography and sputum cytology every 4 months for 6 years. By the end of 6 years of screening, approximately 30% of this cohort had dropped out. The other half of the 10,000 subjects were randomized to the control cohort, in which the usual Mayo recommendation for annual chest radiography was given at the beginning of the study. With this advice, it is not surprising that over 70% had some screening during the study, and so this cohort actually had screening only on an irregular and less intensive basis than the "intervention" cohort. Such protocol non-adherence while not unexpected in any long-term screening study, served to dilute the contrast between the two cohorts.

After 6 years of screening and between 1.5 and 5 years (median 3 years) of follow-up, the cumulative number of deaths from lung cancer from the time of randomization in the "intervention" and "control" cohort were not statistically significant, and thus the "null" hypothesis that the "intervention" was not useful in reducing lung cancer mortality, could not be rejected. Even after long-term follow-up of "more than 76,000 person-years, there was no statistically significant difference in lung cancer mortality" (Marcus et al. 2000). It is also expected that additional follow-up after the termination of screening dilutes the contrast between the two cohorts.

Further investigations by Flehinger and Kimmel (1987), Miettinen (2000) and Sobue et al. (1992a, 1992b) showed that screening with chest radiography propably provided a benefit and that the results of the MLP were misleading and misinterpreted. We provided added evidence as to why this study design led to misleading results (Henschke et al. 2003) and also showed how a similar randomized design led to misleading results in assessment of mammographic screening for breast cancer (Miettinen et al. 2000a, 2000b). In fact, the continuing controversy about mammography shows that the numerous randomized, controlled trials comparing screening with no screening, of more than a half-million women in over 40 years of study, did not provide definitive answers about the benefit of screening for breast cancer (Gøtzsche and Olsen 2000).

The catastrophic failure of these many randomized trials comparing screening with no screening should lead to serious reconsideration by experts of the theoretical underpinnings of randomized controlled trials for studying screening. When the results of these randomized trials comparing screening with no screening keep pointing to negative results that are counterintuitive (EDDY 1989), and these counterintuitive results are explained by reasons, such as extensive overdiagnosis (PARKIN and MOSS 2000; BLACK 2000), which have been shown to be wrong (FLEHINGER et al. 1992; MIETTINEN 2000a; SOBUE et al. 1992; HENSCHKE et al. 2003; MIETTINEN et al. 2002a, 2002b; YANKELEVITZ et al. 2003), the most obvious recourse is to question the principles underlying the study design. Randomized trials came into prominence in medicine in the 1940s for comparing alternative treatments, particularly for tuberculosis, and they provided a powerful tool for evaluation of treatment effectiveness (HILL 1990; MEDICAL RESEARCH COUNCIL 1948). The diagnostic community later embraced this paradigm without recognizing the fundamental differences between evaluation of diagnostic tests and treatments (FRYBACK and THORNBURY 1991; HILLMAN 1994); however, it should be becoming clear by now that this same paradigm used for assessment of treatment leads to misleading results when applied for the assessment of diagnostic tests (MIETTINEN et al. 2003).

9.3 National Lung Screening Trial

The promising results of ELCAP led to the funding of the National Lung Screening Trial (NLST), the most expensive screening study ever done (NATIONAL LUNG SCREENING TRIAL). Its design is based on the traditional view that a randomized trial is necessary to evaluate lung cancer screening. This randomized, controlled trial compares CT screening with chest radiographic screening and its designers envision that it will provide an answer about the benefit of CT screening, or lack thereof, in approximately 10 years. As no critical reevaluation of the ideas underpinning the randomized controlled trial comparing screening with no screening has occurred since it was used for the MLP (MIETTINEN et al.2003), the National Lung Screening Trial (NLST), based on a similar design, has similar flaws.

In the NLST, there will only be three rounds of screening with follow-up up to 5 years (D.R. Aberle et al. 2002). As the lead time of CT over chest radiography for cancer diagnosis is approximately 4–5 years, and as deaths typically occur several years after cancer diagnosis on chest radiography, the ratio of deaths should only start to decrease approximately 7 years after randomization. But, as we illustrated in a prior publication (HENSCHKE et al. 2003), and again in Fig. 9.1, screening will have stopped after 3 years, so that the full effect of screening will never be identified. Other concerns about the NLST included the comparability of the ascertainment of death in each cohort (BLACK et al. 2002) and the effectiveness of the randomization procedure (BENSON and HARTZ 2000; CONCATO et al. 2000; GORLOVA et al. 2001). There also are serious concerns about the applicability of the screening test being evaluated, as in a randomized trial the test procedure cannot easily be updated and thus will not be relevant for future practice due to methodology drift, particularly in view of the long time required to perform the study and analyze its results. From our own simulations, we believe the sample size is insufficient for the NLST as well (GORLOVA et al. 2001; M. Kimmel et al., submitted). Considerable protocol non-adherence should be anticipated in the NLST, in light of the MLP experience. In fact, we anticipate it will be even higher for NLST for many reasons. The control cohort is being screened using chest radiography, yet the ELCAP baseline results showed that chest radiographic screening identified larger nodules, approximately half of which were false positives (HENSCHKE et al. 1999). Within the NLST, those with suspected nodules on chest radiography will surely have CT, and most likely some of these CTs will lead to the diagnosis of small lung cancers which were not identified on the chest radiograph; thus, incidental CT-detected cancers will be found, and so, in reality, the NLST is comparing annual CT screening with "annual chest radiographic and random CT screening." Consider the extreme scenario where every person randomized to the chest radiography cohort had their chest radiograph interpreted as having an abnormality and thus were recommended to have CT. The study would then consist of two cohorts, one having an immediate CT and the other having a chest radiograph followed by CT, so that no real difference would exist between the two groups.

Figure 9.2 shows the decrease in the difference in the case-fatality rates in the NLST by using chest radiography in the control arm, protocol non-adherence, and limited rounds of screening on being able to detect the benefit of CT screening for lung cancer, even when focusing on the relevant parameter during the relevant period in which the benefit can be seen. We had already illustrated this for CT screening for lung cancer (HENSCHKE et al. 2003) and mammography screening for breast cancer (MIETTINEN 2002a, 2002b). The use of cumulative deaths rather than the case-fatality during the relevant time period will further obscure any ben-

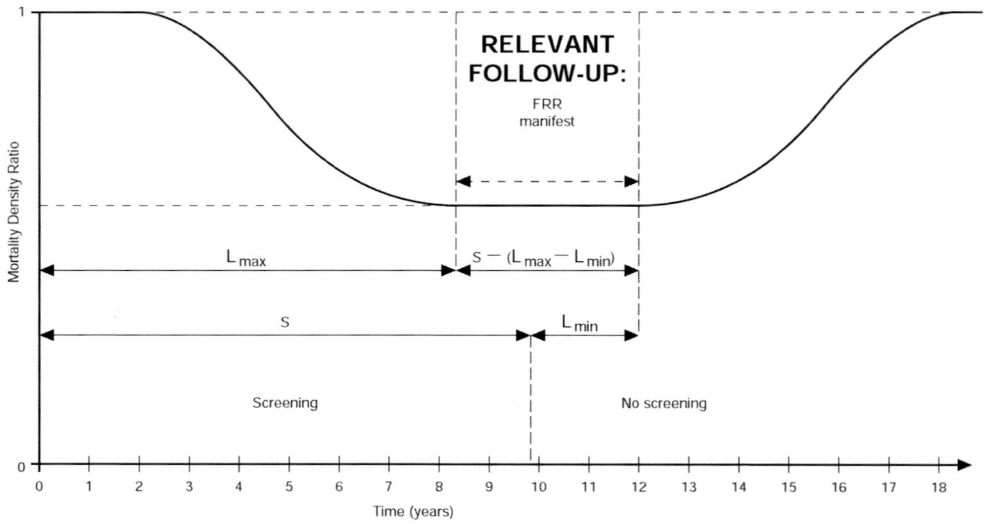

Fig. 9.1. Follow-up experience in a randomized controlled trial comparing screening for cancer with no screening with respect to cause-specific mortality: interrelations of parameters. At any given point in the follow-up there is a particular mortality density (MD) among the screened and the not screened; for an interval of t to t+dt, with dC cases expected in it, MD_t=dC/Pdt, where P is the size of the population. Contrasting the screened with the not screened, there is the corresponding mortality-density ratio (MDR). This ratio is depicted as a function of time since entry into the trial. The early excess mortality among the screened is not shown, since the focus is on the intended result of reduced fatality rate (FR) quantified in terms of fatality-rate ratio (FRR). The MDR coincides with FRR in a particular interval of follow-up time if the duration of screening, S, exceeds the difference between the maximum, L_{max}, and minimum, L_{min}, of the time lag from early diagnosis to the death prevented by early intervention but not by late intervention (i.e., in the absence of screening). (From Miettinen et al. 2002b)

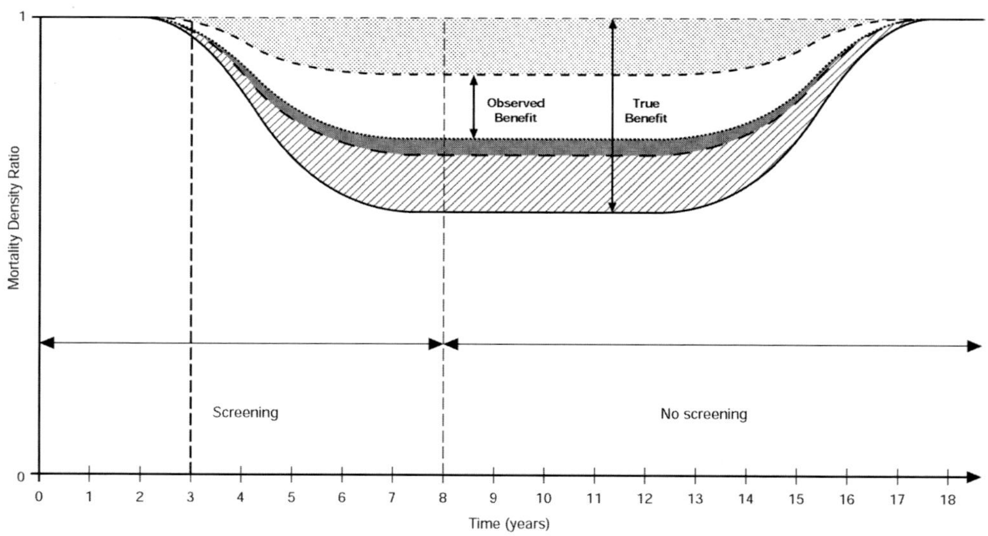

Fig. 9.2. Figure 1 adapted for the National Lung Screening Trial design in which screening is performed for 3 years only. The difference between CT screening and no screening as shown in Fig. 1 is decreased because the control arm is given chest radiographic screening (shown by the *slanted lines*). There is further decrease in the difference due to protocol non-adherence (in the CT (*darkly shaded area*) and in the chest radiographic (*lightly shaded area*) cohorts. Note that after 3 years of screening, the decrease in the deaths in the CT arm are just beginning to be seen, but it would require at least 8 years of continuous screening to reach the maximum observable benefit. When screening stops, e.g., after 3 years, the deaths in the CT screening arm start to increase. Screening would need to continue for at least 8 years to reach the maximum observable benefit, but would need to continue for some time longer to show any statistical significant difference

efit. Note that extending the period of follow-up only serves to further dilute the difference between the two cohorts, as the period during which the benefit due to screening occurs will have passed.

To avoid a misleading result of the NLST, similar to that of the MLP, the NLST, already the most expensive screening study ever done, would need to become even more expensive. Screening would need to continue for at least 10 years, and more people would need to be enrolled to compensate for the anticipated protocol non-adherence. The designers of NLST also designed the Prostate, Lung, Colorectal and Ovarian (PLCO) randomized screening trial in which they recognized that many subjects would need to be screened. The PLCO trial began in 1993, completed enrollment of 150,000 people by 2000, and is anticipated to complete its analyses circa 2014 (Chirikos et al. 2002).

9.4 The Ethical Dilemma

Many physicians have steadfastly refused to accept the idea that lung cancer diagnosed in an asymptomatic person as a result of chest radiographic screening or CT screening has the same curability as a cancer detected late after symptoms are present. The physician knows that CT screening for lung cancer provides for earlier diagnosis and thereby for earlier intervention, and that by now this has been demonstrated by ample evidence. This attitude is acknowledged in the NLST protocol itself, which states that it is "apparent at this time: CT screening will detect more cancers, cancers of earlier stage and smaller cancers than are routinely detected by [chest radiography] or symptoms" (D.R. Aberle et al. 2002). Several analyses of the cost justification of CT screening for lung cancer have demonstrated that it is cost-effective (Miettinen 2000b, Chirikos et al. 2002), including one based on actual data (Wisnivesky et al. 2002), although another paper based on hypothetical data suggested that this might not be true (Mahadevia et al. 2003).

What should the physician do when faced with a person at high risk for lung cancer and with otherwise suitably long life expectancy, especially if the person asks for screening, and particularly since the physician understands that the NLST will not provide an answer for many years, if ever? To more sharply focus the debate, consider the following case: A CT for evaluation of coronary artery disease is done in a healthy 60-year-old man with a history of heavy smoking, and a suspicious nodule is identified. Biopsy is performed and the diagnosis of adenocarcinoma of stage I is made. The physician recommends early, immediate resection. No serious consideration is given to delaying the surgery until symptoms and/or signs appear, because the physician knows that resection of stage-I lung cancer results in far fewer deaths than when the stage is higher (Mountain 1997; Inoue et al. 1998). In fact, the failure to recommend immediate treatment would be the basis of a lawsuit.

The ethical dilemma is illustrated by the initial policy of the Mayo Clinic which stated that CT screening for lung cancer should not be done in a practice setting (Swensen 2002). Since the start of their participation in the NLST, the Mayo Clinic has suggested a major shift in their policy to one that does allow screening in the practice setting (Earnest et al. 2003) as they state "… This position, this middle ground or third path, is the informed consent. … Informed consent will provide patients with correct information about the benefits, risks and alternatives for screening as we currently understand them and will positively influence the practice of all who would choose to offer CT screening examinations." Thus, the revised Mayo policy proposal focuses on patient autonomy, with this deference superceding the prior concerns. This new Mayo policy proposal accords with the one of the principles, the *Principle of patients' autonomy,* in the recently advanced Charter on Medical Professionalism ABIUM Foundation 2002). D.F. Yankelevitz (submitted) in his response pointed out that this is only one of three principles in the charter. The other principles imply that the physician has the responsibility to decide whether providing screening for lung cancer actually serves the cause of the patient's welfare. Merely asking for something, even in the context of being informed, is not cause enough to provide it. Even if the physician agrees with the informed potential screenee that screening is indicated, the necessary conditions for providing the service are not thereby met. The physician needs to be certain that the necessary radiological, pathological, and surgical services are available, and at the requisite level of competence. Yankelevitz et al. (submitted) point out that the informed consent must provide all of the available information and much of this is lacking in the informed consent for NLST.

9.5 The Alternative Approach to Evaluation of the Benefit of Screening

We suggest that a different approach be taken, one that separates the diagnostic concerns from those of the subsequent intervention. This approach avoids the ethical dilemma discussed previously as it provides state-of-the-art screening to all (including informed consent) with continual updates and allows for the evaluation of the benefit of screening at the same time. Screening after all is a process which requires constant updating in response to technologic and knowledge-based advances.

Screening is defined as pursuit of early diagnosis in an asymptomatic person with the aim of providing for early intervention (Miettinen 2001). The pursuit of early diagnosis of a cancer is defined by a *regimen of screening*, not simply by the initial screening test. The regimen starts with the initial test, and if this test is positive, a well-defined diagnostic algorithm is followed to rule in the diagnosis of cancer. If the test result is negative or the diagnostic algorithm does not lead to a diagnosis of cancer, the person is referred to the next routinely scheduled screening. Each screening cycle starts with the initial screening test and ends before the next routinely scheduled repeat screening. The timing of the repeat screening is defined by the regimen. The definition of a positive result of the initial screening test and the diagnostic algorithm used in the pursuit of rule-in diagnosis may be different for the first (baseline) cycle of screening and for subsequent (repeat) cycles of screenings. It is this regimen of screening, including the initial test, the definition of a positive result of screening, and the consequent diagnostic work-up, which determines how early malignancy is diagnosed.

Any malignancy diagnosed as a result of recommendation for biopsy/surgery according to the regimen of screening is by definition a *screen*-diagnosed cancer and is attributed to the cycle during which the recommendation is made even though the person and/or referring physician may only implement the recommendation at some later time. If a cancer is diagnosed prompted by symptoms within 12 months after a negative repeat screening, it is considered to be interim-diagnosed and is attributed to the cycle of screening during which it is diagnosed.

Malignancies diagnosed under a particular screening regimen can be tabulated as a frequency distribution by relevant prognostic factors (e.g., stage, size, histology). We call this frequency distribution the *diagnostic distribution* under screening, as it includes all malignancies diagnosed in a given cycle of screening – both screen- and interim-diagnosed ones. Such distributions were provided, for example, in the ELCAP baseline and annual repeat results (Henschke et al. 1999; Henschke et al.). The diagnostic distribution of the malignancies by relevant prognostic factors, such as stage, size, histology, and biomarkers as produced by a given regimen of screening, can be compared to the diagnostic distribution of another regimen, so that the performance of different screening regimens and the screening tests on which they are based can be compared.

9.6 Updating the Regimen

Helical CT scanning has rapidly advanced in the past 5 years from the single-slice scanner to those that can acquire 4, 8, 16, and soon even more slices simultaneously. Images of the lungs with a slice thickness of less than 1 mm can now be obtained in a single breathhold as compared with those with 10 mm using single-slice scanners. As resolution improves with thinner slices, it is not surprising that many more lung nodules are being detected, primarily those less than 5.0 mm in diameter. These technologic advances require updating of the screening regimen, particularly with regard to the definition of a positive result. Similarly, as additional diagnostic modalities, such as CT/PET scanners, become more widely available, their use may require updating of the diagnostic algorithm.

In the initial planning for ELCAP, our working definition of a positive result of screening was the identification of a solitary non-calcified nodule, but we soon recognized that with CT screening many individuals were found to have multiple nodules. Since we could not discriminate among them, we changed the definition to one to six non-calcified nodules. In addition to the number of pulmonary nodules, the experience of baseline screening of the initial 1000 high-risk individuals in the ELCAP led us to identify a new type of nodule which we termed a *sub-solid* nodule. A sub-solid nodule is one that does not completely obscure the lung parenchyma in which it resides as compared with the solid nodule (Henschke et al. 2002). Small sub-solid nodules had not been recognized on chest radiographs, nor was their importance understood initially in CT screening. The sub-solid nodule has been further sub-classified as *part* solid if there is a solid component within it; otherwise it is a *non*-solid nodule. On review of the ELCAP baseline results, we noted that approximately half of the malignancies were found in sub-solid nodules. In particular, the part-solid nodules had a threefold higher malignancy rate as compared with solid or non-solid ones.

Additional experience has led to further changes in the definition of a positive result of baseline screening. After analysis of approximately 3000 baseline screenings, we found that no malignancy was diagnosed within the first year of screening in nodules less than 5.0 mm (C.I. Henschke, in press). Although we recognized that there were some malignancies among the many non-calcified nodules of this size range, their growth was only recognized on subsequent annual repeat screenings; thus, the definition of a positive result of the initial CT on baseline screening has updated since the original ELCAP in terms of number, type, and size of nodules (I-ELCAP). The current definition is: one or more non-calcified solid or part-solid nodules 5.0 mm or larger, or a non-solid nodule 10.0 mm or larger. Using this updated definition, we found that the percentage of positive results on baseline screening has been reduced to approximately 10–15%, a reduction of approximately 55% from that in the original ELCAP protocol without a concomitant increase in the false-negative rate.

Increased knowledge of the prevalence of malignancy by nodule size has caused us to change the diagnostic algorithm for nodules detected on baseline screening. While the first 1000 individuals screened in ELCAP were a very high-risk group, we subsequently reduced the age criterion for screening to 40 years. We then found that the prevalence of malignancy was lower among nodules less than 15 mm in diameter than in our original cohort, whereas it remained high among those with nodules 15 mm or larger; thus, when risk factors (in this example, age) are changed, the diagnostic algorithm may require modification. In the latest protocol, immediate biopsy is no longer recommended for nodules less than 15 mm found on the initial CT on baseline screening. The rationale for this change is that the prevalence of malignancy for nodules in this size range was low, so that additional non-invasive testing was recommended before proceeding to biopsy. Specifically, analysis of our results indicates that documented growth on follow-up short-term CT or PET scan positivity were the most useful indicators of malignancy.

In considering updates to the diagnostic algorithm, it is important to note that in the ELCAP regimen of screening, the algorithm has always been different for nodules identified at baseline than for those on annual repeat screening. A positive result on annual repeat, by definition, is a nodule that has already demonstrated growth over 1 year and thus requires a more rapid evaluation than those at baseline. It follows that the diagnostic algorithm has not changed significantly for a positive result of repeat screening.

Future technologic improvements which enhance the accuracy of growth assessment, particularly of smaller nodules, will most likely lead to further changes of the definition of a positive result and of the diagnostic algorithm. Concomitantly, it can be expected that ELCAP-like research will provide diagnostic distributions of screen-detected lung cancers under particular screening regimens, as well as their prognosis, and treatment implications which, in turn, will lead to further refinements of the diagnostic algorithm and treatment interventions.

9.7 Diagnostic Sub-Typing of Cancer

An important aspect of the diagnostic process is the identification of subtypes of cancer based on imaging (e.g., solid, sub-solid), cytology, and biomarker findings that might have different prognostic implications. As information is obtained about the prognostic implications of these findings, relevant intervention questions will be framed.

9.8 The Critical Interventive Questions

The critical question to be answered about early intervention following early diagnosis is whether deaths due to lung cancer are reduced. An additional question which arises in the context of screening is whether the screen-diagnosed cancers are genuine ones, i.e., whether these cancers are fatal if not resected. Thus, by definition, the fatality rate of genuine lung cancers in the absence of resection is 100%. This fatality rate is defined as the proportion of deaths from lung cancer among those diagnosed with lung cancer. A cancer which is not genuine is an overdiagnosed cancer as it is not fatal in the absence of treatment (if not interrupted by death from some other cause); thus, the fatality rate of overdiagnosed cancers is 0%. The degree to which the fatality rate for screen-diagnosed but untreated cases is more than 0% which indicates the extent of overdiagnosis. The answer to the second question of the genuineness of the screen-diagnosed lung cancers is critical in answering the first question as to whether the deaths from lung cancer are reduced. After all, if screen-diagnosed cancers are not genuine cancers, then the deaths due to lung cancer might appear to be reduced simply because we are finding more non-genuine lung cancers.

To answer these two questions, we need a set of individuals with screen-diagnosed lung cancers, some of whom undergo immediate resection and others who do not. The topic of how best to choose these two subsets (those with and without resection) is considered later. For now, let us simply assume that we have two such subsets. In each subset of individuals, the deaths from lung cancer and the deaths from competing causes are tabulated together with the time to death following the diagnosis of cancer. The lung cancer deaths adjusted for competing causes of death can be presented as illustrated in Fig. 9.3 using the Kaplan-Meier methodology (Cox and Oakes 1984). In Fig. 9.3, the upper curve shows the deaths from lung cancer over time for screen-diagnosed cases who had immediate resection and the lower curve shows this for the screen-diagnosed but untreated cancers. If this lower curve reaches zero, then the disease is uniformly fatal when not treated. When this curve does not reach zero, as shown in the example, it indicates the extent of overdiagnosis.

As each group is followed, the resulting curve will level off and the cumulative survival at this point is called the asymptote of the Kaplan-Meier survival curve. This value is the *cure rate* for that group in the absence of competing causes of death as it provides the proportion of cancers which are cured.

To answer the question as to whether deaths due to lung cancer are reduced, we need to determine the complement of the cure rate, the *case-fatality rate* (case-fatality rate = 1 – cure rate). The case-fatality rate is the proportion of those who die of lung cancer in the absence of competing causes of death; thus, a reduced case-fatality rate would mean that early intervention of screen-diagnosed cancers saves lives.

The cure rate of the untreated cases, $cure_N$, in the example above is obtained from the asymptote of the lower curve and represents the proportion of cases with overdiagnosed lesions found by screening. If $cure_N$ were equal to zero, there would be no overdiagnosed lesions. Since, in this example, $cure_N$ is not equal to zero, there are overdiagnosed cases and thus it is reasonable to assume that there would also be such cases in the resected group. In this situation, the cure rate of the resected cases, $cure_R$, is an overestimate (biased estimate) of the cure rate of

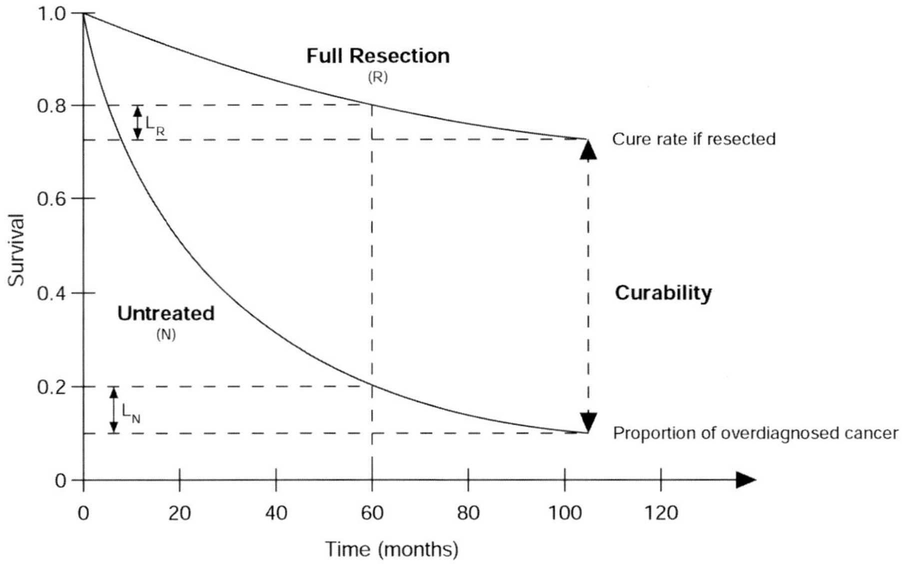

Fig. 9.3. Kaplan-Meier curves for those with screen-diagnosed lung cancers that are resected (*R*) and for those that are not resected (*N*). The asymptote of each curve provides the cure rate for the resected or unresected, respectively. If the asymptote of the curve N does not reach zero, then there are overdiagnosed cases. The curability of screen-diagnosed and resected lung cancers is shown. The lead-time bias of the 5-year survival rate is represented by L_R. This lead-time bias is the overestimation of the cure rate, $cure_R$. Similarly, the 5-year survival rate of the untreated group overestimates the cure rate, $cure_N$, by the amount represented by L_N

genuine, truly fatal cancers, represented by $cure_G$. To determine the cure rate of genuine cancers, $cure_G$, the asymptotic value from the Kaplan-Meier curve of the resected group, $cure_R$, must be decreased. We call this corrected cure rate the *curability* rate, $cure_G$, and it can be defined in terms of the cure rates (or case-fatality rates) obtained from the Kaplan-Meier curves shown in Fig. 9.3:

$$cure_G = \frac{\text{(case-fatality rate without intervention – case-fatality rate with early diagnosis and early intervention),}}{\text{case-fatality rate without intervention}}$$

Thus, the curability rate is the proportional reduction in deaths from lung cancer achieved by early diagnosis and early treatment when compared with no treatment. The above equation can be rewritten in the following two ways:

$$cure_G = 1\text{–(case-fatality rate with early diagnosis and early intervention/case-fatality without intervention),}$$

$$cure_G = 1-[(1-cure_R)/(1-cure_N)] = (cure_R - cure_N)/(1-cure_N).$$

When there is no overdiagnosis ($cure_N$=0), the cure rate obtained from the Kaplan-Meier curve, $cure_R$, is equal to the curability rate, $cure_G$. The curability rate has no overdiagnosis bias even if the case-fatality rates (cure rates) do, as the curability rate is the ratio of the two valves as shown in the foregoing equations.

This approach allows for estimation of the extent of overdiagnosis and by what proportion deaths from lung cancer can be reduced by early diagnosis and treatment. These two questions should not be answered globally for all screen-diagnosed cancers; instead, they need to be answered separately for each diagnostic subtype of cancer as they may be very different for small-cell, squamous-cell, or adenocarcinoma, and different even within these subtypes of lung cancer. Such knowledge for particular subtypes of cancer will provide important information in selecting the appropriate treatment for each subtype. The overall rates are then the weighted averages of the rates for each of the constituent subtypes.

Kaplan-Meier methodology is used to obtain the asymptote of each survival curve. The annual survival rates are not used. Yet, whenever survival curves are shown, the question of lead-time bias is typically raised. There is lead-time bias when survival rates are used. For example, in Fig 9.3, the lead-time bias of the 5-year survival rate is shown as it is an overestimate of the cure rate; thus, the 5-year survival rate of the resected group overestimates the cure rate, $cure_R$, by the amount represented by L_R and the 5-year survival rate of the untreated group overestimates the cure rate, $cure_N$, by the amount represented by L_N. Note that the lead-time bias decreases as 6-, 7-, and 8-year survival rates are used and, in fact, the longer the follow-up time, the closer the particular survival rate is to the cure rate; thus, 7-year survival rates have less lead-time bias than 5-year survival rates. It is important to understand that neither the cure rate nor the case-fatality rate have *lead-time* bias, as the asymptote of the curve is used and not any particular annual survival rate.

The answers to these questions do not depend on the number of screening cycles, as does the NLST, as long as baseline and at least a single annual repeat screening are done. The accuracy of the estimates depends on the total number of resected and unresected cancers.

9.9 Formation of the Two Groups of Resected and Unresected Screen-Diagnosed Cancers

In the foregoing section we assumed that we had an unresected and resected group. In this section we address the methodology used to create these two groups. The key principal in creating these two groups is that all extraneous determinants (i.e., confounders) of the cure rates need to be suitably balanced in both groups (Miettinen 1974, 1985). This requirement of having comparable groups with respect to the confounders determines how the two groups should best be created. If the confounders are known, then their effect on cure rates can be accounted for by the analysis. Alternatively, individuals can be assigned to one of the two groups in such a way that these confounders are balanced.

The randomized controlled trial (RCT) provides one mechanism to attempt to balance confounders in each of the two groups by randomly assigning individuals to the two groups upon diagnosis. In such a random assignment, further balance can be created by randomly assigning the individuals within strata of known confounders (e.g., age, stage of cancer) with the hope that unknown confounders are more likely to be balanced within each stratum between the interventions being compared. It should be recognized, however, that randomization enhances the likelihood but does not assure that the known and unknown confounders are equally distributed.

If pertinent confounders can be identified, then randomization is not needed and patients can self-select as long as all the information is recorded on the potential confounders at the time the choice is made. Such an approach is useful when randomization is not ethically possible or otherwise infeasible. This type of approach, called the quasi-experimental approach, has been used in a variety of designs including the two examples which follow.

9.10 Lung Cancer Curability and Overdiagnosis Without Screening

Previously, we had shown that the curability of screen-diagnosed with chest radiography was 67%, and that at most 10% might be overdiagnosed cancers. Furthermore, we had shown similar results for small stage-IA lung cancers diagnosed under usual care without screening (Henschke et al. 2003). For tumors of size 5–15 mm, we found that the curability rate was 71%, for those of size 16–25 mm it was 67%, and for 26–30 mm it was 55%. Curability thus decreases with increasing tumor size.

When using the quasi-experimental approach as illustrated above, it should be understood that the cure rates are not distorted by unequal comorbidity among the two groups. The Kaplan-Meier methodology mathematically accounts for such inequities by treating deaths from causes other than lung cancer as censored observations. A censored observation is one which cannot be followed for long enough to see if the person dies of lung cancer; thus, a greater comorbidity in one group simply accentuates the frequency of censoring in that group but does not bias its asymptote, the cure rate. It is commonplace to bring up comorbidity as a matter of "selection bias," but at issue really is potentially confounding and the Kaplan-Meier methodology adjusts for such confounding factors.

9.11 Conclusion

We present the current status of CT screening for lung cancer. Its promise has led to the initiation of the NLST, a randomized controlled trial contrasting CT with chest radiographic screening. Grave concerns about the NLST design were identified, particularly in light of the previous similar trials of chest radiographic and mammographic screening. We described how previous randomized trials about diagnostic tests led to falsely negative and thus misleading results.

We present an alternative approach to the evaluation of CT screening for lung cancer. This approach allows for the screening regimen to be updated as needed so that it remains at the state of the art and makes the screening test available to all involved in the research required to determine its effectiveness. The methodology provides for direct estimates of the proportion of deaths prevented by screening as well as the proportion of overdiagnosed cases, the latter being an issue that needs to be addressed when a screening test/regimen is being evaluated. We show that the proportion of overdiagnosed cases and the proportion of deaths prevented by immediate resection of screen-diagnosed cancers can be estimated without lead time and overdiagnosis bias. We also stress that the interest should not be so much on the overall values, but that these proportions should be determined for relevant subtypes of lung cancer for all lung cancers. For example, it is to be expected that these values will be very different for small-cell, squamous-cell, and adenocarcinomas.

We already know that CT screening for lung cancer provides for earlier diagnosis of lung cancer, as a result of the ELCAP and other screening studies of more than 20,000 subjects. Physicians who provide screening need to know how much more curable lung cancer is as a result of the early diagnosis. To that end, the International Early Lung Cancer Action Program (IELCAP) has already provided a protocol for the screening regimen (I-ELCAP) that can be used in both a research and practice setting (made available to the public on a regularly updated website) and which allows the resulting data to be pooled. These data will provide the information on the case-fatality rate of all relevant subtypes of lung cancer, together with the extent to which overdiagnosis exists for each subtype, as for each of these subtypes the answer may be different.

References

Aberle DR, Black WC, Goldin JG et al. Contemporary screening for the detection of lung cancer protocol, May 10, 2002. American College of Radiology Imaging Network (ACRIN #6654) available at http/www.acrin.current-protocols

American Cancer Society (1980) Cancer of the lung. Ca Cancer J Clin 30:189–206

Benson K, Hartz AJ (2000) A comparison of observational studies and randomized, controlled trials. N Engl J Med 342:1878–1886

Black WC (2000) Overdiagnosis: an underrecognized cause of confusion and harm in cancer screening. Editorial. J Natl Cancer Inst 92:1–6

Black WC, Haggstrom AD, Welch HG (2002) All-cause mortality in randomized trials of cancer screening. JNCI 94: 167–173

Chirikos TN, Hazelton T, Tockman M, Clark R (2002) Screening for lung cancer with CT: a preliminary cost-effectiveness analysis. Chest 121:1507–1514

Concato J, Shah N, Horwitz RI (2000) Randomized, controlled trials, observational studies, and the hierarchy of research designs. N Engl J Med 342:1887–1892

Cox DR, Oakes D (1984) Analysis of survival data. Chapman and Hall, London

Earnest F, Swensen SJ, Zink FE (2003) Respecting patient autonomy: screening at CT and informed consent. Radiology 226:633–634

Eddy DM (1989) Screening for lung cancer. Ann Intern Med 111:232–237

Epler GR (1990) Screening for lung cancer. Is it worthwhile? Postgrad Med 87:181–186

Flehinger BJ, Kimmel M (1987) The natural history of lung cancer in a periodically screened population. Biometrics 43:127–144

Flehinger BJ, Kimmel M, Melamed MR (1992) Survival from early lung cancer: Implications for screening. Chest 101:13–18

Fontana RS, Sanderson DR, Woolner LB, Taylor WF, Miller WE, Muhm JR (1986) Lung cancer screening: the Mayo program. J Occup Med 28:746–750

Fryback DG, Thornbury JR (1991) The efficacy of diagnostic imaging. Med Decis Making 11:88–94

Gorlova OY, Kimmel M, Henschke C (2001) Modeling of long-term screening for lung cancer. Cancer 92:1531–1540

Gøtzsche PC, Olsen O (2000) Is screening for breast cancer with mammography justifiable? Lancet 355:129–134

Henschke CI, McCauley DI, Yankelevitz DF, Naidich DP, McGuinness G, Miettinen OS, Libby DM, Pasmantier MW, Koizumi J, Altorki NK, Smith JP (1999) Early Lung Cancer Action Project: overall design and findings from baseline screening. Lancet 354:99–105

Henschke CI, Yankelevitz DF, Smith JP, Miettinen OS (2002a) In: DeVita VT, Hellman S, Rosenberg SA (eds) The use of spiral CT in lung cancer screening. Progress in Oncology 2002. Jones and Barlett, Sudbury, Massachusetts

Henschke CI, Yankelevitz DF, Mirtcheva R, McGuinness G, McCauley D, Miettinen OS (2002b) CT screening for lung cancer: frequency and significance of part-solid and non-solid nodules. AJR 178:1053–1057

Henschke CI, Wisnivesky JP, Yankelevitz DF, Miettinen OS (2003a) Small stage I cancers of the lung: genuineness and curability. Lung Cancer 39:327–30

Henschke CI, Yankelevitz DF, Kostis WJ (2003) CT screening for lung cancer. Semin Ultrasound CT MRI 24:23–32

Henschke CI, Naidich DP, Yankelevitz DF, McGuinness G, McCauley DI, Smith JP, Libby DM, Pasmantier MW, Koizumi J, Vazquez M, Flieder D, Altorki NK, Miettinen OS (2001) Early Lung Cancer Action project: initial findings from annual repeat screening. Cancer 92:153–159

Henschke CI, Yankelevitz DF, Naidich D, McCauley DI, McGuinness G, Libby DM, Smith JP, Pasmantier MW, Miettinen OS. CT screening for lung cancer: Significance of nodules at baseline according to size. Radiology 2003 in press

Hill AB (1990) Suspended judgment. Memories of the British Streptomycin Trial in Tuberculosis. The first randomized clinical trial. Control Clin Trials 11:77–79

Hillman BJ (1994) Outcomes research and cost-effectiveness analysis for diagnostic imaging. Radiology 193:307–310

I-ELCAP protocol. http://ICScreen.med.cornell.edu

International Early Lung Cancer Action Project. http://www.IELCAP.org

Inoue K, Sato M, Fujimura S, Sakurada A, Usuda K, Kondo T, Tanita T, Handa M, Saito Y, Sagawa M (1998) Prognostic Assessment of 1310 patients with non-small-cell lung cancer who underwent complete resection from 1980 to 1993. J Thorac Cardiovasc Surg 116:407–411

International Conferences on Screening for Lung Cancer. Consensus statements. http://ICScreen.med.cornell.edu

Kaneko M, Eguchi K, Ohmatsu H, Kakinuma R, Naruke T, Suemasu K, Moriyama N (1996) Peripheral lung cancer: screening and detection with low-dose spiral CT versus radiography. Radiology 201:798–802

Kimmel M, Gorlova OY, Henschke CI. Modeling lung cancer screening. In: Quantitative Methods for Cancer and Human Health Risk Assessment, eds: L. Edler and C. Kitsos), Wiley and Sons. 2004 In press

Mahadevia PJ, Fleisher LA, Frick KD, Eng J, Goodman SN, Powe NR (2003) Lung cancer screening with helical computed tomography in older adult smokers: a decision and cost-effectiveness analysis. J Am Med Assoc 289:313–322

Mandel JS, Bond JH, Church TR, Snover DC, Bradley GM, Schuman LM, Ederer F (1993) Reducing mortality from colorectal cancer by screening for fecal occult blood. Minnesota Colon Cancer Control Study. N Engl J Med 328: 1365–1371

Marcus PM, Bergstrahl EJ, Fagerstrom RM, Williams DE, Fontana R, Taylor WF, Prorok PC (2000) Lung cancer mortality in the Mayo Lung Project: impact of extended follow-up. J Natl Cancer Inst 92:1308–1316

Medical Research Council (1948) Streptomycin treatment of pulmonary tuberculosis. Br Med J ii:769–782

Miettinen OS (1974) Confounding and effect-modification. Am J Epidemiol 100:350–353

Miettinen OS (1985) Theoretical epidemiology. Wiley, New York

Miettinen OS (2000a) Screening for lung cancer: Can it be cost-effective? Can Med Assoc J 162:1431–1436

Miettinen OS (2000b) Screening for lung cancer. Radiol Clin North Am 38:479–486

Miettinen OS (2001) The modern scientific physician, vol 6. The useful property of a screening regimen. CMAJ 165: 1219–1220

Miettinen OS, Henschke CI, Pasmantier MW, Smith JP, Libby DM, Yankelevitz DF (2002a) Mammographic screening: no reliable supporting evidence? Lancet 359:404–405

Miettinen OS, Henschke CI, Pasmantier MW, Smith JP, Libby DM, Yankelevitz DF (2002b) Mammographic screening: no reliable supporting evidence? http://www.lancet.com

Miettinen OS, Yankelevitz DF, Henschke CI (2003) Evaluation of screening for a cancer: annotated catechism of the Gold Standard creed. J Eval Clin Pract 9:145–150

Mountain CF (1997) Revisions in the international system for staging lung cancer. Chest 111:1710–1717

National Cancer Institute (2000) Screening. Cancer control objectives for the nation: 1985–2000. Division of Cancer Prevention and Control, National Cancer Institute, Greenwald P, Sondik EJ (eds), Monograph, Chap. 3, pp 27–32

National Lung Screening Trial. http://www.nci.nih.gov/nlst/

Newcomb PA, Norfleet RG, Storer BE, Surawicz TS, Marcus PM (1992) Screening sigmoidoscopy and colorectal cancer mortality. J Natl Cancer Inst 84:1572–1575

New York Early Lung Cancer Action Project. http://www.NYELCAP.org

Olsen O, Gotzsche PC (2001) Cochrane review of screening for breast cancer with mammography. Lancet 358:1340–1342

Parkin DM, Moss SM (2000) Lung cancer screening: improved survival but no reduction in deaths – the role of "overdiagnosis". Cancer 89:2369–2376

Prostate, Lung, Colorectal and Ovarian Cancer Screening Trial (PLCO). http://www.cancer.gov/prevention/plco

Sobue T (2000) A case-control study for evaluating lung cancer screening in Japan. Cancer 89 (Suppl 11):2392–2396

Sobue T, Suzuki T, Naruke T (1992a) A case-control study for evaluating lung-cancer screening in Japan. Japanese Lung-Cancer-Screening Research Group. Int J Cancer 50: 230–237

Sobue T, Suzuki R, Matsuda M, Kuroishi T, Ikeda S, Naruke T (1992b) Survival for clinical stage I lung cancer not surgically treated. Cancer 69:685–692

Sone S, Takashima S, Li F et al. (1998) Mass screening for lung cancer with mobile spiral computed tomography scanner. Lancet 351:1242–1245

Swensen SJ (2002) CT screening for lung cancer. Am J Roentgenol 179:833–836

ABIM Foundation. American Board of Internal Medicine; ACP-ASIM Foundation. American College of Physicians-American Society of Internal Medicine; European Federation of Internal Medicine (2002) Medical professionalism in the new millenium: a physician charter. Ann Intern Med 136:243–246

U.S. Preventive Services Task Force (1989) Guide to clinical preventive services. Screening for lung cancer. U.S. Preventive Services Task Force, Washington, D.C., pp 45–47

Vazquez M, Flieder D, Travis W, Carter D, Yankelevitz D, Miettinen OS, Henschke CI (2002a) Early Lung Cancer Action Project Pathology Protocol. Lung Cancer

Vazquez M, Flieder D, Travis W, Carter D, Yankelevitz D, Miettinen OSM, Henschke CI (2002b) Early Lung Cancer Action Project Pathology Protocol. http://ICScreen.med.cornell.edu

Wisnivesky JP, Mushlin A, Sicherman N, Henschke CI (2002) Cost-effectiveness of baseline low-dose CT screening for lung cancer: preliminary results. Chest 2003; 124:614–621

Yankelevitz DF, Kostis WJ, Henschke CI, Heelan RT, Libby DM, Pasmantier MW, Smith JP (2003) Overdiagnosis in chest radiographic screening for lung cancer: frequency. Cancer 97:1271–1275

10 MDCT Screening for Lung Cancer: Current Controversies

F. L. Jacobson

CONTENTS

10.1 Lung Cancer: The Opportunity for Screening

Lung cancer is currently the most common cause of cancer death in men and women in the United States (Travis et al. 1996). Approximately 171,900 new cases of lung cancer will be diagnosed in the United States in 2003 and 157,200 individuals are expected to die of the disease (American Cancer Society 2003). Despite the development of effective multimodality treatments, mortality from primary lung cancer has continued to rise over the past three decades; approximately 85% of those who develop lung cancer die from it (Fry et al. 1996). More Americans die from lung cancer than colon, breast, and prostate cancers combined.

Small-cell lung cancer accounts for approximately 25% of lung cancers. Small-cell lung cancer is usually a systemic disease at initial presentation due to its aggressive nature with early dissemination throughout the body. Outcome is not improved by screening.

F. L. Jacobson, MD, MPH
Department of Radiology, Brigham and Women's Hospital, 75 Francis Street, Boston, MA 02115, USA

Non-small cell lung cancer (NSCLC) accounts for approximately 75% of all lung cancers. The prognosis in patients with NSCLC follows surgical stage at the time of diagnosis. Overall 5-year survival from lung cancer remains less than 15% (Fry et al. 1996); however, patients with surgically resected early stage NSCLC have 5-year survival rates of up to 70% or more (Martini et al. 1995). Five-year survival in a cohort of 598 patients with surgically resected stage I tumors was recently reported as 75%; however, when stratified by TNM tumor classification, patients with T1 tumors fared better than those with T2 tumors, with 5-year survival rates of 82% and 68%, respectively (Martini et al. 1995; Flehinger et al. 1992). Small tumor size at time of diagnosis and treatment is associated with longer survival, particularly when tumors are less than 1 cm in diameter. This improvement in survival forms the primary rationale for the early detection of lung cancer using multi-detector CT (MDCT) screening.

10.2 Prevention of Lung Cancer

Cigarette smoking is associated with 85% of lung cancers and is the single most important risk factor for lung cancer (Doll and Peto 1981; US Department Of Health, Education And Welfare 1979; Burns 1994; Strauss et al. 1995; Reizenstein et al. 1994). Although the prevalence of smoking has decreased in the 30 years since the first report by the United States Surgeon General on the causal relationship between smoking and lung cancer in men, the annual cancer statistics of the American Cancer Society have only recently begun to show any decrease in lung cancer incidence in men and, in fact, continue to demonstrate increasing incidence of lung cancer in women. Women are entering a period of increased risk based on the 20 to 30 year latency period measured from the introduction of filtered cigarettes marketed specifically to women (American Cancer Society 2003).

More than 50% of lung cancers are now diagnosed in former smokers. For this population, primary prevention, in the form of smoking cessation, is not adequate to prevent deaths due to lung cancer. The selection of criteria for screening is based upon the relative risk of lung cancer as influenced by duration of smoking, intensity of exposure, and duration of smoking cessation in ex-smokers. Risk increases in rough proportion to the number of cigarettes smoked per day (Hammond 1966; Rogot and Murray 1980). Duration-specific risks increase steadily, but are most significant beyond 20 years of smoking duration. Cancer risk remains elevated in former cigarette smokers, declining significantly beyond 5 years from cessation. Lung cancer occurs primarily in patients between ages 50 and 80 years. The relative risk of lung cancer is also influenced by family history, occupational exposures, and the presence of airflow obstruction (Tockman et al. 1987; Nomura et al. 1991). Lung cancer prevalence is high among individuals with minimum 30–40 pack year histories of smoking and airflow obstruction, defined by FEV1/FVC less than 70% of predicted value and FEV1 less than 70% of predicted value (Kennedy et al. 1996). Airflow obstruction is associated with a 4–5-fold increase in lung cancer (Tockman et al. 1987; Nomura et al. 1991). Cancer risk is presumably increased by poor clearance of carcinogens. The correlation between small size of tumor and localized disease may not be as simple as selecting early stage disease however (Patz et al. 2000).

Individuals with previously resected stage I NSCLC are at the highest risk for the development of primary bronchogenic carcinoma (Flehinger et al. 1992; Jones et al. 1995; Marcus et al. 2000). The second lung cancer may be of the same or a different histology; the latter case increasing confidence that the tumor is indeed due to a metachronous primary and not a metastasis of the original primary.

10.3 Criticisms of Lung Cancer Screening

Lung cancer screening is criticized in different ways by ethicists, epidemiologists, and cancer biologists. The ethical question of whether it should be performed outside of a clinical trial is subject to change. The position of epidemiologists can be presented with the history of screening studies. The biases with which they are concerned are of importance also to individual patients and do warrant attention as presented in the following paragraphs. Tumor biology is incompletely understood and far more complex than previously thought. The possibility of preclinical disease in an asymptomatic individual already having metastasized challenges the basic assumptions made when screening. It may not be easy or straightforward to determine who will benefit from MDCT screening for lung cancer, at least until we have complementary biomarker screening tests.

Lung cancer screening with chest radiographs has been studied fairly extensively, beginning with studies in the 1950 s and including mass screening studies in the 1970 s. The Mayo Lung Project (MLP) has now followed every participant to a mortality specific outcome (Marcus et al. 2000; Marcus and Prorok 1999). Forty-six excess, largely early stage, lung cancers occurred in the screened group. Late stage cancers were not decreased and nor was lung cancer-specific mortality. The excess lung cancers in the screened participants have been explained by: over-diagnosis of lung cancer in the screened group and under-diagnosis of lung cancer in the control group. This misclassification of the cause of death is difficult to avoid in such a trial when the experimental group receives greater scrutiny than the control group. The contention that the risk profiles of the two groups were not equivalent is not supported by the recent re-analysis of the risk-defining features of the two groups (Marcus et al. 2000; Marcus and Prorok 1999).

Despite the historical lung cancer screening trials and the reevaluation of the Mayo Clinic MLP data after the death of all of the subjects in that trial, there is currently no recommendation by any national organization for lung cancer screening (Marcus et al. 2000). The National Cancer Institute has initiated a large randomized population trial using MDCT and PA chest radiographs for lung cancer screening to determine whether screening can reduce lung cancer-specific mortality by at least 20%. The National Lung Screening Trial (NLST) has begun enrolling 50,000 subjects through the American College of Radiology Imaging Network (ACRIN) and the Prostate-Lung-Colon-Ovarian (PLCO) Intramural study groups.

Randomized population trials overcome the biases of lead-time, length-time and over-diagnosis by allocating known and unknown factors randomly to both of the groups. Lead-time bias refers to the lengthened survival without alteration in mortality when disease is detected earlier but death is not delayed. Length bias pertains to the tendency of screening to detect slow growing cancers as slow growing cancers have a longer preclinical phase. Such tumors may have more indolent biology and growth potential compared with fast growing tumors that are less likely to be detected by screening. Over-diagnosis bias refers to the detection of a lung cancer that would have remained undetected during the patient's lifetime, prior to death from other causes. When diagnosed, such tumors are referred to as "pseudo-disease." Small studies indicate that individuals with clinical stage I lung cancer who have not been treated by surgical resection, experience 80% mortality at 10 years. However, high mortality does not imply that all lung cancers are lethal, only that clinically known lesions are lethal (Sobue et al. 1992). Published reports have documented unexpected "surprise" lung cancers at autopsy in individuals who have died from conditions such as coronary artery disease. Also, it is well known that small lung lesions less than 2 cm in diameter may be easily overlooked at autopsy due to sampling error. The reported necropsy "surprise" detection rates suggest that there may be a significant reservoir of asymptomatic lung cancer.

10.4 MDCT and Lung Cancer Screening

MDCT is the catalyst in low dose CT screening for lung cancer. Spiral (helical) CT allowed imaging of the thorax with a single breath using 8–10 mm thick images obtained in a single breath-hold. With repeated hyperventilation, patients with significant pulmonary pathology are able to hold their breath for 30 seconds. Spiral CT demonstrates smaller and smaller nodules with each incremental improvement in technology. The threshold of visibility for nodules has decreased to 2–3 mm. Optimum imaging of nodules this small requires scan thickness in the 1–2 mm range, thus the thin section images so readily available with MDCT are a fundamental requirement for lung cancer screening. Overlapping reconstruction of images and review on a workstation, rather than film, are also first principles in the performance of lung cancer screening with MDCT. A bit of math will reveal the order of magnitude increase in the number of images generated by an individual MDCT examination. As this is counterintuitive for a screening examination, the management and efficient manipulation of large image data sets is the current focus of industrial interest, research and development. The near isotropic pixel resolution of even four-row systems allows thin section overlapping reconstructions necessary for image processing and computer aided detection. Computer-aided detection and more broad applications fostering computer-aided diagnosis will hopefully ease the burdens imposed upon the radiologist in performance of MDCT for lung cancer screening in the future. Even now, we see promise in the use of alternative display strategies such as Maximum Intensity Projections (MIP) with thicker slab presentations from which very small nodules are readily identified.

10.5 Low-Dose CT Screening Program

A successful lung cancer screening program can be modeled from a successful breast cancer screening program. The service is provided to asymptomatic individuals who are at risk of developing a specific disease. Just as mammography is performed with risk assessment so should lung cancer screening. The patient also appreciates being given an indication of the preliminary result, when possible, at the conclusion of the examination. The involvement of primary care physicians may vary depending on whether referral is required. In any center that accepts self-referral, follow-up responsibilities will remain with the radiology practice. Of course, scanning, any supportive image processing and image interpretation remain at the core of the radiology practice. Financial arrangements for the examination may be handled differently than for diagnostic radiology services as insurance reimbursement is limited to interested HMOs. Advanced Beneficiary Notices may be required depending on the institution. A separate brochure that presents an overview of the lung cancer screening, process, risks, and benefits can be helpful to patients deciding if they want to have this test. It is important for the physician and patient as well as the radiologist to understand that current knowledge is limited (Berlin 2002). The consensus statement of the Society of Thoracic Radiology provided conservative criteria by which clinical screening services may be undertaken outside of clinical trials, in the absence of a mandate for mass lung cancer screening (Aberle et al. 2001).

10.6 CT Scanning Parameters

MDCT scanning for lung cancer screening requires consideration of technical scanning parameters (Table 10.1). With hyperventilation, patients hold

Table 10.1. MDCT Technical Parameters

MDCT parameter	Lung cancer screening
Detector collimation	<or=to 1 mm
Gantry rotation time	0.5–0.8 second
Table speed (mm/rotation)	12–25 mm
Pitch	1.5
kV	120–140
Effective mA	20–80
Nominal slice width	1.25–2 mm
Reconstruction interval	<or=to 1 mm
Reconstruction algorithm	Standard/lung
CTDI vol (dose in mGy)	3–4 mGy
Scan time	7–20 seconds

their breath in maximal inspiration for 20–30 seconds without difficulty. Dose may be reduced significantly when imaging the lungs, with 120–140 kV and 20–80 mAs resulting in satisfactory studies. Collimation of 1 mm with field of view limited to the lungs will produce high quality images. Reconstruction kernel should be chosen to minimize artifact-simulating calcification as well as provide the edge enhancement preferred for lung images. Thin section images should be reconstructed with 20–50% overlap. It is helpful to also keep standard thickness images for future comparison with diagnostic CT scans, as the best comparison is between images of the same scan thickness.

10.7 MDCT Imaging Findings

Many of the findings seen on low dose MDCT reflect the disease processes seen in individuals who smoke without alteration due to the reduction in dose. Section thickness affects appearance of images in the same manner as on full dose MDCT. The areas in which the dose reduction is noticeable are the mediastinum and soft tissues, particularly of the upper abdomen.

Apical scarring frequently has both pleural and parenchymal components. The parenchymal components frequently include nodular opacities, particularly inferiorly, although these may often be understood in 3D as the inferior aspect of a linear feature. Thin section examination frequently reveals calcification in an associated granuloma not appreciated on thicker sections. The benign nature of a scar is best confirmed by documenting stability over time. Conversely, changes in scars can be the primary sign of the development of lung cancer. This can take the form of a convex mass or thickening of a linear structure in an area of emphysema. An additional area in which linear scars or bands or atelectasis are frequently found is the lung bases, particularly in the regions of the costophrenic sulci.

Emphysema and chronic inflammatory changes are also frequent findings. When studies are performed only when patients are in "their best usual state of health," acute inflammatory changes are less frequently encountered. Bronchiectasis and bronchial wall thickening without dilatation are often seen and can be complicated by mucous simulating a nodule. Centrilobular opacities usually have a characteristic appearance with ill-defined margins (Fig. 10.1). The nodule will measure less than 4 mm in diameter and may be of soft tissue or, more commonly, ground-glass density. This type of opacity may be visible only on thin section images.

Intrapulmonary lymph nodes are frequently found as non-calcified ovoid soft tissue nodules in subpleural regions. A very characteristic location is along the posterolateral aspect of the lower lobes. Diagnosis is more difficult when the location is less typical or the nodule grows (Fig. 10.2). Remember too that the ovoid characteristic may be expressed in the z-axis direction.

Smoothly marginated nodules are benign by radiographic criterion only when they exhibit the solid or central calcification characteristic of calcified granulomas (Fig. 10.3). Such nodules do not require further CT follow-up, whether this is determined on an initial or subsequent CT scan, or even if well seen measuring less than 5 mm in diameter on a high kV radiograph. Thinner sections are definitely more helpful in this regard as well.

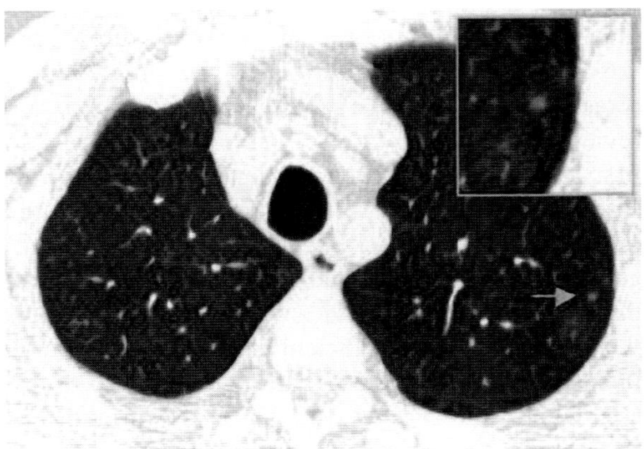

Fig. 10.1. 2 mm CT image demonstrating characteristic small centrilobular ground-glass opacity (GGO) with ill-defined margins. Opacity was not visible on 5 mm image

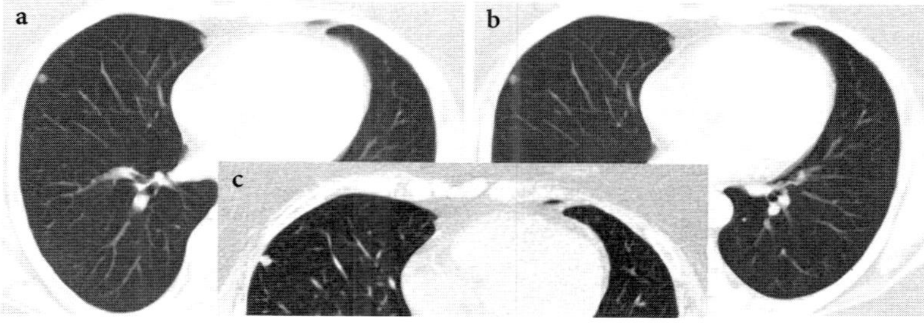

Fig. 10.2. a, 8 mm CT image 2 years prior to screening b, 5 mm image 1 year prior to screening and c is 2 mm CT image from low-dose CT screening. The nodule was resected due to question of growth raised largely due to comparison between images of different scan thickness. Nodule proved to be an intrapulmonary lymph node. A lymph node can grow without indicating malignancy

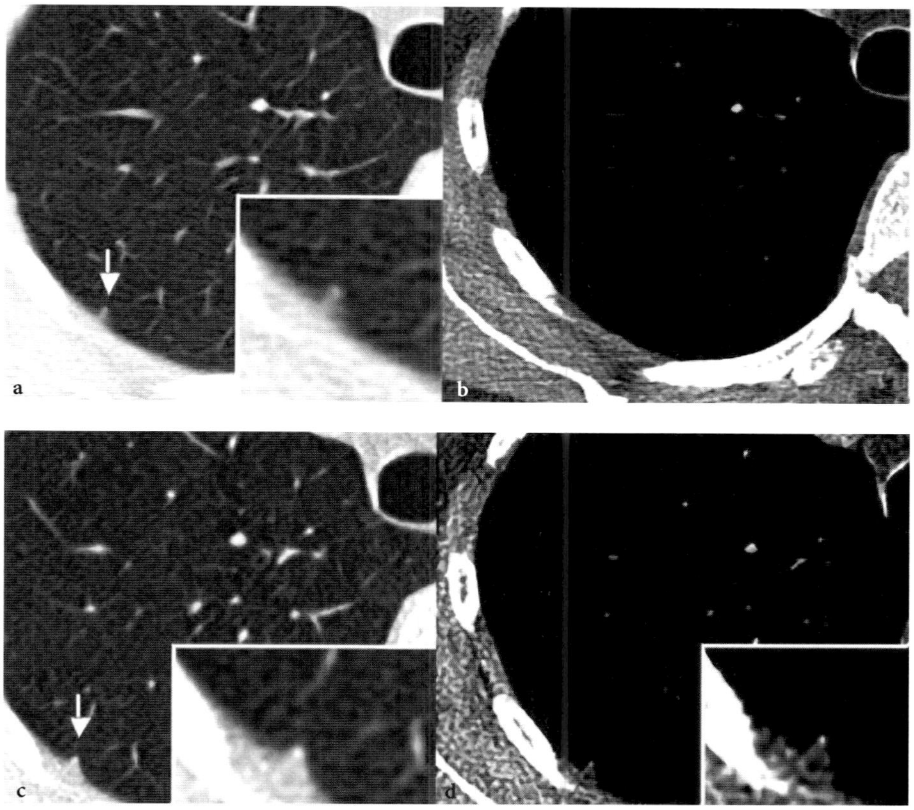

Fig. 10.3. a and b lung and mediastinal windows of 5 mm images revealing a tiny subpleural nodule in right upper lobe without demonstration of calcification. c and d lung and mediastinal windows of 2 mm images at the same table position demonstrating calcification in the same tiny subpleural nodule, confirming it is a calcified granuloma. When calcification is identified, no further follow-up is required

Non-calcified soft tissue nodules are indeterminate and can be benign or malignant regardless of margins, although spiculated borders suggesting desmoplasia are clearly more worrisome for tumor. Evaluation is dependent upon size, appearance of the lesion and the surrounding lung as well as the location and its accessibility for biopsy.

Ground-glass opacity, on MDCT for lung cancer screening, can be difficult to judge when no vessel may be immediately adjacent to the opacity that should not be obscured by it. This is frequently the result of partial volume effect upon a tiny soft tissue, or "solid" nodule. Transient inflammatory opacities can have this appearance as can opacities below the level of resolution by the imaging system, as seen with interstitial lung disease and honeycombing. This designation is also used for opacities that may have structure without mass, making them more worrisome for bronchoalveolar cell carcinoma (Fig. 10.4). Patients may have multiple lesions, with both adenocarcinomas and bronchoalveolar cell carcinomas. Recent reports in the literature indicate potential for tumor and persistent presence without progression or other evidence of significant abnormality (Kodama et al. 2002).

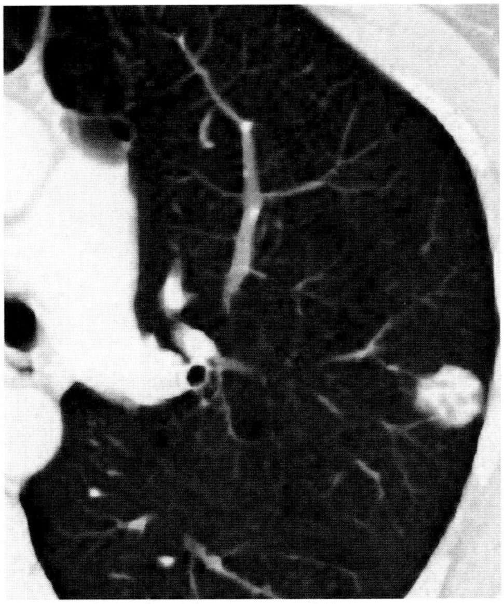

Fig. 10.4. 2 mm image reveals a peripheral nodule with air bronchograms. This proved to be an adenocarcinoma with areas of bronchoalveolar carcinoma

The most controversial category of opacities currently recognized in reporting MDCT for lung cancer screening is the part-solid mixed with ground glass opacity (Fig. 10.5). This may be symmetric or asymmetric. The association with cancer is high compared with solid only and ground-glass only nodules (Henschke et al. 2002). It too can be influenced by slice selection and scan thickness however.

10.8 Interpretation of Screening CT

Technological improvements leading to multi-detector CT and the prevalence of small benign nodules in normal individuals suggest that the use of strict criteria for screening will result in increasing numbers of patients having positive screening CT studies (Swensen 2002). The concept of choosing criteria by which to focus on a subset of study abnormalities is not a new concept. In the Early Lung Cancer Action Program (ELCAP), the large numbers of nodules, beginning with more the 6, were classified differently, as they were more likely related to a process such as prior granulomatous infection than lung cancer. The National Lung Screening Trial (NLST) does not catalog, nodules measuring less than 4 mm in diameter that will not undergo interim follow-up imaging between annual screening CT examinations. At this time, these are decisions made for specific protocols. Given the large number of small benign nodules that are found in the periphery of normal lungs, future incorporation of some as yet unspecified minimum size for nodule follow-up in the standard of care would be helpful to radiologists providing lung cancer screening CT.

Measurement remains cumbersome. Automated measurement tools are not yet widely available and do not perform all of the required measurements under all conditions. Opacities that are not composed of solid nodules, whether due to spiculations or components of ground glass opacities may continue to challenge these tools. The radiologist may be more consistent than an automated measurement tool when measuring ground glass opacities. Adjacent structures ranging from vessels to the mediastinum and the chest wall continue to create ambiguity for measurement although automated measurement will usually more consistently select such a margin than the radiologist.

The overlap between benign and malignant lesions by appearance may be greater in clinical practice than in the early clinical trials such as ELCAP. Reports may seem dated before the next time the patient reports for screening. Many patients choose not to return for screening on a continuing basis, based on current information.

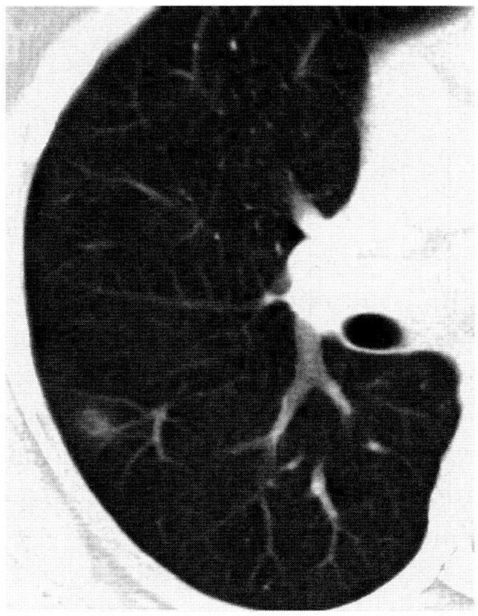

Fig. 10.5. 5 mm image reveals solid opacity and ground-glass opacity. This type of opacity may be associated with benign or malignant disease. This one resolved on a subsequent study

10.9 Algorithms for Follow-up

Follow-up algorithms have been a recent focus of controversy and should be expected to continue to change, even perhaps before the first follow-up exam would be scheduled for a patient having a positive screening CT today. The most definitive benign finding in a very small pulmonary nodule will remain calcification.

Demonstration of characteristic, solid or central, calcification associated with a granuloma, does prove that a nodule is benign. This is true whether this is the first or any subsequent CT. Thinner sections and differences in slice selection result in demonstration of calcification in different nodules on different examinations.

Solid, non-calcified nodules remain indeterminate. When suspicion for malignancy is low, follow-up to demonstrate 2 years of stability remains the current standard of care. Most conservatively, this results in follow-up CT in 3 months, 6 months, 12 months and 24 months. This is based upon the model used in diagnostic examinations. In the case of a patient reporting for screening as an asymptomatic person without known disease, rather than a patient with a known tumor who might have metastases, consideration for follow-up in 6 months, 12 months and 24 months may also be appropriate. The provision of the technological ability to accurately and reproducibly detect small amounts of growth in small nodules in the clinical environment may alter these strategies in the future.

The National Lung Screening Trial will not be doing interim follow-up, at less that 12 months, for most nodules measuring less than 4 mm. While arbitrary, it does eliminate many classes of known benign opacities, including centrilobular opacities, many granulomas, and many micronodules. Lung nodules in this size range that actually represent cancers that have not yet exhibited malignant features, even if due to the limitations of the imaging system, would of necessity have to have a slow to moderate growth rate in order to benefit from screening by being found based upon growth a year later. These characteristics would be necessary for the lesion to be one to benefit from early detection as well.

While tumors can metastasize at any size, it is helpful to review tumor growth in terms of screening and the opportunity to identify preclinical disease.

Part-solid and ground-glass opacities represent more active biological entities that may represent inflammation, or, as demonstrated in the ELCAP experience, early lung cancer. The significance of cancers detected by screening is less well understood than more advanced stage lung cancers that present with clinical signs and symptoms.

For low dose CT to provide successful lung cancer screening, the appropriate individuals will need to be selected. Examinations will need to be performed at specifically chosen intervals with carefully designed follow-up protocols. We do not yet have the necessary data to optimize detection while minimizing morbidity and mortality associated with evaluation of false positive nodules identified at screening. Decrease in lung cancer specific mortality from early detection through screening could be completely offset by morbidity and mortality associated with workup of false positive nodules and "pseudo-disease" that would not have become apparent during the normal lifetime of the patient.

Spiculated lesions and those larger than one centimeter require standard clinical investigation. PET-FDG imaging scan, biopsy, and surgical resection have roles in such lesions. The burden of work-up for false positive nodules will vary with location, generally between 25-and 50%. The health care cost and attendant morbidity and mortality require careful consideration and the most conservative management possible. Biomarker assays may contribute more to the decision process in the future.

10.10 Patient Expectations

It is critically important for the radiologist to communicate with the patient regarding the imperfect state of our knowledge regarding the value of lung cancer screening. It is not a substitute for primary prevention of lung cancer through smoking cessation. It is not known whether earlier identification of lung cancer can reduce the chance of dying from lung cancer. The patient needs to understand the possibility of further tests and even surgery being recommended, with attendant complications of morbidity and mortality, as a result of having the test, even if no benefit is ultimately realized.

10.11 Current Status

Low-dose CT screening is being performed in both clinical and research settings. Targeted populations include heavy smokers and those with occupational exposures to substances such as asbestos.

In baseline and 2 follow-up annual low-dose CT screening examinations of 1520 individuals, the Mayo Clinic has identified 2832 nodules in 1,049 individuals (89%). Forty cases of lung cancer diagnosed included 20 at prevalence screen and 10 at each subsequent annual incidence screening CT examination. Thirty-eight cases were diagnosed by CT alone and 2 were diagnosed by sputum cytology alone. Two interval cancers were not detected by the screening examinations. The stages included 22 stage IA, 3 stage IB, 5 Stage II, 5 Stage II, and 1 Stage IV. All cell types were represented. Individuals in this trial were at least 50 years of age with a minimum 20 pack-year smoking history (Swensen et al. 2003). The results of this study provide realistic data regarding the confounding factors in populations with significant benign nodule forming exposures such as encountered in areas of endemic granulomatous diseases. Despite the high rate of granulomatous disease in this population, this CT screening project has been successful epidemiologically with a very low rate of interval cancers. The data regarding sputum cytology suggests we should continue to seek roles for inexpensive screening tests in conjunction with CT.

These data encourage our screening efforts while we wait for the results of the National Lung Screening Trial, now midway through its baseline, prevalence screen of 50,000 individuals. From this randomized population trial, we expect to finally learn whether early detection of lung cancer decreases lung cancer specific mortality. This has remained the missing piece of information amid increasing enthusiasm for offering the potential opportunity to escape the very poor prognosis of lung cancer. It is intuitive to think that, as with other forms of cancer, early detection will allow effective treatments to provide long-term control and true cure. We have not yet proved we are not identifying cases of lung cancer that would not otherwise come to clinical attention and limited life, a significant concern incidental lung cancer necropsy rates of 16%. Many of the early trial that have allowed us to reach our current level of enthusiasm are subject to lead-time bias by reporting survival as a surrogate for mortality benefit. Tumor biology is complex and we have barely scratched the surface in understanding the interaction between individual nodules. In any case screening will select for relatively indolent disease as the most aggressive tumors should be expected to present as interval cancers. Determining the true frequency of this event in large populations undergoing widespread screening for lung cancer will also be important for providing proper understanding of the limit of what screening can provide to the public.

Finally, our diagnostic methods will have to keep pace with our screening dilemmas. Non-invasive testing and more rapid ways of confirming the benign nature of nodules on baseline screening examinations will also allow earlier identification of the few nodules that represent early lung cancers. As we learn to sort nodules more specifically new screening, diagnostic and therapeutic strategies will probably emerge. Change is still needed to optimize our efforts using low-dose CT for lung cancer screening.

10.12 Current Controversies

Should we screen for lung cancer? After 50 years, this question has still not been answered. The studies looking at the ability of chest radiographs to decrease lung cancer mortality in the 1970 s, including the one done at The Mayo Clinic that has recently had follow-up mortality data obtained for all participants, failed to find a decrease in mortality. In part, this represents limitations in study design, such as power, and flaws that allowed the study and control groups to become more similar. Some limitations are simply unavoidable such as the difference in detailed cause of death information for individuals in the two arms of the study. The depth of information is just not there regarding control subjects.

The urge to screen stems from the continued dismal prognosis of lung cancer, with 15% 5-year survival despite the improvements in treatment over the past 30 years. Lobectomy for Stage 1 A lung cancer provides at least 70% 5-year survival. How to identify the patients who will benefit from this surgery has been controversial because of the shift in tumor cell type to adenocarcinoma and its ability metastasize before reaching 7 mm in diameter. Surgery is not an adequate treatment for tumor that has already metastasized. While no patient who has had a Stage 1 A lung cancer removed has ever been willing to have the tumor put back in his body, we have not yet proved that the incidentally discovered early tumors are the same tumors that would have gone on to kill the patients. It is for this purpose that we await the primary outcome data of the National Lung Screening Trial designed to determine whether screening with either PA chest radiograph or low-dose multidetector CT scan will decrease lung cancer mortality.

Once the mortality issue is better understood, the accumulating data will also point the next direction in creating an integrated screening program. CT is expensive for use as a screening test. As such, it would be best if it could be used like colonoscopy, at milestone ages and relatively long intervals. Other tests, based on body fluids, may well be used for more frequent monitoring and determining when to perform repeat imaging. In this way, we may ultimately need to deviate from the annual imaging model of Mammography that has served us well in beginning to screen for lung cancer. Molecular imaging is an important horizon that should be incorporated into our screening and evaluation algorithms.

10.13 Conclusion

Lung cancer screening remains controversial because no decrease in lung cancer specific mortality has yet been demonstrated through early detection of disease. The National Lung Screening Trial (NLST) has recently begun enrolling 50,000 smokers and former smokers, ages 55–74, in order to answer this important question. Lung cancer screening CT can be of benefit to selected patients. Communication between radiologist, patient and physician is critical to successful low dose CT screening for lung cancer.

Until a standard of care is established, who should be screened, when, and by what modality will remain a subject of debate and variability. CT may ultimately be used in conjunction with an inexpensive screening test performed on urine or blood. Criteria are needed that will maximize the identification of asymptomatic lung cancers and decrease lung cancer deaths with the least burden on radiologists, patients and the health care system.

References

Aberle DR, Gamsu G, Henschke CI et al (2001) A consensus statement of the Society of Thoracic Radiology. Screening for Lung Cancer with Helical Computed Tomography. J Thorac Imaging16:65–68

American Cancer Society (2003) Department of Epidemiology and Surveillance Research. Cancer: facts and figures 2003. Atlanta, Georgia. Available online at http://www.cancer.org/downloads/STT/CAFF2003PWSecured.pdf

Berlin L (2002) Liability of performing CT screening for coronary artery disease and lung cancer. AJR 179:837–842

Burns DM (1994) Tobacco smoking. In: Samet JM (ed) Epidemiology of lung cancer. Dekker, New York, pp 15–19

Doll R, Peto R (1981) The causes of cancer. J Natl Cancer Inst 66:1191–1308

Flehinger BJ, Kimmel M, Melamed M (1992) The effect of surgical treatment on survival from early lung cancer. Chest 101:1013–1018

Fry WA, Menck HR, Winchester DP (1996) The National Cancer Data Base report on lung cancer. Cancer 77:1947–1955

Hammond EC (1966) Smoking in relation to the death rates of one million men and women. Natl Cancer Inst Monogr 19:127–133

Henschke CI, Yankelevitz DF, Mircheva R et al (2002) CT screening for lung cancer: frequency and significance of part-solid and nonsolid nodules. AJR 178:1053–1057

Johnson BE, Cortazar P, Chute JP (1997) Second lung cancers in patients successfully treated for lung cancer. Semin Oncol 24:492–499

Jones AS, Morar P, Phillips DE et al (1995) Second primary tumors in patients with head and neck squamous cell carcinoma. Cancer 75:1343–1354

Kennedy et al (1996) Cancer Res 56:4673–4678

Kodama K, Higashiyama M, Yokouchi H, Takami K et al (2002) Natural history of pure ground-glass opacity after long-term follow-up of more than 2 years. Ann Thor Surg 73:386–393

Marcus PM, Prorok PC (1999) Reanalysis of the Mayo Lung Project data: the impact of confounding and effect modification. J Med Screen 6:47–49

Marcus PM, Bergstralh EJ, Fagerstrom RM, Williams DE, Fontana R, Taylor WF, Prorok PC (2000) Lung cancer mortality in the Mayo Lung Project: impact of extended follow-up. J Natl Cancer Inst 92:1308–1316

Martini N, Bains MS, Burt ME et al (1995) Incidence of local recurrence and second primary tumors in resected stage I lung cancer J Thorac Cardiovasc Surg 109:120–129

Nomura A, Stemmermann Gnk, Chyou P-H et al (1991) Prospective study of pulmonary function and lung cancer. Am Rev Respir Dis 144:307–311

Patz EF, Rossi S, Harpole DH et al (2000) Correlation of tumor size and survival in patients with stage IA non-small cell lung cancer. Chest 117:1568–1571

Reizenstein P, Moden B, Kuller LH (1994) The quandary of cancer prevention. J Clin Epidemiol 47:575–581

Rogot E, Murray JL (1980) Smoking and causes of death among US veterans: 16 years of observation. Public Health Rep 15: 213–217

Sobue T, Suzuki T, Matsuda M et al (1992) Survival for clinical stage I lung cancer not surgically treated. Comparison between screen-detected and symptom-detected cases. The Japanese Lung Cancer Screening Research Group. Cancer 69:685–692

Strauss G, DeCamp M, Dibiccaro E et al (1995) Lung cancer diagnosis is being made with increasing frequency in former cigarette smokers. Proc ASCO 14:362

Swensen SJ (2002) CT screening for lung cancer. AJR 179: 833–836

Swensen SJ, Jett JR, Hartman TE (2003) Lung cancer screening with CT: Mayo Clinic Experience. Radiology 226:756–761

Tockman MS, Anthonisen NR, Wright EC et al (1987) Airway obstruction and the risk for lung cancer. Ann Intern Med 106:512–517

Travis WD, Lubin J, Ries L et al (1996) United States lung carcinoma trends: declining for most histologic types among males, increasing among females. Cancer 77:2464–2470

US Department of Health, Education and Welfare (1979) Smoking and Health. A report of the Surgeon General. Public Health Service. DHEW Publ no PHS 79–50066

11 MDCT Imaging of Focal Lung Disease

D. P. Naidich and J. P. Ko

CONTENTS

11.1 Introduction

Few problems have vexed clinicians as thoroughly as the evaluation of pulmonary nodules. Through a fortuitous combination of recent developments, however, our understanding of factors affecting both the detection and characterization of nodules has undergone a profound transformation. These factors include: the introduction of multi-detector CT (MDCT), including scanners with up to 16 rows of detectors providing as many as 600 to a thousand images per study; the widespread availability of picture archiving systems (PACS) as well advanced image processing workstations capable of a wide variety of tasks, including automatic nodule segmentation and volume assessment; and the growing interest in the use of computer assisted diagnosis (CAD) for image analysis. Coupled with these developments is the recent introduction of low-dose lung cancer screening. Although currently lacking in general acceptance, there is no denying that the potential use of CT screening has proved a major stimulus to a more thorough understanding both of the natural history of pulmonary nodules as well as factors affecting their detection and characterization. It is the purpose of this chapter to review these subjects with particular emphasis on these more recent contributions.

D. P. Naidich, MD
Professor of Radiology and Medicine, New York University Medical Center, 560 1st Avenue, New York City, NY 10016, USA
J. P. Ko, MD
Assistant Professor of Radiology, New York University Medical Center, 560 1st Avenue, New York City, NY 10016, USA

11.2 Lung Nodule Detection

Although CT has repeatedly been documented to be superior to plain chest radiographs for detecting pulmonary nodules, there are well known limitations. As documented by Ambrogi et al, for example, in their study of 22 patients undergoing video-assisted thoracic surgery using a transxiphoid approach for resection of pulmonary metastases, preoperative single detector helical CT identified only 46 (79%) of 58 surgically documented nodules. Overall, occult disease was detected in one third of patients. Similar results have been reported in the surgical literature regarding the preoperative limitations of CT in assessing candidates for lung volume reduction surgery (LVRS). As noted by Hazzelrigg et al. (1997), in their study of 281 patients undergoing LVRS, 17 (22%) of 78 resected nodules proved malignant including 14 false negative CT studies. Recently, additional documentation regarding the limitations of CT has emerged from lung cancer screening studies. As documented by Kakinuma et al. (1999), in their study of 5,418 CT exams in 1,443 smokers, 7 of 22 lung cancers were retrospectively identifiable. Similarly, in a report of follow-up incidence screening, Henschke et al. (2001) found that 22 of 63 newly identified nodules were retrospectively identifiable.

In fact a number of factors have proved of critical importance in the detection of lung nodules on CT including technical parameters, variability in nodule characteristics and factors related to observer variability.

11.2.1 Technical Factors

Technical factors that have been shown to affect nodule detection include slice thickness, reconstruction interval, pitch and dose as well as differences in the methods of viewing. Also critical are differences between single and multi-detector CT scanners.

Compared with multi-detector CT scanners, the effect of pitch on nodule detection is far greater with single detector CT (SDCT). Although SDCT allows volumetric data acquisition, increasing the pitch to allow greater anatomic coverage may result in considerable broadening of the slice profile with resulting decrease in nodule conspicuity (Wright et al. 1996). In distinction, with multi-detector CT scanners, slice sensitivity profiles are either less affected or independent of pitch (Klingenbeck-Regn et al. 1999). Furthermore, with the introduction of newer 16 detector CT scanners, it is now possible to obtain near isotropic voxels, the effect of which should be to further improve nodule conspicuity. Most important, using 1 mm collimators MDCT scanners allowing both prospective and retrospective reconstruction of both thick and thin high-resolution images without the need to rescan patients (Fig. 11.1).

Numerous studies to date have shown that nodule detection is markedly improved with the use of overlapping reconstructions (Buckley et al. 1995; Diederich et al. 1999; Wormanns et al. 2000). These may be obtained either prospectively or retrospectively, and hence do not affect patient dose. As documented by Diederich et al. (1999) use of overlapping reconstructions both enhances detection of nodules, especially those less than 5 mm, as well as improving diagnostic confidence. Wormanns et al. (2000) in a study of 23 patients with 286 nodules found that readers could identify only 205 nodules using contiguous 5 mm sections versus 230 when 5 mm sections were reconstructed every 3 mm. These authors also found that the use of overlapping reconstructions significantly improved reader confidence especially for small lesions less than 5 mm in size.

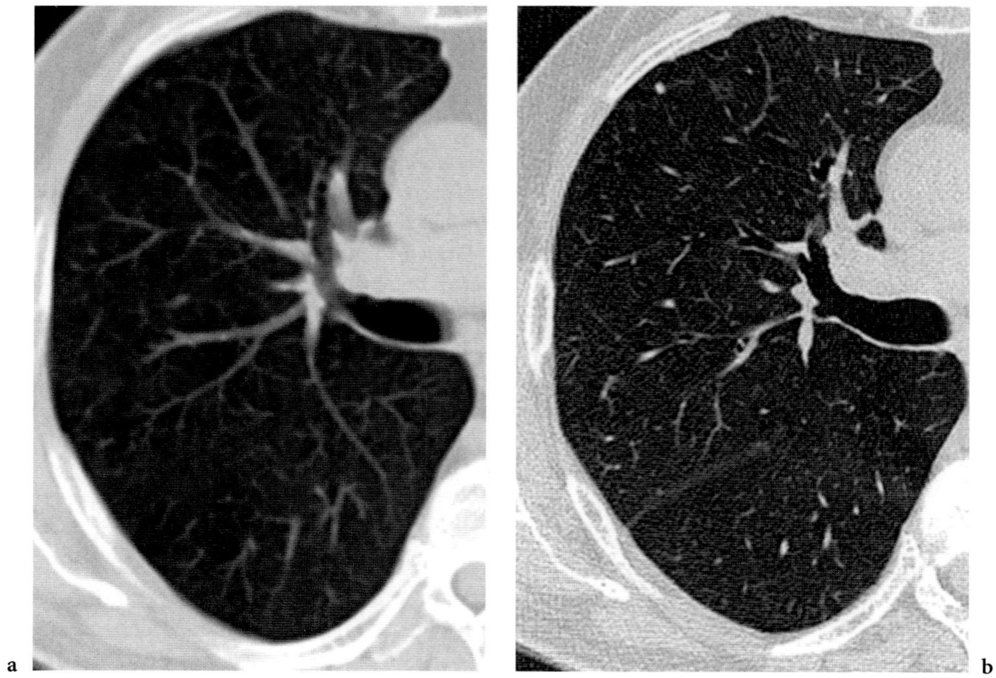

Fig. 11.1a, b. Effect of collimation and density on lesion conspicuity. **a** Target reconstruction of a 7 mm section at the level of the right upper lobe bronchus shows a small 3 mm subpleural nodule in the lung periphery. **b** Target reconstruction of a 1 mm section retrospectively reconstructed from the original scan data at the same level as shown in **a**. Note that in addition to improving the conspicuity of the subpleural nodule it is also apparent that this represents a calcified granuloma. In addition, there is also now evidence of a small ground glass nodule medially, virtually impossible to identify on the initial 7 mm section

Methods of viewing scan data are also of importance. Lung nodule detection has been shown to be compromised when image size is decreased using a fixed viewing distance (Seltzer et al. 1998). Of still greater importance is the use of "cine viewing" of image data on a workstation. As documented by Seltzer et al. (1995), cine viewing is of particular value by facilitating differentiation of nodules from adjacent blood vessels, especially when less than 5 mm in size or centrally located. Recently, in addition to viewing routine axial reconstructions it has been shown that alternate methods of image reconstruction may further enhance nodule detection (Coakley et al. 1998; Gruden et al. 2002). Using maximum intensity projection imaging (MIPS), Gruden et al. (2002) found significantly more nodules due to improved delineation of small peripheral blood vessels (Fig. 11.2).

In distinction to reconstruction intervals and viewing methodology, the use of low dose has considerably less impact on nodule detection. In an initial study comparing low dose with standard CT technique, Rusinek et al. (1998) showed no significant difference in the identification of 3 to 5 mm nodules on 10 mm sections using 20 mAs. More recently, Gartenschlager et al. (1998) in a prospective comparison of nodule detection on 8 mm sections reconstructed every 8 mm using 30 and 200 mA, respectively, found both techniques to be comparable, with the sensitivity and specificity of low dose technique equaling 85% and 93%, respectively.

11.2.2 Morphologic Factors

In addition to technical factors a number of morphologic features are important factors determining nodule conspicuity. These include, among others, size, density, contour, and location.

The most important factor determining nodule conspicuity is size: predictably, smaller lesions, especially those less than 5 mm in size, prove hardest to detect (Fig. 11.1). Rusinek et al. (1998) in an early study employing computer generated nodules found that using 10 mm collimation only 37% and 62% of 3 mm and 5 mm nodules, respectively, could be identified by experienced readers. This poor sensitivity in part reflects the result of partial volume averaging due to the use of 10 mm thick sections. Kakinuma et al. (1999), based on their evaluation of missed lung cancers using low dose CT concluded that the threshold for detection of early lung cancer is between 7 and 9 mm's. In addition to size, location is also a crucial determinant of conspicuity, with nodules located adjacent to blood vessels, as well as those lying centrally near the pulmonary hila or diaphragms particularly difficult to identify. While this represents one extreme point of view, it is apparent that small nodules potentially representing early cancers may be easily missed, especially when contiguous thick sections only are employed (Fig. 11.3).

Nodule density is also a key factor affecting detection. So-called ground-glass or sub solid nodules, in

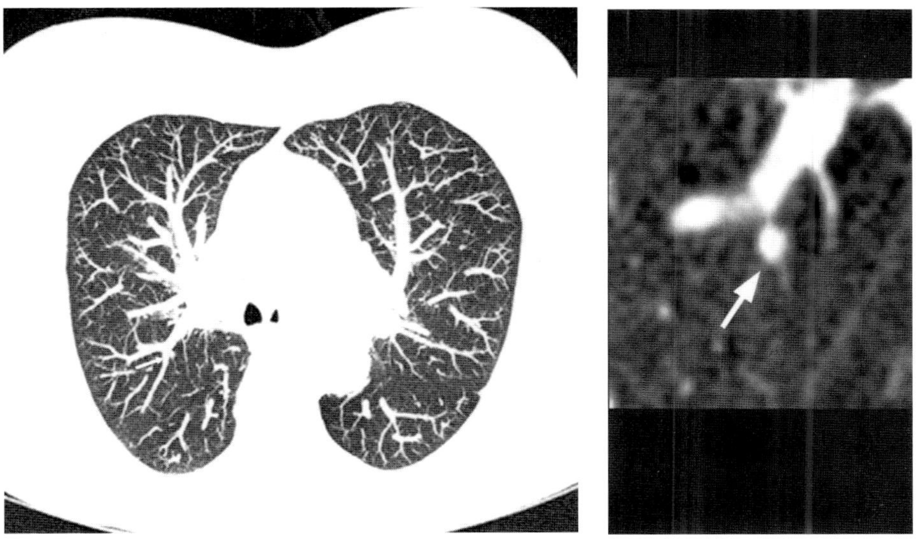

a b

Fig. 11.2a, b. Maximum intensity projection imaging. **a** Maximum intensity projection image (MIP) obtained from 5 contiguous 1 mm axial images shows a subtle perihilar nodule (*arrows*). This was initially missed when routine axial images only were evaluated. **b** Enlargement of representative axial image through the nodule shown in A. MIPs are of greatest utility in identifying small centrally located nodules

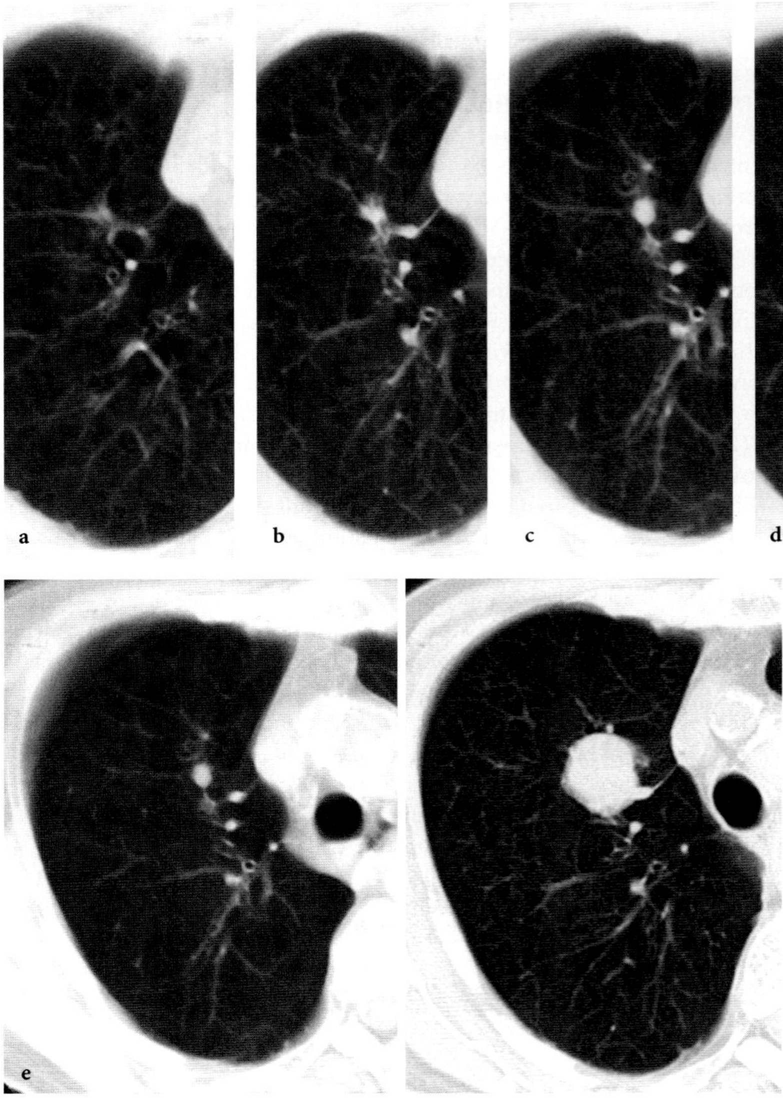

Fig. 11.3a–e. Missed lung cancer. **a–d** Magnified 7 mm images through the right upper lobe show a subtle nodule easily missed due to close proximity to a central vessel. 3 E. Section at the same level as **c** obtained several months later showing a large tumor mass. Biopsy proved non-small cell lung cancer

particular when small, are especially difficult to identify unless high- resolution thin sections are obtained (Fig. 11.1) (KAKINUMA et al. 1999). Another factor is the relationship between nodules and adjacent anatomic structures. In addition to blood vessels, it has also been observed that nodules may be overlooked especially when endobronchial in location (WHITE et al. 1996).

11.2.3 Observer Variability

To date, considerable inter-observer variability has been reported in detecting pulmonary nodules. WORMANNS et al. (2000), for example, assessing interobserver variation in a study of 23 patients with 286 nodules between 2 and 40 mm in size noted that only 103 of 286 nodules were identified by both readers. NOVAK et al. (2002) assessing 10 consecutive low-dose screening studies found that of a total of 26 true nodules, only eight were detected by all 3 readers. In addition to variations in levels of interpretive skill, factors contributing to observer variation include so-called "satisfaction of search," defined as a lessening of diagnostic suspicion following identification of at least one abnormality, as well as reader fatigue. Less easily measured but likely as important are marked variations in individual reader's definitions of what constitute "true" lung nodules.

11.3 Lung Nodule Characterization

Despite recent advances in imaging technology, accurate lung nodule characterization remains elusive. Recent attention has focused on improved morphologic assessment, more accurate densitometry, with special emphasis on the role of intravenous contrast enhancement, and in particular, the potential to obtain precise measurements of changes in nodule volumes over time.

11.3.1 Morphologic Evaluation

Traditionally, nodules have been characterized by a number of criteria, including: definition (sharply defined versus poorly defined); shape (round or irregular); contour (smooth or speculated); density (ground glass, solid or cavitary), and location (including relationship to blood vessels (the "feeding vessel sign"), airways (the "positive bronchus sign'), and pleural surfaces including the fissures) (Milne and Zerhouni 1987; Seemann et al. 1999; Siegelmann et al. 1980, 1986; Zerhouni et al. 1986; Zwirewich et al. 1991). Additional features reported as diagnostically valuable include the presence of surrounding ground glass density (the so-called "halo" sign) (Gaeta et al. 1992, 1999; Kim et al. 1999; Primack et al. 1994) as well as the presence of dilated airways within lesions and the finding of both cavitation and "pseudocavitation" (Nambu et al. 2002). Unfortunately, to date, none of these signs has proved sufficiently predictive to provide reliable clinical management in individual cases. Zerhouni et al. (1986), for example, reported that while 73 (61%) of 120 primary lung cancers – a small majority – proved to have spiculated margins, 41 of 130 nodules classified as smooth and 26 of 48 nodules classified as lobulated proved to be either primary or secondary neoplasms. Seemann et al. (1999) using select signs to characterize 104 consecutive patients with solitary nodules reported a sensitivity of 91.4%, a specificity of 56.5% and an overall accuracy of 83.7% only for correctly identifying malignant nodules. An important exception is the finding of feeding vessels and draining veins in patients with arteriovenous malformations (AVM's). In this setting, CT has proved a reliable guide not only for diagnosis but patient management including providing an anatomic roadmap prior to angiographic intervention (Remy et al. 1994).

Recently it has been suggested that in addition to assessing routine morphologic characteristics nodules may be better evaluated using more sophisticated quantitative measurements. McNitt-Gray et al. (1999), for example, have proposed using not only size, shape and density but the distribution of attenuation and texture analysis as well to differentiate benign from malignant disease. In an evaluation of a training set of 31 cases proved cases, including 14 benign and 17 malignant nodules, these authors used these features to correctly classify 28 (91%) of 31. While intriguing, this approach will require further validation.

11.3.1.1 Size

Although less commonly used as a criterion to distinguish benign from malignant nodules, most tiny lesions in the lung prove to be benign, usually representing either small granulomas of intrapulmonary lymph nodes (Fig. 11.3) (Bankoff et al. 1996; Miyake et al. 1999; Yokomise et al. 1998). It has also been assumed traditionally that the smaller the neoplasm the earlier the stage. Recently, however, it has been suggested that the size of a malignant lesion in itself may not accurately correlate with tumor stage. Patz et al. (2000), in a retrospective study of 510 patients with T1N0M0 lesions (by definition less than 3 cm in size) found no statistical relationship between survival and tumor size. It should be noted that only 26 patients (5%) in this study had lesions less than 1 centimeter in size. Furthermore, despite variation, the five year survival for all groups in this study still proved to be greater than 80%. Nonetheless, the notion that small size per se correlates with a better prognosis remains to be established, especially for nodules less than 1 cm in size.

11.3.1.2 The Sub-Solid Nodule

The introduction of multi-detector CT scanners allowing high resolution 1 to 1.25 mm sections to be obtained throughout the thorax in a single breath-hold period coupled with recent data largely derived from lung cancer screening trials has led to a growing understanding of the significance of ground-glass or sub-solid pulmonary nodules (Henschke et al. 2002).

In distinction to the above mentioned criteria for differentiating benign from malignant lesions, characterizing lesions as ground glass or sub-solid appears to have promising value both as a marker for the histologic spectrum of adenocarcinoma as well as an accurate predictor of prognosis. In particular, there appears to be close correspondence between current pathologic classifications (Travis et al. 1999) and high-resolution CT findings (Aoki et al. 2000). According to the most recent World Health Organization (WHO), bronchoalveolar cell carcinoma (BAC) is limited to include only those tumors with a pure alveolar growth pattern without stromal, vascular, or pleural invasion (Travis et al. 1999). In distinction, three additional types of adenocarcinoma are recognized: acinar, papillary and solid carcinoma with mucous formation. This is similar to the pathologic classification proposed by Noguchi et al. (1995), in which adenocarcinomas are classified into 6 subtypes, A through F. In this classification, at one end of the spectrum are lesions defined as localized bronchoalveolar cell carcinomas (BAC), with and without structural collapse (Types A and B, respectively), or with foci of active fibroblastic proliferation (Type C) - where Types A - C reflect progressive replacement of alveolar lining cells by tumor and fibrosis (Fig. 5a–d). In distinction, Types D - F represent poorly differentiated, tubular, or papillary invasive adenocarcinomas, respectively, having in common no evidence of bronchoalveolar elements (Fig. 11.4e). While Type A and B lesions

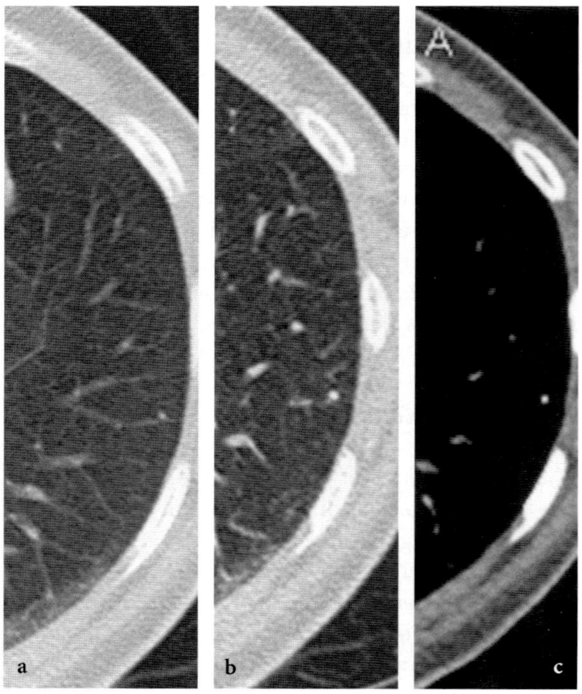

Fig. 11.4a–c. Effect of thin versus thick CT sections: calcified granuloma. **a** A 7 mm target reconstructed section through the left mid lung shows a small (3 mm) nodule in the lung periphery. **b, c** 1 mm target reconstructed section at the same level as in **a** imaged with wide and narrow windows, respectively. Note that the lesions is now considerably more conspicuous and clearly calcified

show no evidence of nodal metastases and a reported five -year survival of 100%, Type C lesions frequently present with nodal metastases and correspondingly lower reported 5 year survivals of 75%, even when small-sized.

As reported by Aoki et al. (2000), close correspondence has been established between the spectrum of CT findings and the Noguchi classification, with pure ground glass nodules more likely representing BAC with predominant lepidic growth and solid components more likely reflecting the presence of invasive carcinoma (Fig. 11.5). Similar correspondence has been shown by Nakata et al. (2002) who also found that the presence of ground glass attenuation in nodules closely correlated with adenocarcinoma: of 43 patients with ground glass nodules less than 2 cm's in size surgically resected, 23 represented bronchoalveolar cell carcinomas while 11 represented invasive adenocarcinomas and 9 proved to be foci of atypical adenomatous hyperplasia.

This latter entity typically presents as a pure ground glass nodule and is now considered a precursor to BAC (Travis et al. 1999). Histologically, these lesions are frequently identified incidentally at the time of surgical resection of lung cancers, and are marked by hyperplasia of single-layered alveolar cuboidal cells. It has been suggested that the presence of these lesions in association with Stage IA adenocarcinomas may indicate a favorable prognosis (Takigawa et al. 1999). Although differentiation between AAH and BAC pathologically may be difficult, as a rule AAH has been shown to have a smaller mean nuclear diameter, less nuclear atypia and smaller cell size than BAC. With CT both appear to have ground glass density; however, AAH typically are smaller (Fig. 11.5a) (Kitamura et al. 1995, 1996). In a report of 9 cases of surgically resected AAHs, Kawakami et al. noted that these lesions typically are round, pure GGOs ranging between 6 and 17 mm (mean of 8.8 mm) with smooth, well-defined borders without evidence of pleural indentation (Kawakami et al. 2001).

Recent evidence based on studies of tumor markers such as mutations in the p53 tumor suppressor gene and the k-ras oncogene identified through immunohistochemical and molecular analysis of biopsy specimens confirm that AAH is now properly classified along with squamous dysplasia/carcinoma in situ and diffuse idiopathic pulmonary neuroendocrine cell hyperplasia in the category of "preinvasive lesions" (Travis et al. 1999). Based on this data, it has been suggested that pure GGOs, especially when small (less than 1 to 1.5 cm's), represent an early stage of BAC

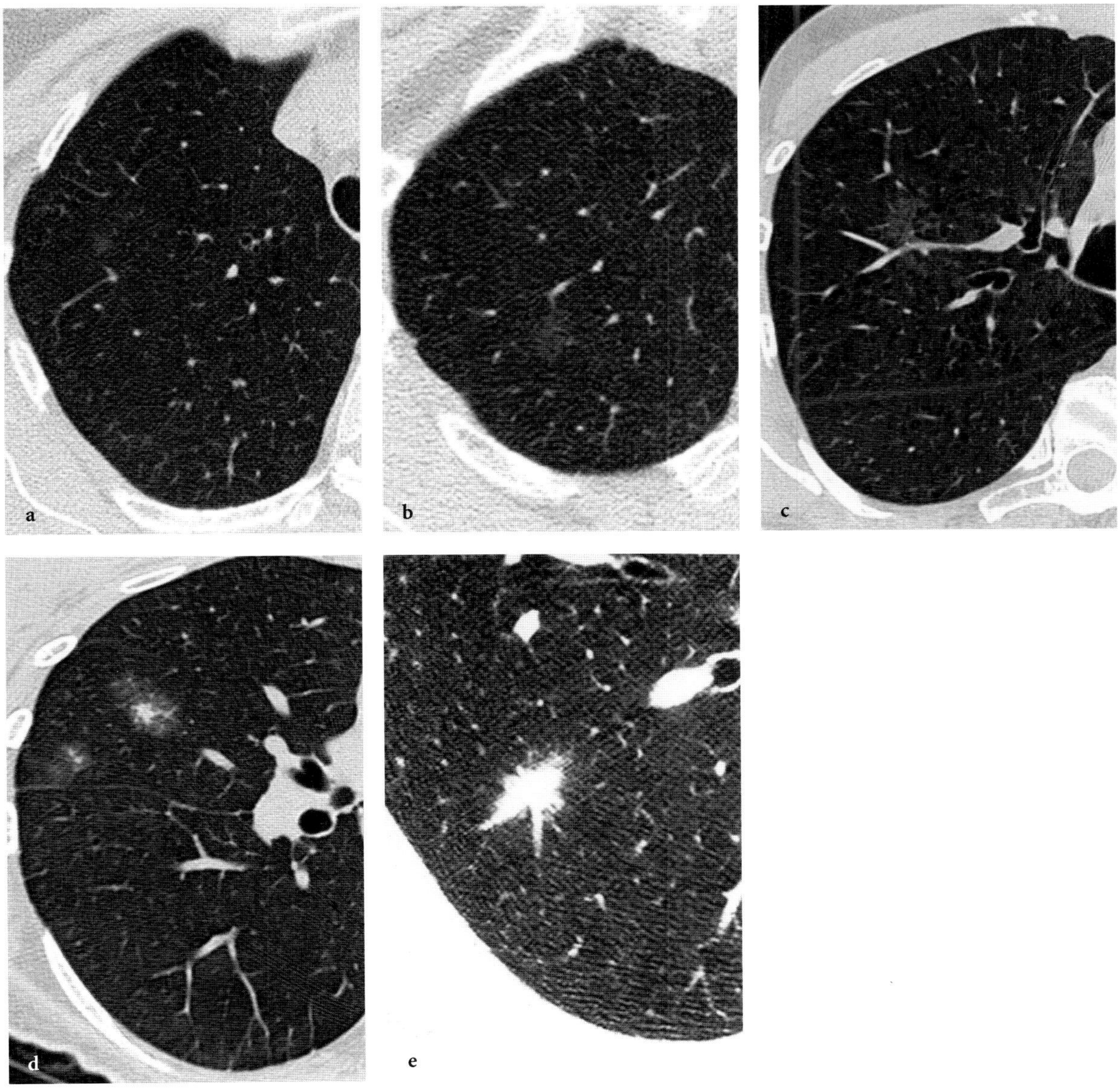

Fig. 11.5a–d. Adenocarcinoma of the lung: CT appearances. **a, b** One-millimeter target reconstructions through the right upper lobe in two separate patients, respectively show characteristic appearance of well defined pure ground glass nodules. The smallest of these is consistent with an incidental focus of atypical adenomatous hyperplasia while the larger raises the possibility of an early bronchoalveolar cell carcinoma, corresponding to Noguchi type A adenocarcinoma (localized bronchoalveolar cell carcinoma). 5 C. 1 mm target reconstruction through the right upper lobe in a different patient than shown in **a, b.** A poorly defined ground glass nodule is identifiable in the mid portion of the lung. This appearance corresponds to Noguchi type B adenocarcinoma. **d** One-millimeter target reconstruction through the middle lobe in a different patient than shown in **a–c.** There are two separate sub-solid nodules present both with clearly definable solid components. This appearance corresponds with Noguchi type C adenocarcinoma in this case in a patient with documented multifocal bronchoalveolar cell carcinomas. **e** One-millimeter target reconstruction through the right lower lobe in a different patient than shown in **a–d.** In this case there is a spiculated predominantly solid nodule surrounded by faint ground glass attenuation. This appearance corresponds with Noguchi types D–F invasive adenocarcinoma, subsequently verified surgically

with progression to more invasive disease marked by an increase in size (typically greater than 1.5 – 2 cm's), as well as the appearance of solid elements, consolidation, lymphatic obstruction and pseudocavitation (Jang et al. 1996). Support for this contention has also been reported by Kitamura et al. (1995, 1996). In an evaluation of the proliferative potential of atypical adenomatous hyperplasia (AAH) and early stage BAC, these authors documented that while low-grade AAH tended to be small (usually less than 5 mm in size) without evidence of nuclear p53 staining and few Ki-67 antigen positive cells (a marker for active cell proliferation), with progression to high grade AAH and AAH-like cancers, lesions appear larger with evidence of progressively greater cell proliferation and more prominent nuclear p53 staining.

Rarely identified prior to the introduction of multidetector CT scanners it is now commonplace to identify small ground glass nodules, especially on low dose lung cancer screening studies. Henschke et al. (2002), in an early study using low dose CT to screen high risk cigarette smokers found that 44 (19%) of 233 nodules initially detected proved to be sub-solid. Interestingly, the finding of a sub-solid nodule in this population proved a better indicator of likely neoplasia than solid nodules with 15 (34%) of 44 proving malignant versus only 7% of solid nodules ($p = 0.000001$). Furthermore, the cancer rate for this subset of nodules remained significantly greater than for solid nodules despite standardizing for size. Not surprisingly, all represented either BAC or adenocarcinomas ($P = 0.0001$).

In an attempt to further define features differentiating bronchoalveolar cell carcinoma (BAC) from adenocarcinomas with bronchoalveolar components (ACB), Mirtcheva et al. classified sub-solid nodules into four separate categories as previously proposed by Gaeta et al. (1998): pure ground glass nodules (GGOs), GGOs with a solid component, well-defined GGOs mixed with consolidation, and GGOs with superimposed lymphangitis. Additional features described included the location, size and margins of lesions as well as the presence of air-bronchograms and/or bubble like radiolucencies (pseudocavitation). Of 29 patients with BAC and 15 with ACB, pure GGOs and/or GGOs with solid components proved most predictive of BAC, while GGOs mixed with consolidation and/or evidence of lymphangitis were more likely to represent ACB. These findings are in keeping with the suggestion that there is a continuum of CT findings from pure ground glass attenuation to solid lesions corresponding to increasing invasiveness.

In this regard, it has been shown that the extent of ground glass density within pulmonary nodules has prognostic value. As reported by Higashiyama (1999), the smaller the ground glass component on CT, the greater the stage and the poorer the survival. Similarly, Kodama et al. (2002) have shown in a study of 104 surgically resected adenocarcinomas less than 2 cm in size, that lesions with greater than 50% ground glass density had no evidence of nodal metastases or postoperative recurrences. Recently it has been suggested that the CT appearance of peripheral adenocarcinomas may be sufficiently diagnostic to determine appropriate management. Suzuki et al. (2002), in a retrospective study of 69 lung cancers with a large (greater than 50%) ground glass component showed that 47 (68%) were BACs while 22 (32%) were minimally invasive adenocarcinomas, none demonstrating lymphatic invasion or nodal metastases. Based on these data, these authors suggest that sub-solid nodules that show no interval growth over three months may either be conservatively managed by continued observation or successfully managed with only limited surgical resection. It should be emphasized that decisions regarding appropriate management of these lesions is complex involving consideration not only of the clinical history but factors affecting the efficacy of additional diagnostic modalities including transthoracic needle aspiration biopsy (TTNBx), contrast enhanced CT, and positron emission tomography (FDG-PET).

That the CT appearance of lesions has prognostic value is especially important in the light of recent data suggesting that the histologic appearance of adenocarcinomas per se may be less important than the clinical pattern and pathologic stage of disease (Ebright et al. 2002). Ebright et al. (2002), in a study of 100 consecutive surgically treated patients found no correlation between survival and histology when lesions were classified as either pure BAC, BAC with focal invasion, or adenocarcinoma with BAC features, with an overall survival of 74% reported. In distinction, a poorer prognosis was documented for lesions presenting either as pneumonic consolidation or with higher pathologic stage, with 5 year survivals for stage I/II and III/IV lesions reported of 84% and 60%, respectively. Interestingly, in this study, excellent long-term survival was reported even for patients with multifocal disease.

11.3.2 CT Densitometry

From the outset, a potential role for volumetric CT to perform CT densitometry has been noted (Kalender et al. 1990). With the introduction of multidetector CT, the ability to acquire contiguous high resolution thin CT sections through even small nodules has been considerably simplified, obviating previous problems related to respiratory and cardiac motion, in particular (Fig. 11.4). As characterizing lesions as benign requires demonstration of the presence of either calcification or fat, the ability to reliably obtain multiple thin sections through the center of lesions eliminating partial volume averaging is a critical advantage. Unfortunately, while CT densitometry can make an important contribution to nodule characterization, it is well established that calcifications per may occur both in benign and malignant lesions (Fig. 11.6). Approximately 10% of documented lung cancers will have CT evidence of calcifications. Although typically eccentric, punctate or stippled in appearance, in rare cases malignant nodules may even be diffusely calcified. This is especially true in patients with metastatic disease from a variety of primary tumors, including mucinous adenocarcinomas arising from the breast (Swensen et al. 1991). Of course, in this setting, lesions are typically multiple. While the presence of fat within nodules is characteristic of pulmonary hamartomas, this occurs in less than half of cases (Fig. 11.7) (Siegelmann et al. 1986). Although liposarcomas can lead to nodular metastases with fat, their occurrence is predictably rare (Webb 1990).

As a consequence of these limitations, attention has focused on the use of contrast enhancement to further characterize pulmonary nodules. Initially suggested by Littleton et al. using conventional tomography, the use of CT for this purpose has been pioneered by Swensen et al. (1992, 1995, 1996, 2000). Based on the assumption that the degree of enhancement within nodules is a function of nodule vascularity, which in itself is indicative of malignancy, Swensen et al. (1995) initially evaluated patterns of contrast enhancement in a total of 163 patients with solitary nodules less than 4 cm in size using a single detector CT scanner. Following a bolus of 100 cc of intravenous contrast media injected at a rate of 2 cc's per second, six serial thin-section 3 mm images were obtained through nodules at 30-second intervals up to 2 minutes, beginning 60 seconds after the onset of the injection. In each case a representative CT number was then obtained for user-determined regions of interest (ROIs) in order to derive a measurement of peak nodule enhancement. Using this technique, these authors found that malignant neoplasms (median, 40 HU) enhanced to a greater extent than benign lesions (median 12 HU). Furthermore, using 20 HU units as a threshold for identifying a malignant nodule, sensitivity proved to be 100%, specificity, 76.9%, positive predictive value, 90.2%, negative predictive value, 100%; and accuracy, 92.6%.

a

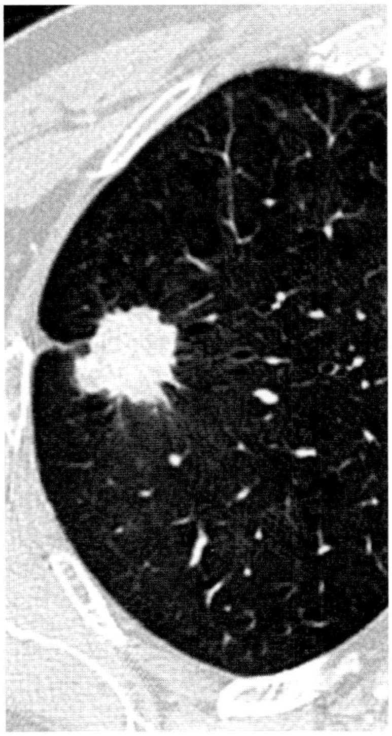

b

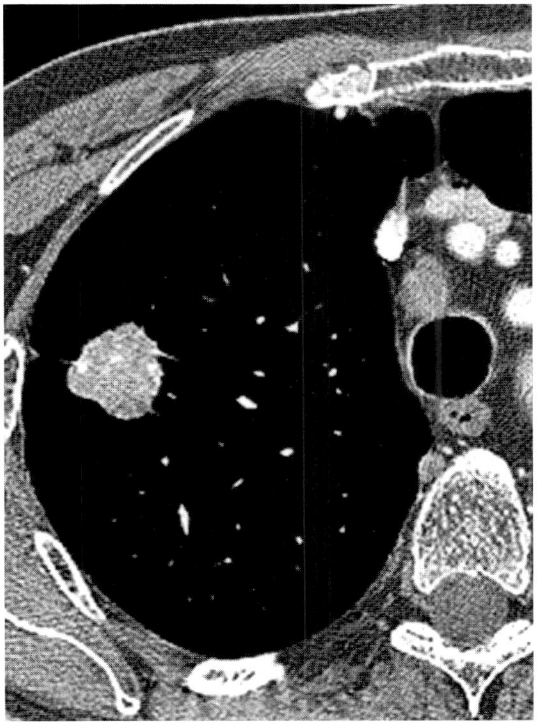

Fig. 11.6a, b. Lung cancer: dystrophic calcification. One-millimeter target reconstructions through the right upper lobe imaged with wide (**a**) and narrow (**b**) windows show an irregular, spiculated tumor in the lung periphery subsequently documented to be a non-small cell lung cancer. Note that there are multiple punctate calcifications within this lesion, presumably representing dystrophic calcification. Note as well the presence of an enlarged right paratracheal node

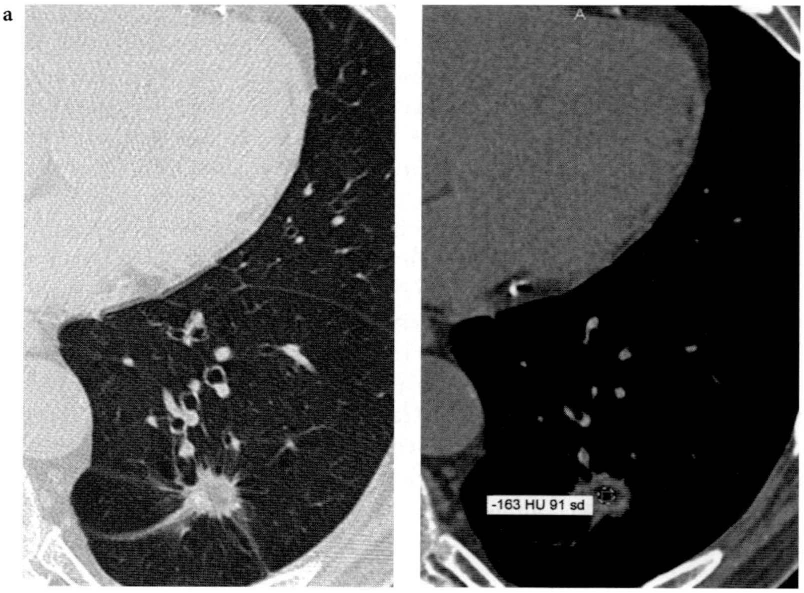

Fig. 11.7a, b. Pulmonary hamartoma. One-millimeter target reconstruction through the left lower lobe imaged with wide (**a**) and narrow (**b**) windows shows a spiculated nodule within which fat density is clearly identifiable. Despite speculated margins, this proved on biopsy to be a hamartoma

More recently, this same approach has been validated in a larger multi-institutional trial. Again using single detector CT scanners, Swensen et al. (2000) showed a significant difference in the degree of enhancement between malignant and benign nodules. In this study, a total of 356 homogenously enhancing nodules were evaluated ranging between 5 and 40 mm in diameter. Of these 48% proved malignant with a median enhancement of 38 HU (range 14 - 165 HU) while 52% proved benign with a median enhancement of 10 HU (range 0 to 96 HU). Using 15 HU as a threshold this time, CT proved to have a sensitivity of 98% (167 of 171 malignant nodules), a specificity of 58% (107/185 benign nodules), a positive predictive value of 68%, a negative predictive value of 96% and an accuracy of 77%. It should be emphasized that since both benign and malignant lesions may show considerable overlap in the degree of contrast enhancement, the true value of this technique is in identifying lesions that fail to demonstrate significant enhancement, as this occurs almost exclusively in benign lesions lacking neo-vascularity. An exception is the rare case of a mucinous carcinoma (Fig. 11.8).

Unfortunately, although frequently of value, technical pitfalls limit the clinical utility of this technique. Small lesions, in particular those less than 8 mm in size, are particularly difficult to assess as these require thin (1.5 - 3 mm) sections to avoid partial volume averaging (Fig. 11.9). The result is considerable image noise, limiting determination of a meaningful representative CT number. Also problematic are lesions that show heterogeneous patterns of enhancement as these have considerably less specificity. In addition, while rare, occasional malignant lesions, especially those with extensive mucous as may occur in bronchoalveolar cell carcinomas, may fail to show significant enhancement leading to a false negative interpretation. Finally, it should be noted that obtaining images at sixty second intervals is not truly representative of either tissue perfusion or permeability. For this purpose, it would be necessary to inject considerably greater volumes of contrast material (on the order of 5 to 7 mm's per second) while obtaining data within seconds following contrast administration. Although this is not currently feasible with 4 detector CT scanners, a more accurate estimate of tissue perfusion may be possible with the use of 16 detector CT scanners.

Although outside the intended scope of the present review, it should be noted that in place of contrast enhancement, increasingly nodules are being evaluated by use of positron emission tomography (PET), especially with 2-[fluorine-18]-fluoro-2-deoxy-D-glucose (FDG). To date a number of studies have documented that FDG-PET is an effective method for evaluating pulmonary nodules with sensitivities reported as high as 96% with specificity and accuracy in the range of 88% and 94%, respectively (Albes et al. 2002; Coleman 2001; Haberkorn and Schoenberg 2001; Keith et al. 2002; Salminen and MacManus 2002; Wong et al. 2001). An important advantage of FDG-PET is the ability to perform whole body imaging (Fig. 11.10). Despite limitations, including a tendency to obtain false negative studies

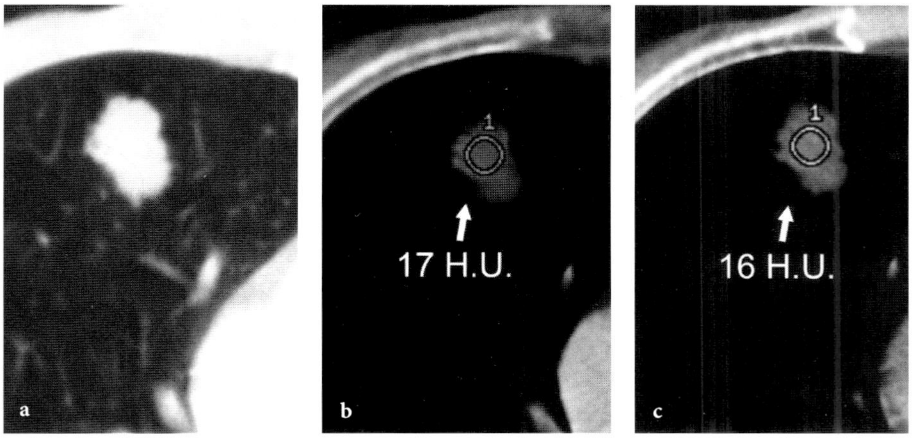

Fig. 11.8a–c. False negative contrast enhanced nodule study. **a** Magnified view of a lobulated middle lobe nodule imaged with wide windows. **b, c** Sections through the same nodule first without and then at 3 minutes following a bolus of intravenous contrast material. Note that there is virtually no enhancement within this lesion. A similar appearance was noted at 1, 2, and 4 min. At surgery this proved to be mucinous carcinoma, accounting for the lack of contrast enhancement. Case courtesy of Jeffrey Klein, University of Vermont Medical Center

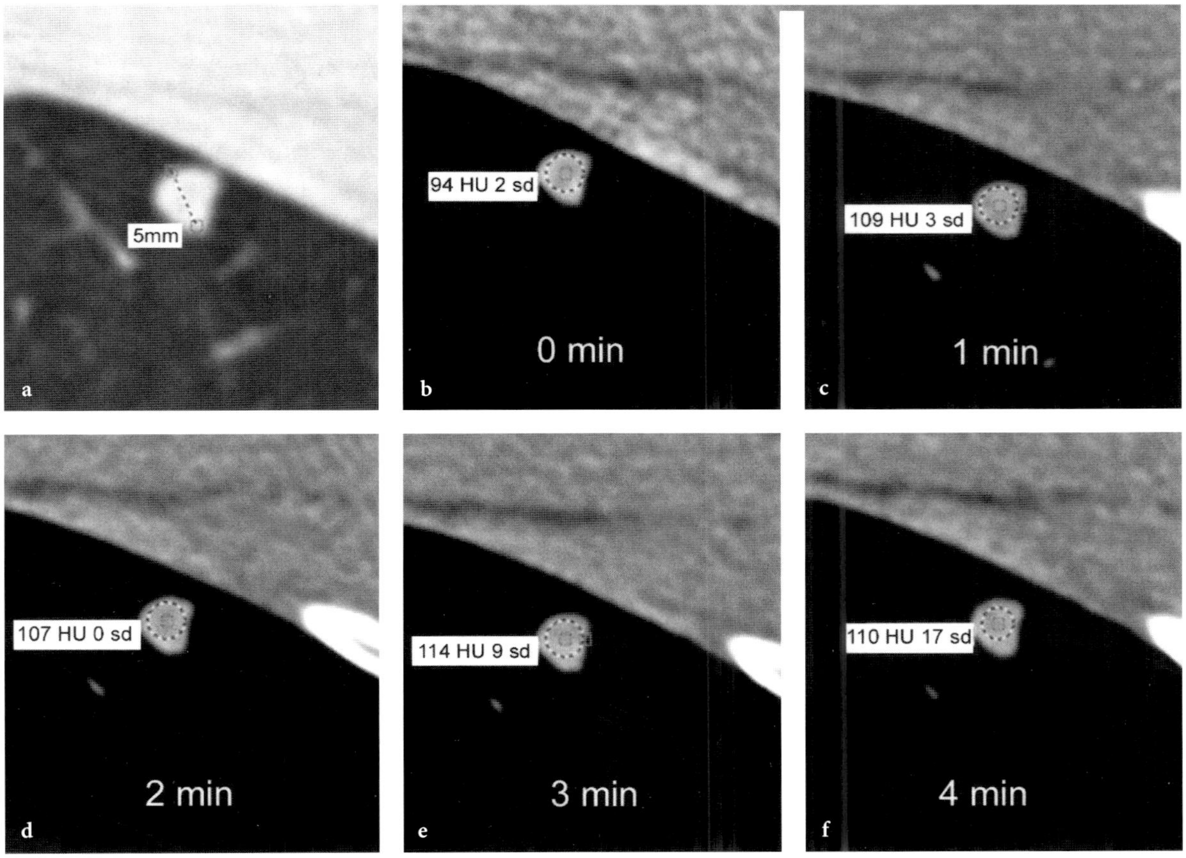

Fig. 11.9. Nodule enhancement. **a** 3 mm target reconstruction through the lingual shows a well defined 5 mm nodule. **b–f** Representative 3 mm sections at the same level selected from repeated volume acquisitions through the nodule in **a** using a multidetector CT scanner first without and then following a bolus of intravenous contrast material. Note that this lesion enhances by 20 HU at 3 min. Although 15 HU has been reported as an accurate threshold differentiating benign from malignant lesions, in this case it was opted to follow this nodule conservatively. Subsequent scans have documented no growth over 2 years

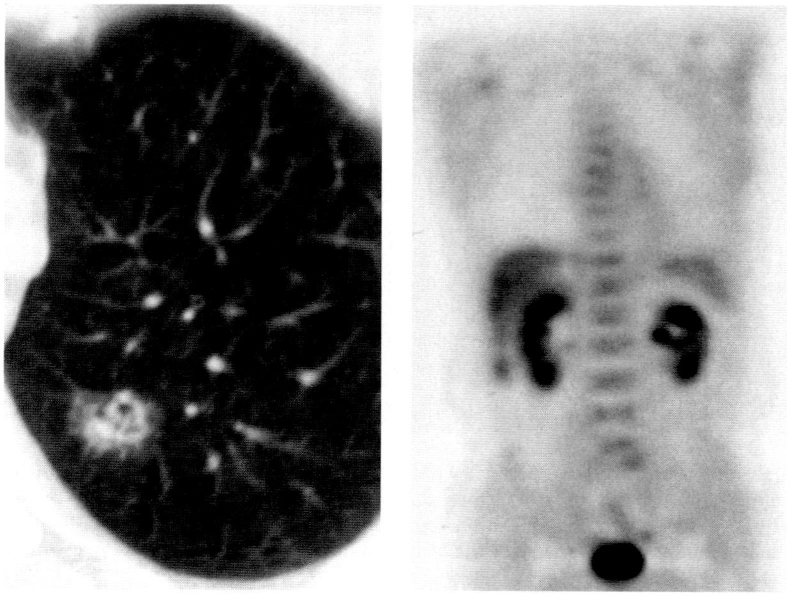

Fig. 11.10a, b. FDG-PET: Stage 1 non-small cell lung cancer. **a** Axial image through the right upper lobe shows an elongated nodule adjacent to bullae. **b** Whole body coronal view from a corresponding FDG-PET study shows intense uptake of tracer in the right upper lobe lesion. Note the presence of normal activity in the heart, and renal collecting system. No other foci of increased uptake are apparent. An obvious advantage of FDG-PET for evaluating nodules is the ability to more accurately stage tumors by visualizing remote lesions otherwise not identified by routine CT. Subsequently pathologically proved Stage 1 non-small cell lung cancer

in patients with bronchoalveolar cell carcinoma (Yap et al. 2002), it is likely that the use of FDG-PET imaging will increase dramatically, especially with the increasing availability of PET-CT scanners allowing advanced fusion imaging to be performed.

11.3.3 Growth Assessment

Given the limitations in definitively assessing lung nodules described above, it is not surprising that considerable interest has focused on the assessment of interval growth as a means for differentiating between benign and malignant disease (Lillington 1991; Nathan et al. 1962). Measurement of growth typically is expressed in terms of "tumor volume doubling time" (VDT). This approach reflects the assumption that cancer cells grow exponentially, providing a means to differentiate benign from malignant disease. For a cancer cell 10 microns to grow into a 1 mm nodule, for example, requires 20 doubling times; for the same nodule to grow first to 5 mm then to one centimeter would require 25 and 30 doublings, respectively (Collins et al. 1956). Measurement of VDT assumes that nodules are essentially spherical: once nodule diameters are converted to volumes, VDT can then be calculated if the time difference (t), initial volume (V_0), and volume at time t (V_t) is known using the formula VDT = $[t \times \log 2]/\log (V_t/V_0)$ (Yankelivitz et al. 2000).

From earlier radiographic studies, VDT's for lung cancer were shown to range between 20 and 400 days (Collins et al. 1956; Lillington 1991; Nathan et al. 1962; Steele and Buell 1973). In distinction, benign nodules typically have VDT's either less than 20 days, especially when the result of acute infection, or greater than 400 days, as occurs in patients with hamartomas or granulomas. Based on these observations, despite some controversy, it is now standard clinical practice to assume that any lesion that is radiographically stable over a two year time period may be considered benign (Yankelevitz and Henschke 1997).

CT, by virtue of its ability to provide direct visualization of lesions without the superimposition of overlying structures, allows considerably more precise measurements than routine radiography, especially of smaller lesions. Considerable impetus to develop accurate methods for assessing the growth of small nodules, especially those less than 8 mm in size (the size typically cited as a cut-off for reliable identification on chest radiographs) has come in recent years from the introduction of low-dose CT screening (Yankelevitz et al. 1999, 2000). In particular, CT has shed new light on the use of 2 years as a cut-off for differentiating benign from malignant growth rates. Recent studies have shown, for example, that the mean VDT's of localized BACs may be in the order of 800 to as long as 1,400 days (Aoki et al. 2000; Yankelevitz and Henschke 1997).

In fact, accurate assessment of growth rates in small lung nodules is often problematic, even with CT. This is especially true of small nodules less than 5 mm in size, those most frequently identified on low-dose screening studies, particularly when bidimensional perpendicular measurements are used to assess growth as recommended both by the world Health Organization and the more recently published Response Evaluation Criteria in Solid Tumors Guidelines (Fig. 11.11) (THERRASSE et al. 2000). For a nodule to double in volume, for example, its diameter must increase by one fourth. A 3 mm nodule, therefore, will have doubled in volume when it reaches 3.75 cm in diameter, and doubled again when it measures 4.7 cm (Fig. 11.12). In principle this means that a nodule with a doubling time of 200 days will be identifiable in 40 days: however, in routine clinical practice, it is difficult to reach this degree of accuracy when assessing small nodules, even when electronic calipers are used, due to even slight differences in scan location or even variations in respiratory excursion between studies (SCHARTZ et al. 2000; WORMANNS et al. 2000). This becomes even more problematic for slower growing nodules with doubling times in the range of 800 days, for which visually perceptible changes in size may require as much as 4 years to identify.

For these reasons, considerable interest has focused recently on the potential for obtaining automated or semi-automated volume quantification in place of measuring cross-sectional diameters as a means for assessing nodule growth (YANKELEVITZ et al. 2000). While of considerable promise, it should be noted that regardless of the methodology employed, accurate and reproducible assessment of the volume of small nodules remains problematic (Ko et al. 2001, 2003). For example, assuming 1 mm collimation, 1/3 of a 4 mm nodule's voxels actually lie on the surface rendering them unusable due to partial volume averaging: For 2 mm nodules virtually all of their voxels lie on the surface rendering accurate assessment virtually impossible with current techniques. These limitations are further compounded by difficulties in assessing the true dimensions of nodules that lie adjacent to vessels or pleural surfaces or are present in patients with underlying emphysema or infiltrative lung disease (Fig. 11.13). Although it has been suggested that the accuracy of volume measurements may be

a b

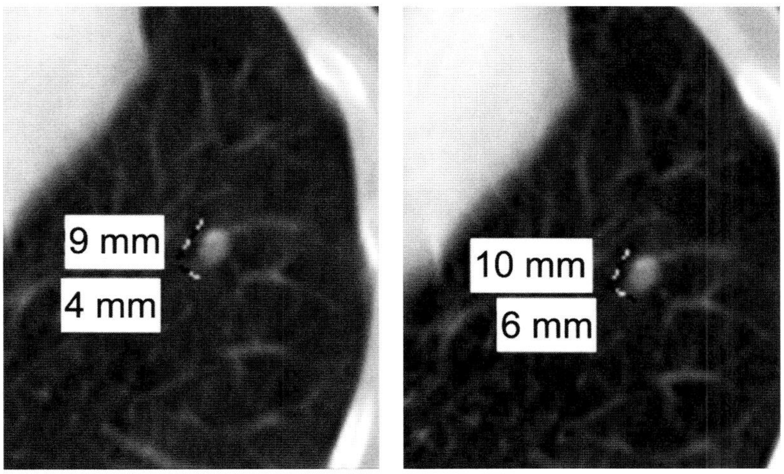

Fig. 11.11a, b. Growth assessment. Identical magnified views of a nodule in the left lower lobe. Note that in **a** this lesion measured 9 by 4 mm (product = 36) and in **b**, 10 by 6 mm (product = 60). It is apparent that for small nodules obtaining consistent measurements may be problematic, even with the use of electronic calipers

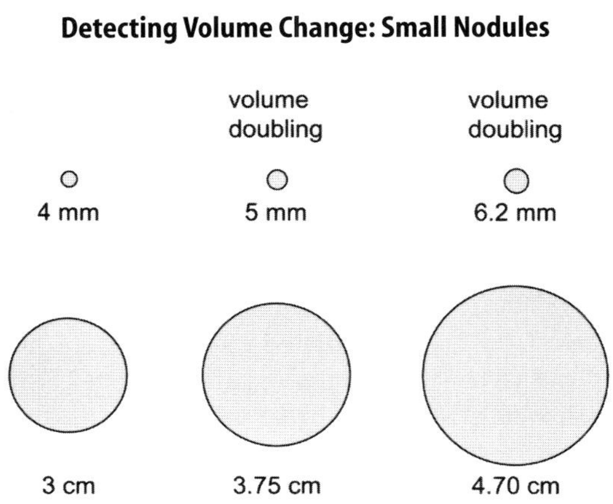

Fig. 11.12. Diagrammatic representation of the 2-dimensional appearance of lesions sequential doubling in time, beginning with a nodule measuring 4 mm at baseline. Note that detection of volume doubling using bidimensional measurements is far more difficult for smaller than larger lesions. It may be imaging that this represents a near impossibility for lesions under 3 mm in size, especially without the use of computer-assisted evaluation

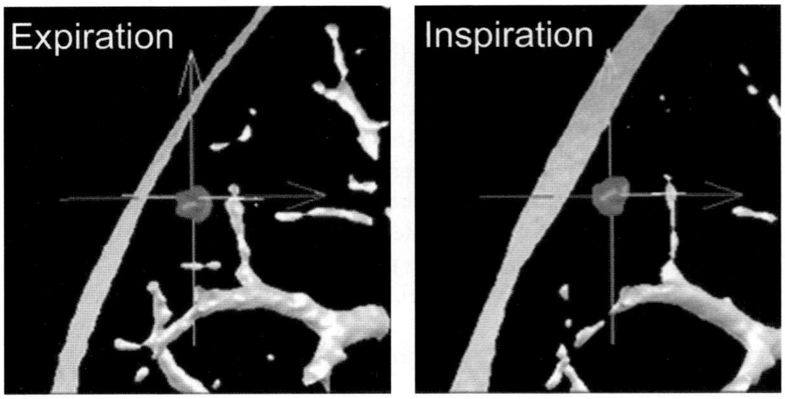

a b

Fig. 11.13a, b. Volume assessment: variations with respiration. Computer generated 3D renderings of a small nodule in the lung periphery obtained in inspiration (**a**) and then in expiration (**b**). Although visually these images appear identical, in fact the diameter of the nodule in inspiration measures 3.2 mm in widest dimension with a volume of 10.3 mm^3 using a threshold of –624 HU; in distinction, the diameter of this same nodule measured in expiration is 4.0 mm with a volume of 12.0 mm^3. This represents a nearly 15% change in volume. It is apparent the accuracy and especially the reproducibility of volume measurements of small nodules remains to be validated. Images courtesy of Carol Novak, PhD. Siemens Corporate Research, Inc., Princeton, New Jersey

assessed within two percentage points, this remains to be definitively determined in a large clinical cohort (Yankelevitz et al. 2000).

Recently, Reeves et al. (1997) have proposed replacing VDT's with measurements of growth rate (GR). Defined as the increase in volume measured over time, these authors, using 365 days to define a 100% growth rate, found that while 5 malignant nodules had GRs of 17 to 141%, 11 benign lesions had a maximum GR of only 2.2% leading them to conclude that measuring GR is superior to VDT as a method for evaluating the likelihood of malignancy. Although appealing in its simplicity, this approach also remains to be further assessed.

11.4 Clinical Management

With the introduction of multidetector CT scanners providing markedly improved spatial resolution for even routine CT examinations, the number of lung nodules identified has grown exponentially. Unfortunately, there is currently no generally agreed upon algorithm defining appropriate clinical management. Despite a lack of consensus, there is a growing realization that some standardization governing the work-up of small lung nodules, in particular, is necessary. Considerations most importantly include the clinical context in which nodules are detected as well as the varieties of available means for further assessing those discovered (Ginsberg et al. 1999). Variables that require consensus include the size of "actionable" nodules appropriate follow-up intervals and a definition of an acceptable range of radiation dose.

It is from the sphere of lung cancer screening that such standardization is likely to emerge. To date, a number of algorithms have been proposed which have in common a focus on the need for close monitoring of small incidentally identified nodules (Henschke et al. 1999, 2001; Nawa et al. 2002; Swensen et al. 2002; Wang et al. 2000). As proposed by the I-ELCAP (International Early Lung Cancer Action Program), recommendations are restricted to those individuals with fewer than six nodules. All non calcified nodules documented by appropriate high resolution 1 to 1.5 mm sections equal to or greater than 3 mm require further evaluation as follows: nodules between 3 and 5 mm in size should be reassessed in 6 months, while those between 5 and 10 mm require reevaluation in 3 months. For nodules greater than 10 mm in size, the following options are available: conservative therapy with antibiotics with subsequent repeat CT in another month; evaluation with additional imaging studies including contrast enhanced CT or FDG-PET; or biopsy.

An alternative approach for managing nodules detected by low dose CT screening has been proposed by the recently initiated National Lung Screening Trial (NLST) sponsored by the National Cancer Institute. In distinction to I-ELCAP, the NLST proposes using 4 mm as a cut-off for "actionable" lung nodules. Of particular interest, nodules identified on incidence screening are defined either as "indeterminate" (defined as newly identified nodules between 4 and 10 mm in size, or growing nodules less than 7 mm in size) or "abnormal" (defined as new nodules greater than 10 mm in size, or growing nodules greater than 7 mm in size). Indeterminate nodules are then monitored by follow-up CT studies at 3, 6, 12 and 24 months, while abnormal nodules similar to I-ELCAP recommendations are evaluated either by contrast enhanced CT, FDG-PET or biopsy.

Others have recommended that actionable nodules be still greater in size than proposed by either I-ELCP or NLST. WANG et al, for example, in a study of cancer growth rates in a population identified by low-dose CT screening concluded that for lesion less than 5 mm in size, interval yearly follow-up CT exams would be acceptable (WANG et al. 2000).

Additional uncertainty surrounds the definition of an appropriate radiation dose, especially in a screened population. Following the initial ELCAP protocol, which required a high resolution CT study of nodules initially discovered at baseline, with subsequent follow-up studies using routine technique at 3, 6 12 and 24 months, the total radiation dose has been considered prohibitive by some (GOODMAN 2002). It is worth emphasizing, however, that these observations do not take into account the use of multidetector CT scanners obviating acquisition of additional high-resolution images to initially characterize nodules, as well as the use of low-dose technique for all subsequent CT studies. Clearly, consideration should be given to using the lowest possible radiation dose for evaluating nodules, regardless of the clinical indication.

11.5 Future Directions

11.5.1 Workflow Optimization

The introduction of multi-detector CT scanners capable of generating hundreds of images in a single breath-hold period has placed considerable strain on daily clinical practice. In response, most manufacturers have developed a series of tools to facilitate routine interpretation of thoracic CT images using advanced workstation capabilities. Ideally, there should be seamless real-time transitions available between routine axial, coronal or sagittal images as well as the use of sliding maximum intensity projection or volumetrically rendered images. The user interface should allow instantaneous transitions between thick and thin sections. Furthermore, and perhaps most importantly, there should be access to additional imaging tools, including among others, the use of a 180 degree cine "fly-around" or "cartwheel" projection as well as real-time 3D cine segmentation with instantaneous volume assessment. Finally, for those cases for which follow-up CT studies are indicated to assess growth, there should be nearly instantaneous registration between studies of different dates allowing rapid identification and comparison of lesions.

To date, preliminary data has shown that use of these tools is effective in facilitating nodule identification and characterization (DAS et al. 2002; FAN et al. 2002; NOVAK et al. 2001, 2002). Using an experimental interactive (ICAD) interface, NOVAK et al. (2001), for example, have shown in a study of 10 low dose CT screening studies first evaluated using a 4 point scale to assess thick section CT images followed by a reassessment of these same nodules using the full range of potential imaging tools outlined above reported a significant shift toward improved confidence of interpretation with 82 potential nodules rated either as "certain" or "excluded" compared with only 44% using 7 mm sections ($p < 0.0001$) (NOVAK et al. 2001). Use of CAD to automatically identify nodules on follow-up CT studies has also been reported (NOVAK et al. 2002; SHEN et al. 2002). NOVAK et al. using real time automatic matching (RAM) evaluated 16 patients scanned with 1 mm collimation at two separate times and found that of a total of 170 focal lung abnormalities, RAM could predict the location exactly on corresponding studies 63.5% of the time, and proved to be within five 1 mm axial slices 88.2% of the time (NOVAK et al. 2002). Furthermore, the time to perform each correspondence averaged less than 1 second. The implications for optimizing follow-up scan interpretations in patients with small parenchymal nodules in particular is apparent.

11.5.2 Computer-Assisted Diagnosis

It is clear from the foregoing discussions that the evaluation of pulmonary nodules has become increasingly complex. With the introduction of newer 10- and 16-detector CT scanners allowing generation of between 600 and 1,000 images per study it is apparent that routine scan interpretation will be still more problematic. Initially introduced as a second reader for screening mammography, and more recently approved for use in computed chest radiography by the Food and Drug Administration (FDA), it may be anticipated that computer-assisted diagnosis (CAD) will likely gain widespread acceptance for interpreting thoracic CT studies, especially as a potential aid to lung cancer screening studies as well as for surveying patients with known malignancies.

Although initial research into the use of CAD for nodule detection with CT began a decade ago, recent interest has increased considerably as a result of growing interest in low-dose screening (Armato et al. 1999, 2001, 2002; Brown et al. 1997, 2001; Kanazawa et al. 1998; Ko et al. 2001; Wormanns et al. 2002). Although a description of the various CAD methodologies lie outside the intended scope of the present chapter, these approaches have in common the overall goal of automatically identifying "candidate" nodules as accurately as possible in a clinically timely fashion. To date results have proved promising.

Kanazawa et al. (1998) using 10 mm thick sections evaluated a total of 230 nodules in 450 patients: each case was evaluated by three separate interpreters with each nodule identified rated on a 4-point scale. Overall, counting all nodules identified even if only by one interpreter, CAD successfully identified 90% of 167 nodules rated as highly suspicious for malignancy (Kanazawa et al. 1998). Revealingly, only 11 of 167 nodules rated as suspicious were identified by all three interpreters. Altogether there were six false negative studies, the main causes of which were lesions with poorly defined boundaries, presumably representing ground glass nodules, small nodules less than 4 mm in size, and those located near the pulmonary hila. For an average data set of 35 slices, the authors further noted 8.6 false positives per case.

Gurcan et al. (2002) have reported similar results. Using 5 mm sections these authors evaluated 34 patients with 63 lung nodules identified by a single chest radiologist, including 8 proved malignant nodules. Using a combination of rule-based classifiers and linear discriminant analysis, CAD sensitivity proved to 84% (53/63 nodules) with a false positive rate of 1.74 objects per slice. For this study, the average nodule size was reported as 9 mm (range 2 – 25 mm's): only 15 of these measure less than 4 mm in size.

Armato et al. (2002) in a study of 38 low-dose CT scans with 50 nodules included 31 malignant nodules not identified on a total of 38 examinations (a total of 38 malignant nodules counting both initial and follow-up studies). While CAD detected 40 (80%) of 50 nodules, most importantly, CAD correctly identified 18 (78%) of 23 cancers missed due to detection errors, and 14 (93%) of 15 lesions missed due to interpretive errors, for a combined sensitivity of 84% with one false-positive nodule identified per section. Of the 6 missed cancers, four proved to be pure ground glass nodules, while the other two were mixed ground glass/solid lesions.

As promising as these data are, it should be emphasized that they all reported results based on the use of initial thick 5 to 10 mm sections. With the introduction of multidetector scanners, however, it is now possible to routinely acquire 1 mm sections through the entire thorax. As reported by Novak et al. (2002), the use of overlapping high-resolution images may result in a dramatic increase in sensitivity with a corresponding decrease in the number of false positive findings. In their study of 10 consecutive low dose screening studies evaluated by three experienced chest radiologists initially using thick 7 mm sections only 8 (31%) of 26 nodules were detected by all three readers. While the three readers only identified 1.4 to 2.1 nodules per patient, a total of 3.2 nodules were identified per patient using CAD representing an increase in sensitivity by 114 to 207%. Not surprisingly, most of these additional nodules proved either to be less than 4 mm in size or centrally located.

Given these data, it is reasonable to assume that CAD may someday become a routine part of the clinical evaluation of all CT studies. It may be further anticipated that this function may then be expanded to that of an integrated computer system that will not only support a variety of functions including nodule size, location and morphology but the creation of database to document and manage findings. Ultimately, integration of the results of computer analysis with a database management system may allow identification of otherwise obscure associations between various nodule characteristics and the rate of malignancy, for example. It is this expectation that underlies the NCI funded initiative to create a MDCT database for researching CAD applications. It only remains to validate the clinical utility of these systems in routine practice.

References

Albes JM, Dohmen BM, Schott U et al (2002) Value of positron emission tomography for lung cancer staging. Eur J Surg Oncol 28:55–62

Aoki T, Nakaata H, Watanabe H (2000) Evolution of peripheral lung adenocarcinomas: CT findings correlated with histology and tumor doubling times. AJR 174:763–768

Armato SG, Giger ML, Moran CJ et al (1999) Computerized detection of pulmonary nodules on CT scans. Radiographics 19:1303–1311

Armato SG, Giger ML, MacMahon H (2001) Automated detection of lung nodules in CT scans: preliminary results. Medical Physics 28:1552–1561

Armato SG, Li F, Giger ML et al (2002) Lung cancer: performance of automated lung nodule detection applied to cancers mssed in a CT screening program. Radiology 225:685–692

Bankoff MS, McEniff NJ, Bhadelia RA et al (1996) Prevalence of pathologically proven intrapulmonary lymph nodes and their appearance on CT. AJR 167:629–630

Brown MS, McNitt-Gray MF, Makovich NJ (1997) Method for segmenting chest CT image data using an anatomical model: preliminary results. IEEE Trans Med Imaging 16:828–839

Brown MS, McNitt-Gray MF, Goldin JG (2001) Patient-specific models for lung nodule detection and surveillance in CT images. IEEE Trans Med Imaging 20:1242–1250

Buckley JA, Scott WW, Siegelman SS et al (1995) Pulmonary nodules: effect of increased data sampling on detection with spiral CT and confidence in diagnosis. Radiology 196:395–400

Coakley FV, Cohen MD, Johnson MS et al (1998) Maximum intensity projection images in the detection of simulated pulmonary nodules by spiral CT. Br J Radiol 71:135–140

Coleman RE (2001) PET in lung cancer staging. Quart J Nucl Med 45:231–234

Collins VP, Loeffler RK, Tivey H (1956) Observations on growth rates of human tumors. AJR 76:988–1000

Das M, Jacobson FL, Judy PF et al (2002) Computer aidede detection (CAD) of lung nodules on mulidetector-row CT (MDCT): impact on readers with variable levels of experience. Radiology 225:476

Diederich S, Lentschig MG, Winter F et al (1999) Detection of pulmonary nodules with overlapping vs non-overlapping image reconstruction at spiral CT. Eur Radiol 9:281–286

Ebright MI, Zakowski MF, Martin J et al (2002) Clinical pattern and pathologic stage but not histologic features predict outcome for bronchioloalveolar carcinoma. Ann Thorac Surg 74:1640–1647

Fan L, Novak CL, Naidich DP et al (2002) Improving optimal radiologic interpretation of low-dose multi-slice lung CT studies using ICAD. Radiology 225:475

Gaeta M, Volta S, Stroscio S et al (1992) CT "halo sign" in pulmonary tuberculoma. J Comput Assist Tomogr 16:827–828

Gaeta M, Caruso R, Barone M et al (1998) Ground-glass attenuation in nodular bronchioloalveolar carcinoma: CT patterns and prognostic value. J Comput Assist Tomogr 22:215–219

Gaeta M, Blandino A, Scribano E et al (1999) Computed tomography halo sign in pulmonary nodules: frequency and diagnostic value. J Thorac Imag 14:109–113

Gartenschlager M, Schweden F, Gast K et al (1998) Pulmonary nodules: detection with low-dose vs conventional-dose spiral CT. Eur Radiol 8:609–614

Ginsberg MS, Griff SK, Go BD et al (1999) Pulmonary nodules resected at video-assisted thoracoscopic surgery: etiology in 426 patients. Radiology 213:277–282

Goodman PC (2002) Radiation risk in CT screening for lung cancer. Radiology 225:233

Gruden JF, Ouanounou S, Tigges S (2002) Incremental benefit of maximum-intensity-projection images on observer detection of small pulmonary nodules revealed by multidetector CT. AJR 179:149–157

Gurcan MN, Sahiner B, Petrick N et al (2002) Lung nodule detection on thoracic computed tomography images: preliminary evaluation of a computer-aided diagnosis system. Med Phys 29:2552–2558

Haberkorn U, Schoenberg SO (2001) Imaging of lung cancer with CT, MRT and PET. Lung Cancer 34:S13–S23

Hazzelrigg SR, Boley TM, Weber D, Magee MJ, Naunheim KS (1997) Incidence of lung nodules found in patients undergoing lung volume reduction. Ann Thorac Surg 63: 303–306

Henschke CI, Naidich DP, Yankelevitz DF (2001) Early lung cancer action project: initial findings on repeat screeings. Cancer 1:1533–1159

Henschke CI, Yankelevitz DF, McCauley D (1999) Early lung cancer action project: overall design and findings from baseline screenings. Lancet 354:99–105

Henschke CI, Yankelevitz DF, Mirtcheva RM (2002) CT screening for lung cancer: frequency and significance of part-solid and nonsolid nodules. AJR 178:1053–1057

Higashiyama M (1999) Ann Thorac Surg 68

Jang HJ, Lee KS, Kwon OJ et al (1996) Bronchioloalveolar carcinoma: focal area of ground-glass attenuation at thin-section CT as an early sign. Radiology 199:485–488

Kakinuma R, Ohmatsu H, Kaneko M (1999) Detection failures in spiral CT screening for lung cancer: analysis of CT findings. Radiology 212:61–66

Kalender WA, Seissler W, Klotz E et al (1990) Spiral volumetric CT with single-breath-hold technique, continuous transport, and continuous scanner rotation. Radiology 176:181–183

Kanazawa S, Kawata Y, Niki N (1998) Computer-aided diagnosis for pulmonary nodules based on helical CT images. Comput Med Imaging Graph 22:157–167

Kawakami S, Sone S, Takashima S (2001) Atypical adenomatous hyperplasia of the lung: correlation between high-resolution CT findings and histopathologic features. Eur Rad 11:811–814

Keith CJ, Miles KA, Griffiths MR et al (2002) Solitary pulmonary nodules: accuracy and cost-effectiveness of sodium iodide FDG-PET using Australian data. Eur J Nucl Med Mol Imaging 29:1016–1023

Kim Y, Lee KS, Jung KJ et al (1999) Halo sign on high resolution CT: Findings in spectrum of pulmonary diseases with pathologic correlation. J Comput Assist Tomogr 23: 622–626

Kitamura H, Kameda Y, Nakamura N (1996) Atypical adenomatous hyperplasia and bronchoalveolar lung carcinoma. Analysis by morphometry and the expression of p53 and carcinoembryonic antigen. Am J Surg Pathol 20:553–562

Kitamura H, Kameda Y, Nakamura N (1995) Proliferative potential and p53 overexpression in precursor and early stage lesions of bronchioloalveolar lung carcinoma. Am J Pathol 146:876–887

Klingenbeck-Regn K, Schaller S, Flohr T (1999) Subsecond multi-slice computed tomography: basics and applications. Eur J Radiol 31:110–124

Ko EJ, Betke M (2001) Chest CT: automated nodule detection and assessment of change over time: preliminary experience. Radiology 218:267–273

Ko JP, Rusinek H, Jacobs E et al (2003) Volume measurement of small pulmonary nodules on chest CT: a phantom study. Radiology 228:864–870

Kodama K, Higashiyama M, Yokouchi H et al (2002) Natural his-

tory of pure ground-glass opacity after long-term follow-up of more than 2 years. Ann Thorac Surg 73:386–392
Lillington GA (1991) Management of solitary pulmonary nodules. Dis Mon 37:271–318
McNitt-Gray MF, Hart EM, Wyckoff NE (1999) A pattern classification approach to characterizing solitary pulmonary nodules imaged on high-resolution CT: preliminary results. Med Phys 26:880–888
Milne ENC, Zerhouni EA (1987) Blood supply of pulmonary metastases. J Thorac Imag 2:15–23
Miyake H, Yamada Y, Kawagoe T et al (1999) Intrapulmonary lymph nodes: CT and pathological features. Clin Radiol 54:640–643
Nakata M, Saeki H, Takata I et al (2002) Focal ground-glass opacity detected by low-dose helical CT. Chest 121:1464–1467
Nambu A, Miyata K, Ozawa K et al (2002) Air-containing space in lung adenocarcinoma: hgh-resolution computed tomography findings. J Comput Assist Tomogr 26:1026–1031
Nathan MH, Collins VP, Adams RA (1962) Differentiation of benign and malignant pulmonary nodules by growth rate. Radiology 79:221–231
Nawa T, Nakagawa K, Kusano S (2002) Lung cancer screening using low dose spiral CT. Chest 122:15–20
Noguchi M, Morikawa A, Kawasaki M et al (1995) Small adenocarcinoma of the lung: histologic characteristics and prognosis. Cancer 75:2844–2852
Novak CL, Naidich DP, Fan L et al (2001) Improving radiologist' confidence of interpreting low-dose multi-slice lung CT screening studies using an interactive CAD system. Radiology 22(p):497
Novak CL, Qian J, Fan JP et al (2002) Inter-observer variations on interpretation of multi-slice CT lung cancer screening studies, and the implications for computer-aided diagnosis. In: Chakraburty DP, Krupinski EA (eds) Medical imaging: Image perception, observer performance, and technology assessment. Proceedings SPIE; vol 4686: pp 68–79
Novak CL, Shen H, Odry B et al (2002) Performance of an automatic system for nodule correspondence in follow-up CT studies of the lung. Radiology 225:476
Patz EF Jr (2000) Correlation of tumor size. Chest 117
Primack SL, Hartman TE, Lee KS et al (1994) Pulmonary nodules and the CT halo sign. Radiology 190:513–515
Reeves AP, Zhao B, Yankelevitz DF et al (1997) Characterization of three-dimensional shape and size changes of pulmonary nodules over time from helical CT images. Radiology 205:396
Remy J, Remy-Jardin M, Giraud F et al (1994) Angioarchitecture of pulmonary art eriovenous malformations: clinical utility of three-dimensional helical CT. Radiology 191:657–664
Rusinek H, Naidich DP, McGuinness G et al (1998) Pulmonary nodule detection: low-dose versus conventional CT. Radiology 209:243–249
Salminen E, MacManus M (2002) FDG-PET imaging in the management of non-small-cell lung cancer. Ann Oncol 13: 357–360
Schwartz LH, Ginsberg MS, DeCorato D (2000) Evaluation of tumor measurements in oncology: use of film-based and electronic techniques. J Clin Oncol 18:2179–2184
Seemann MD, Staebler A, Beinert T et al (1999) Usefulness of morphological characteristics for the differentiation of benign from malignant solitary pulmonary lesions using HRCT. Eur Radiol 9:409–417
Seltzer SE, Judy PF, Adams DF et al (1995) Spiral CT of the chest: comparison of cine and film-based viewing. Radiology 197:73–78
Seltzer SE, Judy PF, Feldman U et al (1998) Influence of CT image size and format on accuracy of lung nodule detection. Radiology 206:617–622
Shen H, FAN l, Qian J et al (2002) Real-time correspondence between lung nodules in follow-up multi-slice high resolution CT studies. Radiology 225:407
Siegelman SS, Khouri NF, Leo FP et al (1986) Solitary pulmonary nodules: CT assessment. Radiology 160:307–312
Siegelman SS, Khouri NF, Scott WW et al (1986) Pulmonary hamartoma: CT findings. Radiology 160:313–317
Siegelman SS, Zerhouni EA, Leo FP et al (1980) CT of the solitary pulmonary nodule. AJR 135:1–13
Steele JD, Buell P (1973) Asymptomatic solitary pulmonary nodules. Host survival, tumor size, and growth rate. J Thorac Cardiovasc Surg 65:140–151
Suzuki K, Asamura H, Kusumoto M et al (2002) "Early" peripheral lung cancer: prognostic significance of ground glass opacity on thin-section computed tomographic scan. Ann Thorac Surg 74:1635–1639
Swensen SJ, Brown LR, Colby TV et al (1995) Pulmonary nodules: CT evaluation of enhancement with iodinated contrast material. Radiology 194:393–398
Swensen SJ, Brown LR, Colby TV et al (1996) Lung nodule enhancement at CT: prospective findings. Radiology 201: 447–455
Swensen SJ, Harms GF, Morin RL et al (1991) CT evaluation of solitary pulmonary nodules: value of 185-H reference phantom. AJR 156:925–929
Swensen SJ, Jett JR, Sloan JA et al (2002) Screening for lung cancer with low-dose spiral computed tomography. Am J Respir Crit Care Med 165:508–513
Swensen SJ, Morin RL, Schueler BA et al (1992) Solitary pulmonary nodule: CT evaluation of enhancement with iodinated contrast material – a preliminary report. Radiology 182: 343–347
Swensen SJ, Viggiano RW, Midthun DE et al (2000) Lung nodule enhancment at CT: multicenter study. Radiology 214:73–80
Takigawa N, Segawa Y, Nakata M et al (1999) Clinical investigation of atypical adenomatous hyperplasia of the lung. Lung Cancer J Iaslc 25:115–121
Therrasse P, Arbuck SG, Eisenhauer EA (2000) New guidelines to evaluate the response to treatment in solid tumors. European Organization for Research and Treatment of Cancer, National Cancer Institute of the United States, National Cancer Institute of Canada. J Natl Cancer Inst 92:205–216
Travis WD, Colby TV, Corrin B et al (1999) Histologic typing of lung and pleural tumors. In: WHO World Health Organization Pathology Panel (ed) WHO international histological classification of tumors, 3rd edn. Springer, Berlin Heidelberg New York, pp 46–55
Wang JC, Sone S, Li F (2000) Rapidly growing small peripheral lung cancers detectged by screening TC: correlation between radiological appearance and pathological features. Br J Radiol 73:930–937
Webb WR (1990) Radiologic evaluation of the solitary pulmonary nodule. AJR 154:701–708
White CS, Romney BM, Mason AC et al (1996) Primary carcinoma of the lung overlooked at CT: analysis of findings in 14 patients. Radiology 199:109–115
Wong CYO, Nunez R, Bohdiewicz P et al (2001) Patterns of abnormal FDG uptake by various histological types of non-

small cell lung cancer at initial staging by PET. Eur J Nucl Med 28:1702–1705

Wormanns D, Diederich S, Lentschig MG (2000) Spiral CT of pulmonary nodules: interobserver variation in assessment of lesion size. Eur Radiold 10:710–713

Wormanns D, Fiebich M, Saidi M (2002) Automatic detection of pulmonary nodules at spiral CT: clinical application of a computer-adied diagnosis system. Eur Radiol 12:1052–1057

Wright AR, Collie DA, Williams JR et al (1996) Pulmonary nodules: effect on detection of spiral CT pitch. Radiology 199:837–841

Yankelevitz DF, Gupta R, Zhao B et al (1999) Small pulmonary nodules: evaluation with repeat CT-preliminary experience. Radiology 212:561–566

Yankelevitz DF, Henschke C (1997) Does 2-year stability imply that pulmonary nodules are benign? AJR 168:325–328

Yankelevitz DF, Reeves AP, Kostis WJ (2000) Small pulmonary nodules; volumetrically determined growth rates based on CT evaluation. Radiology 217:251–256

Yap CS, Schiepers C, Fishbein MC et al (2002) FDG-PET imaging in lung cancer: how sensitive is it for bronchioloalveolar carcinoma? Eur J Nucl Med Mol Imaging 29: 1166–1173

Yokomise H, Mizuno H, Ike O et al (1998) Importance of intrapulmonary lymph nodes in the differential diagnosis of small pulmonary nodular shadows. Chest 113: 703–706

Zerhouni EA, Stitik FP, Siegelman SS et al (1986) CT of the pulmonary nodule: a cooperative study. Radiology 160:319–327

Zwirewich CV, Vedal S, Miller RR et al (1991) Solitary pulmonary nodule: high-resolution CT and radiologic-pathologic correlation. Radiology 179:469–476

12 MDCT Strategies for the Non-Invasive Work-Up of the Indeterminate Pulmonary Nodule

P. Herzog, M. Das, M. F. Reiser

CONTENTS

12.1 Introduction

Pulmonary nodules are one of the most common findings on chest radiographs and CT scans of the thorax (Schoepf et al. 1999, 2001). As an incidental finding they often cause a cascade of diagnostic procedures including biopsy or surgery which, in many cases, is neither beneficial for the patient nor in any way cost-effective (Miller 2002).

Nodules found at CT follow-up scans in patients with malignant disease have a higher likelihood to represent metastatic spread and require adequate therapeutic measures. The risk of a lung nodule to represent lung cancer is greater in the presence of particular underlying diseases (Kishi et al. 2002) or predisposing behavioral factors; however, there is an abundance of incidental nodular findings at chest CT in patients without known underlying malignancy, e.g. those undergoing CT angiography to exclude pulmonary embolism (Fig. 12.1). Lately, a plethora of indeterminate incidental findings in patients undergoing lung cancer screening aggravates this general phenomenon (Diederich et al. 2003; Garg et al. 2002; Li et al. 2002; Swensen 2002). The clinicians, on the other hand, expect a final and hopefully correct diagnosis from the radiologist, which is hard to establish without invasive work-up (Mazzone and Stoller 2002) or with lacking information about actual and past clinical history (Zhang et al. 2002).

P. Herzog, MD
Institute of Clinical Radiology, University of Munich, Klinikum Grosshadern, Marchioninistrasse 15, 81377 Munich, Germany
M. F. Reiser, MD
Institute of Clinical Radiology, University of Munich, Klinikum Grosshadern, Marchioninistrasse 15, 81377 Munich, Germany
M. Das, MD
Department of Radiology, University Hospital, RWTH Aachen, Pauwelsstrasse 30, 52074 Aachen, Germany

12.2 Classic Procedure for Work-Up

Some incidental indeterminate pulmonary nodules can be compared with previous scans or radiographs and classified as longstanding and unchanged; however, classifying a nodule as "unchanged" can be treacherous ground. When evaluating nodules with diameters below 5 mm, a doubling in volume within 3 or 6 months, suggesting malignant growth, cannot be diagnosed by simply measuring the diameter of the lesion in two dimensions. This is due to the fact that the volume increases with the third power of the diameter. This is also the reason why a significant increase in volume can go along with only a minor increase in diameter, which often times cannot be measured on a 2D image, particularly in a thick-slice data set. Also, it is important to keep in mind that a nodule can grow unevenly in different dimensions. It can grow by filling out little furrows or wrinkles on its surface, which would be challenging to detect in a two-dimensional image, or it can grow only in the Z-direction, which would be missed when evaluating thick sections only.

Nodules can show distinct patterns of calcifications and thereby can be classified as inflammatory or post-specific (Fig. 12.2). Such nodules tend to be granulomatous in nature when histology is obtained (Hartman 2002).

If there are no previous examinations to compare or if the nodule is new, showing no signs of benignity, many clinical algorithms call for immediate invasive work-up of the lesion, such as CT-guided biopsy or

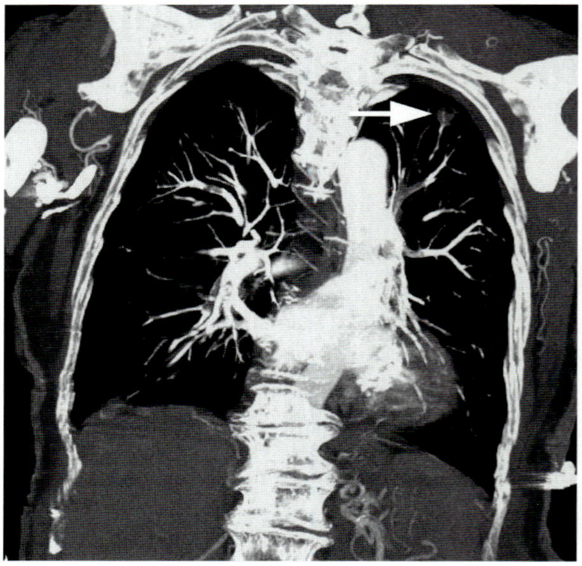

Fig. 12.1. Indeterminate pulmonary nodule in the left upper lobe of the lung in a patient with acute multiple pulmonary embolism as an incidental finding. Subsequent work-up revealed small cell lung cancer

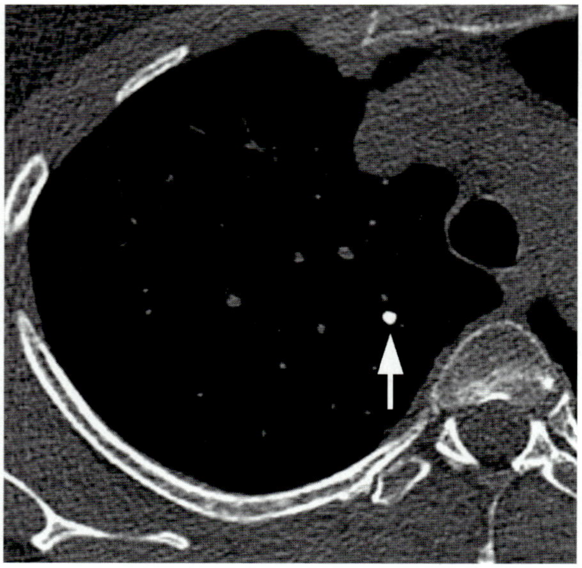

Fig. 12.2. Pulmonary nodule showing complete, diffuse calcification as a sign of benignity, typical for post-inflammatory lesions

even surgery (Fig. 12.3; Okajima et al. 2002; Wallace et al. 2002).

Marcus et al. in a re-evaluation of the initial Mayo Lung Project show that in a screening program in which every soft tissue nodule is evaluated by invasive means, the screening arm has no advantage regarding mortality or morbidity compared to a population in which no screening and invasive work-up of suspicious findings was performed (Marcus et al. 2000). This is due to the low percentage of cancer in this population and the morbidity and even mortality incurred by the invasive procedures (Fig. 12.4; Baldwin et al. 2002). Also direct surgical resection suffers from a certain rate of complications (Cooper 2002; Decamp 2002). Positron emission tomography scanning is probably useful in nodules >10 mm in diameter but expensive and less available than competing modalities (Fletcher 2002).

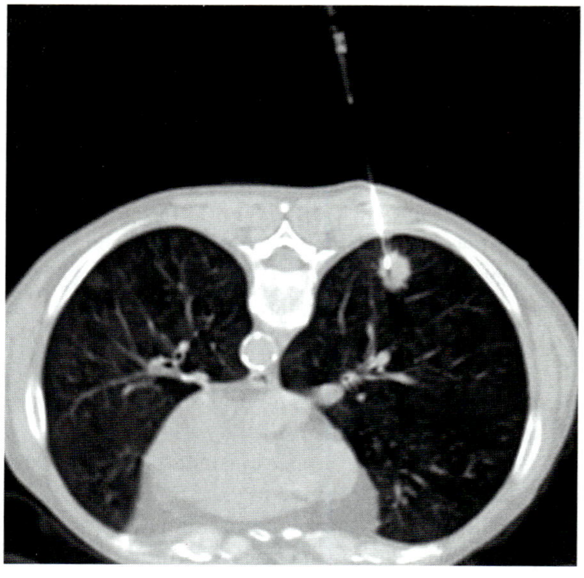

a

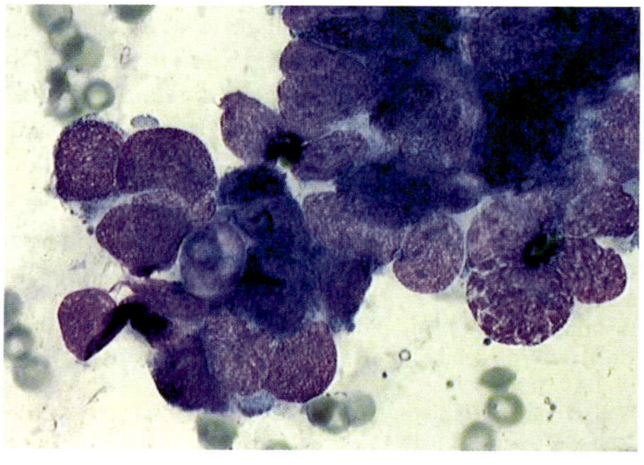

b

Fig. 12.3. Highly suspicious pulmonary nodule. Work-up with CT-guided biopsy. Histology reveals small cell lung cancer

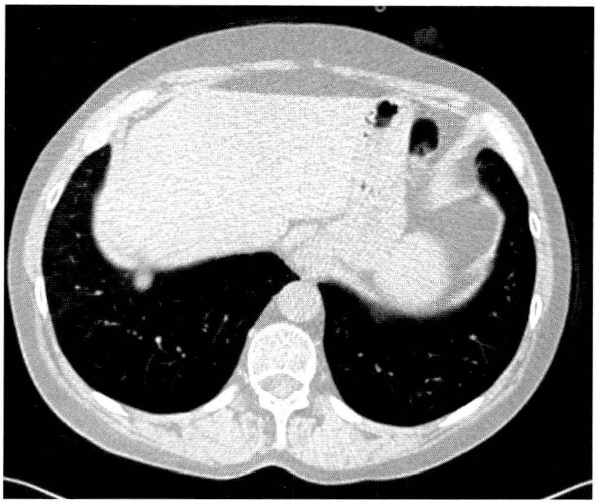
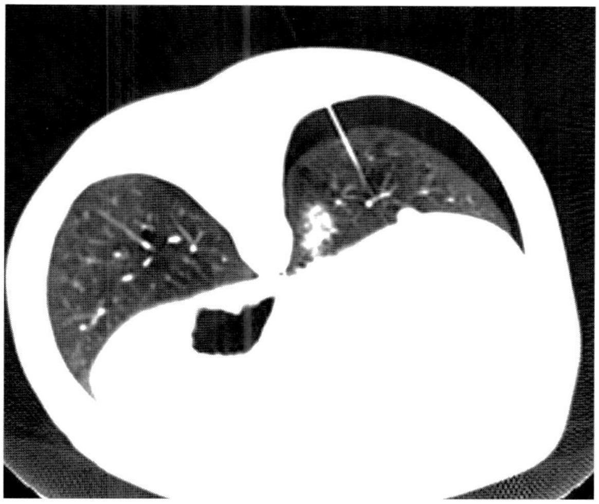

Fig. 12.4. Indeterminate pulmonary nodule in a patient with emphysema, on the waiting-list for lung transplantation. Biopsy was required to rule out malignant disease as a contraindication for lung transplantation. Pneumothorax occurred as a complication of the invasive approach

12.3 Advanced MDCT Strategies

Multi-slice CT (MSCT), with the ability of examining the whole thorax with thin slice sections in one breath hold aids us in the non-invasive evaluation of indeterminate pulmonary nodules. Therefore a collimation of 1 mm or less should be selected for scanning. Pitch can be increased up to 1.75, depending on the capabilities of the scanner and the number of detector rows. Scan time should not exceed 25 s for a comfortable breathhold time. If only the lung parenchyma is to be evaluated for pulmonary nodules, tube current and the resulting radiation dose can be drastically reduced compared to a staging CT of the thorax (Swensen et al. 2002). In such cases no contrast material needs to be administered. For appropriate evaluation of the mediastinum and the chest wall, standard radiation dose settings and intravenous contrast administration is needed. A tube voltage of 120 kV is appropriate for examining the thorax in most cases. In some cases (e.g. screening) a lower tube voltage of 100 or 80 kVp can be used to further decrease the radiation dose (Huda et al. 2002; Huda 2002). Reconstruction should be performed using a medium sharp lung kernel and an overlapping increment. Reconstructed slice thickness should be slightly greater than collimation to reduce noise and to smooth pitch artifacts. With recent generations of MSCT scanners this often times results in datasets of 500–600 axial images. A second reconstruction with a greater section thickness (e.g. 6 mm) can be performed to generate a second data set with a reasonable number of images suited for filming or printing.

Reading should be performed on a workstation. To avoid reading of an excessive number of individual axial slices (500–600) image by image, a thin sliding MIP, MPR or VRT reconstruction can be used for more effective reading. Thin sliding MIPs have already proven to be the most suitable visualization method of all secondary reconstruction techniques for delineating small pulmonary nodules and distinguishing them from pulmonary vessels.

As mentioned above, typical patterns of calcification or fatty areas in a previously indeterminate nodule can be used as approximate markers for benignity or malignancy.

Thin slices better enable the reader to evaluate the internal structure of a nodule while thick slice thickness often obscures fatty or small calcified areas due to partial-volume effect (Fig. 12.5); however, those subtle features are often an important sign or even proof of benignity, e.g. in the case of hamartomas.

Subtle features of benignity, comprising only a few hyperdense calcified voxels or hypodense fatty areas, can also be evaluated and quantified by using a histogram analysis determining the number of voxels with this particular density versus the overall density of the lesion.

Histogram analysis is available on most types of PACS workstation viewing platforms.

Appropriate histogram analysis can only be performed based on thin-slice data because of the absence

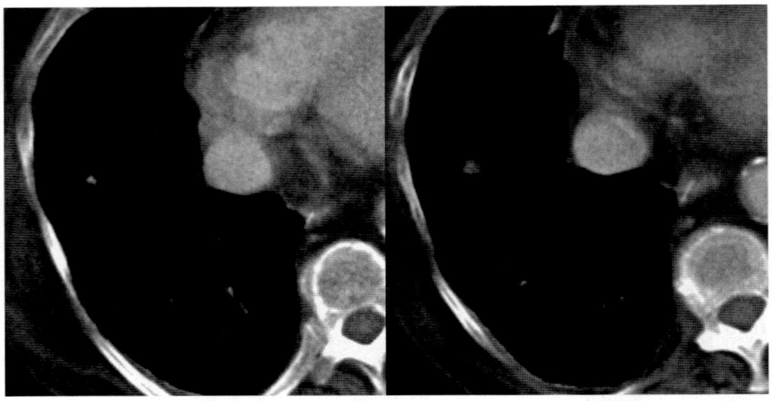

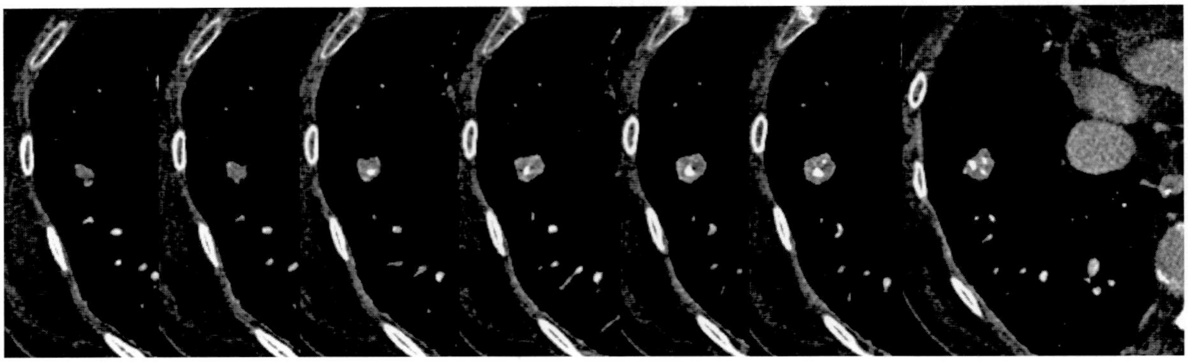

Fig. 12.5. Indeterminate nodule on 10-mm slices *above* and 1-mm slices *below*: calcification and fatty components allow ruling out malignancy when the nodule is interrogated using thin slices. Signs of benignity are obscured by volume averaging on thicker slices

of considerable partial-volume effects. A histogram of a thick-slice data set of the same nodule would show only average densities around soft tissue values due to partial-volume effects. The best way to obtain such histograms is to apply the algorithm generating the histogram to a *segmented* 3D data set. When using segmented data, the histogram will contain only data from the nodule. Using 3D data ensures that the histogram contains data from the entire nodule and not only from individual slices in which relevant areas may not be included (Fig. 12.6). Generating segmented data sets and applying them to histogram analysis requires dedicated software that is not yet implemented in standard PACS environments.

The segmentation of 3D data sets is a mathematical process that divides the data set into areas with the same properties. When segmenting pulmonary nodules, each voxel of the data set is evaluated and classified as being part of the nodule or not. In that process the gray-scale image data is transformed into a binary image (two-value image). The algorithm determines the borders (surface) of the nodule based on Hounsfield densities of the individual voxels, the reason for which the segmentation process is based primarily on thresholding processes. A threshold of –200 HU has been proven to be most efficient for the segmentation of round pulmonary lesions. While a solid soft tissue mass has higher Hounsfield densities than –200 HU (most commonly around 70–80 HU if not calcified), even with thin-slice isometric data a higher threshold would cause underestimation of the nodule size or shape due to partial-volume effects. This algorithm, of course, can only segment a nodule that has no contact with other non-nodular structures; therefore, the segmentation of lesions that are attached either to vessels, bronchi or the pleura is a considerable challenge for all segmentation algorithms. Such structures should be identified and then separated from the nodule. One possible solution is to use an algorithm that aims at fitting a spherical outline into each identified structure and reducing its radius until both structures are separated. This method has the disadvantage of changing the number of voxels defining the nodule, thereby also changing the volume of the nodule. Another more suitable method is to use a morphological opening filter to smooth the surface of a nodule and to eliminate structures connected to its surface. This is a quite common method in digital image processing but has not yet found widespread use in the context of medical imaging. Using mathematical operators, irregularities of the contour are eliminated by erosion and the "shrinking" of the volume is compensated by a final

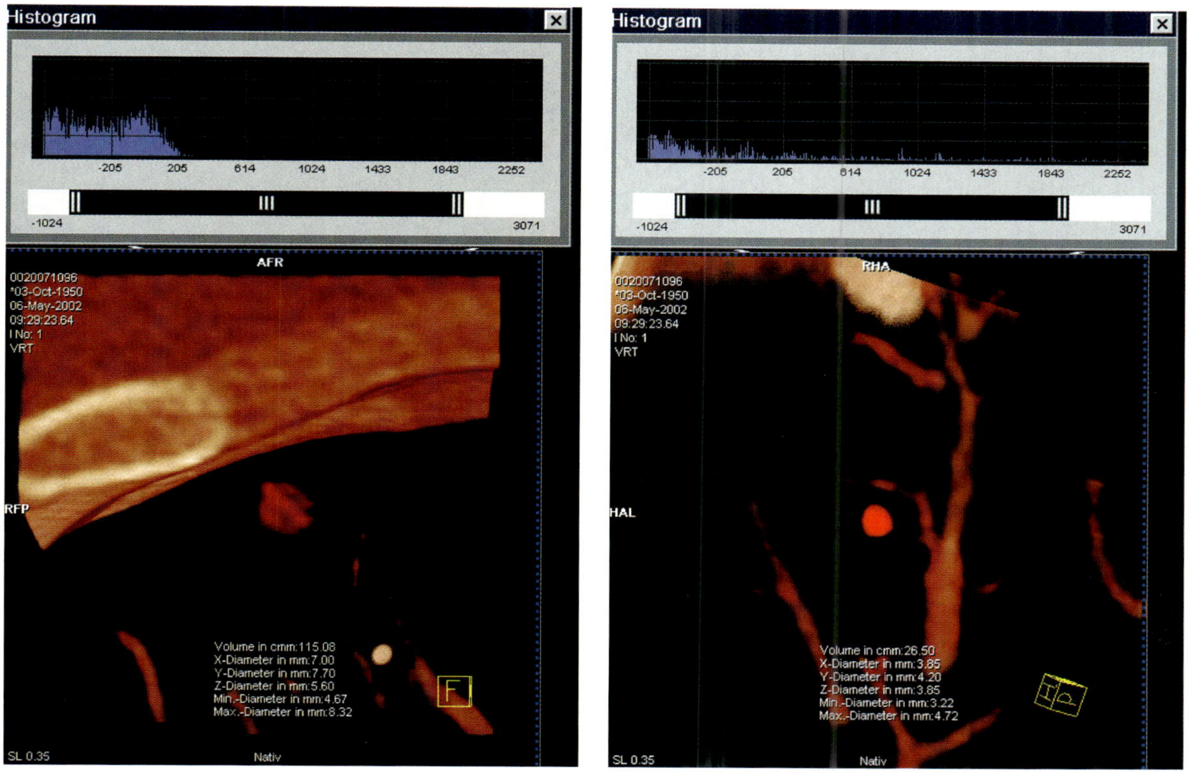

Fig. 12.6. Histograms showing the number of voxels vs their Hounsfield density calculated based on segmented data: soft tissue nodule on the left and granuloma with tiny calcifications on the right. Calcification of the granuloma not seen on axial images

dilatation procedure. See Fig. 12.7 as an example using a 2D matrix.

Using this method as an iterative procedure, the surface is modulated until the lesion becomes a compact structure. The compactness factor is used to determine how compact a structure is. For a sphere the compactness factor (CF) is 1 or 100%, for a plane it is 0 or 0%.

If the CF exceeds a predetermined value, the iterative process is stopped and the contour can be saved for further evaluation.

This, potentially, is a simple, albeit-effective, way of distinguishing between nodules and surrounding structures, and to eliminate the latter. This way, most of the lesions attached to vessels, bronchi or the pleura can be separated correctly (Fig. 12.8). Other

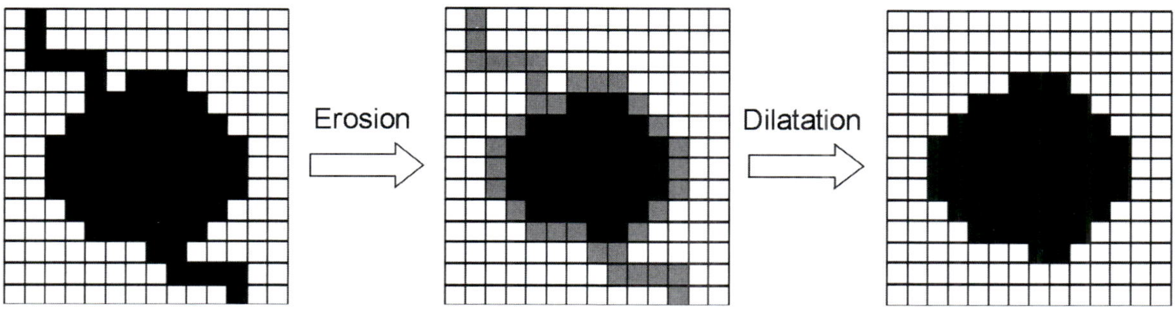

Fig. 12.7. Morphological opening filter for the smoothing of surfaces: first a layer of voxels (gray pixels) is eroded (*Erosion*). Finally, a layer of the same number of voxels is added again to regain the original diameter of the lesion (*Dilatation*)

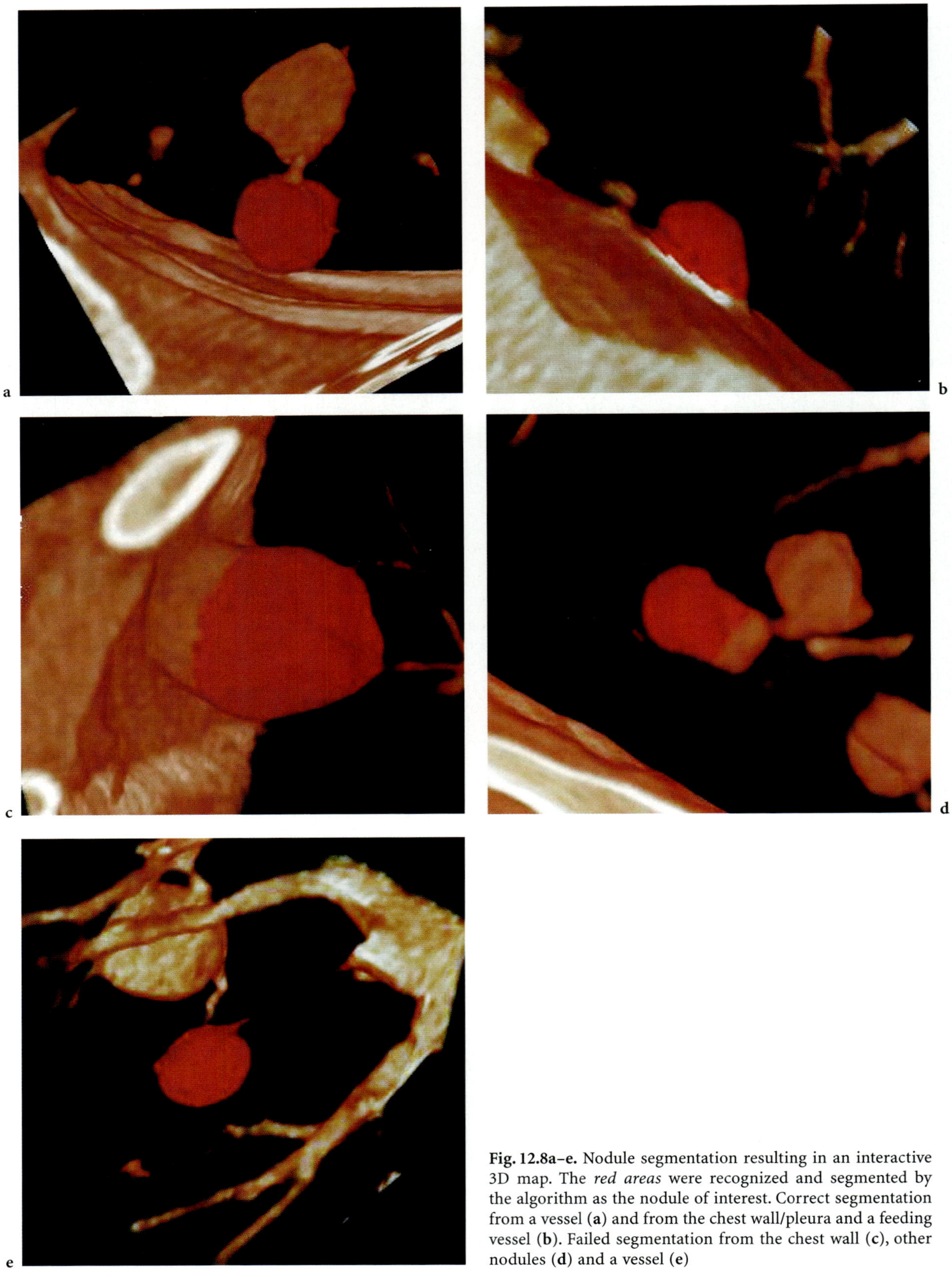

Fig. 12.8a–e. Nodule segmentation resulting in an interactive 3D map. The *red areas* were recognized and segmented by the algorithm as the nodule of interest. Correct segmentation from a vessel (**a**) and from the chest wall/pleura and a feeding vessel (**b**). Failed segmentation from the chest wall (**c**), other nodules (**d**) and a vessel (**e**)

algorithms have been developed and are already in the process of clinical evaluation that may further facilitate segmentation of pulmonary nodules from surrounding structures (Kido et al. 2002).

A nodule without fat or calcium as obvious signs of benignity still has to be considered as indeterminate because only a small portion of all incidental nodules are malignant and an invasive evaluation in every case would do more harm than good; therefore, other methods of non-invasive evaluation have to be considered.

12.4 Contrast Uptake

Contrast media uptake has been used for sensitive differentiation between benign and malignant lesions. Contrast media uptake can be determined by means of an actual perfusion study with multiple repetitive scans (up to 80 times) at the same table position encompassing the lesion. Another option is to perform an unenhanced scan before and four scans every minute after contrast enhancement. This way, more than one nodule can be evaluated with a total of five scans without a further increase in radiation exposure. After those five scans, the mean Hounsfield densities in the unenhanced scan are subtracted from the corresponding enhanced scans in all suspicious nodules. A threshold of enhancement of 15 HU has been found to be a sensitive (98%) but unspecific (55%) marker for differentiating between benign and malignant lesions.

12.5 CT Volumetry

Maybe the most efficient way to evaluate the dignity of an indeterminate nodule is to assess lesion growth. Active malignancy should exhibit a certain growth pattern depending on the tissue type, especially when untreated. Small cell lung cancers have the highest growth rate with a doubling time of approximately 70 days. Lung cancers other than small cell lung cancer tend to have an intermediate growth rate with a doubling time of approximately100 days, whereas adenocarcinomas exhibit slower growth rate with a doubling time of approximately 130–160 days. Nodules with faster growth rates and doubling times of less than 50 days usually represent acute inflammatory lesions, which should recede under antimicrobial therapy (Figs. 12.9, 12.10). Nodules with doubling times of more than 300–500 days usually represent benign or sub-acute inflammatory lesions when histology is obtained.

Based on thin-slice MDCT data, accurate CT volumetry can be performed based on automated segmentation algorithm as described above. Since growth is the very hallmark of malignancy, such tools may be the most suitable method for the non-invasive characterization of lung lesions in the future and may help avoid unnecessary invasive procedures with the morbidity and mortality inherent to them (Fig. 12.11).

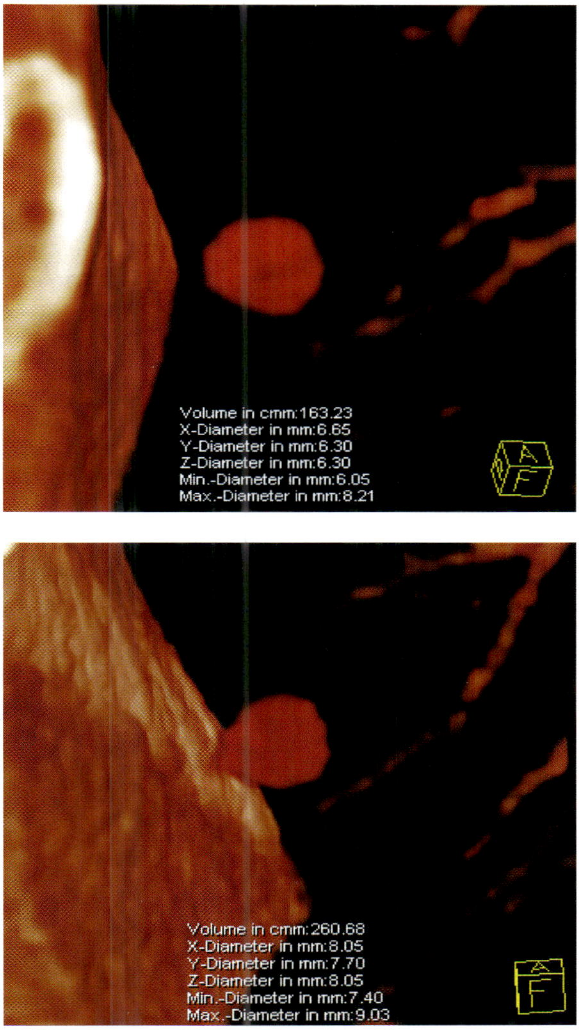

Fig. 12.9. Squamous cell carcinoma. Initial scan on the upper and 3 months follow-up on the lower image panel. The lesion exhibits a malignant growth pattern with an increase from 160 mm^3 to 260 mm^3

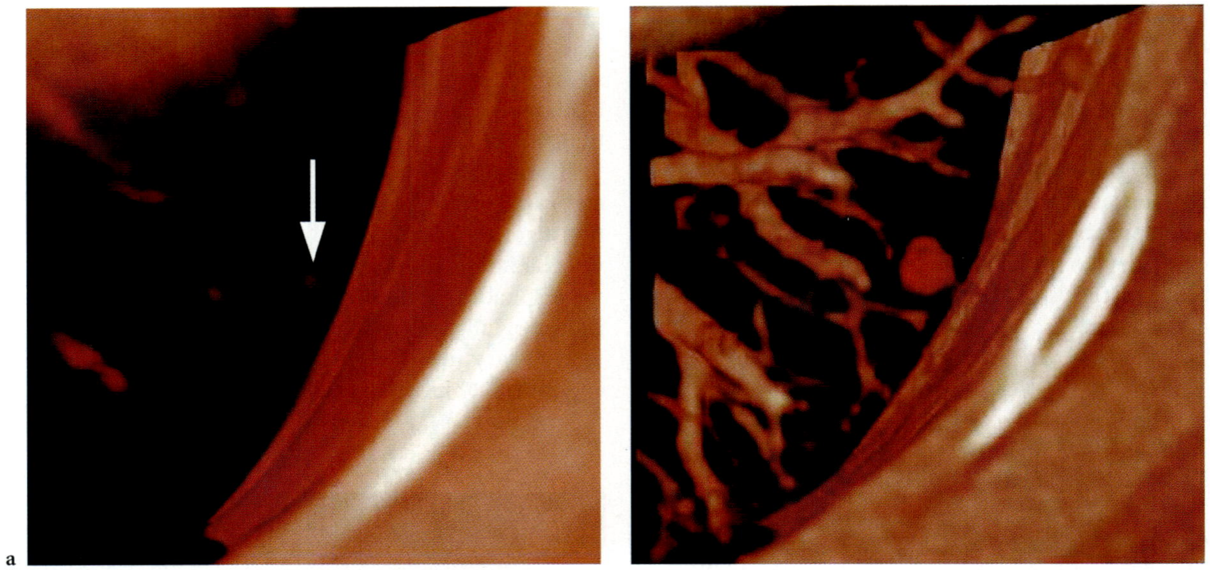

Fig. 12.10. Small cell carcinoma. Initial scan (37 mm^3) on the left with 6 months follow-up (152 mm^3) on the right

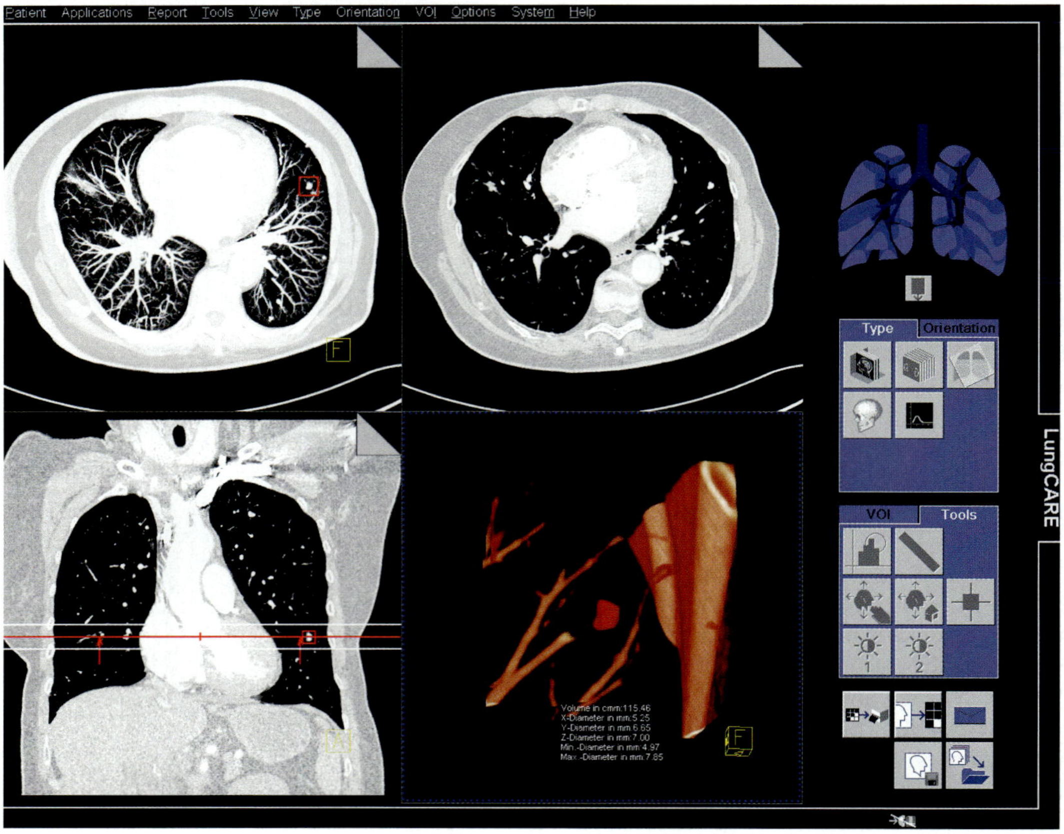

Fig. 12.11. Example of a dedicated software platform for visualization and analysis of focal lung disease: The LungCARE (Siemens, Erlangen, Germany) software platform enables intuitive visualization of focal lung disease using MIP, VRT or MPR reconstructions in various imaging planes. If focal lung disease is found, accurate lesion volumetry can be performed, based of the principles described herein

References

Baldwin DR, Eaton T et al. (2002) Management of solitary pulmonary nodules: How do thoracic computed tomography and guided fine needle biopsy influence clinical decisions? Thorax 57:817–822

Cooper JD (2002) Management of the solitary pulmonary nodule: directed resection. Semin Thorac Cardiovasc Surg 14:286–291

Decamp MM Jr (2002) The solitary pulmonary nodule: aggressive excisional strategy. Semin Thorac Cardiovasc Surg 14: 292–296

Diederich S, Wormanns D et al (2003) Lung cancer screening with low-dose CT. Eur J Radiol 45:2–7

Fletcher JW (2002) PET scanning and the solitary pulmonary nodule. Semin Thorac Cardiovasc Surg 14:268–274

Garg K, Keith RL et al (2002) Randomized controlled trial with low-dose spiral CT for lung cancer screening: feasibility study and preliminary results. Radiology 225:506–510

Hartman TE (2002) Radiologic evaluation of the solitary pulmonary nodule. Semin Thorac Cardiovasc Surg 14:261–267

Huda W (2002) Dose and image quality in CT. Pediatr Radiol 32: 709–713, 751–754

Huda W, Ravenel JG, Scalzetti EM (2002) How do radiographic techniques affect image quality and patient doses in CT? Semin Ultrasound CT MR 23:411–422

Kido S, Kuriyama K et al. (2002) Fractal analysis of small peripheral pulmonary nodules in thin-section CT: evaluation of the lung-nodule interfaces. J Comput Assist Tomogr 26:573–578

Kishi K, Gurney JW et al. (2002) The correlation of emphysema or airway obstruction with the risk of lung cancer: a matched case-controlled study. Eur Respir J 19:1093–1098

Li F, Sone S et al. (2002) Lung cancers missed at low-dose helical CT screening in a general population: comparison of clinical, histopathologic, and imaging findings. Radiology 225:673–683

Marcus PM, Bergstralh EJ et al. (2000) Lung cancer mortality in the Mayo Lung Project: impact of extended follow-up. J Natl Cancer Inst 21:321–323

Mazzone PJ, Stoller JK (2002) The pulmonologist's perspective regarding the solitary pulmonary nodule. Semin Thorac Cardiovasc Surg 14:250–260

Miller DL (2002) Management of the subcentimeter pulmonary nodule. Semin Thorac Cardiovasc Surg 14:281–285

Okajima Y, Tajima H et al. (2002) Clinical application of a CT-guided lung biopsy system: core needle biopsy at the IVR center. J Nippon Med Sch 69:434–444

Schafer JF, Vollmar J et al. (2002) Imaging diagnosis of solitary pulmonary nodules on an open low-field MRI system: comparison of two MR sequences with spiral CT. Rofo Fortschr Geb Rontgenstr Neuen Bildgeb Verfahr 174: 1107–1114

Schoepf UJ, Bruning R et al. (1999) Imaging of the thorax with multislice spiral CT. Radiologe 39:943–951

Schoepf UJ, Bruening RD et al. (2001) Multislice helical CT of focal and diffuse lung disease: comprehensive diagnosis with reconstruction of contiguous and high-resolution CT sections from a single thin-collimation scan. Am J Roentgenol 177:179–184

Swensen SJ (2002) CT screening for lung cancer. Am J Roentgenol 179:833–836

Swensen SJ, Jett JR et al. (2002) Screening for lung cancer with low-dose spiral computed tomography. Am J Respir Crit Care Med 165:508–513

Wallace MJ, Krishnamurthy S et al. (2002) CT-guided percutaneous fine-needle aspiration biopsy of small (£1-cm) pulmonary lesions. Radiology 225:823–828

Zhang L, Wang M et al. (2002) Clinico-pathological study of 98 patients with pulmonary solitary nodule. Zhonghua Zhong Liu Za Zhi 24:491–493

13 Transthoracic Needle Biopsy of Lung Nodules

D. F. Yankelevitz, D. Shaham, M. Vazquez, C. I. Henschke

CONTENTS

13.1 Introduction

Transthoracic needle biopsy (TNB) has become a widely used technique to evaluate pulmonary nodules. In part, the increased use of this technique has come about through the emergence of improved image guidance with CT scanning and most recently with CT fluoroscopy. Performance of this procedure requires the skills of the radiologist to obtain the sample and the skills of a pathologist to interpret the sample provided. The performance of the procedure starts with careful consideration of the indications and contraindications, followed by choice of image guidance, technical considerations in performance of the procedure, risk reduction techniques and finally, interpretation of the specimen along with considerations for appropriate follow up. In this chapter we will discuss each of the above considerations in the chain of events that are involved in the performance of this procedure. As this chapter focuses on biopsy of pulmonary nodules we will not discuss the related topics of mediastinal or hilar biopsy.

13.2 Indications and Contraindications

The indication for performance of this procedure is the presence of a pulmonary nodule. This can either be the presence of a solitary nodule that is indeterminate or the presence of multiple nodules where metastatic disease is considered. The procedure can be used to confirm either malignant or benign conditions. In terms of nodule size and location there are no absolute contraindications to the performance of the procedure. It is clear however that both of these factors can influence the technical difficulty in the performance of the procedure. These factors must be weighed by the radiologist in terms of his/her own skill level in deciding whether to perform the procedure. Contraindications to the performance of TNB are for the most part only relative. The only absolute contraindication is an uncooperative patient (Lalli et al. 1978). In cases where a patient is unable to remain still or follow instructions, the procedure cannot be performed. In special situations, where a diagnosis is considered imperative, the procedure could be performed while the patient is sedated. The other relative contraindications include the following:

D. F. Yankelevitz, MD, Professor of Radiology;
M. Vazquez, MD, Associate Professor of Clinical Pathology;
C. I. Henschke, PhD, MD, Professor of Radiology;
Weill Medical College of Cornell University, 525 East 68th Street, New York, New York 10021, USA
D. Shaham, MD
Lecturer in Radiology, Hadassah University Hospital, Kiryat Hadassah, Jerusalem 91120, Israel

1. Bleeding diathesis with international normalized ratio (INR) >1.3 or platelet count <50,000: When necessary, these can be corrected with transfusion even on an emergent basis (Klein and Zarka 2000).
2. Severe pulmonary dysfunction including emphysema or bullous disease: In these cases, careful selection of biopsy path to minimize crossing of severely damaged lung is helpful. Ultimately, these underlying conditions increase the risk of pneumothorax; therefore it is necessary to apply appropriate risk reduction techniques and be familiar with treatment of complications.
3. Contralateral pneumonectomy: The risk in this situation is the development of pnuemothorax in the remaining lung. Again careful attention to risk reduction and treatment when necessary are the main concerns.
4. Suspicion of hydatid cyst: Rupture of a hydatid cyst can cause widespread dissemination within the lung and pleural space (Stampfel 1982).
5. Difficulty in positioning: On occasion patients may have difficulty maintaining a position that allows the easiest access to the nodule. In general the shortest path to the nodule is chosen for the procedure, however on occasion the position may be uncomfortable and it may not be possible to maintain for the duration of the procedure. Careful attention to patient comfort prior to the start of the procedure, and once positioned performing the procedure as quickly as possible helps to alleviate this problem. Occasionally patients must be positioned so that they are more comfortable even though this necessitates an alternative path for the needle to travel that may be longer and more difficult than the original.
6. Medications with anticoagulant effects: These include coumadin, aspirin and non steroidal anti-inflammatory agents. These should generally be discontinued five days prior to the procedure, in order to avoid excessive bleeding into the lung (Hirsh et al. 1989).

13.3 Alternative Diagnostic Tests

The choice of workup for pulmonary nodules can be quite challenging. It requires an understanding of the complex relationship of several probabilities. In the case of solitary nodules, this requires an understanding of what the probability of malignancy is for a given nodule based on the initial evaluation of radiologic and clinical findings, as well as an understanding of how this initial assessment can be altered based on the results of additional diagnostic tests. Additional considerations in regard to the workup include the availability of equipment and personnel, costs for various procedures, skill of the operator and risk of complications. These factors are quite complex and it seems likely that there is no single paradigm for the work up of a nodule that is appropriate in all situations. Workup will vary from case to case and even different approaches for an identical nodule may be necessary at different institutions.

Several diagnostic tests are often considered in the workup of pulmonary nodules. They range from totally non-invasive to minimally invasive to invasive. Under the category of non-invasive, the commonly considered diagnostic alternatives include contrast enhanced CT scanning and PET scanning. There is a large body of literature describing these tests. However, the literature can be confusing with wide ranges reported for their respective sensitivities and specificities. Some general conclusions about these two approaches can be made. They both have diminished accuracy for sub-centimeter nodules. Both are prone to be false positive with active inflammatory processes, and both tend to be false negative with low-grade cancers. Nevertheless, both of these procedures continue to be improved and are active areas of research and development. Newer high-resolution multi-detector CT scanners should impact both of these tests and allow for more accurate diagnosis of smaller nodules. In the case of nodule enhancement, it will allow for higher resolution images of the nodule to be obtained quickly, and for PET scanning, mapping the PET images to high resolution images obtained with CT may allow for additional attenuation correction.

Under the category of minimally invasive, bronchoscopy is often considered as an alternative to TNB. However, the published reports of the accuracy of bronchoscopy are nearly uniformly lower than that of TNB. Bronchoscopy is generally limited to those cases where there is a positive bronchus sign. This implies that a bronchus is seen leading into the nodule. However, even with this favorable sign present, the procedure is still less accurate than TNB (Yankelevitz et al. 2000c).

Invasive procedures include thoracoscopic biopsy and thoracotomy. The obvious advantage of these procedures is that they obtain a larger amount of tissue. However, as a diagnostic procedure, thoracotomy should generally be avoided. This is a major surgical procedure with attendant risks and morbidity associated with it (YANKELEVITZ et al. 2000c). When necessary, thoracoscopy generally suffices to yield enough tissue and can be converted into a thoracotomy if necessary. While claims of one hundred percent sensitivity and specificity have been attributed to thoracoscopy, the increasing use of this procedure to diagnose small nodules that are difficult for the surgeon to palpate have led to revision of this belief (Fig. 13.1).

One of the newer approaches being used to evaluate small nodules relies on estimating their growth rates using serial CT scans (YANKELEVITZ et al. 2000c). This technique leverages the unique ability of CT scanning to make accurate measurements. Once the volume can be accurately measured and the time between scans is known, it is relatively straight forward to estimate doubling times (Fig. 13.2). This technique is still relatively new and more work needs to be done to fully integrate its role into the diagnostic process.

13.4 Prebiopsy Procedure

The majority of TNB's are performed on an outpatient basis. The ideal situation is to have the films reviewed by the radiologist prior to scheduling the case. Once it is decided that the procedure is warranted, the patient can be placed on the schedule. The patient should be informed about what to expect prior to coming for the procedure. This includes a discussion of the risks and benefits, eating instructions, medications to either be continued or temporarily be discontinued, and to be prepared for the possibility of staying overnight in the event of complications. It is also helpful to have written material that can be sent to the patient that contains information regarding the procedure so that they can have any questions or concerns answered for them before they come. Laboratory tests are generally required prior to the procedure to confirm that there are no serious problems related to bleeding. The pathology department is made aware of the biopsy schedule in advance so that they are ready to evaluate the specimen. In addition, many institutions are now requiring documentation of a recent history and physical examination. This can be obtained from the patients referring physician and must be recent. The radiologist generally obtains informed consent immediately before the procedure begins. The elements of informed consent include a discussion of the risks and benefits, including details about the frequency of pneumothorax, hemmorahage and infection. Alternatives are also discussed with the patient.

13.5 Biopsy Prucedure

13.5.1 Choice of Image Guidance

The majority of TNB are now performed under CT guidance. Flouroscopic guidance is also available, but is used less frequently at present. Occasionally, ultrasound can be used for guidance, but this is generally limited to nodules that abut the chest wall or for

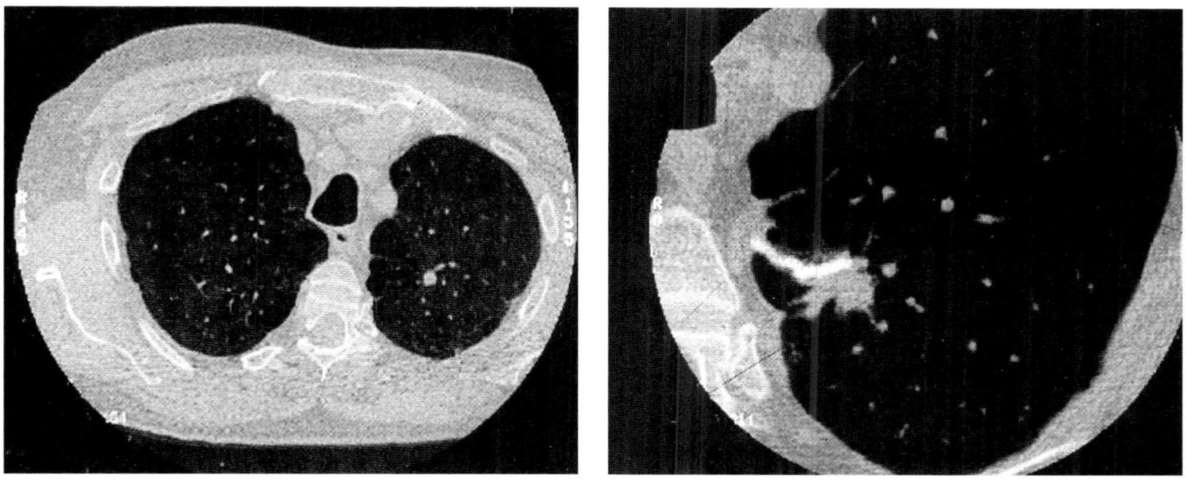

a b

Fig. 13.1. **a** High resolution CT image of a nodule prior to attempted thoracoscopic resection. **b** High resolution CT image post attempted thoracoscopic resection shows the nodule still present adjacent to the suture line

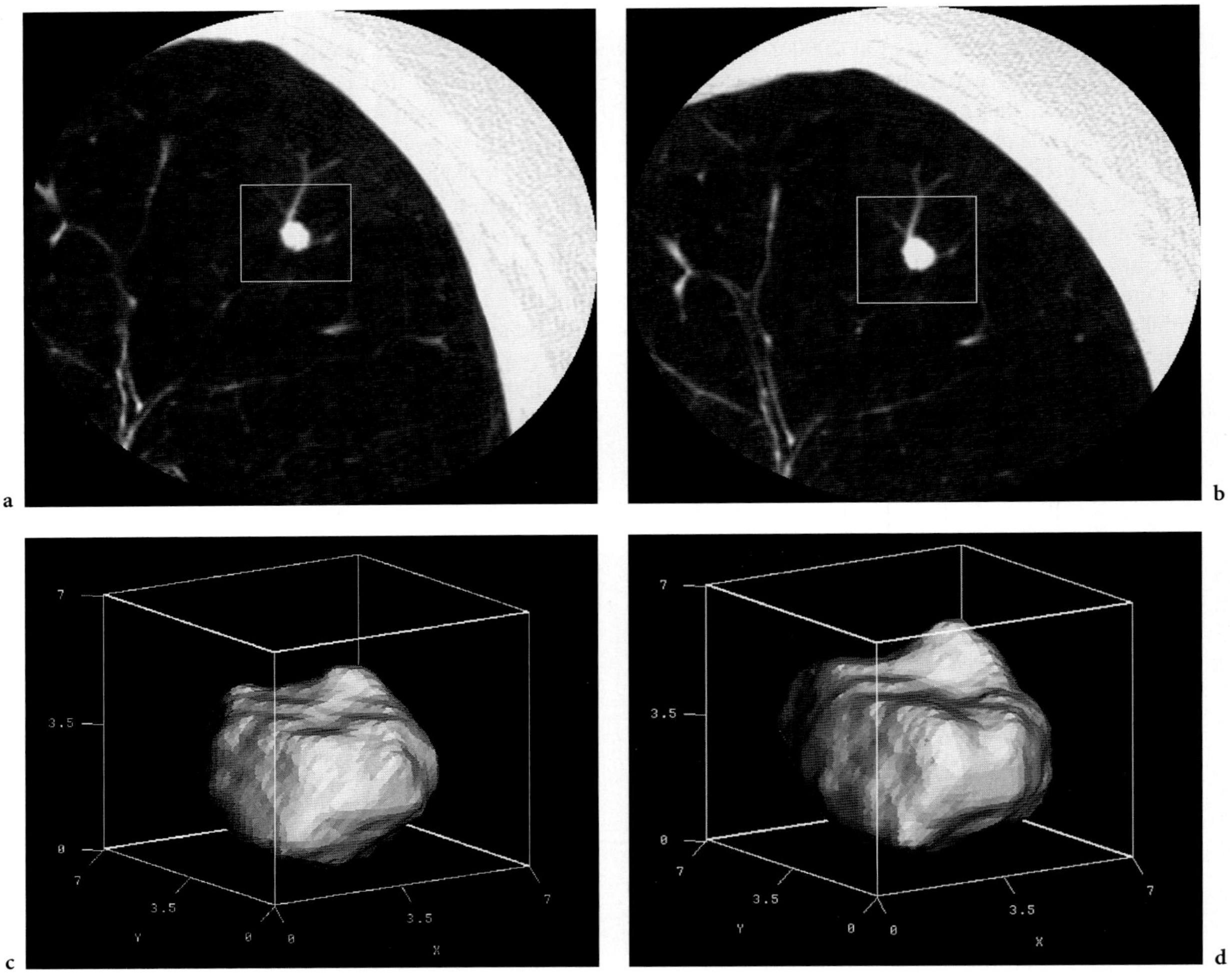

Fig. 13.2. (**a**) High resolution CT image of a small nodule. (**b**) High resolution CT image of the nodule obtained at a later time. (**c, d**) Comparison of the 3-D renderings of the nodules respectively. Based on the time between scans and the change in volume, an estimate of the nodule volume doubling time can be easily performed

mediastinal lesions (Gupta et al. 1999). In regard to the choice of fluoroscopy or CT, there are advantages and disadvantages when compared to each other. It is generally faster to perform the procedure under fluoroscopic guidance. With bi-plane fluoroscopy the depth of the needle in relation to the nodule can be visualized and there is the benefit of real time performance. However, CT can identify lesions that are not well identified with fluoroscopy and documentation of the needle tip within the nodule can be done with more confidence using CT. Ultimately, weighing the relative merits of these approaches is often done on a case-to-case basis and rests in part with the radiologists experience and preference. CT fluoroscopy has recently been introduced. This technology allows for some of the advantages previously only found with routine fluoroscopy, notably real time evaluation, to now be available in the performance of CT guided procedures (White et al. 2000). CT fluoroscopy is particularly useful in those cases where the nodule is small and poorly visualized by fluoroscopy and for nodules that are located near the diaphragm where there is considerable motion and routine real time evaluation is helpful.

13.5.2 Patient Positioning

Patient positioning is generally done to allow for the most direct route to the nodule. There are however numerous considerations that can alter this. The choice of positions is either supine, prone or decubitus. Prone position is advantageous for several reasons, the primary one being that there is less chest wall motion in this position. The ribs are attached to vertebral bodies in their posterior aspects and thus the posterior aspect does not move in the vertical plane when the patient breathes. Instead, it rotates in plane. This has been likened to the motion of the handles of a bucket. When the patient is supine, the anterior portions of the ribs move in the vertical plane and this causes motion of the needle with each breath. The decubitus position has the largest amount of motion associated with it. In this case, the dependent lung is relatively motionless and the majority of motion occurs in the non dependent lung, which is generally the lung being biopsied. Another reason to prefer the prone position is that following the procedure the patient is instructed to lie with the biopsy site in the dependent position. This is useful in reducing the risk of developing a pneumothorax. It is generally much easier for patients to lie on their backs for several hours post procedure than to lie prone. A final reason for preferring the prone position is that the patients do not have to visualize the needle actually entering them. While many patients simply close their eyes to avoid seeing this, for some it can be quite anxiety provoking.

Other considerations in terms of positioning relate to gaining the best access to the nodule. On occasion there may be structures blocking the path of the needle. This includes bony structures such as the scapula or ribs as well as vascular structures such as the great vessels. Proper positioning is a major component in planning the procedure and time spent on optimizing this is well worth it. The scapula can be rotated out of the way by placing the patients arm at their side and internally rotating the shoulder (Yankelevitz et al. 2000b). This generally moves the scapula laterally (Fig. 13.3). On occasion, it is helpful to place a pillow or folded sheet under the chest so as to allow the shoulder to rotate even further and move the scapula laterally. This technique is also sometimes helpful in spreading the ribs to allow for direct perpendicular access to the nodule without having to advance the needle on an angle to the scanning plane. Regarding the great vessels and clavicle, it is often not possible to rotate these structures out of the biopsy plane. In cases where a nodule is located near these structures, a prone approach is necessary, even though it may necessitate a longer path (Fig. 13.4).

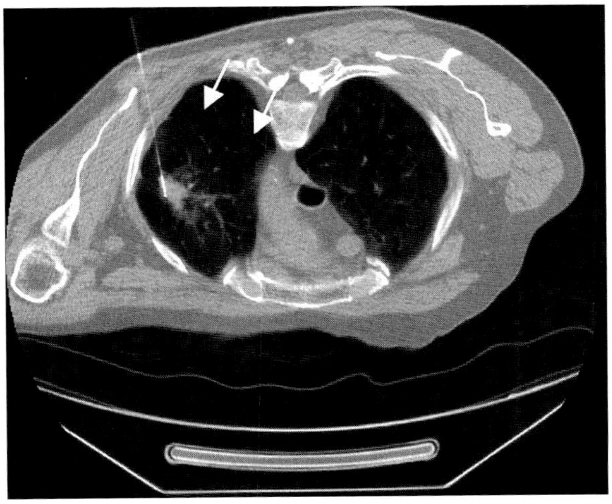

Fig. 13.3. CT image of patient in the prone position. The left arm is located at the patient's side and is rotated internally. This pulls the scapula laterally allowing much greater access to the lateral portion of the lung. Note the difference between the two sides. The lateral positioning of the needle allows it to be placed directly into the left upper lobe. Had the entry site been more medial, the major fissure (arrows) would have had to be crossed and that would have led to an increased chance for pneumothorax

13.5.3 Sedation

In general, conscious sedation is not necessary in the performance of TNB. The majority of patients are calm enough to allow for the performance of the procedure without any additional medication. In addition, it is often desirable to have the patients cooperate with specific breathing instruction during the procedure. However, on occasion, after discussion with the patient, it may be worthwhile to consider giving sedation. In those cases it is necessary to conform to all relevant hospital policies in regard to this administration.

13.5.4 Breathing Instructions

With fluoroscopic guidance, the degree of inspiration can be monitored in real time. This allows for the relationship between the needle and the nodule to be observed and instructions are given to stop breathing when the alignment between them appears correct. Once this occurs, the needle is advanced towards the nodule with continuous observation. With CT guidance, except in the case of CT fluoroscopy, real time observation is not possible, and the needle is advanced without its orientation being directly observed. Each adjustment of the needle is performed based on review of the last set of CT images. The needle is adjusted and a new set of images is

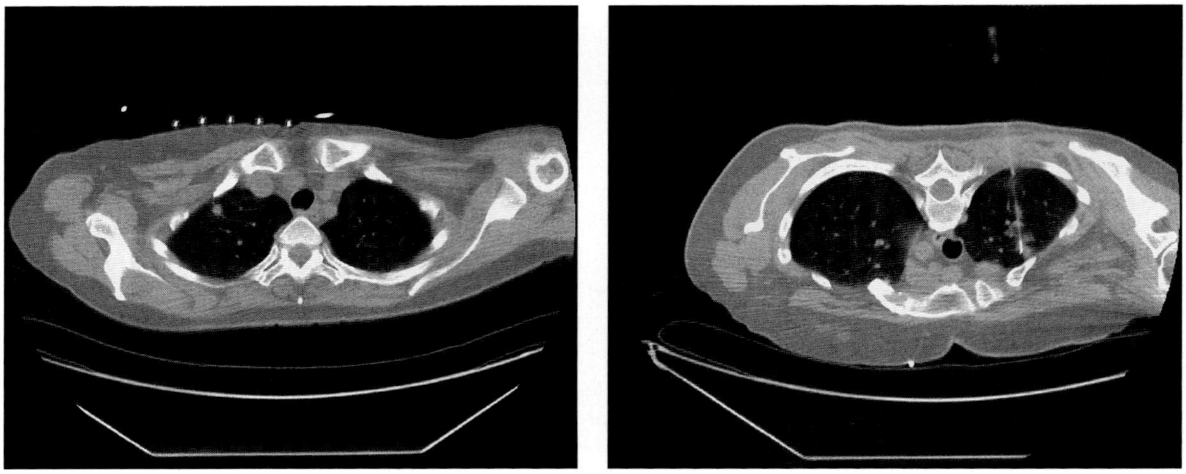

a b

Fig. 13.4. **a** The nodule located in the apex of the right lung is closer to the anterior surface of the lung than to the posterior surface. However, both the first rib and the subclavian vein blocks direct access. **b** The biopsy is performed in the prone position. There is nothing obstructing a direct path toward the nodule, however, the needle must travel a greater distance to reach its target

then obtained. In terms of specific breathing instructions, different instructions are given depending on the situation. When nodules are located in the upper lobes and the patient can be placed in the prone position, the amount of motion in the lungs is quite small and patients are simply requested to breathe gently throughout the procedure. The relationship between the advancing needle and the nodule is sufficiently stable to allow for this approach. In patients where the nodule is located near the diaphragm or when the biopsy is performed with the patient in the supine position, it is often necessary to give specific breathing instructions. The purpose of these instructions is to have the nodule in the identical location each time the needle is being advanced. In the case of CT fluoroscopy, the advancing needle can be visualized in relation to the nodule. However, there are some important differences in comparison to routine fluoroscopy in that only a single axial plane is visualized and there is a slight, approximately 0.5 second, offset for the images to update. Nevertheless, this technique is quite useful in those cases where there is motion due to breathing (White et al. 2000).

13.5.5 Preparation for Needle Insertion

Once the patient has been correctly positioned and instructed, the next step is to mark the skin entry site. With flouroscopy, this can be done by placing a forceps into the imaging plane and observing its location relative to the nodule. Once the tip of the forceps is in the correct location, its location at the skin surface is marked. With CT, a set of images are obtained for initial localization of the nodule. A plane is chosen for the skin entry site. This is not always the image plane that includes the nodule, as there are occasions where planes above or below must be chosen because of a structure blocking a directly perpendicular approach. Next, a set of markers is placed on the patient in the chosen entry plane. These markers can be as simple as a set of blood drawing needles taped together and the purpose is to allow for localization within the scanning plane. A new set of images is now obtained in the scanning plane, with the markers in place. The marker in the optimal location is now chosen. Once the marker is chosen, the laser light on the scanner is turned on to show the scanning plane on the skin surface and now the combination of the laser light and the chosen marker defines the precise entry site. The skin is marked, generally with a felt tip marker.

Once the skin entry site is chosen, the skin is cleansed with antiseptic solution and the surrounding area is covered with a sterile drape. Local anesthesia is now given. It is important to give sufficient anesthesia to make the procedure virtually pain free. This involves numbing by instillation of anesthesia from the skin surface all the way to the parietal pleural surface. There are sensory nerve fibers on the parietal pleural surface, and while it is not necessary to directly insert the needle into it, infusion into adjacent tissue allows for anesthesia to diffuse into the pleura. Documentation of the anesthetic needle adjacent to the parietal pleural surface is useful, and the creation of a small amount of local swelling at the pleural surface caused by the anesthetic agent is helpful in determining that sufficient anesthesia has been given. With experience, operators can actually feel when the needle has reached the parietal pleural surface while they are instilling the anesthetic.

13.5.6 Choice of Biopsy Needle

There are numerous types of biopsy needles. They come in various lengths and gauges. Broadly, however, there are two basic types of needle designs that are used. This includes the co-axial design and the single shaft (non co-axial). Choice between these two is generally a matter of preference. However, each type has certain advantages compared to the other. Using the co-axial technique, multiple samples can be obtained with a single pleural puncture. In this way, if the initial sample is insufficient, additional material can be obtained without the additional risk of puncturing the pleura and causing pneumothorax. The advantage of the single needle is that it is generally of thinner gauge, as it does not require an outer cannula, and is more flexible. The thinner gauge may be helpful in reducing risk of pneumothorax and bleeding, while the increased flexibility is found by some operators to be useful in guiding the needle to the correct location. Additionally, in cases where the initial sample is inadequate it may be useful to move the needle to a very different portion of the nodule where more viable, diagnostic tissue can be obtained. This would offset the benefit of the co-axial approach, where the additional samples are obtained in close proximity to the original sample. However, each additional puncture of the pleural surface increases the risk of pneumothorax.

Another distinction between the types of needles is whether they are of the aspiration type or cutting type. Aspiration needles only obtain material suitable for cytologic interpretation, while cutting needles obtain material that allows for histologic evaluation. Needles suitable for obtaining histologic material have either a circumferential cutting tip, a side slot that acts as a receptacle, or a spring-loaded cutting edge over a side slot. The spring-loaded needles generally have a throw distance of one to two centimeters. In some of the designs, this is adjustable. In general, obtaining cytologic material is sufficient to diagnose malignancy. However, to diagnose benign conditions, it is sometimes helpful to have histologic material. The cytologic criteria necessary to establish benign diagnoses are less well defined, nevertheless, these criteria continue to be refined.

Yet another distinction among the needles relates to the shape of the needle tip. There are two basic types, symmetrical and beveled. Both are sufficiently sharp so as to pass through the skin without first making a small incision. The main difference relates to guidance. Symmetrical tips tend to travel in a straight line whereas beveled tips tend to travel in the direction opposite the bevel. Some have found this later effect useful in guiding or steering the needle.

13.5.7 Choice of Syringe

Once the needle is inserted into the nodule the next step is to aspirate material for cytologic inspection. Attaching a syringe to the needle and creating negative pressure accomplish this. The amount of negative pressure that can be created is the same regardless of the size of the syringe (Yankelevitz et al. 1995). Once a vacuum is created, it creates the full amount of negative pressure possible regardless of whether a 50 cc syringe or a 5 cc syringe is used. The only difference is that it requires more effort to create this vacuum with the larger syringe. For practical purposes, it is easy to use the smaller size syringes. A 10 cc syringe represents a good compromise in size, as it is still relatively easy to create a vacuum, and at the same time, if a small amount of air enters the system during the aspiration, the syringe is usually large enough to still maintain sufficient negative pressure to effectively complete the aspiration.

13.5.8 Targeting the Nodule

Depending on the size of the nodule, it is often quite difficult, if not impossible to directly align the needle in the soft tissue so that it will be on course to directly enter the nodule. As an example, lets assume a situation involving placing a needle into a one centimeter nodule that is ten centimeters deep to the pleural surface. After giving local anesthetic, the biopsy needle is inserted into the soft tissues. If this biopsy needle is off target by as little as two degrees, then by the time it has advanced the full ten centimeters, it will miss the target. For smaller nodules, the degree of accuracy needs to be even higher. Proper alignment of the needle with this degree of accuracy is quite challenging by itself, however when small degrees of

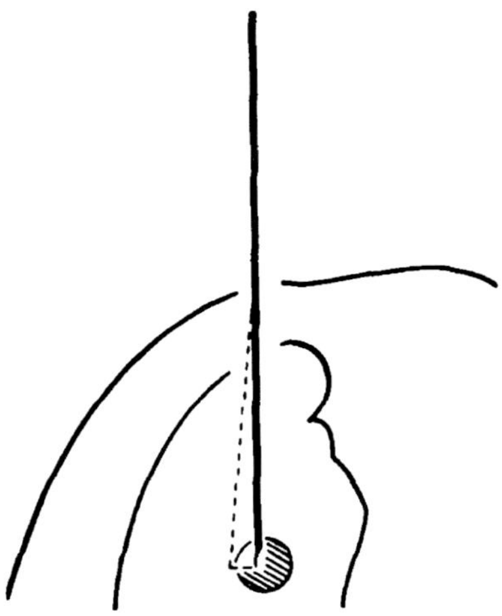

Fig. 13.5. Illustration of a one-cm. nodule 10 cm. beneath the skin surface. If the needle is angled by as little as two degrees away from the line perpendicular to the center of the nodule, the needle will miss the nodule completely. This implies that for nodules that are small and deep, there needs to be a technique to compensate for minor misalignments

patient motion are added, it becomes apparent that directly targeting the nodule from the soft tissues in a straight line is generally not possible (Fig. 13.5). Therefore some mechanism of steering the needle is necessary. A technique that is useful for this purpose is often referred to as 'bevel steering' (Yankelevitz et al. 1996a) (Fig. 13.6). This technique allows for the needle tip to be repositioned without completely withdrawing it, thus avoiding re-puncturing the pleura. After identifying that the tip of the needle will not enter the nodule, the technique involves the following steps

1. The needle is partially withdrawn
2. The bevel is turned so that it faces in the direction opposite to the direction that it must move
3. The needle has pressure placed on it to direct it towards the nodule
4. The skin and soft tissues (to the extent possible) are pulled with the operators free hand to exaggerate the angle of the needle shaft towards the nodule.

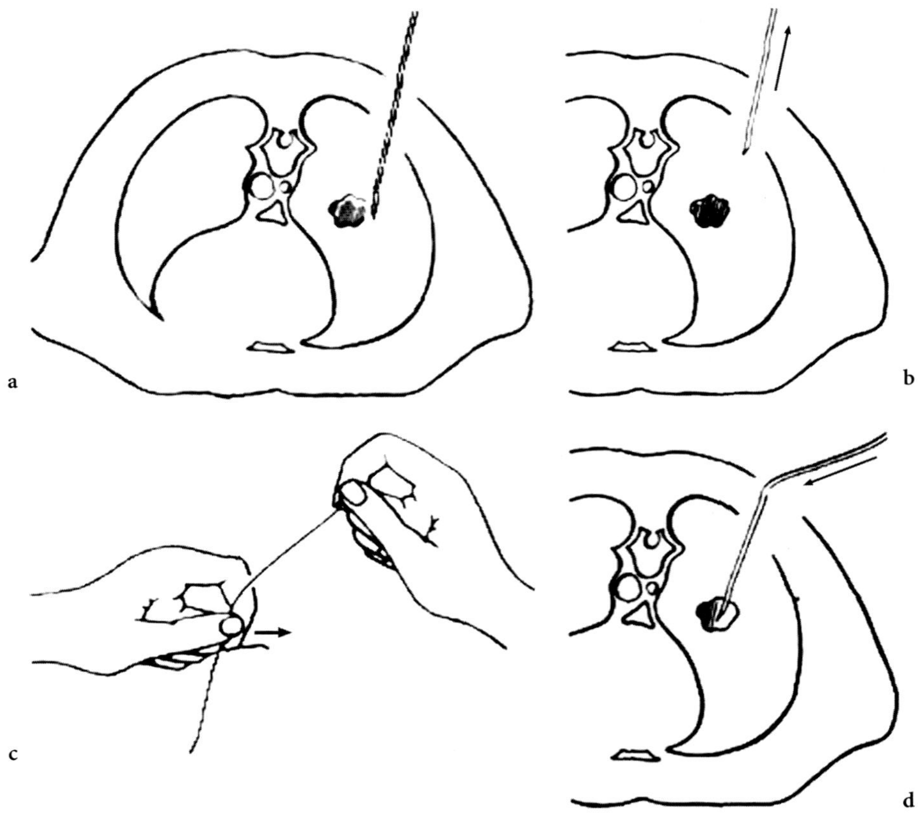

Fig. 13.6. Bevel steering is a technique used to reposition the needle tip without completely removing the needle. It involves several steps. **a** Shows needle has missed the nodule. **b** The needle is partially withdrawn and rotated so that the bevel faces in the direction opposite to its intended course. **c** Torque is applied to the needle and the soft tissues are pulled so as to redirect the needle towards the nodule. **d** The needle is now advanced and the amount that it has been re-directed is assessed. This process may need to be repeated several times

This approach can cause the needle tip to significantly change its location (Fig. 13.7). The degree of effectiveness is influenced by a number of factors. This includes the depth of the lesion and the soft tissue thickness. When these are large, the degree to which the needle tip can be re-positioned may not be sufficient. In addition this approach often requires multiple attempts. The degree to which the needle is withdrawn and the amount of force placed on it can vary each time. Once expertise in using this technique is mastered, it is possible to make fine adjustments to the needle tip location and this becomes indispensable when performing biopsies of small lesions (Fig. 13.8).

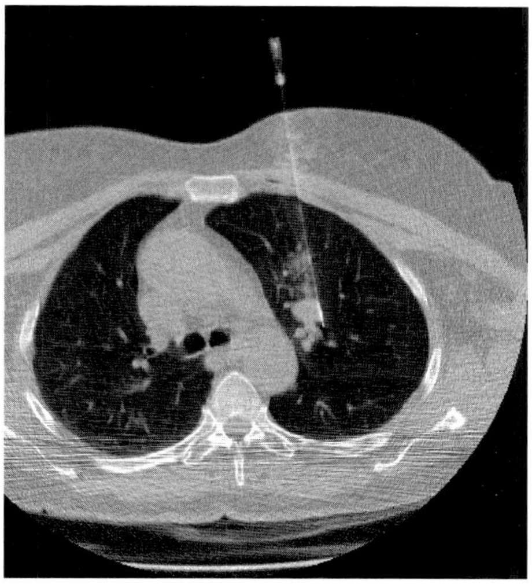

a

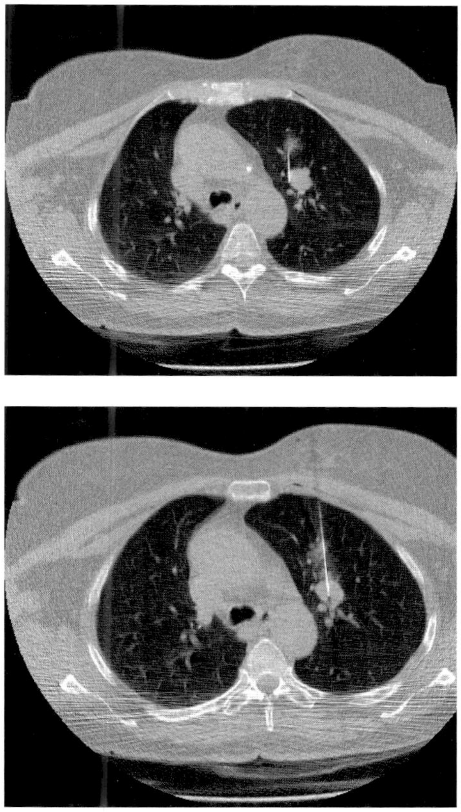

b

c

Fig. 13.7. **a** The needle tip is just lateral to the nodule. **b** Using the technique of bevel steering the needle is re-positioned, however, the degree of adjustment moves the needle to the other side of the nodule. Thus with a single re-adjustment and only partially withdrawing the needle, the tip has moved by over one cm. **c** The process is now repeated, except that steering is now in the opposite direction and to a lesser extent. The tip is now in the center of the nodule. It is often necessary to repeat this process several times to position the needle tip in the desired location

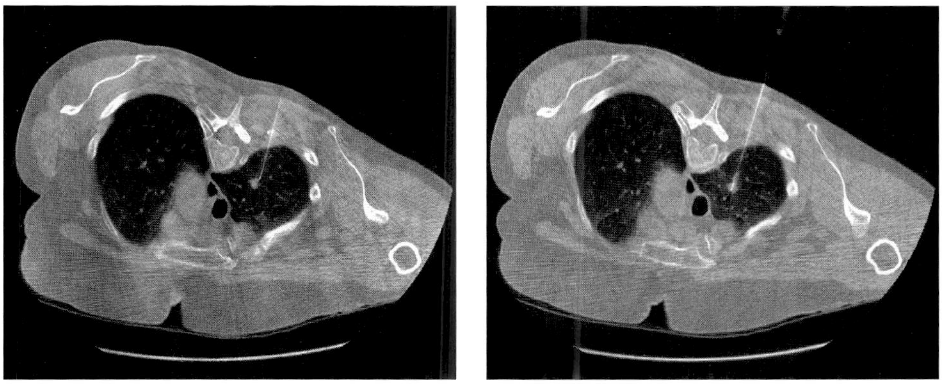

a b

Fig. 13.8. a The needle tip is minimally off course for this small nodule. **b** The technique of bevel steering is applied and the tip has moved several mm. towards the center of the nodule

13.5.9 CT Scan Parameters

This primarily relates to choice of mA and slice thickness. As a general rule, the lowest dose that allows for evaluation of the needle in relation to the nodule is required. With modern scanners this involves an mA setting of 40 or lower. Radiation dose reduction is important because it is often necessary to perform multiple images through the same tissue volume during the course of the procedure.

The slice thickness is generally chosen in relation to the size of the nodule. In order to be certain that a single CT image contains only nodule and is not a combination of lung and nodule, the slice thickness should be less than half the diameter of the nodule. In this way contiguous slices will include at least one image that contains no partial volume effects. A simple, general rule of thumb for choosing slice thickness is as follows:

1. For nodules greater than three centimeter in diameter a CT slice thickness of one centimeter or five millimeters.
2. For nodules between one centimeter and three centimeters a slice thickness of five millimeters
3. For nodules between five millimeters and one centimeter a slice thickness of three millimeters
4. For nodules less than five millimeters a slice thickness of three millimeters for guidance and one millimeter for final localization.

When performing the procedure, CT images are usually obtained in sets of three contiguous images, with the central image located at the point where the needle tip is expected to be located, upon its being advanced. In this way there is an image above and below the needle tip location.

13.5.10 Documentation of Needle Tip Location

This is a critical step in proper performance of TNB, and one that is frequently left out. Perhaps the single most important cause of an inconclusive biopsy result is not having the needle tip located within the nodule. There are a variety of reasons that this can occur. This includes partial volume effects where the tip actually appears to be located in the nodule when in fact it is not (Fig. 13.9). It can also occur when the tip passes through the nodule and may actually be located in a plane beyond the nodule (Fig. 13.10). There are three ways to be certain that the needle tip is actually visualized (Yankelevitz and Henschke 1993) (Fig. 13.11).

1. Identification of a distinctive feature of the tip such as a notch.
2. An intense shadowing artifact emanates from the tip when it is perpendicular to the scanning plan.
3. Images above and below the tip document that no additional portion of the needle is distal to the tip.

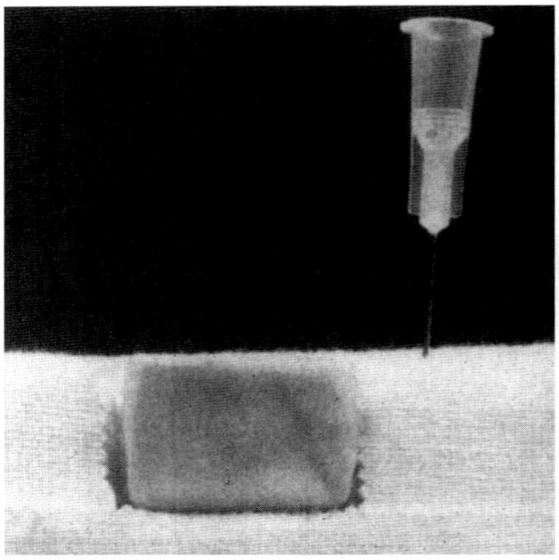
a

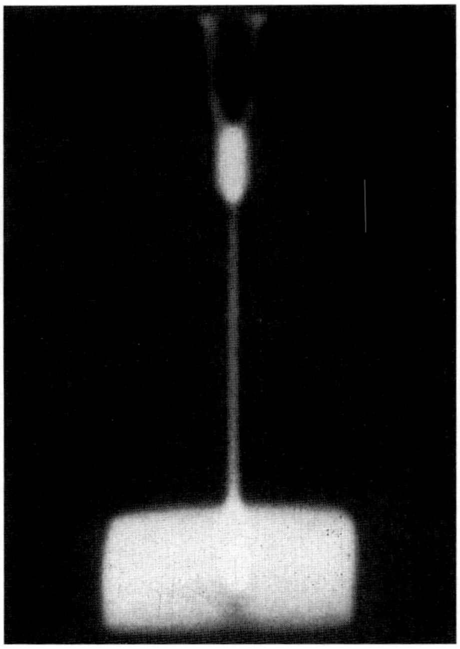
b

Fig. 13.9. a Picture of a needle placed outside of a synthetic nodule (along the z-axis). **b** CT scan of the synthetic nodule and needle gives the appearance of the needle actually being within the nodule. This occurs due to partial volume effect. The CT slice thickness may be wide enough to include both a portion of the nodule as well as the needle

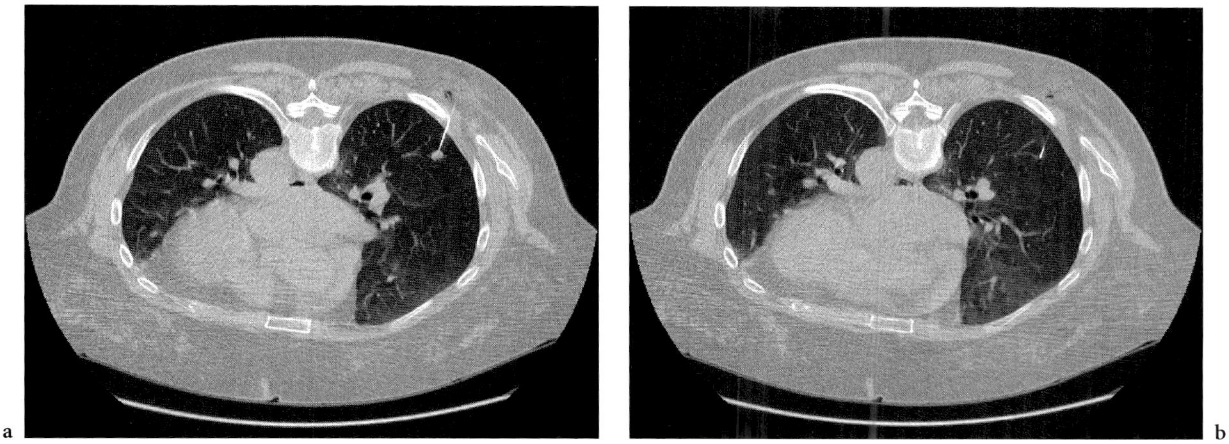

Fig. 13.10. a The needle tip appears to be piercing the nodule on this single image. b However, on the adjacent image, it is apparent that the tip extends beyond the nodule. Had a specimen been obtained at this time, it would have been inadequate. This demonstrates the importance of obtaining images above and below the estimated needle tip location

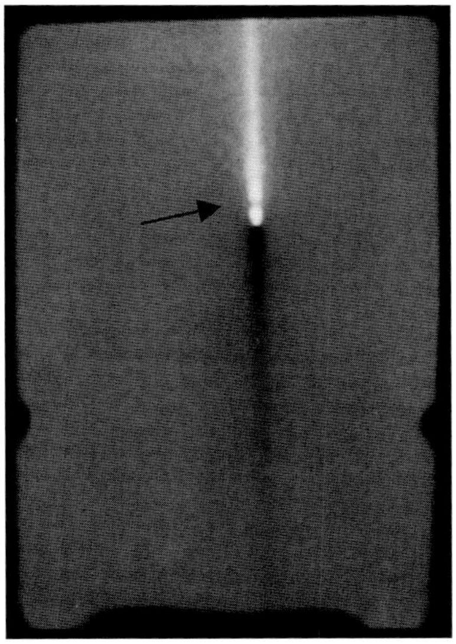

Fig. 13.11. CT image of a side slotted needle aligned with the CT scanning plane and inside a water bottle. The needle tip can be identified with certainty when a distinctive feature, such as the notch (arrow) is visualized or when a shadowing artifact is seen extending from the tip. In this example, both of these features are present

Localization of the tip and documenting that it is inside the nodule by obtaining three images that prove there is no partial volume effect is an essential part of the procedure (Yankelevitz et al. 1993). This is particularly important when indeterminate material is obtained and there is consideration of following a non-specific result. Without confidence that a genuine sample from within the nodule has been obtained, this cannot even be a consideration.

13.5.11 Angled Approach

When possible, a direct approach with the needle directly above the nodule and traveling within the scanning plane is preferable. However, this is not always possible due to overlying bony structures or other impediments, such as large vessels, that make an angled approach necessary in order to avoid these structures. With bi-plane fluoroscopy the relation between the nodule and needle can be observed in real time. Adjustments can be made as the needle is being advanced and its spatial orientation with the nodule is continuously being assessed. In the case of CT (unless CT flouroscopy is used), it is more challenging and an understanding of basic geometric considerations is necessary in order to avoid missing the nodule (Yankelevitz et al. 1995). The most common situation where an angled approach is necessary is when a small nodule is being biopsied and it is located directly beneath a rib. Nodules larger than the width of the rib allow for direct access through an intercostal space. In those that are smaller, the needle must travel on an angle through the intercostal space adjacent to the nodule, but the CT section that includes the intercostal space may not include the nodule. Thus, the length of the needle from skin surface to the nodule is never seen on a single image. The needle passes through successive CT sections until it reaches the nodule. When it becomes necessary to use this approach, it is generally best to start above the rib and angle downwards. In this way, the intercostal vessels that run in a groove on the undersurface of the ribs can be avoided. The correct angle that the needle needs to enter the skin can be determined by counting the number of contiguous sections that the needle will pass through as it advances from the skin entry point until reaching the nodule. This information, along with knowledge of the depth of the nodule relative to the skin entry point allows for estimation of the correct angle (YANKELEVITZ et al. 1995) (Fig. 13.12). When the nodule is directly beneath the skin entry point, then a single image shows the entire length of the needle along with the nodule. When the nodule is located on a slice next to the skin entry point, and when the needle is properly angled and advanced into the nodule the CT images would show half of the needle length in the image containing the entry point and the remaining half of the needle would be visualized in the image containing the nodule. If the skin entry point were two slices over, then each image would contain one third of the length of the needle. The higher the degree of angulation, the smaller the needle length will appear on contiguous slices. The length of needle visualized on each successive CT image will always appear the same, and will begin on each successive image at the same level that it ended on the previous one (YANKELEVITZ et al. 1995) (Fig. 13.13).

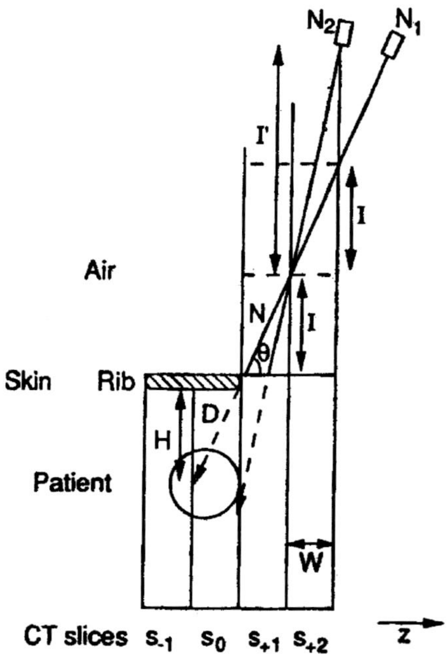

Fig. 13.12. In this illustration, the nodule is located beneath the rib and does not allow for direct access within the scanning planes that contain the nodule (S-1 and S-0). In order to reach the nodule, the needle must be inserted in a different scanning plane (S+1). Needle N1 is properly angled to avoid the rib and reach the nodule. Needle N2, while entering the skin in the same CT scanning plane, is not properly angled and would miss the nodule. The length of N1 in each CT image is represented by the vertical line (I). This length is constant for each scanning plane and is equal to the distance (H) that the nodule is located beneath the rib. For N2 the length seen on each CT image is represented by (r) and thus it can be predicted that when this needle is advanced, it will miss the nodule. On image (S+1) it has length (I) only because it has not yet passed through the entire imaging plane

Angling the CT gantry is an alternative approach to advancing the needle on an angle relative to the scanning plane. It allows for visualizing the needle and the nodule in a single plane while avoiding any overlying structures (STERN et al. 1993). In this way, the CT image plane can be made to align with the intercostal space and the nodule. The needle is then advanced directly along this plane. This approach avoids the need to focus on the relative lengths of the needle seen on successive images, although finding the proper angle so that the needle is parallel to the angled gantry plane during its entire course can also be problematic.

13.6 Complications

The most frequent complication related to TNB is pneumothorax (PTX). The reported rate that this occurs varies greatly, ranging from 15–60% (KLEIN and ZARKA 2000). There are several reasons to account for this wide variation. With the increasing use of CT guidance for TNB, it is possible to detect very small PTX that may not even be visible on chest x-ray. Therefore, depending on the threshold of amount of PTX that is reported, the number of cases reported will vary. In addition, patient populations vary and it can be expected that patients that have a larger degree of emphysema will have a higher rate of PTX (MILLER et al. 1988). The choice of needle will also affect the rate of PTX. Larger gauge needles will cause more PTX than small gauge needles (KLEIN and ZARKA 2000). While the relationship between either overall amount of emphysema or gauge of the needle and the development of PTX is not exactly known, and there have even been reports suggesting a very limited relationship (COX et al. 1999), it is obvious that some relationship must exist and that both of these factors relate to the proportion of patients that develop PTX. Perhaps more important than the frequency of PTX is the proportion of PTX that need to be treated. There has also been wide variation in the range that PTX requiring treatment has been reported as well, ranging from 5%–25% with

a b c d e

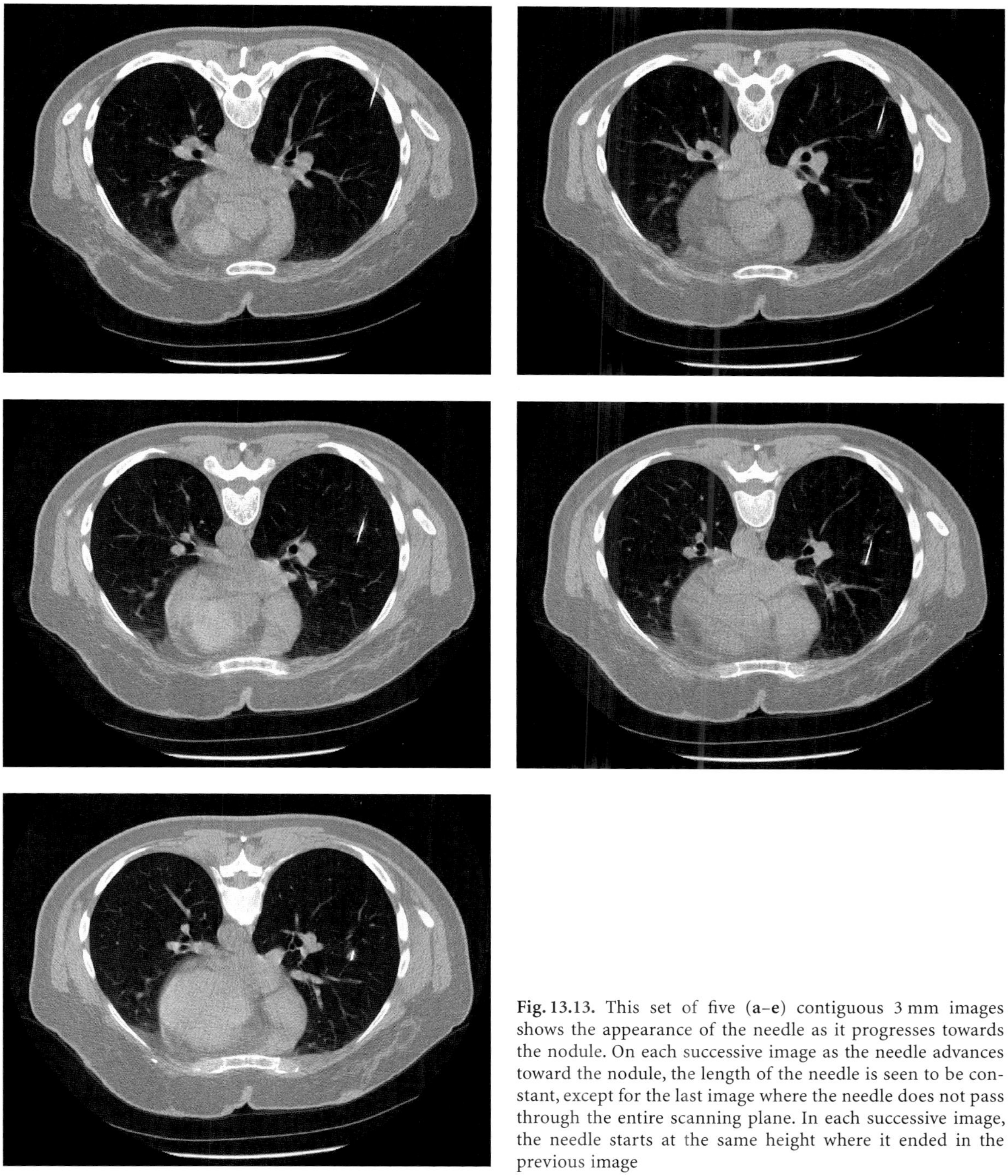

Fig. 13.13. This set of five (**a–e**) contiguous 3 mm images shows the appearance of the needle as it progresses towards the nodule. On each successive image as the needle advances toward the nodule, the length of the needle is seen to be constant, except for the last image where the needle does not pass through the entire scanning plane. In each successive image, the needle starts at the same height where it ended in the previous image

an average of 7% (Klein and Zarka 2000). Treatment of large PTX is generally required once the PTX reaches about 30% or the patient is developing symptoms (Moore 1997). It is generally preferred to treat the PTX with a one-piece self-contained chest tube that can be inserted by the radiologist. These one-piece chest tubes are easily inserted and allow the patients to remain ambulatory once they are in place. Patients are generally admitted to the hospital for one night once these tubes have been inserted.

Hemorrhage is the next most frequently occurring complication. It results in hemoptysis in only 5% of patients, and is generally very limited. Patients should be made aware of the possibility of this occurring before the procedure starts since it can be quite alarming if they are not alerted to its possibility and that it will stop quickly. At least to some extent every patient undergoing TNB develops some degree of hemorrhage. It may be too small an amount to be visualized with fluoroscopy and in some cases may even be difficult to identify with CT. Hemoptysis is usually preceded by a cough. It is generally most severe when large vessels, particularly arteries, are punctured. Although quite rare, particularly with the use of small gauge needles, severe hemorrhage is the most frequent cause of death following TNB (Protopapas et al. 1996).

One of the least frequent, but most severe complications is air embolism. This occurs when air enters the pulmonary venous system and can lead to systemic air embolism. Air embolism can cause myocardial infarction, arrhythmia, stroke and death. Once air embolism is suspected the patient should be placed in the left lateral decubitus position or in Trendelenberg position to prevent residual air in the left atrium from entering the systemic circulation. The patient should be placed on 100% oxygen and general symptomatic support should be provided. Patients may then need to be transferred to hyperbaric oxygen units for further treatment (Klein and Zarka 2000).

Other infrequent complications include malignant seeding of the biopsy track, which has a reported occurrence rate of .012% (Ayar et al. 1998), vasovagal reactions (Moore 1998), and lung torsion following large pneumothorax (Fogarty and Dudek 1995). Inadvertent puncture of the pericardium can lead to hemopericardium (Man et al. 1998).

13.7 Post Biopsy Routine

Following TNB, a routine protocol is useful for reducing the risk of complications. The most common of these complications is PTX. There are several techniques that have been used to try and diminish its likelihood of occurrence. The most useful of these is to place the patient with the biopsy site in the dependent position. This is presumed to be effective for the following reasons. The weight of the lung is now pressing down on the biopsy site and acts to prevent leakage of air (analogous to compressing a bleeding site). In addition, the alveolar air spaces contract in the dependent portion of the lung making leakage of air more difficult, and there is also less movement of the dependent lung during routine breathing. Generally it is suggested that the patient remain in this dependent position for about two hours. During this time the patient is encouraged to breathe normally and remain relatively motionless. One difficulty with this approach is that it is often difficult for patients to remain prone for long periods of time. In those cases, patients are initially placed prone and allowed to turn over into a supine position once they feel uncomfortable. This is one of the reasons that prone position is preferable during the performance of the biopsy, so that the patients can lie supine afterwards.

During the immediate post biopsy period, some patients experience pleuritic type chest pain without actually having a PTX. In these patients the pain typically lasts for less than one hour. It is frequently relieved with minor analgesics.

Post biopsy radiographs are ordered to check for the development of PTX two to four hours post procedure. If symptoms develop prior to this, radiographs are obtained immediately. If patients have no PTX at two hours and are feeling well, they are discharged after being given explicit instructions regarding development of symptoms and what to do and who to contact. They are advised to avoid any activity that will make them breath heavily for at least 24 hours and to avoid strenuous activity for at least three days. In patients that do have a PTX noted on the two-hour radiograph, an additional radiograph can be obtained one hour later to assess for stability, provided the patient is asymptomatic. While there is no absolute cut off in size of a PTX that mandates treatment, it is generally initiated when the PTX reaches approximately 30% or when the patient is symptomatic, as mentioned above.

Several options exist for treatment of PTX although all of these involve the removal of air from the pleural space. In patients that develop PTX while still in the biopsy suite, aspiration of the PTX can be performed with a small removable temporary catheter such as a two inch 18 gauge intravenous catheter (Yankelevitz et al. 1996b). The catheter is attached to a one-way valve and air is aspirated from the pleural space. Patients are placed on nasal oxygen during this time and it is kept on for at least one-hour post procedure. This procedure is nearly always successful in initially removing the PTX and in about half of the patients the PTX either does not recur or recurs to a lesser extent (Fig. 13.14). In those patients where the PTX enlarges or in those that develop it during the recovery period and are becoming symptomatic, chest tube insertion is necessary. While there are many varieties of chest tubes available, the small bore tubes attached to one-way valves are nearly

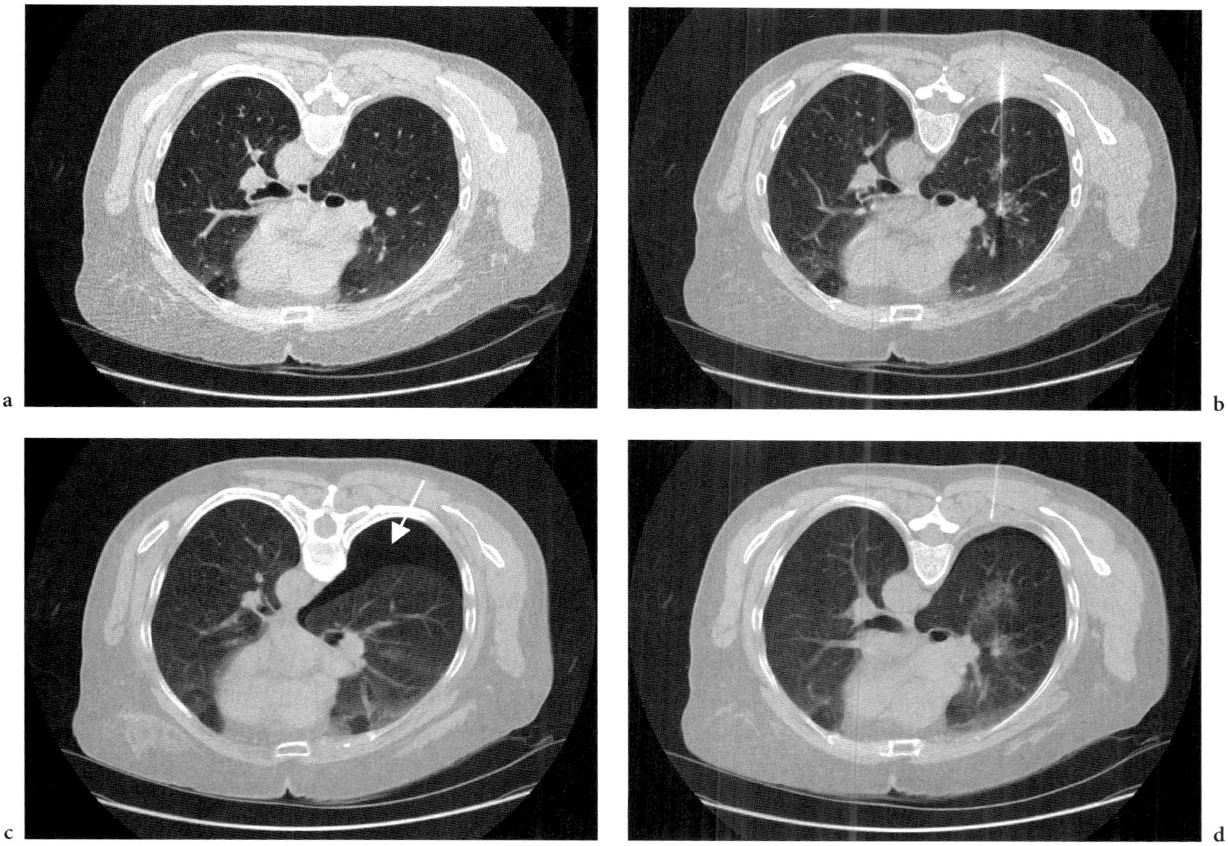

Fig. 13.14. **a** A small right upper lobe nodule with patient in the prone position. It was felt that even though the needle would pass through the fissure, thus increasing the possibility of pneumothorax (PTX), that the likelihood of success would be improved using this approach. **b** Needle tip is seen within the nodule. **c** Several minutes post procedure, a post biopsy CT image shows a moderate size PTX (arrow). **d** Following aspiration of the PTX using a small catheter (a portion of the catheter is seen in the soft tissue) the PTX is almost completely resolved. On follow-up CXR several hours later, only a minimal PTX could be identified, and the patient was subsequently discharged

always sufficient for treatment. Larger tubes, inserted by the chest surgeons are rarely needed.

Aside from instructions about limiting activity, it is advisable to contact the patient the next day to confirm that they are asymptomatic. Generally, the results from the pathology, once they are available, are given to the referring physician so that (s)he can discuss issues related to management and possible follow-up directly with the patient.

13.8 Results

There are three basic categories of results obtained with TNB. This includes diagnosis of malignancy, specific benign diagnosis and non-specific benign diagnosis. For nodules above a threshold size (1–1.5 cm, depending on experience) there is general agreement about the accuracy of TNB in diagnosing malignancy. It is generally considered to be over 90% sensitive, with less than 1% false positive rate (Taft et al. 1980). In one series, among 218 cases for which both cytology as well as tissue diagnosis obtained by biopsy, resection or autospy were available, 11 of the cytology diagnoses were initially thought to be false positives. However, upon re-review of the surgical biopsies, it was felt that they failed to sample the lesion and therefore the aspiration biopsy diagnoses were accurate with a specificity of 100% and (Cagle et al. 1993). With smaller size, the accuracy declines. However, this should not be viewed as a limitation of TNB in making a diagnosis, rather it should be viewed as a technical challenge in placing the tip of the needle in the nodule. Assuming that this can be accomplished, there is no reason that the accuracy for diagnosing malignancy in small nodules should not be equivalent to that of large ones. There is even reason to believe that biopsy of small lesions may be more accurate once the technical factors of performing the biopsy are removed. In small nodules there is generally less necrosis and surrounding inflammation and therefore the nodule is primarily composed of actual tumor cells, thus yielding more reliable specimens.

The diagnosis of specific benign disease is generally more difficult than that of malignancy. In general, this requires a larger amount of tissue for the diagnosis. There are several categories of specific benign diagnosis that can be made. This includes benign tumors such as hamartomas, infectious nodules such as tuberculomas, and non infectious granulomas such as rheumatoid nodules. The literature supporting the accuracy of making these diagnoses with TNB can be quite confusing, with results varying from 16% to 68% (Klein and Zarka 2000). These widely varying results can at least in part be explained by three factors: sampling error, amount of specimen and pathologic interpretation. As benign nodules are generally smaller than malignant ones, it is more likely to miss the nodule and not obtain any representative specimen. Missing the lesion is probably the single most important factor in not obtaining a diagnosis both in benign and malignant nodules (Westcott 1995). The amount of tissue that can be obtained with cutting needles compared to simple aspiration needles can be substantially increased, and in some cases cutting needles provide sufficient additional material to allow for specific benign diagnosis. The extent to which this occurs is not precisely known and is in part related to the skill of the interpreting pathologist. The skill set necessary for making specific benign diagnosis based on cytology is quite high and not always available, thus in many situations larger amounts of tissue may be necessary to allow for diagnosis.

The category of non-specific benign diagnosis is quite controversial. There have been numerous reports that suggest that in the absence of a specific benign diagnosis, malignancy cannot be excluded and therefore a non-specific benign diagnosis cannot be accepted (Liptay 1999). This argument is generally made in the context of ruling out lung cancer, with the implicit recognition that not diagnosing lung cancer early on is quite serious. The counterpoint to this view is that non-specific diagnosis can be accepted as benign with the following conditions (Yankelevitz et al. 1997):

1. That there has been careful documentation of the needle tip within the nodule
2. That when possible, more than a single sample has been obtained from different portions of the nodule
3. That the specimen contain material other than simply blood, such as fibrous tissue or non-specific inflammatory tissue
4. That a careful plan exists for continued follow-up of the nodule to assess for change

When these conditions are met, the proportion of nodules with non-specific TNB results that are ultimately found to be malignant is quite low, on the order of 5–10%.

13.9 Cytology

The interdisciplinary collaboration between the cytologist and the radiologist is imperative to achieve a high diagnostic accuracy. The necessity for proper specimen preparation and immediate microscopic assessment of procured specimens cannot be overemphasized. It is preferable to schedule cases sequentially on the dame day, at a rate of approximately one case per hour. In this way, the same cytologist can be easily scheduled to work with the radiologist for the entire day. An assistant to the cytologist is assigned to place fresh stains and all supplies that the cytologist may require in a designated area in the CT suite by the CT table on a counter adjacent to a sink. The supplies include Diff-Quik® (Dade AG, Dudingen, Switzerland) stains and a jar of fresh water, gloves, slides, slide labeling pens, Coplan jars with alcohol, Cytolyt®, formalin jars, sterile cell medium such as RPMI® (for flow cytometry), needles, a watch glass, cardboard slide holders, and specimen bags. The Diff-Quik® Stain is a water soluble modification of the Wright Stain which is rapidly performed on air-dried smears. The methylene blue component of the Diff-Quik® Stain accounts for a basophilic staining of nucleoli and cytoplasm and the metachromatic (red to purple) staining of the nuclei is due to the azure component. The Eosin component of the stain accounts for the yellow-red staining of the cytoplasm.

Ideally, a multiheaded microscope is utilized onsite for the evaluation of Diff-Quik® stained air-dried smears so that the cytologist and radiologist can view the sample together and decide, based on the evaluation of adequacy, whether an additional biopsy needs to be performed. This decision is not only based on the ability to make a diagnosis but, if benign, whether there is sufficient material for culture and sensitivity studies or, if malignant, for immunochemical studies to assist in determining the primary site of the malignancy. The initial concern when evaluating an aspirate on-site is the identification of cancer and if possible, its classification as small cell or non small cell carcinoma. Small cell carcinoma is composed of small metachromatic cells showing nuclear molding and streaking, granular chromatin, inconspicuous nucleoli, and scant cytoplasm leading to a markedly increased nuclear to cytoplasmic (N/C) ratio (Fig. 13.15). Non-small cell carcinoma is composed of larger cells with enlarged nuclei, conspicuous nucleoli and eccentric cytoplasm which is frequently dense or vacuolated in adenocarcinoma or keratinized in squamous cell carcinoma (Fig. 13.16) (Kamiya et al. 1995). If mucin is identified in the cytoplasm of the cells or is found extracellularly in the background of the smear, a diagnosis of mucinous adenocarcinoma can be confidently made (Roger et al. 1976).

The subtle nuclear morphology seen in low grade carcinomas is best seen on Papanicolaou Stain. Additionally, the Papanicolaou Stain easily identifies the keratinized cells in squamous cell carcinoma by their orangeophilic cytoplasm. Squamous cell carcinoma may show extensive necrosis and the aspirated material shows liquifaction. In these instances, the fluid can be expelled from the syringe along the perimeter of a watch glass so that any cellular particles will adhere to the watch glass. The particles can then be smeared onto a slide and the air-dried smear stained with Diff-Quik® to render an immediate interpretation which is usually diagnostic. The remaining material is best preserved in Cytoloyt® for ThinPrep slides. If necessary, special stains for organisms or immunostains can be performed on additional ThinPrep monolayered cellular preparations from the same sample. The tissue concentration technique utilizing the watch glass can be applied to bloody aspirates as well (Giri and Vazquez 2000). The bloody material is expelled along the perimeter of the watch glass, the particles are collected and smeared, and then the clotted blood is submitted in formalin for a cell block (paraffin embedded blood clot) from which standard H&E stained cut sections are made. In general, if the immediate interpretation of the bloody aspirate is malignant, the cell block will have an abundance of cells for evaluation by immunohistochemistry.

Occasionally, smooth round tumors are aspirated that prove to be carcinoid tumors or hamartomas.

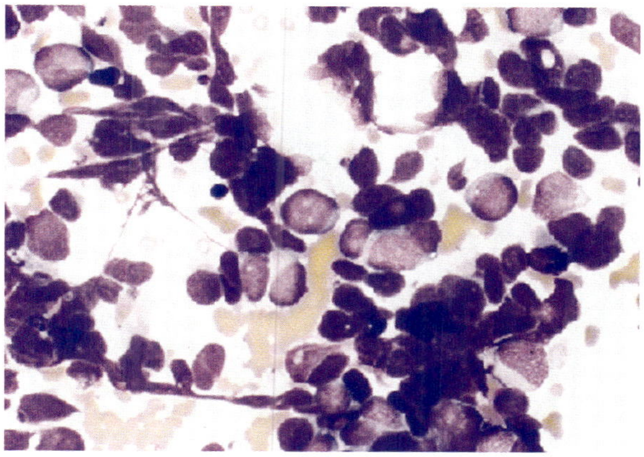

Fig. 13.15. Diff-Quik Stain of small cell cell carcinoma (high power). The aspirate shows a population of small cells with metachromatic nuclei, inconspicuous nucleoli and scant cytoplasm. The nuclei are fragile and show molding and streaking. Note the golden red blood cells in the smear as well

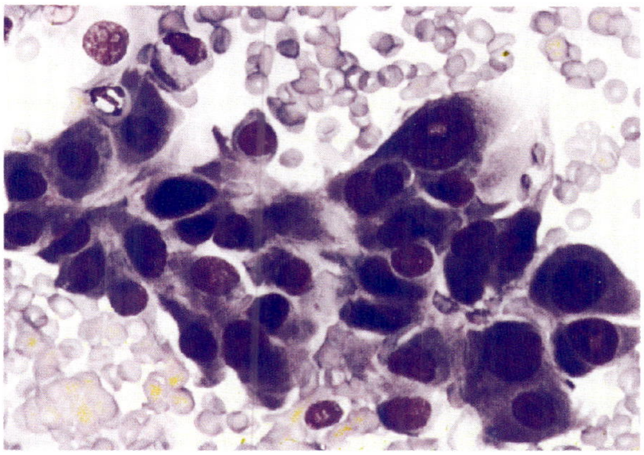

Fig. 13.16. Diff-Quik Stain of non-small cell carcinoma (high power). The aspirate shows clusters of cohesive large cells with pleomorphic metachromatic nuclei, prominent basophilic nucleoli, and abundant basophilic cytoplasm

The former is characterized by a monotonous population of round to spindled cells with granular nuclear chromatin and scant cytoplasm (Fig. 13.17) that can show a neuroendocrine pattern of growth. Vessels can be a prominent feature on the smears and their identification helps to distinguish carcinoid tumors from high grade neuroendocrine carcinoma. Since carcinoid tumors tend to be bloody, a cell block preparation should be made for staining with chromogranin and synaptophysin in order to confirm the cytologic diagnosis. Aspirates of hamartomas show fibrillary myxoid ground substance, variable amounts of fibroadipose tissue and cartilage and clusters of bland ciliated and reactive bronchial cells. When the tumor is composed entirely of the fibrillary

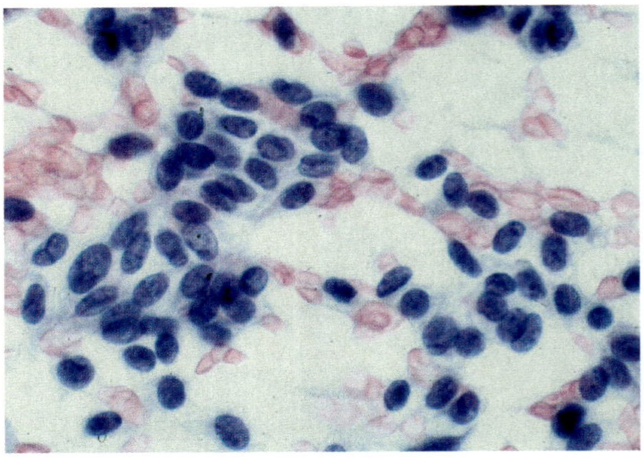

Fig. 13.17. Papanicolaou Stain of a carcinoid tumor (medium power). The aspirate shows small uniform oval to spindled cells with finely granular nuclear chromatin, inconspicuous nucleoli and scant cytoplasm

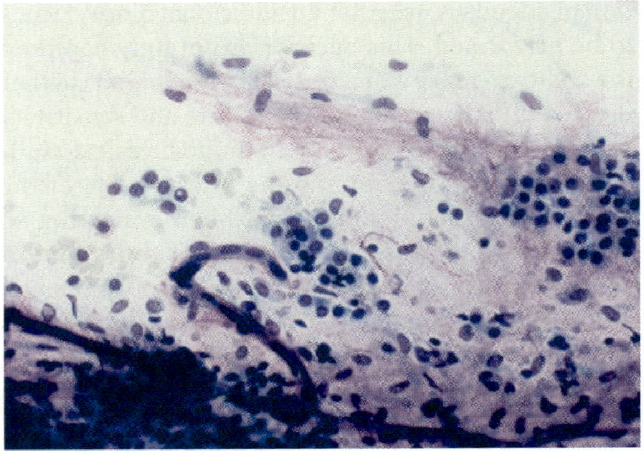

Fig. 13.18. Diff-Quik Stain of a hamartoma (low power). The aspirate shows myxoid stroma with bland mesenchymal cells and delicate vessels. There is an accompanying proliferation of benign bronchioloalveolar cells with uniform nuclei, intranuclear inclusions and smooth round nuclear membranes

myxoid ground substance, its homogeneous appearance on CT scan can arouse suspicion for malignancy. Also, the ground substance can mimic mucin and the proliferation of benign bronchioloalveolar cells, adenocarcinoma (Fig. 13.18). This pitfall must be recognized in order to avoid a false positive diagnosis of mucinous adenocarcinoma.

The most common benign aspirate yields only non-specific findings including alveolar macrophages, inflammatory cells, ciliated bronchial cells and reactive alveolar pneumocytes. Fragments of mesothelium may be aspirated when the nodule is pleural based and these mesothelial sheets must not be falsely interpreted as adenocarcinoma. Sometimes, acid fast orgasnisms and fungal forms can be identified with special stains on smears of necrotizing granulomas. In general however, a nonspecific benign diagnosis on transthoracic aspiration biopsy is not considered definitive for the work-up of a pulmonary nodule. As mentioned above, follow-up is based on presence or absence of growth on subsequent CT scans and other clinical factors, as well as certainty regarding needle tip positioning.

13.10 Conclusion

TNB is a highly accurate procedure for the diagnosis of pulmonary nodules. With careful attention to technical factors, nodules of any size in any location may be biopsied. The close collaboration with a skilled cytologist is essential and it is also quite helpful to develop close working relations with the clinicians so that they have confidence in the results. This is particularly helpful in those cases where non specific results have been obtained. Following the patients with repeat CT scans to assess the nodules for interval change or scheduling them for repeat biopsy may be used to establish the benign nature of a nodule and avoid unnecessary surgery.

References

Ayar D, Golla B, Lee JY et al (1998) Needle-track metastasis after transthoracic needle biopsy. J Thorac Imaging 13:2–6

Cagle PT, Kovach M, Ramzy I (1993) Causes of false results in transthoracic fine needle lung aspirates. Acta Cytol 37: 16–20

Cox JE, Chiles C, McManus CM et al (1999) Transthoracic needle aspiration biopsy: variables that affect risk of pneumothorax. Radiology 212:165–168

Fogarty JP, Dudek G (1995) An unusual case of lung torsion. Chest 108:575–578

Giri D, Vazquez MF (2000) "Pick and Smear" tissue concentration technique for image guided FNA specimens. Acta Cytol 45:889–890

Gupta S, Takhtani D, Gulati M et al (1999) Sonographically guided fine-needle aspiration biopsy of lytic lesions of the spine: technique and indications. J Clin Ultrasound 27:123–129

Hirsh J, Salzman EW, Harker L et al (1989) Aspirin and other platelet active drugs: relationship among dose, effectiveness and side effects. Chest 95:12S–18S

Kamiya M, Uei Y, Shimosato Y (1995) Cytologic features of peripheral squamous cell carcinoma of the lung. Acta Cytol 39:61–68

Klein JS, Zarka MA (2000) Transthoracic needle biopsy. Radiol Clin North Am 38:235–266
Lalli AF, McCormack LJ, Zelch M et al (1978) Aspiration biopsies of chest lesions. Radiology 127:35–40
Liptay MJ (1999) Solitary pulmonary nodule: treatment options. Chest 116 [Suppl 6]:517S–518S
Man A, Schwarz Y, Greif J (1998) Case report: Cardiac tamponade following fine needle aspiration (FNA) of a mediastinal mass. Clin Radiol 53:151–152
Miller KS, Fish GB, Stanley JH et al (1988) Prediction of pneumothorax rate in percutaneous needle aspiration of the lung. Chest 93:742–745
Moore EH (1997) Needle-aspiration lung biopsy: a comprehensive approach to complication reduction. J Thorac Imaging 12:259–271
Moore EH (1998) Technical aspects of needle aspiration lung biopsy: a personal perspective. Radiology 208:303–318
Protopapas Z, White CS, Miller BH et al (1996) Transthoracic needle biopsy: results of a nationwide survey (abstract). Radiology 201:270–271
Roger V, Nasiell M, Linden M et al (1976) Cytologic differential diagnosis of bronchiolo-alveolar carcinoma and bronchogenic carcinoma. Acta Cytol 20:303–307
Saleh HA, Haapaniemi J, Khatib G et al (1998) Bronchioloalveolar carcinoma: diagnostic pitfalls and immunocytochemical contribution. Diagn Cytopathol 18:301–306
Stampfel G (1982) Anaphylactoid reaction – a rare complication after fine needle aspiration of the lung. Radiology 22:329–330
Stern EJ, Webb WR, Gamsu G (1993) CT gantry tilt: utility in transthoracic fine-needle aspiration biopsy. Work in progress. Radiology. 187:873–874
Taft PD, Szyfelbein WM, Greene R (1980) A study of variability in cytologic diagnoses based on pulmonary aspiration specimens. Am J Clin Pathol 73:36–40
Westcott JL (1995) Needle biopsy of chest lesions. In: Taveras JM, Ferrucci JT (eds) Radiology, vol 1, chap 45. Lippincott, Philadelphia
White CS, Meyer CA, Templeton PA (2000) CT fluoroscopy for thoracic interventional procedures. Radiol Clin North Am 38:303–322
Yankelevitz DF, Henschke CI (1993) Needle-tip localization for CT-guided biopsies. J Thorac Imaging 8:241–243
Yankelevitz DF, Henschke CI, Davis SD (1993) Percutaneous CT biopsy of chest lesions: an in vitro analysis of the effect of partial volume averaging on needle positioning. AJR Am J Roentgenol 161:273–278
Yankelevitz DF, Hayt D, Henschke CI (1995) Transthoracic needle biopsy. What size syringe? Clin Imaging 19: 208–209
Yankelevitz DF, Davis SD, Chiarella D et al (1996a) Needle-tip repositioning during computed-tomography-guided transthoracic needle aspiration biopsy of small deep pulmonary lesions: minor adjustments make a big difference. J Thorac Imaging 11:279–282
Yankelevitz DF, Davis SD, Henschke CI (1996b) Aspiration of a large pneumothorax resulting from transthoracic needle biopsy. Radiology 200:695–697
Yankelevitz DF, Henschke CI, Koizumi JH et al (1997) CT-guided transthoracic needle biopsy of small solitary pulmonary nodules. Clin Imaging 21:107–110
Yankelevitz DF, Reeves AP, Kostis WJ et al (2000a) Small pulmonary nodules: volumetrically determined growth rates based on CT evaluation. Radiology 217:251–256
Yankelevitz DF, Vazquez M, Henschke CI (2000b) Special techniques in transthoracic needle biopsy of pulmonary nodules. Radiol Clin North Am 38:267–279
Yankelevitz DF, Wisnivesky JP, Henschke CI (2000c) Comparison of biopsy techniques in assessment of solitary pulmonary nodules. Semin Ultrasound CT MR 21:139–148

14 Staging of Lung Cancer with MDCT

P. M. Boiselle

CONTENTS

14.1 Introduction

Lung cancer is the leading cause of cancer mortality in the United States, with deaths from this disease surpassing the combined total of deaths from cancers of the breast, colon, and prostate combined (Greenlee et al. 2000). Accurate staging of non small cell lung cancer (NSCLC) is of critical importance in order to determine which patients are most likely to benefit from surgical resection, the only true hope for a cure from this disease (Jett et al. 1997). The International System for Staging Lung Cancer, including the TNM subsets and stage groupings (Tables 14.1 and 14.2), provides important information for estimating prognosis and planning appropriate therapy (Mountain 1997). For example, patients with Stage IA disease have a relatively high cure rate following surgical resection, whereas patients categorized as having disease consistent with stages IIIB or IV have a much poorer prognosis and are unlikely to benefit from surgical resection. The staging system also provides helpful information for entering patients into appropriate clinical trials, comparing different treatment regimens, and evaluating new prognostic factors (Mountain 2002).

Despite its recognized limitations, CT is considered the imaging study of choice for the initial staging evaluation of patients with NSCLC (McLoud 2002). The recent advent of MDCT affords significant advantages over single-detector helical CT scanners, including faster scanning, improved resolution, better vascular enhancement and higher quality multiplanar reformation and 3-D reconstruction images (Choi and Boiselle 2002). These advantages have the potential to enhance the ability to accurately stage lung neoplasms. This chapter reviews the potential contributions and relative limitations of MDCT with regard to assessing the T (primary tumor), N (nodal) and M (distant metastases) components of the International System for Staging Lung Cancer.

P. M. Boiselle, MD
Director of Thoracic Imaging, Beth Israel Deaconess Medical Center, Assistant Professor of Radiology, Harvard Medical School, Department of Radiology, 330 Brookline Avenue, Boston, MA 02215, USA

14.2 T-Status

14.2.1 T-1 and T-2 Lesions

MDCT scanners have the potential to enhance the detection of small lung cancers by allowing for the use of narrower collimation than is routinely employed with single detector CT scanners. For example, it has been shown that thin-collimation images are more sensitive than thick-collimation images for detecting small, subcentimeter lung nodules (Nishi et al. 2000).

Thin-collimation images also provide more accurate characterization of nodules than thick-collimation images, especially with regard to the identification of calcification within nodules and the assessment of nodule margins. These are important factors for determining the likelihood that a nodule is either benign or malignant (McLoud 2002). A unique feature of MDCT is the ability to retrospectively create images with a collimation that is narrower than the value that was prospectively employed (Choi and Boiselle 2002). In

Table 14.1. TNM Descriptors

Primary tumor (T)

TX Primary tumor cannot be assessed, or tumor proven by the presence of malignant cells in sputum or bronchial washings but not visualized by imaging or bronchoscopy

T0 No evidence of primary tumor

Tis Carcinoma in situ

T1 Tumor ≤ 3 cm in greatest dimension, surrounded by lung or visceral pleura, without bronchoscopic evidence of invasion more proximal than the lobar bronchus* (*ie*, not in the main bronchus)

T2 Tumor with any of the following features of size or extent:
>3 cm in greatest dimension
Involves main bronchus, ≥ 2 cm distal to the carina
Invades the visceral pleura
Associated with atelectasis or obstructive pneumonitis that extends to the hilar region but does not involve the entire lung

T3 Tumor of any size that directly invades any of the following: chest wall (including superior sulcus tumors), diaphragm, mediastinal pleura, parietal pericardium; or tumor in the main bronchus <2 cm distal to the carina, but without involvement of the carina; or associated atelectasis or obstructive pneumonitis of the entire lung

T4 Tumor of any size that invades any of the following: mediastinum, heart, great vessels, trachea, esophagus, vertebral body, carina; or tumor with a malignant pleural or pericardial effusion,† or with satellite tumor nodule(s) within the ipsilateral primary-tumor lobe of the lung

Regional lymph nodes (N)

NX Regional lymph nodes cannot be assessed

N0 No regional lymph node metastasis

N1 Metastasis to ipsilateral peribronchial and or ipsilateral hilar lymph nodes, and intrapulmonary nodes involved by direct extension of the primary tumor

N2 Metastasis to ipsilateral mediastinal and/or subcarinal lymph node(s)

N3 Metastasis to contralateral mediastinal, contralateral hilar, ipsilateral or contralateral scalene, or supraclavicular lymph node(s)

Distant metastasis (M)

MX Presence of distant metastasis cannot be assessed

M0 No distant metastasis

M1 Distant metastasis present‡

* The uncommon superficial tumor of any size with its invasive component limited to the bronchial wall, which may extend proximal to the main bronchus, is also classified T1

† Most pleural effusions associated with lung cancer are due to tumor. However, there are a few patients in whom multiple cytopathologic examinations of pleural fluid show no tumor. In these cases, the fluid in nonbloody and is not an exudate. When these elements and clinical judgment dictate that the effusion is not related to the tumor, the effusion should be excluded as a staging element and the patient's disease should be staged T1, T2, or T3. Pericardial effusion is classified according to the same rules.

‡ Separate metastatic tumor nodule(s) in the ipsilateral nonprimary-primary lobe(s) of the lung also are classified M1

(From Mountain 1997)

Table 14.2. Stage Grouping – TNM Subjects*

Stage	TNM Subject
c.	Carcinoma in situ
IA	T1NOM0
IB	T2NOM0
IIA	T1N1M0
IIB	T2N1M0
	T3NOM0
IIIA	T3N1M0
	T1N2M0
	T2N2M0
	T3N2M0
IIIB	T4NOM0
	T4N1M0
	T4N2M0
	T1N3M0
	T2N3M0
	T3N3M0
	T4N3M0
IV	Any T Any N M1

* Staging is not relevant for occult carcinoma, designed TXNOMO

(From Mountain 1997)

order to optimally characterize a detected nodule, it is important to retrospectively obtain images through the nodule with the narrowest collimation possible (0.5 mm to 1.25 mm, depending upon the CT manufacturer).

The ability to obtain high quality multiplanar and 3-D reconstruction images from routine MDCT studies has the potential to further improve nodule detection and characterization. For example, it has been demonstrated that multiplanar coronal and sagittal reformatted images increase the rate of lung nodule detection compared to axial images (Fig. 14.1) (Eibel et al. 2000). Moreover, multiplanar reformatted images can also be used to improve accurate localization of nodules. For example, multiplanar reformatted images can be used to aid preoperative localization of small nodules prior to video-assisted thoracoscopic surgery and to enhance accurate staging of primary tumors with respect to fissural involvement (Fig. 14.2). In order to optimize the quality of multiplanar reformatted images, it is important to choose

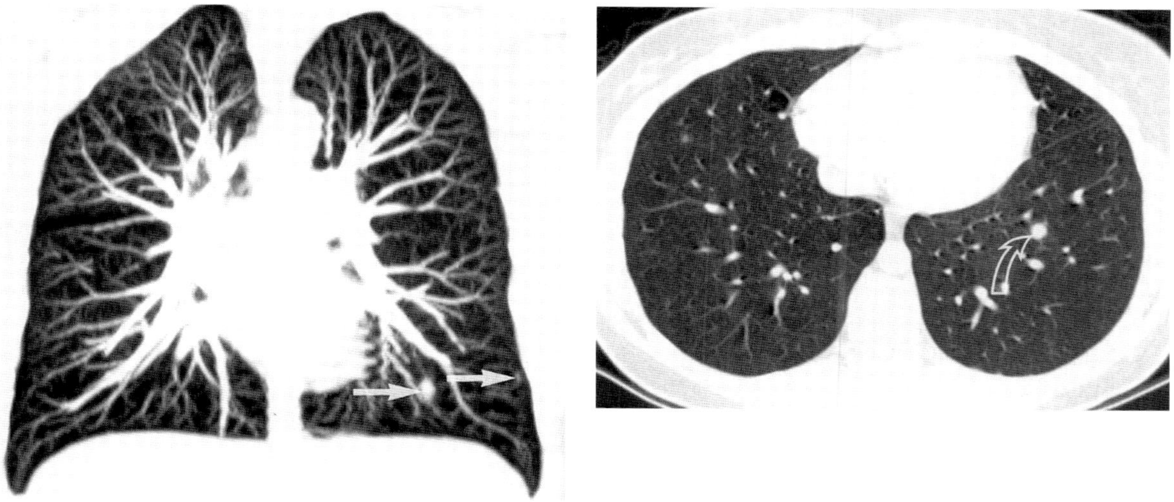

a b

Fig. 14.1. Value of 2-D multiplanar reconstruction images in lung nodule detection. **a.** Coronal reconstruction maximal intensity projection image shows two small lung nodules in left lower lobe (arrows). **b.** Axial image from original CT dataset shows the larger of the two left lower lobe lung nodules located centrally (curved open arrow). This nodule was initially overlooked on the axial image but was readily detected on the reformation images. Centrally located nodules are more easily detected on multiplanar reformation images than on axial images (Reprinted with permission from Choi and Boiselle 2002)

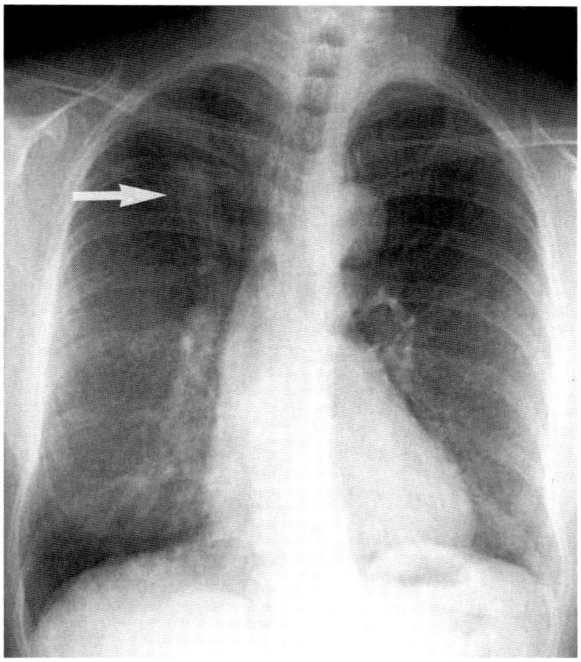

a

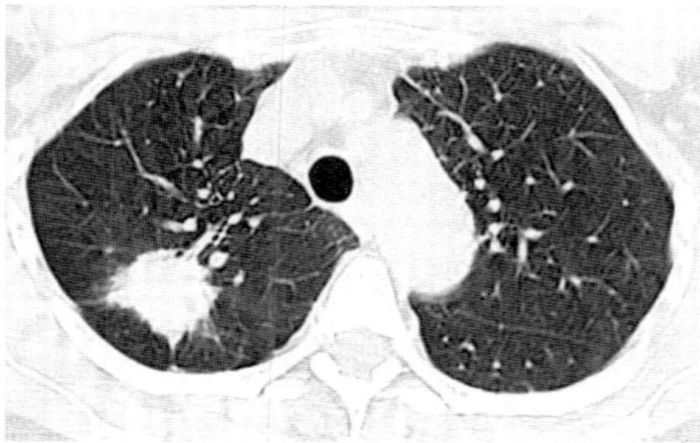

b

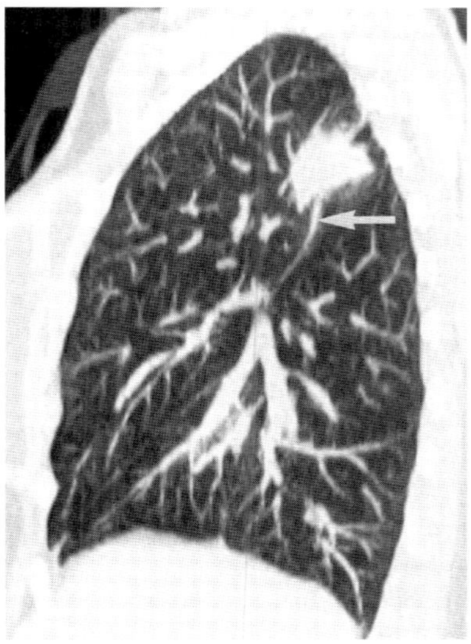

c

Fig. 14.2. Improved assessment of relationship of neoplasm to fissure with multiplanar reformation image. **a.** Frontal chest radiograph shows a nodule in right upper lobe (arrow). **b.** Axial CT image confirms the lung nodule and shows spiculated margins, consistent with neoplasm. Relationship to fissure is not well demonstrated. **c.** Sagittal reformation maximal intensity projection image demonstrates extension of the nodule across the major fissure into the adjacent superior segment of the right lower lobe. Also note fissural thickening (arrow) the narrowest collimation possible and to use at least a 50% overlapping reconstruction interval (Choi and Boiselle 2002).

14.2.2
T-3 and T-4 Lesions

The most important role of imaging in the assessment of the primary tumor (T) is to aid identification of T-3 (potentially resectable) lesions and to accurately distinguish them from T-4 (generally unresectable) lesions (Table 14.1). With regard to T-3 lesions, preoperative identification of chest wall invasion aids surgical planning because such lesions require *en bloc* resection of the lung neoplasm and adjacent chest wall (McLoud 2002).

CT has a limited ability to detect chest wall invasion: The only reliable indicators of chest wall invasion on CT are the identification of rib destruction and the extension of a mass beyond the ribs into the adjacent chest wall (Quint et al. 1995). It is important to be aware that the identification of pleural thickening adjacent to a mass is not necessarily representative of invasion of the parietal pleura by tumor, because a similar appearance may be produced by local fibrous adhesions (McLoud 2002).

Due to its ability to routinely provide thin collimation axial images and high quality multiplanar reformation images, it is likely that MDCT will lead to an improved accuracy for detecting chest wall invasion (Fig. 14.3a). However, future studies are necessary to determine the impact of this new technology on this aspect of staging. Because of its superior contrast resolution, MR has a slight advantage over CT in its ability to accurately predict chest wall invasion (Fig. 14.3b) (McLoud 2002). MR may thus be a helpful second-line problem-solving tool for cases that are indeterminate for chest wall invasion by CT imaging.

Superior sulcus tumors are defined as lung cancers that occur in the extreme lung apex. Such lesions are potentially resectable, unless there is evidence of involvement of the brachial plexus, subclavian artery, or adjacent vertebral body. MR is considered the study of choice for assessing for involvement of these structures, particularly with regard to spinal and brachial plexus involvement (McLoud 2002). However, for patients with contraindications to MR imaging (such as the presence of a pacemaker), the high quality of coronal and sagittal reformatted images provided by MDCT (Fig. 14.4) provide a reasonable imaging alternative. Future studies are necessary to compare the accuracy of multiplanar reformation CT images with direct multiplanar MR images in the staging evaluation of these lesions.

As defined in Table 14.1, a T-4 lesion is defined by invasion of "vital" structures, such as the mediastinum, heart, great vessels, trachea, carina, esophagus, or vertebral body. T-4 lesions are generally considered unresectable, although exceptions are made for certain cases at some highly specialized centers. Although direct

a

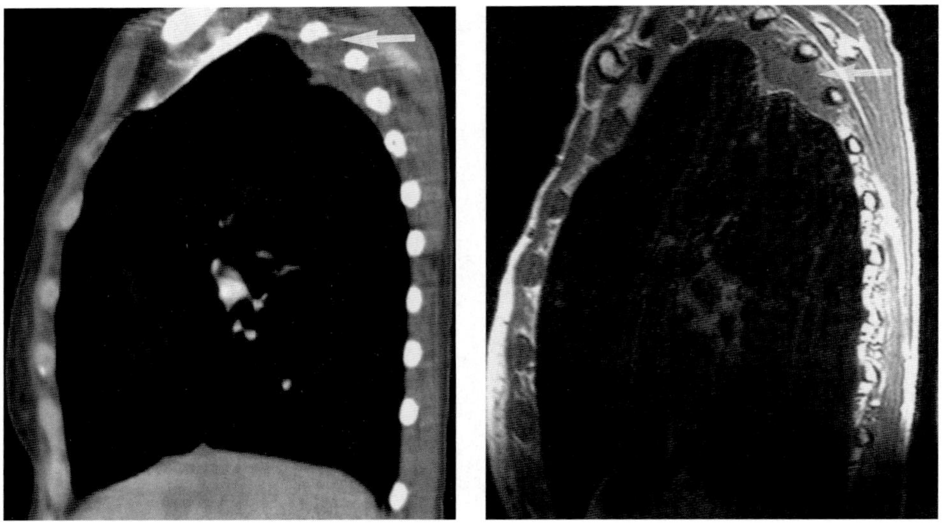

b

Fig. 14.3. Chest wall invasion from peripheral lung cancer on CT and MR imaging. **a.** Sagittal multiplanar reformation CT image demonstrates peripheral mass in right upper lobe, with extension into chest wall (*arrow*) between upper posterior ribs. Chest wall invasion was not well demonstrated on the original axial images. **b.** Sagittal T-1 weighted MR image of same patient. The higher contrast resolution of MR results in slightly better demonstration of the tumor infiltrating the fat between the posterior ribs (arrow)

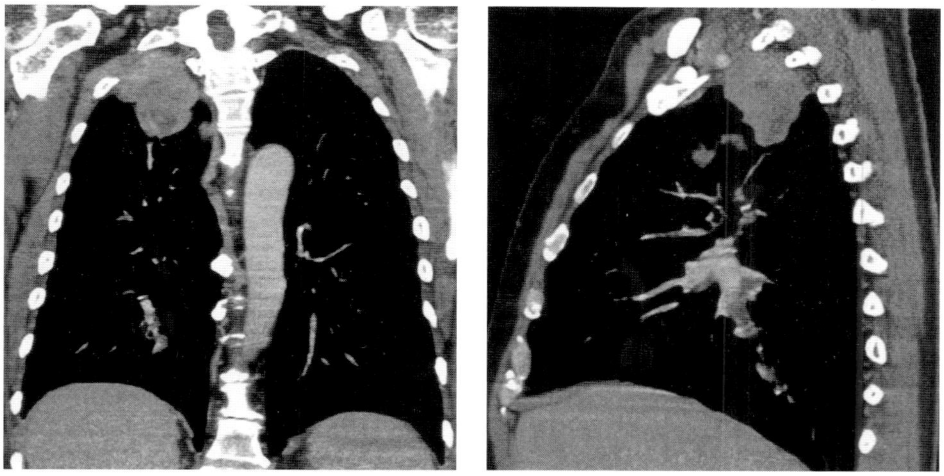

a b

Fig. 14.4. Apical lung tumor. Coronal (**a**) and sagittal (**b**) multiplanar reformation CT images demonstrate a right apical lung mass. The reformation images showed the extent of tumor to greater detail than axial images (not shown). Although MR is the study of choice for superior sulcus tumors, MDCT with multiplanar reformation images is a reasonable alternative for patients with contraindications to MR

invasion of vital structures is sometimes clearly delineated with axial CT images (Fig. 14.5), it is not always possible to distinguish contiguity of tumor with the mediastinum from actual invasion of vital mediastinal structures (McLoud 2002). Several technical factors can enhance the assessment for invasion of vital structures using MDCT, including the use of intravenous contrast enhancement, selection of narrow collimation (less than or equal to 3 mm), and the creation of multiplanar reformation and 3-D reconstruction images (Figs. 14.6–14.8). Despite the important technological advances afforded by MDCT, however, some cases will still remain indeterminate by CT imaging.

Approximately one decade ago, the Radiologic Diagnostic Oncology Group (RDOG) study prospectively compared CT and MR imaging in the preoperative staging evaluation of patients with non small cell lung cancer (Webb et al. 1991). This study showed that MR was slightly more accurate than CT for determining invasion of vital mediastinal vascular structures, although this difference was not statistically significant. MR should be considered as a second-line, problem-solving tool for cases that are indeterminate for mediastinal invasion by CT, especially in patients who have a contraindication to iodinated contrast agents. Indeed, it can be difficult to assess for invasion of vascular structures on unenhanced CT studies. Considering the development of significant advances in both CT and MR in the past decade, a new prospective trial is needed to assess the relative merits and respective roles of these techniques in the staging evaluation of NSCLC.

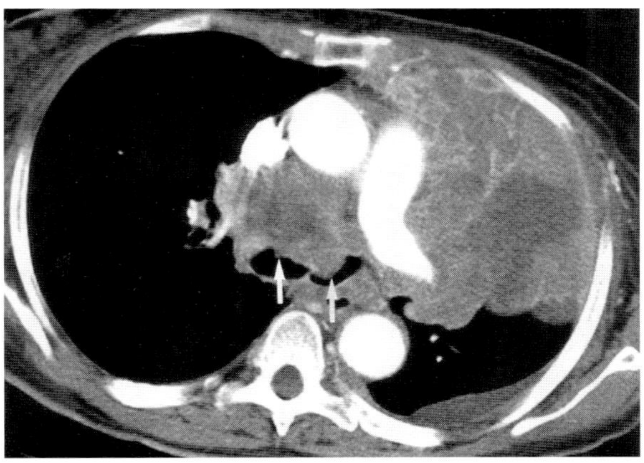

Fig. 14.5. Advanced-stage, inoperable non-small cell lung cancer. Contrast-enhanced axial CT image of patient with extensive non-small cell lung cancer demonstrates extensive mediastinal involvement, including invasion of the airway at level of carina. Note extension of neoplasm into proximal mainstem bronchi (arrows). Also note centrally obstructing tumor, with associated left upper lobe collapse

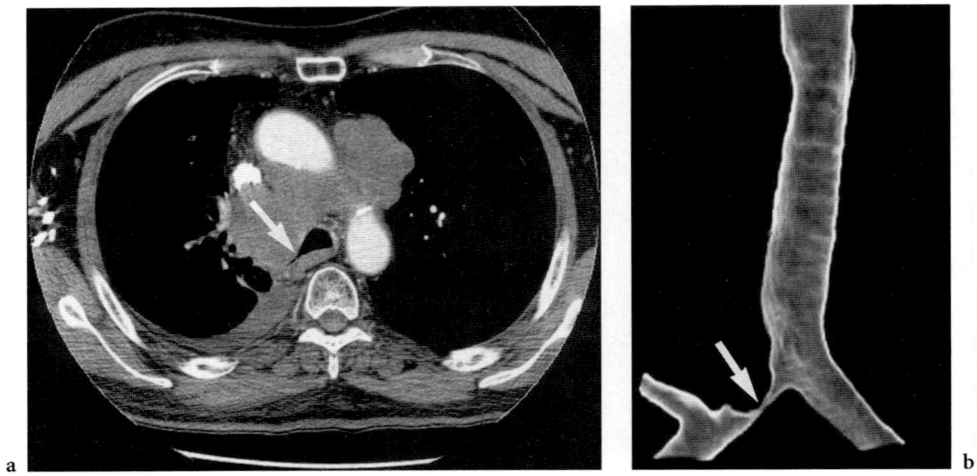

Fig. 14.6. Improved assessment of central airway invasion with 3-D reconstruction image. **a.** Axial, contrast-enhanced CT at level of aorticopulmonary window shows large nodal mass compressing the carina. Origin of right mainstem bronchus (arrow) is severely narrowed but is difficult to fully assess because of its oblique orientation with respect to the axial plane. **b.** 3-D external volume rendering of airway reveals irregular deformity of distal trachea and carina, as well as severe narrowing of proximal right mainstem bronchus (arrow) with distal patency. Compared with axial images, the 3-D images provided a more accurate assessment of the overall extent of airway involvement (Reprinted with permission from Boiselle et al. 2002)

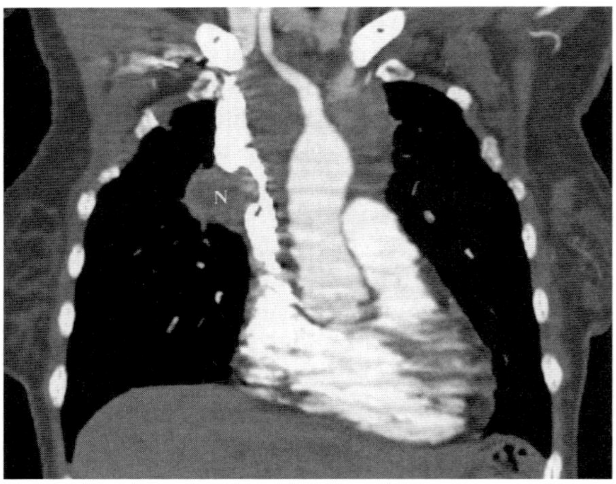

Fig. 14.7. Invasion of superior cava. Coronal reformation image shows central neoplasm (N) invading the superior vena cava, consistent with a T-4 lesion. Also note extensive neoplastic involvement of the mediastinum, encasing the aorta and other vascular structures

14.3
N-Status

The nodal status (N) provides important information for determining prognosis and planning appropriate therapy. For example, a patient with a T-1 or T-2 lesion and no evidence of regional metastatic nodal disease (N0) or distant metastases (M0) has a relatively favorable prognosis (approximately 65% 5-year survival) following surgical resection (Mountain 1997). On the other hand, a patient with a T-1 or T-2 lesion with metastatic disease to contralateral mediastinal lymph nodes (N3) but no distant metastases (M0) has a poor prognosis (less than 10% 5-year survival rate) and is considered inoperable (Mountain 1997).

14.3.1
N-2 and N-3

With regard to the assessment of mediastinal lymph nodes, CT relies upon anatomic features, most notably lymph node size, in order to distinguish between benign and malignant lymph nodes. Although very early investigations with CT suggested sensitivities and specificities comparable to

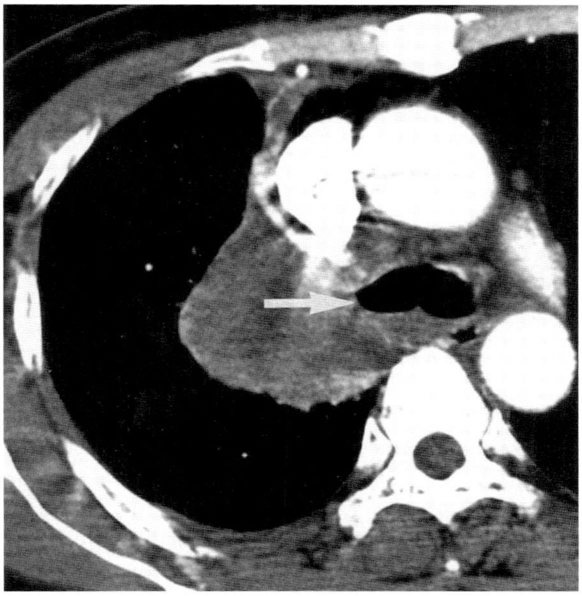

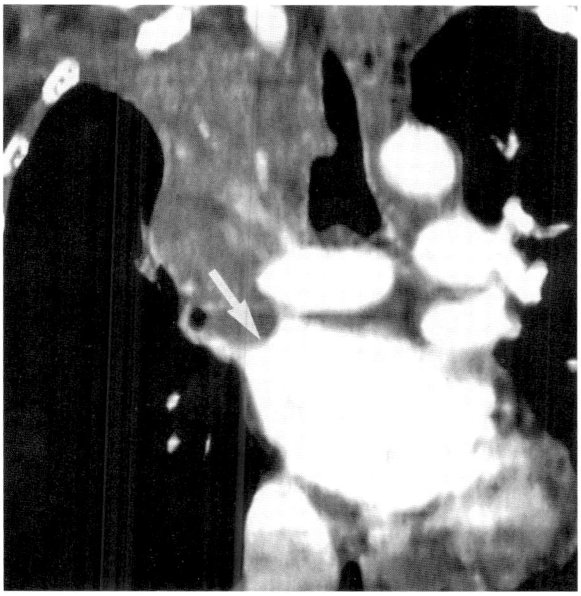

Fig. 14.8. Invasion of left atrium. a. Axial CT image shows central lung cancer resulting in obstruction of right upper lobe bronchus (arrow). b. Coronal reformation image demonstrates invasion of superior aspect of left atrium (arrow) [Case courtesy of Dr. Kyung S. Lee, Samsung Medical Center, Seoul, Korea]

mediastinoscopy, subsequent, more thorough studies have shown that the accuracy of CT is significantly lower (Boiselle 2002). For example, a study that employed extensive nodal sampling and correlative CT imaging of nodal stations showed a relatively low sensitivity (62%) and specificity (64%) for predicting neoplastic involvement using 1 cm as the upper limits of normal size for short axis of lymph nodes (McLoud et al. 1992). These results emphasize the limitations of using nodal size to determine nodal status: Enlarged nodes may be hyperplastic rather than neoplastic, and small nodes may harbor foci of metastatic disease (Boiselle et al. 1998).

Because of the low specificity of CT, enlarged nodes must be biopsied for staging purposes. It is important to be aware that benign nodes as large as 4 cm in diameter have been described in association with bronchogenic carcinoma (Jett et al. 1997). False-positive nodes most often occur in the setting of postobstructive pneumonitis from a centrally obstructing neoplasm (Fig. 14.9).

Similar to CT, MR relies predominantly upon nodal size for predicting neoplastic involvement. Thus, MR has similar limitations to CT in the assessment of mediastinal lymph nodes. Historically, the direct multiplanar imaging capability of MR has offered a relative advantage over axial CT images in the assessment of certain nodal stations, such as the aorticopulmonary window and subcarinal nodal stations (Boiselle et al. 1998). However, with the ability of MDCT to routinely perform high-quality multiplanar reformation images, this is no longer a significant distinction. MR has also historically offered a relative advantage over CT in the assessment of hilar nodes, particularly when intravenous contrast enhancement is suboptimal or absent on CT (Boiselle et al. 1998). With the improved vascular enhancement of hilar vessels afforded by MDCT,

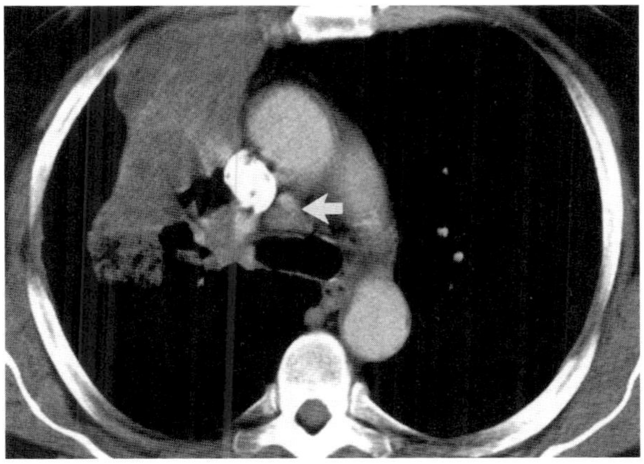

Fig. 14.9. False-positive lymph node. Axial CT image shows a central neoplasm obstructing the right upper lobe bronchus, with associated post-obstructive atelectasis and pneumonitis. Enlarged precarinal lymph node (arrow) proved to be hyperplastic at biopsy, with no evidence of neoplasm

this distinction is no longer relevant. However, for patients who have a contraindication to iodinated contrast agents, MR may be a helpful problem-solving tool if the status of the hilar structures is indeterminate by CT imaging.

Despite its recognized limitations, CT still plays several important roles in nodal staging (Boiselle 2002). First, by identifying and localizing lymph nodes, CT aids the selection of the most appropriate biopsy procedure (mediastinoscopy, mediastinotomy, thoracoscopy, transbronchial needle aspiration, or percutaneous CT-guided biopsy) for staging purposes. For example, aorticopulmonary window lymph nodes are not accessible by cervical mediastinoscopy and thus require another method of biopsy such as anterior or parasternal mediastinotomy (Fig. 14.10).

Second, CT can be used to guide nodal biopsies. Although preliminary studies (Protopapas and Westcott 1997; Zwischenberger et al. 2002) have shown promising results using CT-guided percutaneous biopsy for mediastinal nodal staging, this technique currently plays a limited role compared to other biopsy procedures. In a recent study of 89 patients who underwent CT-guided biopsy of mediastinal lymph nodes greater than 1.5 cm in diameter, a diagnosis was made in 78% of cases (Zwischenberger et al. 2002). Although virtually all nodal stations were accessible with this technique, these investigators emphasize that aorticopulmonary nodes can be difficult to access with this method. Based upon their findings, Zwischenberger et al. concluded that CT-guided biopsy should play a larger role in staging lung cancer.

CT can also be used to guide transbronchial biopsy procedures, either indirectly with virtual bronchoscopy or directly with CT-fluoroscopy. Such guidance has been shown to improve the accuracy and reduce the time of this procedure (Vining et al. 1996; Goldberg et al. 2000).

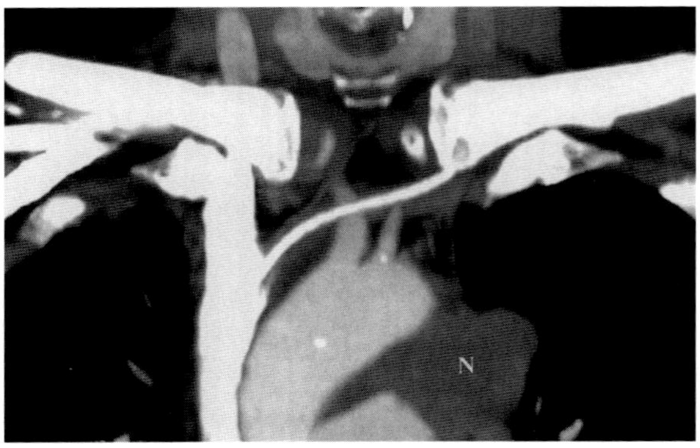

Fig. 14.10. Coronal reformation image shows large nodal mass (N) in the aorticopulmonary window. This nodal station is not accessible by cervical mediastinoscopy

An emerging role of CT involves the provision of complementary anatomic information for correlation with physiologic FDG-PET studies (Boiselle et al. 1998). Several recent studies suggest that combined anatomic and physiologic imaging using CT and FDG PET is more accurate than PET imaging alone (Gupta et al. 1999, Magnani et al. 1999, Vansteenkiste et al. 1997, 1998). For example, in a study that prospectively compared the accuracy of CT scanning, FDG PET imaging blinded to CT, and FDG PET visually correlated with CT in the detection of N2 metastatic mediastinal lymph nodes in patients with NSCLC, the highest diagnostic accuracy was observed when a combined CT-PET approach was employed (Vansteenkiste et al. 1997). Thus, CT and FDG PET should be considered as complementary rather than competitive imaging techniques. Recently, integrated PET-CT has become available and has been shown to be more accurate than CT alone, PET alone, or conventional visual correlation of PET and CT (Lardinois 2003). At present, integrated PET-CT is the most accurate method of nodal staging for non-small lung cancer.

14.3.2 N-1

CT has also been shown to have a low sensitivity and specificity for assessing hilar lymph node metastases. The evaluation of hilar lymph nodes has become an important factor in the selection of patients with early lung cancer and poor pulmonary reserve for minimal resection procedures such as segmentectomy and wedge resection (Boiselle 2002). It has recently been suggested that hilar nodal contour may be a more accurate predictor of metastatic involvement than nodal size (Shimoyama et al. 1997). In a study that assessed the ability of CT to detect hilar nodal metastases, Shimoyama et al. (1997) classified lymph nodes with straight or concave margins to the lung as benign and those with convex margins as malignant. Using this criterion, these investigators reported a relatively high sensitivity (87%) and specificity (88%) for detecting hilar nodal metastases. Future studies involving larger numbers of patients are necessary to confirm these promising results.

14.4 M-Status

Extrathoracic metastases are present in a significant proportion of patients with newly diagnosed NSCLC. In most cases, clinical symptoms or laboratory data abnormalities will signal the presence of distant metastases and guide the imaging evaluation of affected patients. In recent years, the occurrence of clinically "silent" brain metastases has received increasing attention, particularly among patients with adenocarcinoma. At present, the role of imaging in the evaluation of "silent" metastases remains somewhat controversial.

The discussion of extrathoracic metastases in this chapter will be limited to the adrenal gland, an important site of metastatic disease that is generally included on all staging thoracic CT scans. Although the adrenal gland is a relatively common site of metastatic disease in NSCLC, it is important to be aware that the majority of adrenal lesions detected in patients with NSCLC represent benign adenomas (McLoud 2002). For staging purposes, it is critically important to distinguish adenomas from metastases.

A non-invasive diagnosis of adenoma is based primarily upon the presence of large lipid-laden cells within most adenomas. On unenhanced CT scans, adenomas are characterized by a Hounsfield unit (HU) measurement of less than 10. This criterion is associated with a sensitivity of 71% and a specificity of 98% (Mayo-Smith et al. 2001). The specificity approaches 100% when other features such as size (<4 cm), shape (round), and margins (smooth) are also considered (Mayo-Smith et al. 2001). An advantage of MDCT is the ability to retrospectively obtain images with narrow collimation, which may aid the characterization of adrenal lesions with regard to accurately assessing density and margins.

Importantly, about 30% of adenomas will demonstrate HU >10 on CT scans (Mayo-Smith et al. 2001). MR can be helpful for further assessment of such lesions. On MR imaging, the lipid content of adenomas can be demonstrated using chemical shift imaging, which is based upon the different resonance frequency rates of protons in fat and water molecules (Mayo-Smith et al. 2001). Tissues that contain both lipid and water will demonstrate signal loss (dark signal) on out-of-phase images compared to in-phase images. This technique is highly accurate for diagnosing adenomas, with reported sensitivities ranging from 81% to 100% and specificities ranging from 94% to 100% (Mayo-Smith et al. 2001).

14.5 Summary

Despite its limitations, CT remains the initial imaging modality of choice for the staging assessment of patients with NSCLC. MR plays an important complementary role in selected elements of staging, particularly in the evaluation of superior sulcus lesions and in the assessment of chest wall or mediastinal invasion. It may also be helpful as a secondary, problem-solving tool for assessment of the vascular invasion and hilar structures for patients with contraindications to iodinated intravenous contrast. Importantly, both CT and MR are limited by their reliance upon anatomic parameters. Combined anatomic and physiologic imaging with CT and FDG-PET is currently the most accurate non-invasive method available for staging NSCLC.

Considering the development of significant advances in both CT and MR in the past decade, as well as the advent of PET imaging, a prospective trial is needed to assess the relative merits and respective roles of these three techniques in the staging evaluation of NSCLC.

Acknowledgements. I gratefully acknowledge the contribution of Fig. 14.8 from Dr. Kyung S. Lee, Samsung Medical Center, Seoul, Korea and the expert photography of Michael Larson, Beth Israel Deaconess Medical Center, Boston, MA.

References

Boiselle PM (2002) State-of-the-art thoracic lymph node imaging. In: Boiselle PM, White CS (eds) New techniques in thoracic imaging. Dekker, New York, pp 51–69

Boiselle PM, Patz EF, Vining DJ et al (1998) Imaging of mediastinal lymph nodes: CT, MR, and FDG PET. RadioGraphics 18:1061–1069

Boiselle, Reynolds, Ernst (2002) Multiplanar and 3-D imaging of the central airways with multidetector CT. AJR 179:302

Choi RC, Boiselle PM (2002) Multidetector helical CT. In: Boiselle PM, White CS (eds) New techniques in thoracic imaging. Dekker, New York, pp 71–90

Eibel R, Tuerk T, Huber AM et al (2000) Multi-slice thoracic CT for detection of pulmonary nodules: a study on coronal and sagittal STS-MIPS and MPRS (abstract). Radiology 217:384

Goldberg SN, Raptopoulos V, Boiselle PM et al (2000) Improved diagnostic yield for transbronchial mediastinal lymph node biopsy using CT-fluoroscopic guidance. Radiology 216:764–767

Greenlee RT, Murray T, Bolden S et al (2000) Cancer statistics, 2000. CA Cancer J Clin 50:7–33

Gupta NC, Graeber GM, Rogers JS et al (1999) Comparative efficacy of positron-emission tomography FDG and computed tomographic scanning in preoperative assessment of non-small cell lung cancer. Ann Surg 229:286–291

Jett J, Feins R, Kvale P et al (1997) Pretreatment evaluation of non-small cell lung cancer: official statement of the American Thoracic Society and the European Respiratory Society. Am J Respir Crit Care Med 156:320–332

Lardinois D, Weder W, Hany TF, Kamel EM, Korom S, Seifert B, von Schulthess GK, Steinert HC (2003) Staging of non-small-cell lung cancer with integrated positron-emission tomography and computed tomography. N Engl J Med 348:2500-7

Magnani P, Carretta A, Rizzo G et al (1999) FDG/PET and spiral CT image fusion for mediastinal lymph node assessment of non-small cell lung cancer patients. J Cardiovasc Surg 40:741–748

Mayo-Smith WW, Boland GW, Noto RB et al (2001) State-of-the-art adrenal imaging. RadioGraphics 21:995–1012

McLoud TC (2002) Imaging techniques for diagnosis and staging of lung cancer. Clin Chest Med 23:123–136

McLoud TC, Bourgoin PM, Greenberg RW et al (1992) Bronchogenic carcinoma: analysis of staging in the mediastinum with CT by correlative lymph node mapping and sampling. Radiology 182:319–323

Mountain CF (1997) Revisions in the international system for staging lung cancer. Chest 111:1710–1717

Mountain CF (2002) Staging classification of lung cancer. A critical evaluation. Clin Chest Med 23:103–121

Nishi J, Kadota M, Yamashita Y et al (2000) Detection of small lung nodules: the value of retrospective thin slice reconstruction and cine viewing with a multidetector helical CT sytem (abstract). Radiology 217:384

Protopapas Z, Westcott JL (1997) Transthoracic needle biopsy of mediastinal lymph nodes for staging lung and other cancers. Radiology 199:489–496

Quint LE, Francis IR, Wahl RL et al (1995) Preoperative staging of non-small cell carcinoma of the lung: imaging methods. Am J Roentgenol 164:1349–1359

Shimoyama K, Murata K, Takahashi M et al (1997) Pulmonary hilar lymph node metastases from lung cancer: evaluation based on morphology at thin-section, incremental, dynamic CT. Radiology 203:187–195

Vansteekiste JF, Stroobants SG, de Leyn PR et al (1997) Mediastinal lymph node staging with FDG-PET scan in patients with potentially operable non-small cell lung cancer: a prospective analysis of 50 cases. Chest 112:1480–1486

Vansteekiste JF, Stroobants SG, Dupont PJ et al (1998) FDG-PET scan in potentially operable non-small cell lung cancer: do anatometabolic PET-CT fusion images improve localisation of regional lymph node metastases? Eur J Nucl Med 25:1495–1501

Vining DJ, Liu K, Choplin RH et al (1996) Virtual bronchoscopy: relationships of virtual reality endobronchial simulations to actual bronchoscopic findings. Chest 109:549–553

Webb WR, Gatsonis C, Zerhouni EA et al (1991) CT and MR imaging in staging non-small cell bronchogenic carcinoma: report of the Radiologic Diagnostic Oncology Group. Radiology 178:705–713

Zwischenberger JB, Savage C, Alpard S et al (2002) Mediastinal transthoracic needle and core lymph node biopsy. Chest 121:1165–1170

15 MDCT in Mediastinal Imaging

A. R. Hunsaker

CONTENTS

15.1 Introduction

The usefulness of MDCT in imaging vascular, tracheobronchial, lung parenchymal and chest wall lesions has been described in the recent literature by several investigators (Lawler and Fishman 2001; Ravenel et al. 2001; Remy-Jardin et al. 1998a, 1998b; Bhalla et al. 1996; Johnson et al. 1996, 1998; Calhoun et al. 1999; Kauczor et al. 1996). Very little has been written about the usefulness of MDCT in other non-vascular and non-airway mediastinal lesions as we have traditionally studied the mediastinum. In this chapter we show relevant clinical applications of MDCT in mediastinal lesions.

The mediastinum is composed of the heart, vessels, airways, esophagus, fat, lymph nodes and lymphatics, thymic tissue, and nerves. These normal structures, in isolation or in consort, can be involved in a variety of disease processes which originate directly from them, metastasize to them, or invade them from adjacent structures. These disease processes can be fluid, soft tissue, fatty material, or a combination of these. Imaging of the mediastinum, therefore, is aimed at providing relevant information regarding tissue characteristics, enhancement patterns, location of a lesion, and invasion of structures.

Computed tomography (CT) has been deemed the primary modality for imaging the mediastinum (Tecce et al. 1994), particularly the anterior mediastinum; however, magnetic resonance imaging (MRI) has been used as a modality which clarifies ambiguous findings on CT (Bittner and Felix 1998; Webb and Sostman 1992) because of its multiplanar capabilities its ability to image vessels, and its ability to distinguish between different tissues. Prior to the advent of spiral CT imaging in the late 1980s, MR imaging was very comparable to CT for evaluating the mediastinum (Bittner and Felix 1998; Webb and Sostman 1992) but lost equal ground in its use once spiral CT was introduced. Multidetector CT (MDCT) has the potential to put even further distance between it and MR imaging because of its ability to perform isotropic scanning and thin-section imaging through the entire thorax in a very short space of time and the capabilities of applying postprocessing multiplanar reconstructions and three-dimensional (3D) techniques. For this reason, all of the apparent advantages of MRI have been supplanted by MDCT.

15.2 Imaging Techniques

In general, MDCT offers several advantages over single-detector CT. One advantage is that the examination can be performed with thinner sections, leading to higher spatial resolution along the patient z-axis. Additionally, scanning can be performed much faster, resulting in improved temporal resolution and reduced motion artifacts (Rydberg et al. 2000; Berland and Smith 1998). Intravenous contrast material is delivered at a higher flow rate, increasing the vascular enhancement of detected abnormalities. Rydberg et al. (2000) found that these factors combined to improve the spatial, temporal, and contrast

A. R. Hunsaker, MD
Department of Radiology, Brigham and Women's Hospital, Boston, MA 02115, USA

resolution of the images, significantly increasing the diagnostic accuracy of an examination (Rydberg et al. 2000). These advantages are particularly useful for demonstration of subtle areas of tumor enhancement in demonstrating vascular supply of lesions preoperatively (Fig. 15.1). Postprocessing techniques offer a great advantage in that postprocessing techniques can be adapted to the underlying disorder (Schoepf et al. 2001); thus, the focus in planning a CT study is directed away from the data acquisition and towards postprocessing techniques. From a single thin slice MDCT study, 2D multiplanar reformatted images, maximum intensity projection and minimum intensity projection images, and 3D imaging can be attained at a workstation. Interactive displays allow for demonstration of relationship between mass and normal mediastinal structures.

Although many postprocessing techniques are available, only those with potential usefulness in the mediastinum are described in order of their practicality from the least to the greatest. The first techniques to be described are 3D maximum intensity projection imaging (3D MIP) and 3D minimum intensity projection imaging (3D min-IP). The MIP images are created by a series of parallel rays projected through a volume of data. Only the highest attenuation voxels are made part of the image. In the process of creating these images, over 95% of the original data is lost (Ravenel et al. 2001), because only the brightest voxels or voxels with the highest attenuation values along a projection ray are used; thus, there is a tendency to misrepresent spatial relationships. For this reason, it is of limited usefulness in the mediastinum, particularly in imaging mediastinal vessels. The min-IP images are acquired in the same way as MIP images with the exception that the lowest attenuation voxels are projected to create an image.

A second technique is that of 2D multiplanar reformatted images (2D MPR). With this technique MPR images can be created in any plane with the same spatial resolution as the original sections because of the isotropic acquisition of data. Reformatted images in the coronal, sagittal, and axial planes can be created from one spiral acquisition and have the same isotropic spatial resolution as sections from the original acquisition (Rydberg et al. 2000). This type of reconstruction is the simplest and most frequently performed reconstruction and is achieved by stacking the axial images and cutting them in different planes (Ravenel et al. 2001). One simply places a line in either the sagittal or coronal planes and then obtains reformations from these images. Oblique or curved reformatted images can also be applied along the axis of a lumen, thus decreasing interpretive errors (Ravenel et al. 2001). Thin-collimation and overlapping sections also decrease artifacts along the z-axis (Fleischmann et al. 2002). The MPR images are very useful in the mediastinum, as we show later,

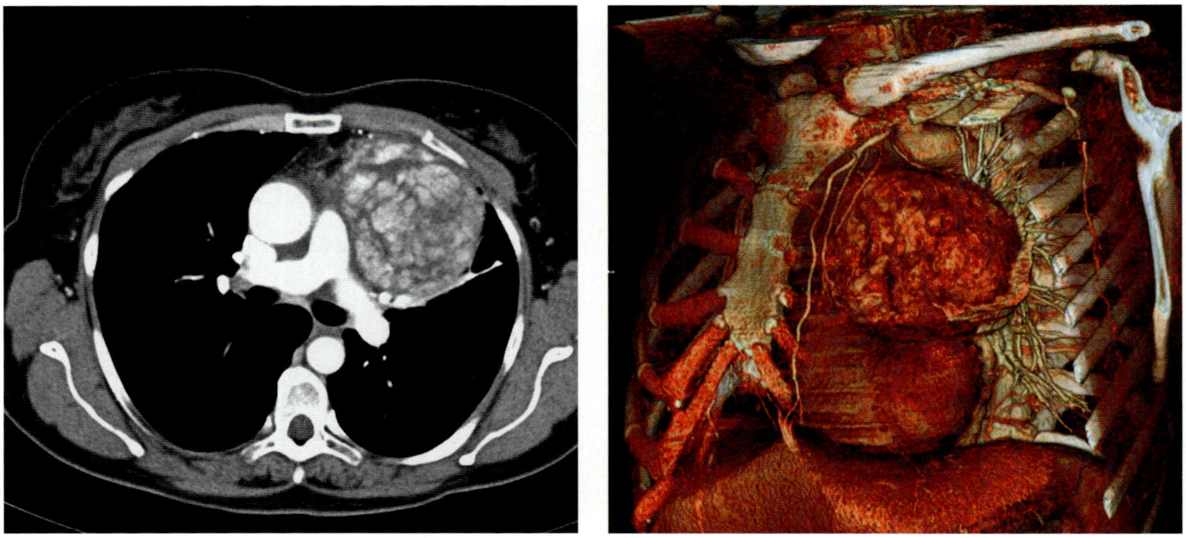

a b

Fig. 15.1a, b. Invasive thymoma. **a** Contrast-enhanced image shows an intensely enhancing nodular mediastinal mass with adjacent atelectasis. **b** Color-enhanced 3D volume-rendered image effectively shows enlarged internal mammary vessels and other thoracic collaterals in this very vascular tumor. This preoperative information was invaluable to surgeons in surgical planning. The extent of vessels were not demonstrated on the axial images in demonstrating craniocaudal extent of disease and possibly origin of disease. Most importantly, MPR images eliminate the need for direct imaging in the sagittal or coronal planes, thus eliminating increased radiation dose to the patient. In a study performed by Honda et al. (2002), the image quality of coronal multiplanar reconstructions from isotropic voxel data obtained using 0.5-mm collimation, with or without overlapping reconstruction, was found to be similar to that of direct coronal thin-section CT scans. This was found to be the case in a previous study by Caldemeyer et al. (1999).

The last technique of value to be discussed in the mediastinum is 3D imaging, which may be either surface-shaded display (3D SSD) or volume rendered. Three-dimensional surface-shaded techniques display a subset of the volumetric data by including voxels in a range of attenuation values to determine surface (Ravenel et al. 2001). These images are acquired by two methods. An attenuation range for reconstruction can be provided and the computer will generate an image, or images can be obtained by manually drawing around an object's boundaries by selecting points in a data set from which the computer will automatically connect these areas (Ravenel et al. 2001). Since this is a shaded surface, one cannot „see through" the images, and like the MIP displays, more than 90% of the data is lost making this technique not as useful as volume-rendering techniques. The 3D volume rendering, in contrast to 3D SSD, uses all the data in creating a final image. Data from all voxels are summed and displayed as a composite image on the monitor. By changing parameters, the data can be segmented by attenuation values to display the area of interest such as vessels, airways, or chest wall (Ravenel et al. 2001). Unlike SSD, one can „see through" with volume rendering.

In imaging a patient for suspected mediastinal disease at our institution, patients are scanned on either a 4- or 16-channel multidetector scanner (Siemens, Malvern, Pa.). Images are acquired with thin sections (1 mm on the 4-channel and 0.75 mm on the 16-channel scanners) through the entire thorax and then reconstructed at 5-mm slice thickness using a mediastinal algorithm. Most of our mediastinal protocols require the intravenous administration of contrast material. We use 100 cc of Ultravist 300 (Wayne, N.J.) injected at a rate of 3 cc per second following a 30-s scan delay. The data are then transferred to a workstation (Voxar, Edinburgh, Scotland, UK) where a trained technologist performs 2D MPR or 3D imaging as requested.

15.3 Clinical Applications

15.3.1 Invasion

Bronchogenic carcinoma is one of the leading causes of cancer death in the U.S. and imaging plays an important role in assessing prognosis and resectability based on metastasis to nodes and local invasion of the mediastinum or chest wall. In a state-of-the-art paper by Webb and Sostman (1992), MR imaging was considered to provide information which was superior to that of CT in certain situations. They suggested that MR should be used as the primary imaging modality in these situations. Lung cancer was one of those situations. Specifically, it was felt that MR may be superior in the diagnosis of chest wall or mediastinal invasion by the primary lung tumor because of better contrast on T1- and T2-weighted images between tumor and fat and vessels in the mediastinum. With the ability to obtain 2D MPR images with very thin sections and with the increase in concentration of intravascular contrast material, MDCT is certainly now at least equal to MR imaging in showing invasion (Figs. 15.2, 15.3) or lack thereof (Fig. 15.4), and likely will be shown to be superior. Because CT is less expensive, more readily available, takes less time to perform, and is now much easier for sick patients to tolerate, it is the imaging method of choice for invasion into the mediastinum. This is likely to be true in the evaluation of not just bronchogenic carcinoma but of malignant mesothelioma. Volume rendering can also aid in determining tumor resectability based on invasion of adjacent structures and pre-operative planning for tumor resection (Calhoun et al. 1999).

15.3.2 Assessment of Lymph Nodes

Lymph nodes are frequently seen in the mediastinum, and when larger than 1 cm in short axis or when many in number, they are a cause for concern as evaluation of mediastinal nodes is important in the work-up of non-small cell lung carcinoma. Routine CT studies of the thorax on single-detector CT (SDCT) scanners usually do not routinely include thin slices through the mediastinum. The MDCT offers an advantage in that by using the smallest collimation (1 mm on the 4-channel and 0.75 mm on the 16-channel scanners) one is able to retrospectively examine a worrisome

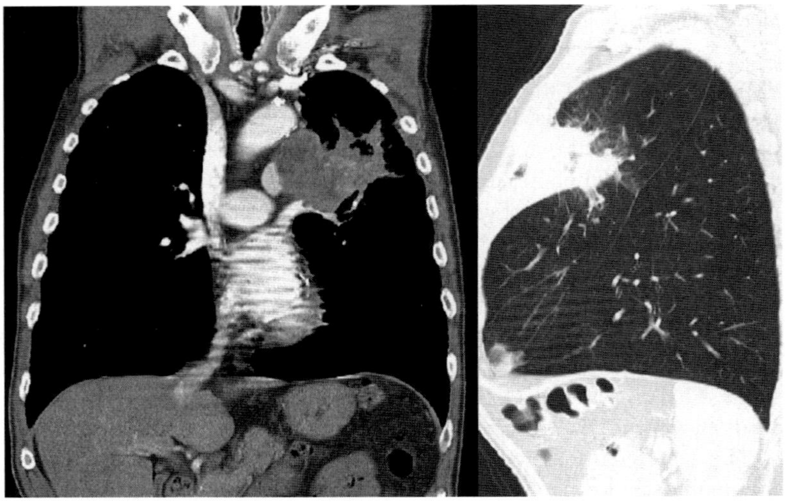

Fig. 15.2. Bronchogenic carcinoma. Contrast-enhanced 2D coronal multiplanar reformatted images (MPR) image demonstrates a large aggressive mass which involves the mediastinum, particularly the left superior pulmonary vein. It also clearly shows complete obstruction of the left upper lobe (LUL) bronchus resulting in partial LUL atelectasis

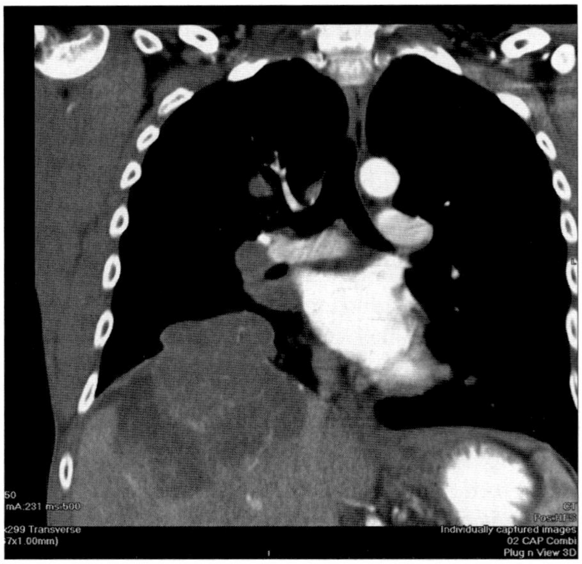

a

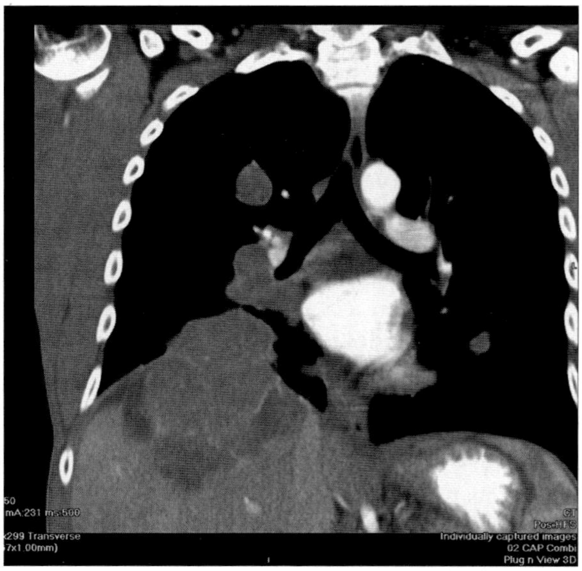

b

Fig. 15.3a, b. Bronchogenic carcinoma. Contrast enhanced 2D coronal images show extensive tumor mass encircling the **a** right lower lobe bronchus and **b** bronchus intermedius. Invasion of the diaphragm is also demonstrated

node to evaluate its tissue content (Fig. 15.5). The ability to obtain thin-section images retrospectively is limited by the collimation; hence, routinely using the smallest collimator can prevent additional unnecessary imaging or invasive procedures. In a study by Boiselle et al. (1998), CT, MRI, and 2-[fluorine-18] fluoro-2-deoxy-D-glucose (FDG) positron emission tomography (PET) were compared for their ability to identify tumor-positive nodes. They concluded that FDG-PET showed improved diagnostic accuracy in nodal status when compared with anatomic imaging with CT and MR. As demonstrated in Fig. 15.5, thin-section MDCT imaging through nodes followed by postprocessing MPR techniques will at least prevent further work-up of nodes which are clearly benign by CT, i.e., nodes which clearly show low-attenuation centers.

15.3.3 Extent and Origin of a Lesion

At times the origin of a lesion within the mediastinum can be confusing if only one plane is provided. By using MPR reconstructions in the sagittal and coronal planes in conjunction with the axial images, a more accurate assessment of a lesion can be made with regard to its origin and possibly its diagnosis (Fig. 15.6).

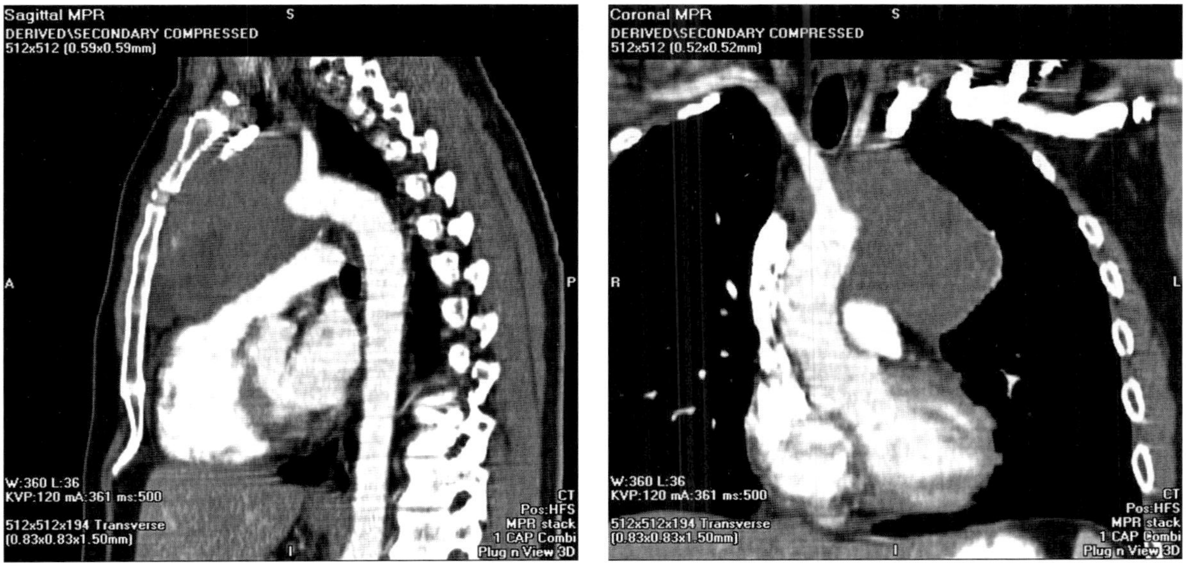

Fig. 15.4a, b. Non-Hodgkin's lymphoma. Contrast-enhanced **a** coronal and **b** sagittal 2D MPR images show a large heterogeneous mass in the anterior mediastinum which is shown to abut rather than invade the vessels. Note the smooth contour of the vessels as opposed to the superior pulmonary invasion shown in Fig. 15.2

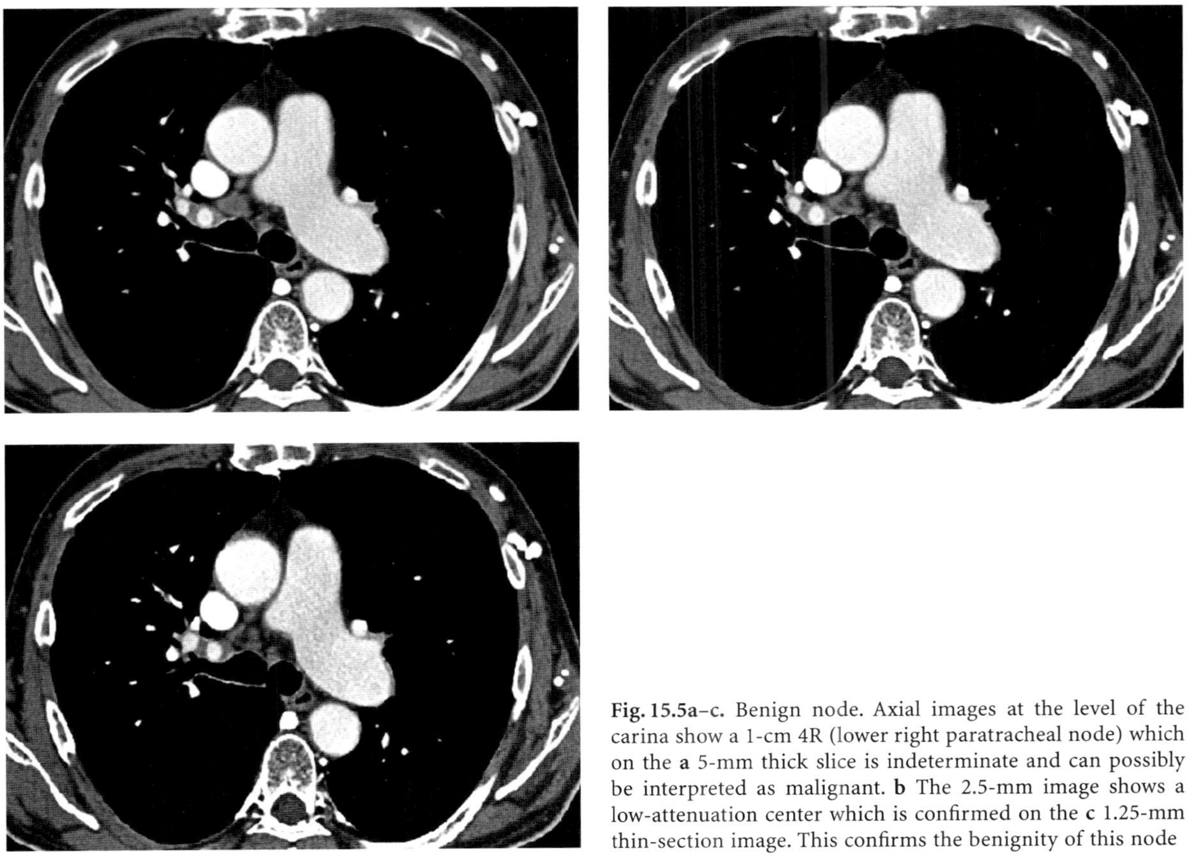

Fig. 15.5a–c. Benign node. Axial images at the level of the carina show a 1-cm 4R (lower right paratracheal node) which on the **a** 5-mm thick slice is indeterminate and can possibly be interpreted as malignant. **b** The 2.5-mm image shows a low-attenuation center which is confirmed on the **c** 1.25-mm thin-section image. This confirms the benignity of this node

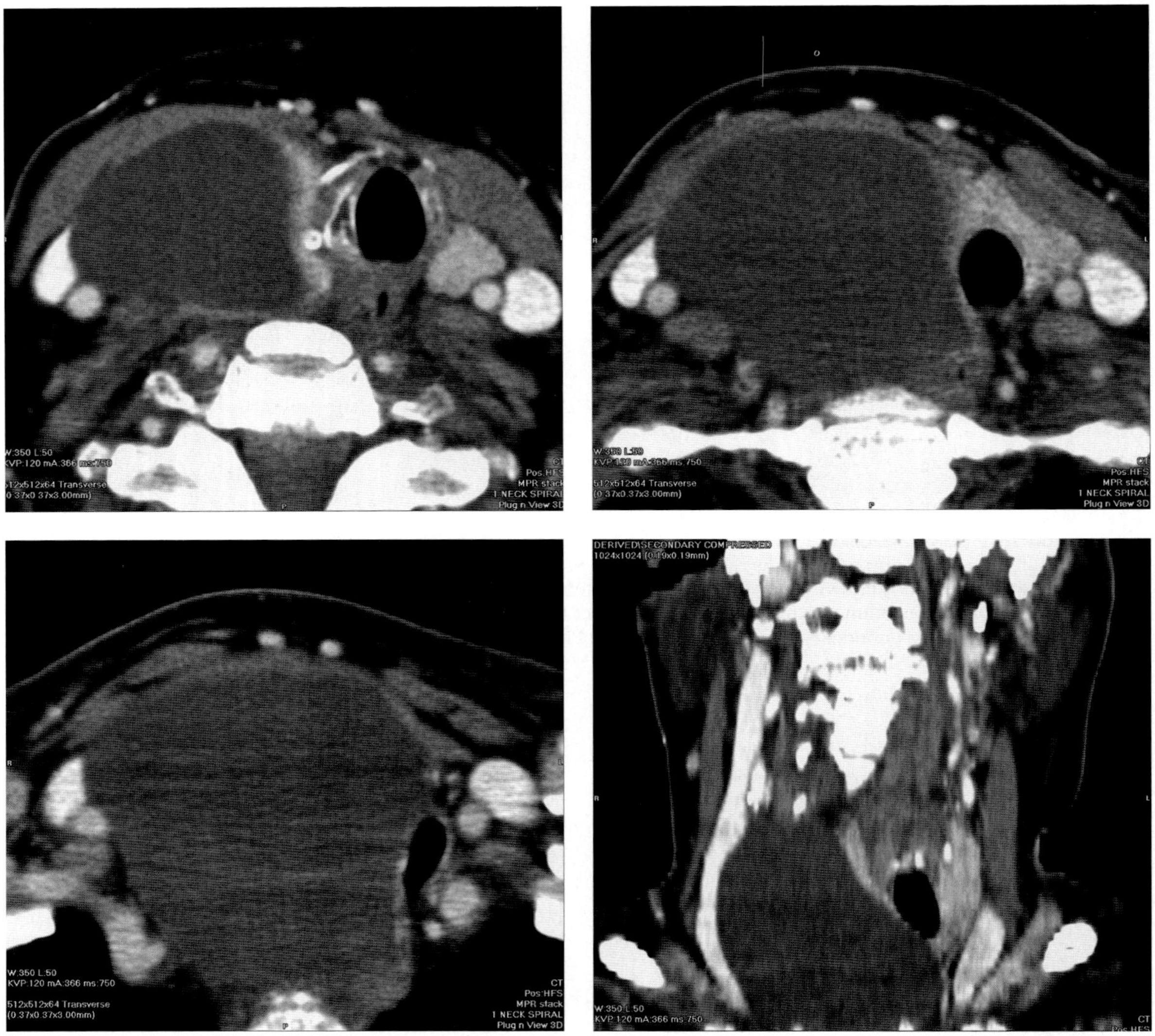

a b c d

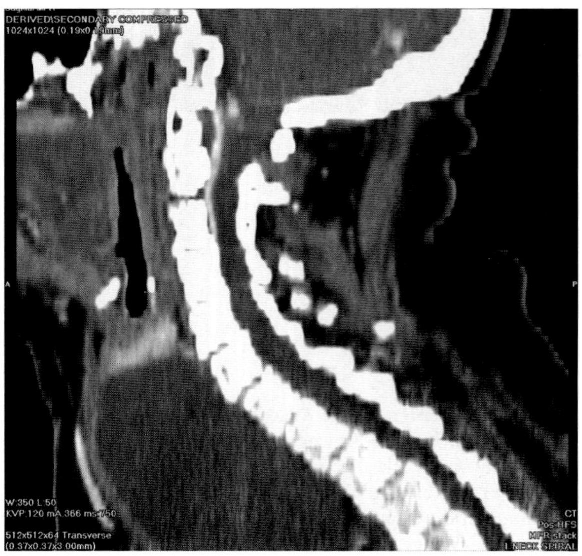

e

Fig. 15.6a–e. Bronchogenic cyst. **a–c** Three contrast-enhanced axial images show a cystic lesion which appears inseparable from the thyroid gland and, in fact, based on these images was thought to be a thyroid cyst; however, **d** coronal and **e** sagittal 2D MRR images strongly suggested otherwise. These images led to a confident preoperative diagnosis that this was not of thyroid origin but rather a mediastinal cyst and probably a bronchogenic cyst. This was confirmed surgically and pathologically

15.3.4 Tissue Characteristics

Many lesions within the mediastinum are of mixed attenuation including teratoma, lymphoma, bronchogenic carcinoma, thymolipomas and other thymic tumors, thyroid lesions, and others. Previous reports have indicated that internal characteristics of a mass as well as invasion into the mediastinum or its relationship to vessels are best shown with MR imaging (Webb and Sostman 1992). Magnetic resonance is felt to be superior for tissue characterization when compared with CT. Because of the improvement in spatial temporal and contrast resolution of the MDCT images, the diagnostic accuracy of CT has been improved when compared with MR imaging (Fig. 15.7). Coronal and sagittal MPR images can be more useful for diagnostic purposes when compared with axial sections. (Rydberg et al. 2000). The 3D techniques may be useful in showing the relationship of lesions to vasculature and the airways (Fig. 15.7).

15.3.5 Airway Masses

A brief description of airway lesions and imaging is presented as the airways are included in mediastinal differential diagnoses. Both 2D and 3D reconstruction techniques provide useful information in evaluation of the central airways (Fig. 15.8), particularly when used with axial imaging (Ravenel et al. 2001; Boiselle et al. 2002). Sagittal and coronal 2D MPR images aid in assessing degree of stenosis as well as craniocaudal extent. Modest improvement in airway analysis is achieved with 3D SSD and volume-rendered images (Ravenel et al. 2001; Boiselle et al. 2002; Remy-Jardin et al. 1998). Boiselle et al. (2002) and Remy-Jardin et al. (1998) concluded that 2D MPR and 3D volume rendering does not create new information but rather presents complementary ways of viewing information already present on the original axial images. Although it has been shown that in the majority of uncomplicated cases 3D images are of minimal usefulness, 3D images are moderately or highly valuable in assessing complex airway lesions (Kauczor et al. 1996; Remy-Jardin et al. 1998). It has been suggested that 2.5- to 3.0-mm-collimation images be used for better definition of multiplanar reformatted and 3D images. This should be done with overlapping reconstruction intervals (Boiselle et al. 2002). The 3D volume-rendered images are useful for extrinsic airway compression as well as a wide variety of complex tracheobronchial anomalies. The 3D images also have the advantage of assessing airways distal to an impassable structure or mass (Ravenel et al. 2001) when compared with bronchoscopy. The 2D MPR images can be displayed in a curved fashion along the axis of an airway, thus better displaying the length of an abnormality.

15.4 Conclusion

Multidetector CT imaging shows great potential in mediastinal imaging, not merely in the vascular, cardiac, and airways lesions, but also in evaluation of more typical mediastinal lesions. Specifically, due to improvement in temporal, spatial, and contrast resolution, and the ability to obtain 2D multiplanar reformations and 3D reconstructions, the ability of CT to characterize tissues and assess for invasion into mediastinal structures may potentially be equal to that of MR imaging. Both 2D and 3D imaging in mediastinal imaging also contribute to surgical planning and to assessing resectability of lesions. The need for 2D multiplanar reformations and 3D reconstructions should be considered at the time of planning the CT scan so that adequate imaging is obtained which will optimize exquisite reconstructions.

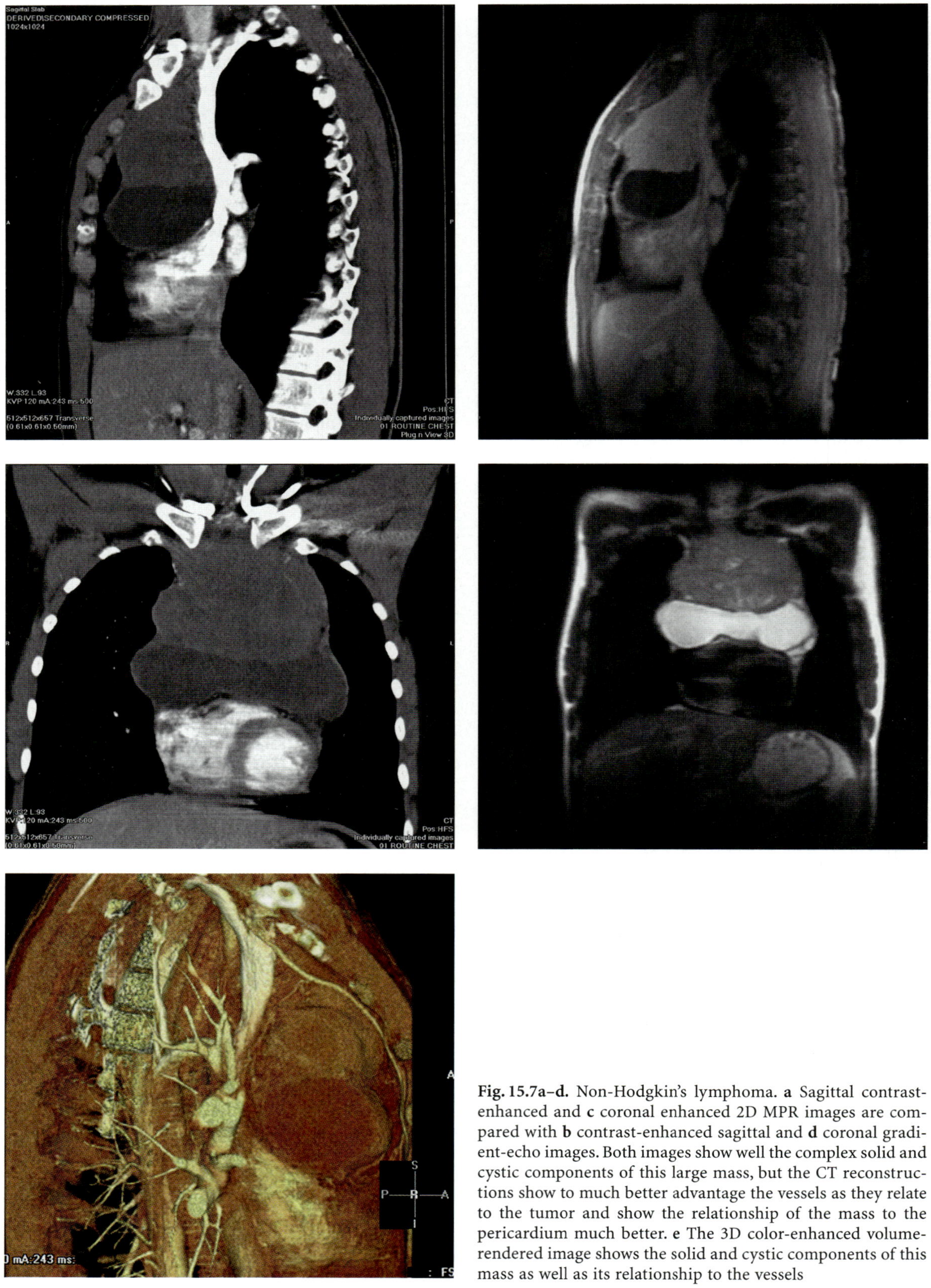

a b c d e

Fig. 15.7a–d. Non-Hodgkin's lymphoma. **a** Sagittal contrast-enhanced and **c** coronal enhanced 2D MPR images are compared with **b** contrast-enhanced sagittal and **d** coronal gradient-echo images. Both images show well the complex solid and cystic components of this large mass, but the CT reconstructions show to much better advantage the vessels as they relate to the tumor and show the relationship of the mass to the pericardium much better. **e** The 3D color-enhanced volume-rendered image shows the solid and cystic components of this mass as well as its relationship to the vessels

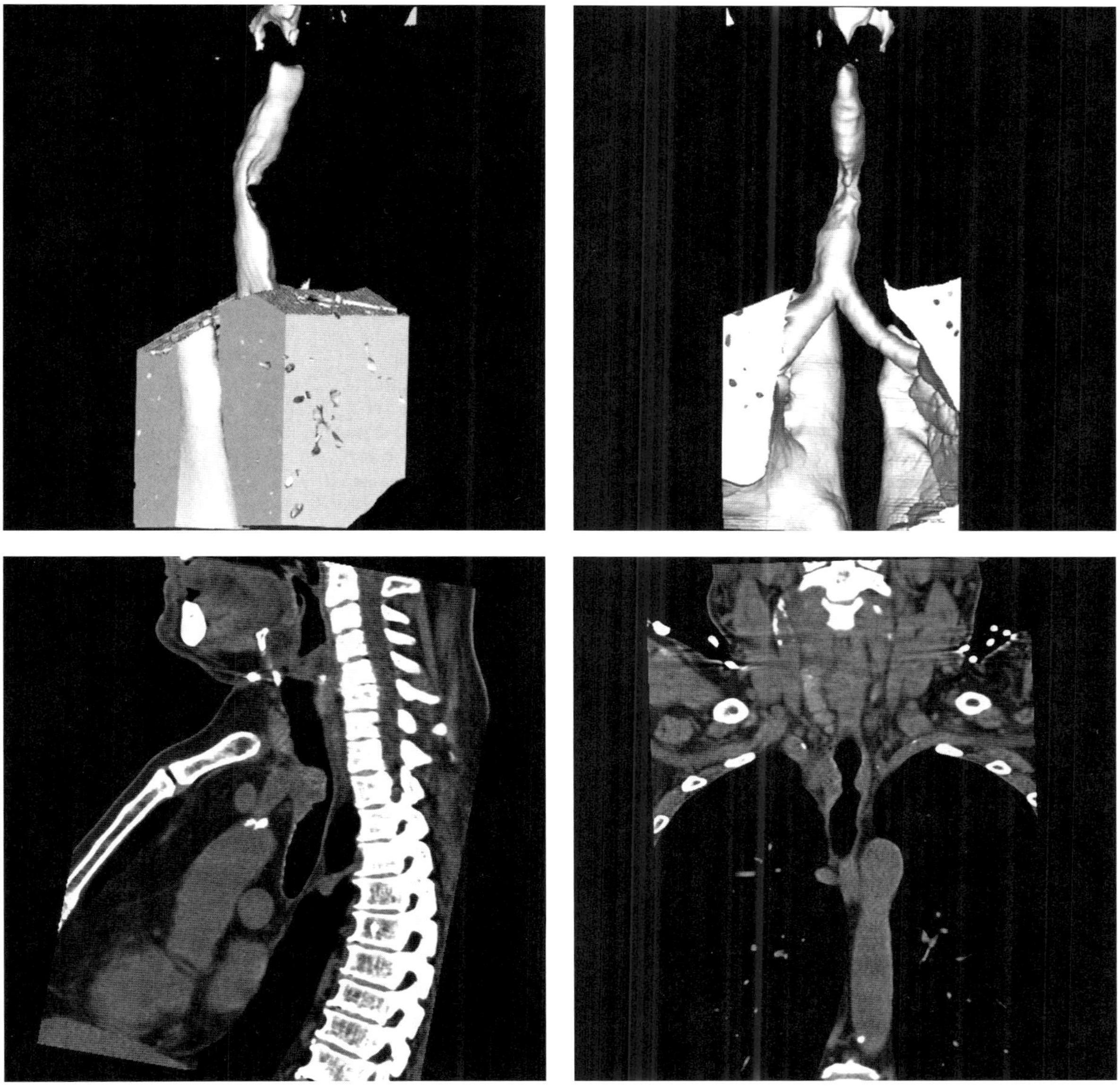

a b c d

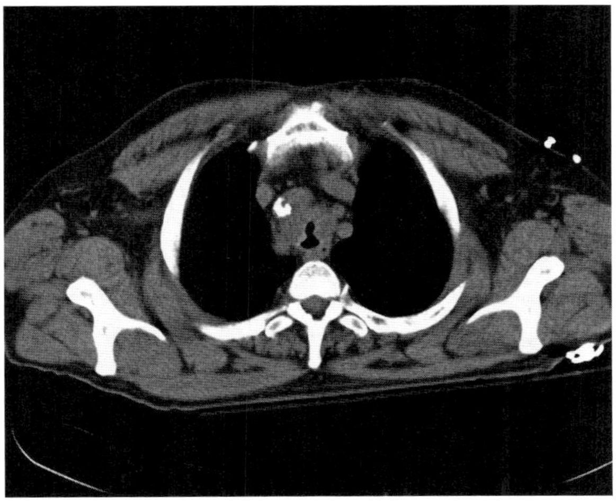

e

Fig. 15.8a–e. Squamous cell carcinoma of trachea. **a** Axial, **b** coronal 2D MPR, and **c** sagittal 2D MPR images interpreted in a complementary fashion show the circumferential and cephalocaudad extent of this tumor. They all show marked narrowing of the trachea; however, the **d** coronal and **e** sagittal 3D volume-rendered sculpted images show more dramatically the extent of airway narrowing relative to the more normal luminal size of the trachea above and below the lesion

References

Berland LL, Smith JK (1998) Multidetector-array CT: once again, technology creates new opportunities. Radiology 209:327–329

Bhalla M, Naidich DP, McGuiness et al. (1996) Diffuse lung disease: assessment with helical CT – preliminary observations of the role of maximum and minimum intensity projection images. Radiology 200:341–347

Bittner RC, Felix R (1998) Magnetic resonance (MR) imaging of the chest: state-of-the-art. Eur Respir J 11:1392–1404

Boiselle PM, Patz EF, Vining DJ et al. (1998) Imaging of mediastinal lymph nodes: CT, MR, and FDG PET. Radiographics 18:1061–1969

Boiselle PM, Reynolds KF, Ernst A (2002) Multiplanar and three-dimensional imaging of the central airways with multidetector CT. AJR 179:301–308

Caldemeyer KS, Sandrasegaran KS, Shinaver CN et al. (1999) Temporal bone: comparison of isotropic helical CT and conventional direct axial and coronal CT. AJR 172: 1675–1682

Calhoun PS, Kuszyk BS, Heath DG et al. (1999) Three-dimensional volume rendering of spiral CT data: theory and method. Radiographics 19:745–764

Fleischman D, Rubin GD, Paik DS et al. (2000) Stair-step artifacts with single versus multiple detector-row helical CT. Radiology 216:185–196

Honda O, Johkoh T, Yamamoto S et al. (2002) Comparison of quality of multiplanar reconstructions and direct coronal multidetector CT scans of the lung. AJR 179:876–879

Johnson PT, Heath DG, Bliss DF et al. (1996) Three-dimensional CT: real-time interactive volume rendering. AJR 167:581–583

Johnson PT, Fishman EK, Duckwall JR et al. (1998) Interactive three-dimensional volume rendering of spiral CT data: current applications in the thorax. Radiographics 18:165–187

Kauczor HU, Wolcke B, Fischer B et al. (1996) Three-dimensional helical CT of the tracheobronchial tree: evaluation of imaging protocols and assessment of suspected stenoses with bronchoscopic correlation. AJR 167:419–424

Lawler LP, Fishman EK (2001) Multi-detector row CT of thoracic disease with emphasis on 3D volume rendering and CT angiography. Radiographics 21:1257–1273

Ravenel JG, McAdams HP, Remy-Jardin M, Remy J (2001) Multidimensional imaging of the thorax. J Thorac Imaging 16:269–281

Remy-Jardin M, Remy J, Artaud D et al. (1998a) Volume rendering of the tracheobronchial tree: clinical evaluation of bronchographic images. Radiology 208:761–770

Remy-Jardin M, Remy J, Artaud D et al. (1998b) Tracheobronchial tree: assessment with volume rendering– technical aspects. Radiology 208:393–398

Rydberg J, Buckwalter KA, Caldemeyer KS et al. (2000) Multisection CT: scanning techniques and clinical applications. Radiographics 20:1787–1806

Schoepf UJ, Bruening RD, Hong C et al. (2001) Multislice helical CT of focal and diffuse lung disease: comprehensive diagnosis with reconstruction of contiguous and high-resolution CT sections from a single thin-collimation scan. AJR 177:179–184

Tecce PM, Fishman EK, Kuhlman JE (1994) CT evaluation of the anterior mediastinum: spectrum of disease. Radiographics 14:973–990

Webb WR, Sostman HD (1992) MR imaging of thoracic disease: clinical uses. Radiology 182:621–630

16 PET/CT of the Thorax

H. C. Steinert and G. K. von Schulthess

CONTENTS

16.1 Basic Aspects of PET/CT Imaging

16.1.1 Introduction

Positron emission tomography (PET)/CT is a new imaging modality. This is true despite the fact that traditionally PET belongs to nuclear medicine and that CT belongs to radiology. As a consequence, both fraternities derive from the respective imaging modality, that they should "own" PET/CT. Looking at PET/CT from this political perspective is not conducive to optimizing the information obtained. Our experience with PET/CT suggests that the CT portion enhances PET's unmatched ability to identify tumor foci; thus, the clinician can relate better to a PET scan when he knows where the foci are located. The PET scans contain little anatomic information, and knowing exactly where a lesion is located is sometimes critical, so the role of CT is not only to make PET more palatable to clinicians. A metastasis of a colorectal carcinoma in the liver hilus is completely different from one in the adjacent liver tissue. In order to clarify the notion that PET/CT is a new modality, observe the following: fluorodeoxyglucose (FDG), the radiopharmaceutical used predominantly in clinical practice is such a good "contrast agent," that many of the routines established in standard CT imaging may be obsolete when designing imaging protocols for PET/CT. Having a small lymph node take up FDG will obviate the necessity to resort to subtle analyses of lesion shape, contrast media enhancement, and size on CT; thus, PET/CT may require less "CT-ology" than the CT specialists are used to, and maybe more PET-driven CT image analysis. As an example, early results suggest that using a low-dose CT without intravenous contrast agent in conjunction with PET may be adequate in most settings of tumor staging (Hany et al. 2002a); thus, the future of PET/CT will rely on imaging specialists who are both competent readers of PET and CT images. To state this drastically, no radiologist has ever had the idea that one specialist should look at T1-weighted MR scans, the other at T2-weighted scans, and the diagnosis is then made in conference! But this is precisely what some departments introducing PET/CT are currently practicing.

Thus, the approach to PET/CT in this chapter tries to avoid political issues and assumes that the readers of PET/CT images are competent in PET imaging and CT imaging. The future will show how this will be achieved politically. We are fortunate enough in the Department of Nuclear Medicine at the Zurich University Hospital to have several board-certified radiologists on the staff, in addition to board-certified nuclear physicians.

H. C. Steinert, MD
Nuclear Medicine, Department of Medical Radiology, University Hospital, 8091 Zurich, Switzerland
G. K. von Schulthess, MD
Professor and Director, Nuclear Medicine, Department of Medical Radiology, University Hospital, 8091 Zurich, Switzerland

16.1.2 PET Imaging

The PET imaging is a nuclear medicine imaging modality, using radiopharmaceuticals such as standard nuclear medicine. The principal difference is that PET uses positron emitters rather than radionuclides, which emit gamma rays or X-rays. The ensuing two sections are a summary. More in-depth information may be obtained from von Schulthess (2003). The positron emitted by a nucleus decays according to a positron decay scheme, i.e., the nuclei of positron emitters, which have a neutron deficit, and the proton decays to a neutron with concomitant emission of a positron. The positron, being a particle of antimatter, is not stable in matter. After emission, it is slowed down and at low kinetic energies it will annihilate with one of the electrons present plentifully in matter. This slow-down process occurs typically within 1–3 mm from the site where the nuclide emitted the positron, and is dependent on the emission energy of the positron. As this emission occurs randomly into any spatial direction, this is one of the main determinants of the lowest spatial resolution achievable in PET imaging. The annihilation reaction results in two gamma rays of 511 keV, which part from the site of annihilation at an angle of almost exactly 180°. This angle is dictated by the physical laws of conservation of energy and momentum: 511 keV is the equivalent energy of the electron (and positron) mass (two such particles annihilate to give rise to two gamma rays), and the angle is a result of momentum conversation. In fact, the angle is not precisely 180° but is determined by the net momentum of the electron and the positron at the time of annihilation and may vary by one or two degrees. This represents a second limit to the theoretical spatial resolution achievable in a PET scanner, which is around 2–3 mm, providing optimal scanner geometry and using F-18 as radiolabel.

In a high-end PET scanner the two gamma rays emitted are subsequently detected by a ring scintillation detector consisting of thousands of detector elements, which are connected by coincidence circuitry. If a detector detects one gamma photon, for a few nanoseconds all other relevant detector elements are ready to detect the second photon from the annihilation event. If indeed a second event is recorded, the radioactive decay of the positron emitter has had to take place on a (almost) straight line connecting the two detector elements responding. The PET is thus a map of lines connecting two detectors. It is intuitively clear that regions where many of these lines intersect correspond to hot spots observed in PET. Not all coincidences are true coincidences, but there are also random coincidences and coincidences of gamma photons where one or both have been Compton scattered. The PET scanners have mechanisms to correct for these "false" events, but a discussion would be beyond the scope of this chapter and the reader is referred to von Schulthess (2003).

The PET, such as single photon emission computed tomography (SPECT) is an emission scanning method. This means that gamma rays from annihilation events buried deep inside the body are less likely to exit the patients' body than those coming from annihilations close to the patients' body surface. In order to obtain homogeneous images and to be able to quantify PET images, a so-called attenuation correction of the PET data, which are called emission data, has to be done. Attenuation in PET is measured by using photons from a radioactive source, which rotates around the patient very much like a CT tube, and uses the gamma detectors of the PET scanner; however, the photon flux of these sources is very low and attenuation correction scans are thus lengthy procedures. The attenuation data to correct the PET emission data are introduced into the image reconstruction process of the emission images and result in attenuation-corrected PET images. This is currently considered state-of-the-art PET imaging. A typical rule of thumb is that the measurement time for attenuation correction in PET systems is approximately half of that used to obtain emission data; thus, a 30-min PET scan is divided into 20-min emission image acquisitions and 10-min transmission image acquisition.

16.1.3 Radiopharmaceuticals

As stated, PET imaging requires radiopharmaceuticals such as conventional nuclear medicine imaging. The standard positron emitters available from cyclotrons of 10–30 MeV are carbon-11, nitrogen-13, oxygen-15, and fluorine-18. C-11, N-13, and O-15 have half-lives of less than 30-min and are impractical for clinical use beyond centers disposing of a cyclotron. Compounds using F-18 as a label have physical half-lives of 110-min; thus, central production and limited-area shipment of F-18 based compounds is possible. By far, the most widely used compound is F-18 FDG, which is a glucose analog. It is taken up into cells and 6-phosphorylated like glucose, but no further metabolism is notable; thus, FDG labels cellular glucose uptake and metabolism, the latter because hexokinase responsible for 6-phosphorylation is the rate limiting enzyme in glycolysis. FDG happens to be an "unbelievably" good molecule to label many malignant tumors and active inflammatory sites, and thus it is FDG-PET, which is currently in predominant use. Glucose is obligatorily used in the brain and excreted by the kidneys, but not substantially accumulated in other organs except the heart. As a result, the lesion-to-background ratio is excellent in most situations except for brain lesions. There is muscular uptake in muscles exercised and uptake into nuchal fat in some patients as recently identified, but the pathophysiological significance of this fat uptake is not known at present (Hany et al. 2002b). The clinical data discussed in this chapter are based on FDG-PET only.

Many other F-18 labeled compounds have been synthesized and are under clinical evaluation. Of interest are a vast array of receptor ligands such as F-18 DOPA, amino acid metabolism tracers, such as F-18 ethyl-tyrosine (FET), F-18-based cell membrane proliferation markers, which are choline derivatives, and DNA synthesis markers such as F-18 thymidine (FLT). The clinical experience with these markers is currently too limited to decide what their future clinical role may be. FET may be a better marker of brain tumors than FDG, because it does not accumulate much in the normal brain, and choline derivatives may have similar properties but in addition may be good markers in prostate carcinoma, where FDG mostly fails to identify lesions.

In units where a cyclotron is available, additional compounds can be used clinically. The most notable are H2O-15 water and N-13H3 ammonia for the quantitative assessment of brain and heart perfusion, respectively. In addition, many C-11 compounds can be used in such units, but the short half-life of 20-min of C-11 makes synthesis of relevant compounds difficult and costly.

16.1.4 PET/CT

There are several good reasons for combining PET and CT into a single in-line imaging system, where the patient is moved from the CT to the PET gantry by simple table motion (Kinahan et al. 1998; von Schulthess 1999).

Such a system provides PET and CT images perfectly co-registered by hardware arrangement provided that the patient does not move. This is of major importance because PET scans of the body provide little anatomic information, and software image co-registration has been shown to be cumbersome and inaccurate by many authors.

At least as important and maybe the main incentive for manufacturers to promote and produce PET/CT scanners is the fact that attenuation correction in a PET/CT scanner can be done as well with the CT data obtained as anatomic reference. This obviates the lengthy standard attenuation procedure used in PET and improves patient throughput by approximately 30%, when a state-of-the-art CT scanner is incorporated into a PET/CT scanner. A CT scan is in fact an attenuation map, albeit measured with 70–140 keV polychromatic X-rays, whereas the PET attenuation scan is obtained with relatively monochromatic photons at 511 keV. Measurements have demonstrated, however, that the Hounsfield CT maps can be transformed into PET attenuation maps with relatively simple transformations requiring minimal computational efforts (Burger et al. 2002). The qualitative and quantitative properties of PET are maintained when CT is used for attenuation correction (Kamel et al. 2002a).

The higher patient throughput of a PET/CT scanner compared with a PET-only scanner may offset the additional equipment cost at least in environments where the number of patients to be scanned per PET scanner is high. A net cost advantage results from the fact that FDG decays rapidly with a half-life of 110-min; thus, faster scanning results in more efficient use of FDG, which may be delivered as an initial dose for several patients.

While a combination of PET and MR is also conceivable, using MR is difficult, because the MR images are not attenuation maps like the CT images. In the brain, where MR is superior to CT for anatomic imaging, software image co-registration is much simpler than with body data, and thus a PET/CT scanner is mainly an instrument which is useful in imaging of the human body from the head down to the feet.

It is likely that these synergistic effects obtained when adding CT to PET are responsible for the almost explosive growth of PET/CT imaging worldwide. One and a half years after the commercial announcement probably close to 100 PET/CT systems are installed and another 100 have been ordered.

16.1.5 Clinical Protocols in PET/CT

As PET/CT is a novel technology, the clinical protocols in PET/CT are subject to fast evolution. At our institution we routinely give diluted bowel contrast agent 1 h prior to scanning (Dizendorf et al. 2002) followed by supine FDG injection and patient rest of at least 30 min. After bladder voiding just prior to scanning, we first perform a low-dose CT scan at 40 mAs (Hany et al. 2002a). This covers 100 cm of axial field of view in less than 30 s with a slice thickness of 4.5 mm, which is matched to the PET slice thickness. The CT scanner is a state-of-the-art 4-slice MDCT with a gantry rotation of 0.5 s minimum. Extensive evaluation of the CT breath-hold breathing pattern best matching the free-breathing pattern of PET data acquisition has led us to conclude that an unforced end-expiratory state is best, during the period where the CT images the regions adjacent to the diaphragm (Goerres et al. 2002); thus, patients are instructed to exhale and hold their breath when the CT scanner scans this body region. As stated, CT scanning is accomplished in less than 30 s. Subsequently, PET scanning is started from the pelvis up. Starting PET scanning in the pelvis rather than the head obviates a potential major PET/CT mismatch in the bladder region. This is due to bladder filling between CT data acquisition and the relatively lengthy PET scan, if started at the head. The PET scan is performed using six to seven table positions. As the PET scanner covers an axial field of view of around 15 cm with 32 slices per table position, approximately 90–105 cm of the patient are covered, which include the anatomic regions from the brain to the upper thighs in almost all patients. With table position imaging times of 3–4 min, typical scan length of a PET/CT partial-body scan covering the patient from the head to the mid-upper thighs is 20–30 min.

After this "baseline" PET/CT data acquisition, additional standard CT protocols can be run depending upon the clinical requirements. As is discussed in the second part dealing with lung tumor imaging, it is desirable in some settings to also perform a CT scan enhanced with i.v. contrast, which can better delineate the lesions in relation to vascular structures. The overall protocol design for such all-encompassing PET/CT examinations is not defined and the next years will have to indicate where and when additional contrast-enhanced CT scanning is useful.

Other groups have advocated the use of i.v. contrast-enhanced CT scans from the beginning and as only CT scan. It is our opinion that this is less than optimal for two reasons: firstly, in many settings, CT contrast is not needed, as FDG is mostly a much better "contrast agent" than the contrast agents used in CT. Secondly, vascular contrast, which for vessel delineation is dense and transient, causes the CT data not to be ideal attenuation maps for the subsequent PET scan. It has to be emphasized that iodinated contrast behaves in a way that it can be difficult to use a scan enhanced with intravenous contrast agent for attenuation correction (Dizendorf et al. 2003); iodine looks like bone at 80–140 keV but like soft tissue at 511 keV; and thus the Hounsfield- to 511 keV transformation used for attenuation correction may not work consistently without segmenting the vessels out of the CT and replacing the vessels with soft tissue density on the CT data). The additional radiation burden to a patient with a low-dose CT at 40 mAs is in the range of 2–3 mSv, that of PET around 10 mSv, thus making a PET/CT examination with the above protocol one with a lower radiation dose or comparable to standard CT.

16.1.6 Critical Appraisal of Clinical PET/CT

Clinical experience with PET/CT is currently limited; however, after performing approximately 3000 clinical scans thus far and having been the first users of a clinical system (an initial prototype combining a low-end PET and CT has been operational at the university of Pittsburgh since 1998), we can confidently appraise at least some aspects of clinical PET/CT.

PET/CT is easy to use and in the overwhelming number of patients, image co-registration is excellent. This is probably due to the fact that oncology patients, who represent the major patient group imaged, are generally cooperative. PET/CT is more specific than PET. To our surprise, routine availability of an anatomic reference frame has led to the identification of various pitfalls not fully appreciated in PET prior to the introduction of PET/CT. The superimposition of an FDG avid focus onto an anatomically identifiable structure makes the image interpreter more confident of what he sees and reduces interobserver variability. This also applies to the use of PET/CT data in radiation planning. The software infrastructure has now been developed which permits transfer of PET and CT data into the planning environment of radiation oncologists by DICOM standard formats. The PET/CT is more sensitive than PET because some lesions, particularly in the lung, which are too small to be noted on PET, are recognized on CT.

Viewing PET and CT images next to each other is not adequate for lesion localization once lesions are below approximately 2 cm, and it is particularly in such lesions where PET excels and where standard morphological criteria of malignancy in CT no longer are very useful; thus, co-registration and fusion or linked cursor viewing are mandatory. All currently available data suggest that the software approach is at least logistically difficult and obviously

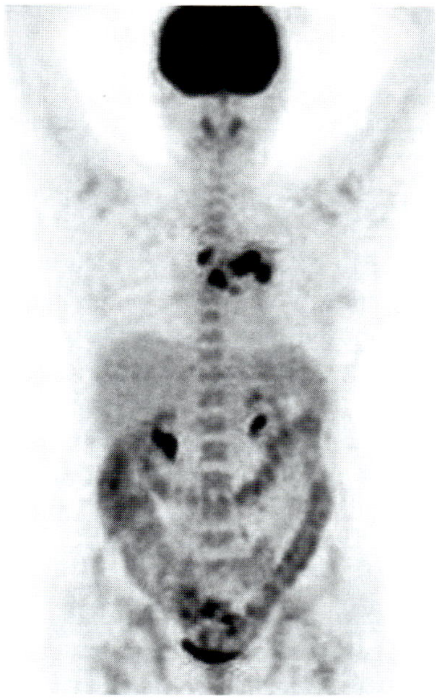

Fig. 16.1a–g. A 55-year-old woman with a large cell carcinoma in the left lung. PET/CT was performed for preoperative staging. **a** Maximum intensity projection (MIP) PET scan, **b, e** axial unenhanced low-dose CT scans, **c, f** axial CT-attenuation corrected PET scans, and **d, g** axial co-registered PET/CT scans. Diagnosis of PET/CT imaging: lung cancer in the left hilar region. Lymph node metastases in the aorto-pulmonary window, subcarinally, and in the contralateral mediastinum, making the patient inoperable

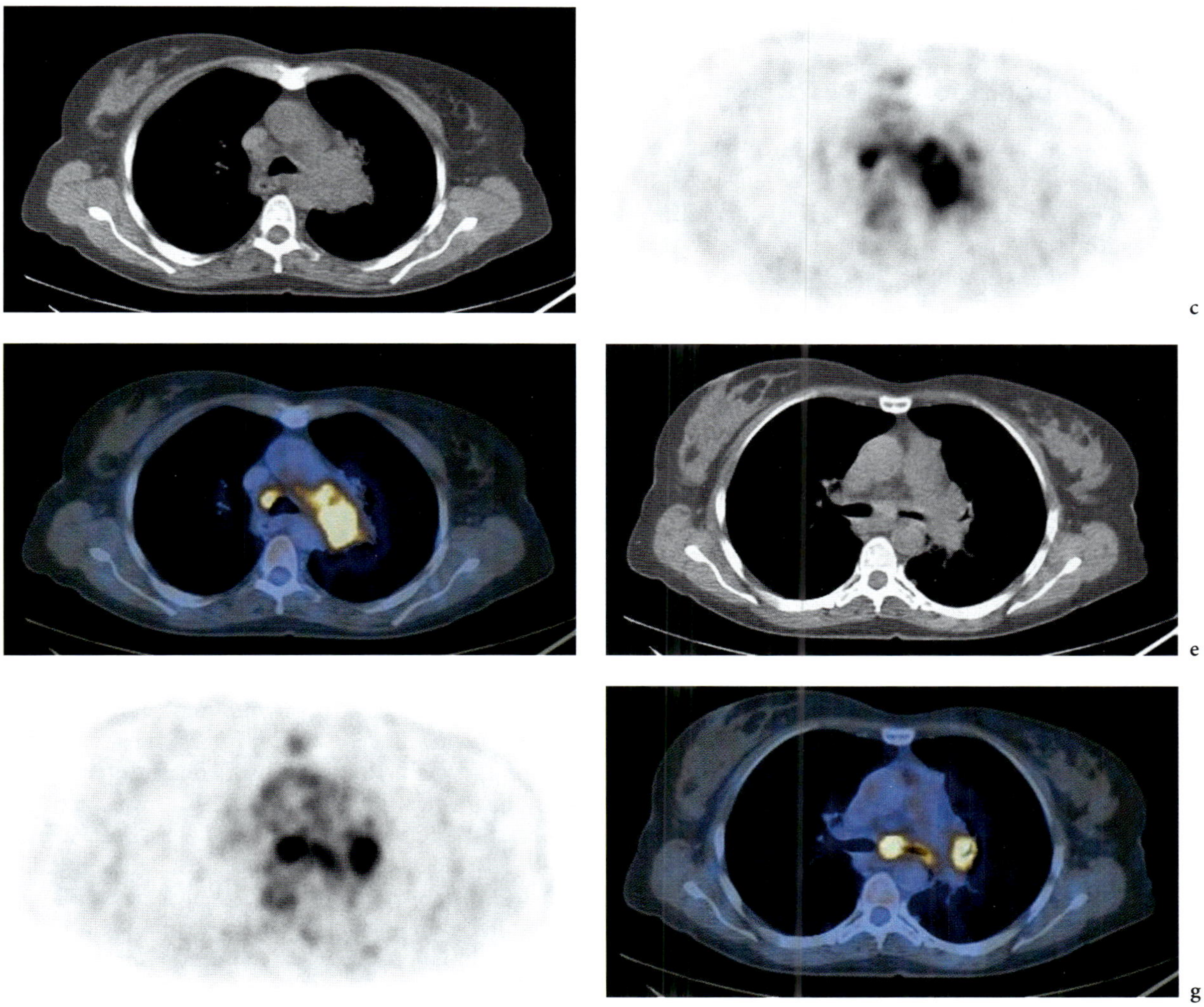

does not provide easily accessible data for attenuation correction.

Any new modality has also new artifacts and pitfalls. The most relevant artifact identified so far are misregistration artifacts around the diaphragm (Fig. 16.2d). They lead to abdominal lesions apparently located in the supradiaphragmatic lung zones and a photon deficit of variable importance overlying the diaphragmatic domes and looking like "bananas" on the coronal CT attenuation corrected PET scans. A second artifact, which may be more prominent in CT-corrected PET scans than PET scans corrected with the standard transmission scan methods, is that arising around metallic implants. Slight misregistrations can lead to overcorrections, which then result in focal or linear regions of apparently increased FDG uptake. The last artifact comes from major misregistration due to patient motion between the acquisition of the two scans.

16.2 Clinical Applications of PET/CT in the Chest

Lung cancer staging is based on the TNM system and requires accurate characterization of the primary tumor (T stage), regional lymph nodes (N stage), and extrathoracic metastases (M stage). Accurate tumor staging is essential for choosing the appropriate treatment strategy. The majority of PET imaging work has been done in non-small cell lung cancer (NSCLC). It has been shown that FDG PET is highly accurate in classifying lung nodules as benign or malignant. Whole-body PET improves the rate of detection of mediastinal lymph node metastases as well as extrathoracic metastases when compared with conventional imaging methods such as CT, MR, ultrasound, or bone scan. Since commercial PET scanners provide nominal spatial resolution of 4.5–6 mm in the center of the axial field of view, even lesions less than 1 cm with an increased FDG uptake can be detected. This represents a critical advantage of PET over CT and MR. Recently, integrated PET/CT scanners have been introduced. Integrated PET/CT enables the exact matching of focal abnormalities on PET to anatomic structures on CT. First clinical results of integrated PET/CT imaging show that PET/CT is superior in diagnostic accuracy in comparison with PET alone, CT alone, and visual correlation of PET and CT (Hany et al. 2002a; Lardinois et al. 2003).

16.2.1 Solitary Lung Nodule

The ability of PET to separate between benign and malignant lesions is high, but not perfect. For benign lesions, a high specificity for FDG PET has been demonstrated. It has been shown that FDG PET is highly accurate in differentiating malignant from benign solitary pulmonary nodules (0.6–3 cm) when radiographic findings were indeterminate (Gupta et al. 1996). In a series of 61 patients, PET had a sensitivity of 93% and a specificity of 88% for detecting malignancy; however, FDG PET may show negative results for pulmonary carcinoid tumors and bronchiolo-alveolar lung carcinoma. Lesions with increased FDG uptake should be considered malignant, although false-positive results have been reported in cases of inflammatory and infectious processes, such as histoplasmosis, aspergillosis, or active tuberculosis. The PET is clinically useful in patients with a solitary pulmonary nodule less than 3 cm in diameter, especially where biopsy may be risky or where the nodule carries a low risk for malignancy based on patients' history or radiographic findings. With integrated PET/CT an additional certainty to the presence or absence of FDG uptake in the pulmonary nodule can be achieved.

16.2.2 T Staging

Without image fusion, the use of PET in T staging lung cancer is limited. Recently, it has been shown that integrated PET/CT is superior to CT alone, PET alone, and visual correlation of PET and CT in T staging of patients with NSCLC (Lardinois et al. 2003). Due to the exact anatomic correlation of the extent of FDG uptake, the delineation of the primary tumor can be defined precisely; therefore, the diagnosis of chest wall infiltration and the mediastinal invasion by the tumor is improved. Lesions with chest wall infiltration are classified as stage T3 and are potentially resectable. Integrated PET/CT provides important information on mediastinal infiltration, too; however, PET/CT imaging is unable to distinguish contiguity of tumor with the mediastinum from the direct invasion of the walls of mediastinal structures. It has been shown that FDG PET is a useful tool for the differentiation between tumor and peritumoral atelectasis. This is particularly important for the planning of radiotherapy in patients with lung cancer associated with atelectasis. The information provided by FDG PET

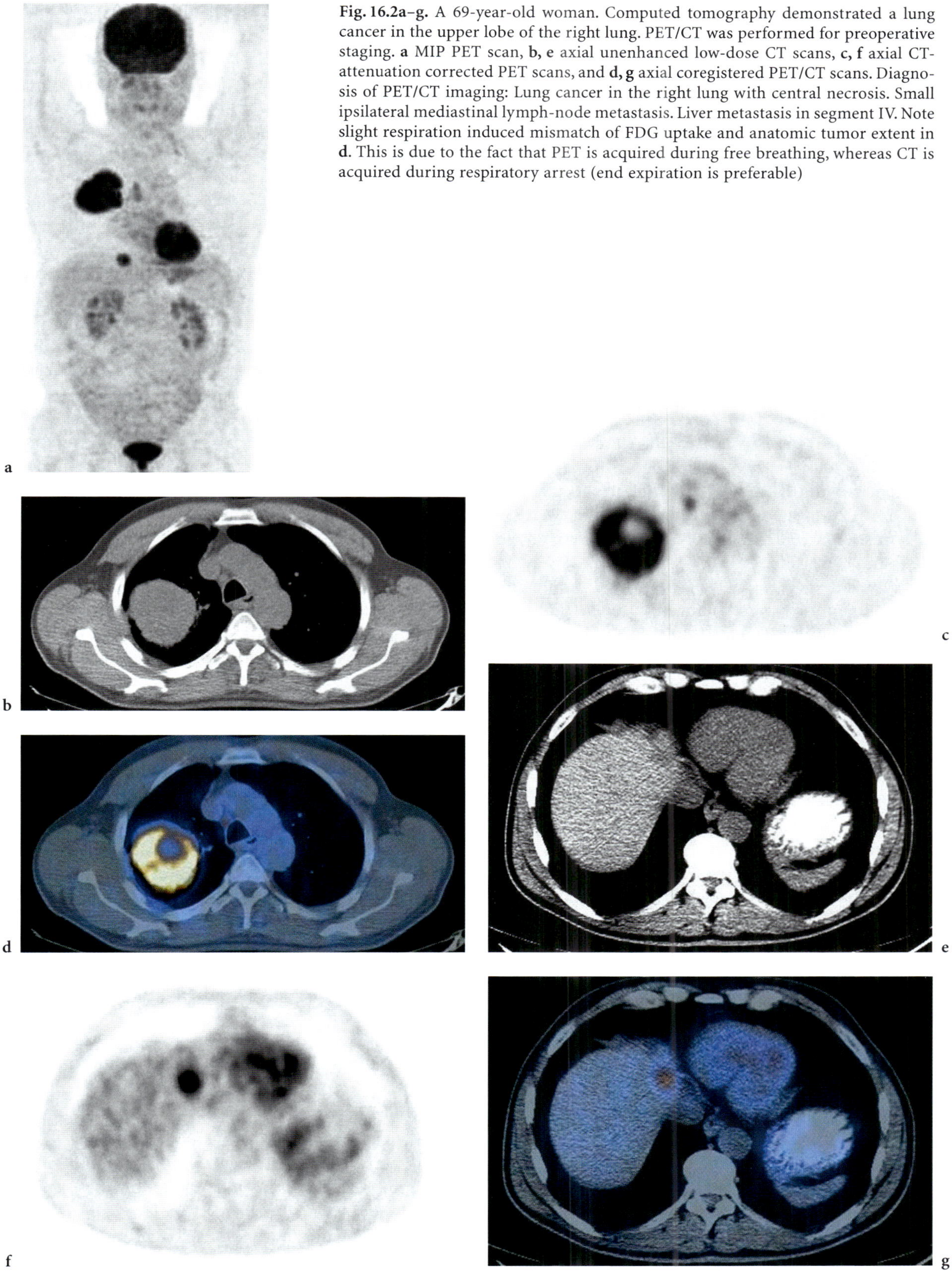

Fig. 16.2a–g. A 69-year-old woman. Computed tomography demonstrated a lung cancer in the upper lobe of the right lung. PET/CT was performed for preoperative staging. **a** MIP PET scan, **b, e** axial unenhanced low-dose CT scans, **c, f** axial CT-attenuation corrected PET scans, and **d, g** axial coregistered PET/CT scans. Diagnosis of PET/CT imaging: Lung cancer in the right lung with central necrosis. Small ipsilateral mediastinal lymph-node metastasis. Liver metastasis in segment IV. Note slight respiration induced mismatch of FDG uptake and anatomic tumor extent in **d**. This is due to the fact that PET is acquired during free breathing, whereas CT is acquired during respiratory arrest (end expiration is preferable)

a b c d e f g

results in a change in the radiation field in approximately 30–40% of patients (Nestle et al. 1999).

16.2.3 N Staging

The PET has proven to be a very effective staging modality for mediastinal nodal staging (Steinert et al. 1997; Vansteenkiste et al. 1998; Dwamena et al. 1999; Pieterman et al. 2000; Hellwig et al. 2001). CT and MR imaging are limited in depicting small mediastinal lymph node metastases. Several studies have demonstrated that FDG PET is significantly more accurate than CT in determination of nodal status (Gupta et al. 1996; Nestle et al. 1999; Steinert et al. 1997). In our own study of 47 patients, PET assigned the correct N stage in 96% of cases and CT was correct in 79% of cases (Steinert et al. 1997). Dwamena et al. (1999) performed a meta-analytic comparison of PET and CT in mediastinal staging of NSCLC. The mean sensitivity and specificity (±95% CI) were 0.79±0.03 and 0.91±0.02, respectively, for PET and 0.60±0.02 and 0.77±0.02, respectively, for CT (Dwamena et al. 1999). These results were confirmed in another meta-analysis with a total of more than 1000 patients (Hellwig et al. 2001).

Even if mediastinoscopy remains the gold standard for mediastinal staging, not all mediastinal lymph nodes are routinely accessed by use of mediastinoscopy, particularly in the para-aortic region and in the aorto-pulmonary window. The limited view through the scope and the single direction in which biopsies can be carried out prevents 100% accuracy. The accuracy of mediastinoscopy is approximately 90% and is surgeon dependent (Patterson et al. 1987). Recently, it has been demonstrated that PET is useful to assist mediastinoscopy. Due to the knowledge of PET information, mediastinoscopy revealed additional mediastinal disease in 6% of patients (Kernstine et al. 2002).

Exact allocation of focal abnormalities on PET to specific lymph nodes is difficult or even impossible due to the poor anatomic information provided by PET alone. The presence and site of lymph node metastases should be recorded according to the revised American Thoracic Society lymph node station-mapping system (Mountain and Dresler 1997). In patients with bulky mediastinal disease or multilevel nodal involvement the assessment of N stage is easy; however, the exact localization of lymph node metastases in the hilus is difficult. Lymph nodes distal to the mediastinal pleural reflection and within the visceral pleura are classified as N1 nodes. Lymph nodes within the mediastinal pleural envelope are classified as N2 nodes. Because the pleura is visible neither in CT nor in PET, the exact classification of a hilar node as N1 node or N2 node remains difficult. The difficulty of PET is the localization of small single nodes, particularly in patients with a mediastinal shift due to an atelectasis or anatomical variants. In our experience, integrated PET/CT imaging will become the new standard of mediastinal staging. The high reliability of integrated PET/CT in the exact localization of extrathoracic vs intrathoracic and mediastinal vs hilar lymph nodes might have very important therapeutic implications.

Until now, our group used non-enhanced CT scans for integrated PET/CT imaging. We could not ethically justify the use of vascular contrast material, because all patients had a conventional contrast-enhanced CT for staging before. In non-enhanced CT scans delineation of vessels was considerably poorer than with contrast enhancement, or impossible; however, in our patient series non-enhanced PET/CT scans are sufficient for planning surgery in approximately 80% of patients. Further evaluation is necessary to define conditions in which the application of intravascular contrast material might have an additional diagnostic impact in integrated PET/CT imaging; however, regarding infiltration of hilar and mediastinal vessels, a relatively low sensitivity, specificity, and accuracy (68, 72, and 70%, respectively) of conventional CT scan with contrast enhancement has been observed (Rendina et al. 1987).

Microscopic foci of metastases within very small lymph nodes cannot be detected with any imaging modality. If there is no increased FDG uptake in PET, integrated PET/CT will not provide further information based on FDG accumulation. Recently, it has been reported that FDG PET after induction therapy is less accurate in mediastinal staging than in staging of untreated NSCLC (Akhurst et al. 2002). The PET overstaged nodal status in 33% of patients, understaged nodal status in 15%, and was correct in 52%. Future studies are required to correlate FDG PET prior to and after treatment.

16.2.4 M Staging

Whole-body FDG PET is an excellent method to screen for extrathoracic metastases (Weder et al. 1998). In a meta-analysis of 581 patients, sensitivity, specificity, and accuracy of FDG PET were 94, 97, and 96%, respectively (Hellwig et al. 2001). Current imaging methods are inadequate for accurate M staging of patients. The PET detects unexpected extrathoracic metastases in 10–20% of patients and changes therapeutic management in approximately 20% of patients. The FDG PET is more accurate than CT in the evaluation of adrenal metastases (Erasmus et al. 1997). Marom et al. (1999) compared the accuracy of FDG PET to conventional imaging in 100 patients with newly diagnosed NSCLC. Comparing bone scintigraphy and FDG PET in detection bone metastases, the accuracy was 87 and 98%, respectively. All hepatic metastases were correctly identified with PET and CT. With CT, however, benign liver lesions were overstaged as metastases; thus, accuracy of PET was superior to CT in the diagnosis of liver metastases.

The clinical significance of a single focal abnormality on PET remains unclear, especially when no morphological alterations occur on CT images. The advantage of integrated PET/CT imaging is the exact localization of a focal abnormality on PET. This was the case in 20% of all patients with extrathoracic metastases in our study on the value of integrated PET/CT (Lardinois et al. 2003).

16.2.5 Recurrent Lung Cancer

A very high accuracy of FDG PET in distinguishing recurrent disease from benign treatment effects has been shown. If PET images demonstrate areas of tumor viability, they can direct biopsy for pathologic confirmation. Patients should be evaluated a minimum of 2 months after completion of therapy. Otherwise post-therapeutic healing processes or radiation pneumonitis may result in false-positive PET findings. These abnormal findings return to normal at variable times without further intervention. In the experience of Inoue et al. (1995), a curvilinear contour of increased FDG accumulation was seen mostly in inflammatory lesions, whereas focal nodular uptake was seen mostly in recurrent tumors. Their data suggest that FDG PET can be clinically used for selecting biopsy sites because of its high sensitivity in detecting recurrent lung cancer.

16.2.6 Pitfalls

False-negative FDG PET results have been reported in pulmonary carcinoid tumors and in bronchioloalveolar carcinomas. Some active infectious or inflammatory lesions may have an increased FDG uptake. Tuberculosis, eosinophilic lung disease, histoplasmosis, aspergillosis, and other infections may have a significant uptake of FDG (Strauss 1996). Furthermore, sarcoid shows a typical bilateral relatively symmetric hilar uptake pattern. Therefore, lesions with an increased FDG accumulation should be histologically confirmed; however, most chronic inflammatory processes do not significantly take up FDG.

It is well known that active muscles accumulate FDG. In some patients with lung cancer an intense focal FDG accumulation is seen in the lower anterior neck just lateral to the midline. Co-registered PET/CT images revealed that the focal FDG uptake was localized in the internal laryngeal muscles (Kamel et al. 2002b). This finding is a result of compensatory laryngeal muscle activation caused by contralateral recurrent laryngeal nerve palsy due to direct nerve invasion by lung cancer of the left mediastinum or lung apices. The knowledge of this finding is important to avoid false-positive PET results.

16.2.7 Small Cell Lung Cancer

The staging procedures for small cell lung cancer (SCLC) do not differ from those for NSCLC. The primary role for imaging is to separate accurately limited disease (LD) from extended disease (ED). Based on the widespread dissemination of SCLC, a battery of imaging tests is performed such as CT of the chest and abdomen, CT, or MRI of the brain and a bone scan. Recently, it has been shown that whole-body FDG PET is a useful tool for staging SCLC (Schumacher et al. 2001). The FDG PET is superior to conventional staging in the detection of all involved sites, and particularly in the assessment of mediastinal lymph node metastases. Our first experience demonstrate that integrated PET/CT imaging in SCLC is a highly valuable tool for planning radiation treatment. It is useful for accurate target definition by reducing the probability of overlooking involved areas.

16.2.8 Malignant Pleural Mesothelioma

Similarly to lung cancer, excellent FDG uptake in malignant pleural mesothelioma (MPM) has been previously described (Marom et al. 2002).

Schneider et al. (2000) demonstrated that PET is particularly valuable for distinguishing between benign and malignant pleural processes. The FDG is not taken up in pleural fibrosis; thus, differential diagnosis of the pleural lesions is possible.

PET imaging is useful in localizing the areas involved with MPM; however, PET and CT are unable to differentiate MPM from pleural adenocarcinoma, so that histology is needed for confirmation.

The role of PET is to document the extent of pleural disease, to establish mediastinal lymph node involvement, to evaluate tumor invasion, and to diagnose recurrence. Our experience demonstrates that integrated PET/CT imaging is an excellent method for staging patients with MPM. With the co-registration of anatomic and metabolic information, the extent of the tumor can be precisely defined. Small mediastinal lymph node metastases can be detected and precisely localized. Integrated PET/CT imaging is helpful in identifying the optimal biopsy site thereby increasing diagnostic accuracy of the histological examination.

References

Akhurst T, Downey RJ, Ginsberg MS et al. (2002) An initial experience with FDG-PET in the imaging of residual disease after induction therapy for lung cancer. Ann Thorac Surg 73:259–266

Burger G, Goerres S, Schoenes A, Buck A, Lonn HR, Schulthess GK von (2002) PET attenuation coefficients from CT images: experimental evaluation of the transformation of CT into PET 511-keV attenuation coefficients. Eur J Nucl Med 29:922–927

Dizendorf E, Hany TF, Buck A, Schulthess GK von, Burger C (in press) Cause and magnitude of the error induced by oral CT contrast agent in CT-based attenuation correction of PET emission studies. J Nucl Med

Dizendorf EV, Treyer V, Schulthess GK von, Hany TF (2002) Application of oral contrast media in coregistrated positron emission tomography–CT. Am J Roentgenol 179:477–481

Dwamena BA, Sonnad SS, Angobaldo JO, Wahl RL (1999) Metastases from non-small cell lung cancer: mediastinal staging in the 1990s – meta-analytic comparison of PET and CT. Radiology 213:530–536

Erasmus JJ, Patz EF, McAdams HP et al. (1997) Evaluation of adrenal masses in patients with bronchogenic carcinoma using 18F-fluorodeoxyglucose positron emission tomography. AJR 168:1357–1362

Goerres GW, Kamel E, Heidelberg TN, Schwitter MR, Burger C, Schulthess GK von (2002) PET–CT image co-registration in the thorax: influence of respiration. Eur J Nucl Med 29: 351–360

Gupta NC, Maloof J, Gunel E (1996) Probability of malignancy in solitary pulmonary nodules using flurine-18-FDF and PET. J Nucl Med 37:943–948

Hany TF, Steinert HC, Goerres GW, Buck A, Schulthess GK von (2002a) Improvement of diagnostic accuracy of PET imaging using a high performance in-line PET–CT system: preliminary results. Radiology 225:575–581

Hany TF, Gharehpapagh E, Kamel EM, Buck A, Himms-Hagen J, Schulthess GK von (2002b) Brown adipose tissue: a factor to consider in symmetrical tracer uptake in the neck and upper chest region. Eur J Nucl Med 29:1393–1398

Hellwig D, Ukena D, Paulsen F, Bamberg M, Kirsch CM (2001) Metaanalyse zum Stellenwert der Positronen-Emissions-Tomographie mit F-18-Fluorodesoxyglukose (FDG-PET) bei Lungentumoren (in German). Pneumologie 55: 367–377

Inoue T, Kim E, Komaki R et al. (1995) Detecting recurrent or residual lung cancer with FDG-PET. J Nucl Med 36: 788–793

Kamel E, Hany TF, Burger C et al. (2002a) CT vs 68Ge attenuation correction in a combined PET/CT system: evaluation of the effect of lowering the CT tube current. Eur J Med 29:312–318

Kamel E, Goerres GW, Burger C, Schulthess GK von, Steinert HC (2002b) Detection of recurrent laryngeal nerve palsy in patients with lung cancer using PET–CT image fusion. Radiology 224:153–156

Kernstine KH, McLaughlin KA, Menda Y et al. (2002) Can FDG PET reduce the need for mediastinoscopy in potentially resectable nonsmall cell lung cancer? Ann Thorac Surg 73:394–402

Kinahan PE, Townsend DW, Beyer T, Sashin D (1998) Attenuation correction for a combined 3D PET/CT scanner. Med Phys 25:2046–2053

Lardinois D, Weder W, Hany TF, Kamel EM, Korom S, Seifert B, von Schulthess GK, Steinert HC (2003) Integrated PET/CT imaging improves staging on non-small-cell lung cancer. N Engl J Med. 348(25):2500–2507

Marom EM, McAdams HP, Erasmus JJ (1999) Staging non-small cell lung cancer with whole-body PET. Radiology 212:803–809

Marom EM, Erasmus JJ, Pass HI, Patz EF Jr (2002) The role of imaging in malignant pleural MPM. Semin Oncol 29: 26–35

Mountain CF, Dresler CM (1997) Regional lymph node classification for lung cancer staging. Chest 11:1718–1723

Nestle U, Walter K, Schmidt S, Licht N et al. (1999) 18F-deoxyglucose positron emission tomography (FDG-PET) for the planning of radiotherapy in lung cancer: high impact in patients with atelectasis. Int J Radiat Oncol Biol Phys 44:593–597

Patterson GA, Ginsberg RJ, Poon PY et al. (1987) A prospective evaluation of magnetic resonance imaging, computed tomography, and mediastinoscopy in the preoperative assessment of mediastinal node status in bronchogenic carcinoma. J Thorac Cardiovasc Surg 94:679–684

Pieterman RM, van Putten JWG, Meuzelaar JJ et al. (2000) Preoperative staging of non-small-cell lung cancer with positron-emission tommography. N Engl J Med 343: 254–261

Rendina EA, Bognolo DA, Mineo TC et al. (1987) Computed tomography for the evaluation of intrathoracic invasion by lung cancer. J Thorac Cardiovasc Surg 94:57–63

Schneider DB, Clary-Macy C, Challa S et al. (2000) Positron emission tomography with F18-fluorodeoxyglucose in the staging and preoperative evaluation of malignant pleural MPM. J Thorac Cardiovasc Surg 120:128–133

Schumacher T, Brink I, Mix M et al. (2001) FDG-PET imaging

for the staging and follow-up of small cell lung cancer. Eur J Nucl Med 28:483–488

Steinert HC, Hauser M, Allemann F et al. (1997) Non-small cell lung cancer: nodal staging with FDG PET versus CT with correlative lymph node mapping and sampling. Radiology 202:441–446

Strauss LG (1996) Fluorine-18 deoxyglucose and false-positive results: a major problem in the diagnosis of oncological patients. Eur J Nucl Med 23:1409–1414

Vansteenkiste JF, Stroobants SG, de Leyn PR et al. (1998) Lymph node staging in non-small cell lung cancer with FDG PET scan: a prospective study on 690 lymph node stations from 68 patients. J Clin Oncol 16:2142–2149

Schulthess GK von (ed) (2003) Clinical molecular anatomic imaging: PET, PET/CT and SPECT/CT. Lippincott Williams and Willkins, New York

Schulthess GK von (200) Cost considerations regarding an integrated CT–PET system. Eur Radiol 10:S377–S380

Weder W, Schmid R, Bruchhaus H, Hillinger S, Schulthess GK von, Steinert HC (1998) Detection of extrathoracic metastases by positron emission tomography in lung cancer. Ann Thorac Surg 66:886–893

Pulmonary Embolism / Thoracic Vessels

17 Multidetector-Row CT Angiography of the Pulmonary Circulation

U. J. Schoepf, J. M. Martensen, P. Costello

CONTENTS

17.1 Introduction

The introduction of multidetector-row CT (MDCT) into clinical radiology has decisively reemphasized and reinvigorated the cardinal role of CT as the premier imaging modality for imaging the pulmonary circulation. The specific requirements of diagnostic imaging in the high-resolution environment of the chest, with fast moving organs and the need for image acquisition during apnea, are ideally met by multidetector-row CT technology. The scan speed of current generation MDCT scanners translates into the ability of scanning the entire chest within a few seconds. Despite sub-millimeter resolution, this results in motion-free images even in the sickest of patients. Use of thin slices was shown to significantly improve the detection of minute vascular pathology, such as small peripheral pulmonary emboli (Ghaye et al. 2001; Schoepf et al. 2002). For a comprehensive diagnosis of focal and diffuse lung disease, both, contiguous images and high-resolution CT can be reconstructed from the same single acquisition, without scanning the patient twice (Schoepf et al. 2001). ECG synchronization with MDCT is a valuable tool to improve image quality and diagnostic accuracy by reducing motion artifacts as potential sources of diagnostic error (Schoepf et al. 1999); however, while MDCT provides innumerable opportunities, its unique characteristics also pose hitherto unknown challenges to its users. The large-volume data sets generated by current and future generations of high-resolution CT scanners are a logistical problem that threatens to overburden the radiologist with diagnostic information. Also, although MDCT can be used in ways which result in a reduction of patient radiation dose, with many applications the patient dose is likely to increase if no adequate precautions are taken. Solutions, however, are on the horizon and are comprehensively discussed throughout this book. The practice of radiology is quickly adapting to novel concepts of data visualization embracing 2D and 3D display techniques. Effective means for reducing radiation dose are being implemented. Tools for facilitating the analysis of large-volume MDCT data sets for accurate detection of pathology are continuously being refined. Herein we discuss specific improvements, novel challenges, and sophisticated solutions, which the advent of ever faster MDCT acquisition techniques has brought about for imaging of the pulmonary circulation.

U. J. Schoepf, MD
Department of Radiology, Brigham and Women's Hospital, Harvard Medical School, 75 Francis Street, Boston, MA 02115, USA
J. M. Martensen, MD
Department of Radiology, Brigham and Women's Hospital, Harvard Medical School, 75 Francis Street, Boston, MA 02115, USA
P. Costello, MD
Department of Radiology, Brigham and Women's Hospital, Harvard Medical School, 75 Francis Street, Boston, MA 02115, USA

17.2 Multidetector-Row CT Angiography of Pulmonary Embolism

17.2.1 Imaging Pulmonary Embolism: The Paradigm Is Shifting

Although increasingly sophisticated clinical algorithms for "bed-side" exclusion of pulmonary embolism (PE) are being developed, based mainly on a negative d-dimer test (Wells et al. 2001; Kruip et al. 2002; Dunn et al. 2002; Brown et al. 2002), there is a high and seemingly increasing demand for imaging tests for suspected PE.

Invasive pulmonary angiography is still regarded by some as the gold standard technique but in reality is rarely ever used as such (Schluger et al. 1994; Khorasani et al. 1997; Crawford et al. 2001; Prologo and Glauser 2002). The main reason for the latter appears to be the invasiveness of this procedure, although the incidence of complications with contemporary technique is low (Stein et al. 1992; Zuckerman et al. 1996). More importantly, there is mounting evidence for the limitations of this technique for the unequivocal diagnosis of isolated peripheral pulmonary emboli: at two recent analyses the inter-observer agreement rates for detection of subsegmental emboli by selective pulmonary angiography ranged between only 45 and 66% (Diffin et al. 1998; Stein et al. 1999). Given such limitations, use of this test as an objective and readily reproducible tool for the verification of findings at competing imaging modalities as to the presence or absence of PE seems questionable and the status of pulmonary angiography as the standard of reference for diagnosis of PE is tarnished.

Use of nuclear medicine imaging, once the first study in the diagnostic algorithm of PE, appears to be declining (Schibany et al. 2001; Leveau 2002) due to the high percentage of indeterminate studies (73% of all performed; PIOPED Investigators 1990) and poor inter-observer correlation (Blachere et al. 2000). Revised criteria for the interpretation of ventilation–perfusion scans (Stein et al. 1996; Stein and Gottschalk 2000) and novel technologies in nuclear medicine, such as single photon emission tomography (SPECT; Palmer et al. 2001; Bajc et al. 2002), can decrease the ratio of indeterminate scintigraphic studies, but cannot offset the limitations inherent to a mere functional imaging test (Garg et al. 1998).

Contrast-enhanced magnetic resonance (MR) angiography has been evaluated for the diagnosis of acute PE (Meaney et al. 1997; Roberts et al. 1999; Gupta et al. 1999; Oudkerk et al. 2002); however, the acquisition protocols that are currently available for MR pulmonary angiography lack sufficient spatial resolution for reliable evaluation of peripheral pulmonary arteries (Gupta et al. 1999; Oudkerk et al. 2002). More importantly, this modality has not seen widespread use in the acutely ill patient with suspected PE due to lack of general availability, relatively long examination times, and difficulties in patient monitoring.

This leaves us with computed tomography (CT), which for most practical purposes has become the first-line imaging test after lower-extremity ultrasound for the assessment of patients with suspected PE in daily clinical routine. The most important advantage of CT over other imaging modalities is that both mediastinal and parenchymal structures are evaluated, and thrombus is directly visualized (Fig. 17.1; Gurney 1993; Woodard 1997). Studies have shown that up to two-thirds of patients with an initial suspicion of PE receive another diagnosis (Hull et al. 1994), some with potentially life-threatening diseases, such as aortic dissection, pneumonia, lung cancer, and pneumothorax (van Rossum et al. 1998; Fig. 17.2). Most of these differential diagnoses are amenable to CT visualization, so that in many cases a specific etiology for the patients' symptoms or important additional diagnoses can be established (Garg et al. 1998). The inter-observer agreement for CT is better than for scintigraphy (van Rossum et al. 1998). In a recent study inter-observer agreement for the diagnosis of PE was excellent for spiral CT angiography (=0.72) and only moderate for ventilation–perfusion lung scanning (=0.22; Blachere et al. 2000). Computed tomography also appears to be the most cost-effective modality in the diagnostic algorithm of PE compared with algorithms that do not include CT, but are based on other imaging modalities (ultrasound, scintigraphy, pulmonary angiography; van Erkel et al. 1996). Also, there is some indication that CT may not only be used for evaluating thoracic anatomy in suspected PE but could also to some degree allow deriving physiologic parameters on lung perfusion at single-slice, electron-beam, and multidetector-row CT (Groell et al. 1999; Schoepf et al. 2000; Wildberger et al. 2001). The main impediment for the unanimous embrace of CT as the modality of choice for the diagnosis of acute PE have been limitations of this modality for the accurate detection of small peripheral emboli. Early studies comparing single-slice CT to selective pulmonary angiography demonstrated CT's high accuracy for the detection of PE to the segmental arterial level (Remy-Jardin et al. 1992, 1996; Teigen et al. 1995; Goodman et al. 1995) but suggested that subsegmental pulmonary emboli may be overlooked by CT

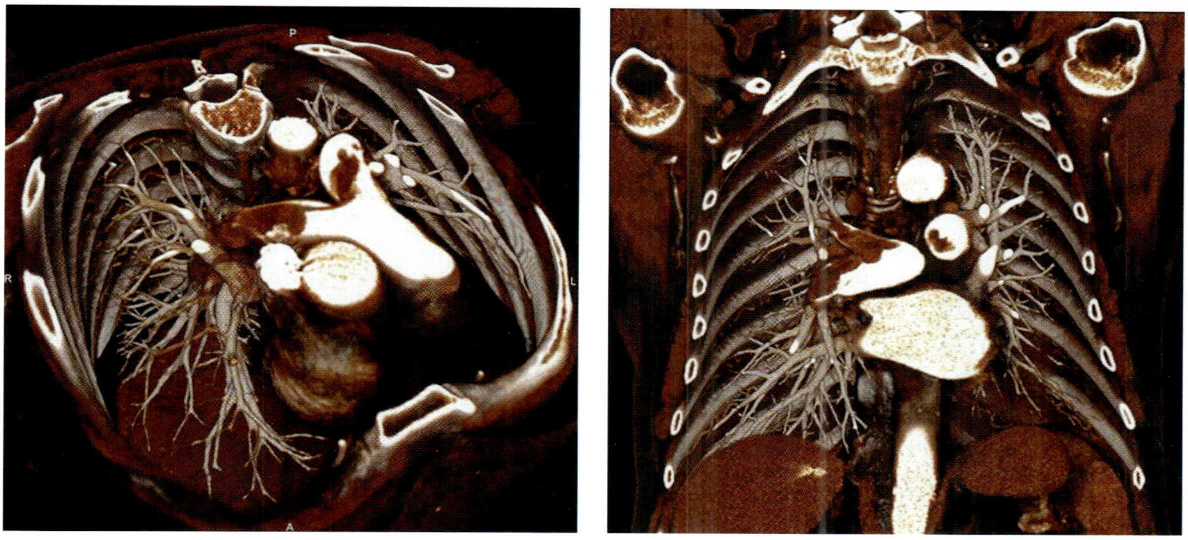

Fig. 17.1a, b. A 72-year-old man with extensive, acute central pulmonary embolism with "saddle embolus" extending into both central pulmonary arteries. Contrast enhanced 16-slice CT examination. Colored volume-rendering technique seen from a frontal cranial (**a**) and coronal (**b**) perspective allows intuitive visualization of location and extent of embolism and facilitates communication with referring physicians

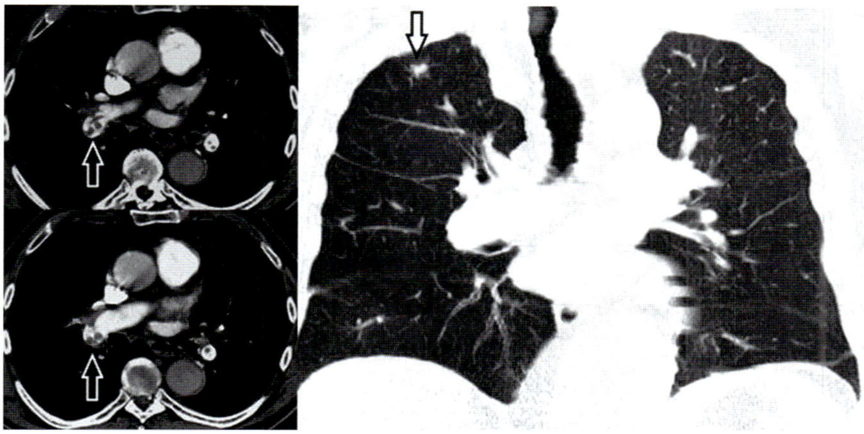

Fig. 17.2. Incidentally found T1 peripheral adenocarcinoma (*arrow, right panel*) in the right upper lobe of a patient with central pulmonary embolism (*arrows, left panels*). Contrast-enhanced 4-slice MDCT study. Axial sections (*left panels*) and coronal multiplanar reformat (*right panel*). Direct visualization of emboli and relevant alternative or additional disease is the key advantage of CT over competing modalities for the diagnosis of pulmonary embolism (PE)

scanning. The degree of accuracy that can be achieved for the visualization of subsegmental pulmonary arteries and for the detection of emboli in these vessels with single-slice, dual-slice, and electron-beam CT scanners was found to range between 61 and 79% (Goodman et al. 1995; Remy-Jardin et al. 1997; Qanadli et al. 2000; Schoepf et al. 2000).

17.2.2 Advantages of Multidetector-Row CT for PE Imaging

In the past few years CT has seen decisive dynamic developments, mainly brought about by the advent of multidetector-row CT technology (McCollough and Zink 1999; Hu et al. 2000). The current generation of 4-slice, 8-slice, and16-slice CT scanners now allows for acquisition of the entire chest with 1-mm or sub-millimeter resolution within a short single breath hold of now less than 10 s in the case of 16-slice CT (Fig. 17.3). The ability to cover substantial anatomic volumes with high in-plane and through-plane spatial resolution has brought with it a number of decisive advantages. Short breath-hold times were shown to benefit imaging of patients with suspected PE and underlying lung disease and should reduce the percentage of non-diagnostic CT pulmonary angiography investigations (Remy-Jardin et al. 2002). The near isotropic nature of high-resolution multidetector-row CT data lends

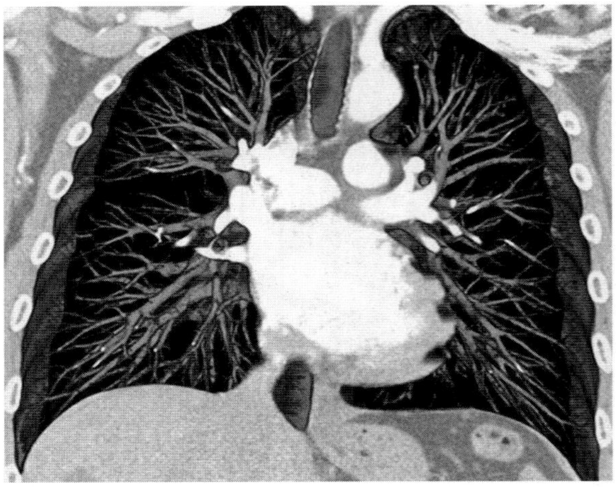

Fig. 17.3. Normal pulmonary vessels in a 56-year-old man presenting with mild chest pain after a long-distance flight. Contrast-enhanced 16-slice CT examination covers the entire chest within a scan time of 10 s allowing analysis of even the most peripheral pulmonary vessels with fine detail

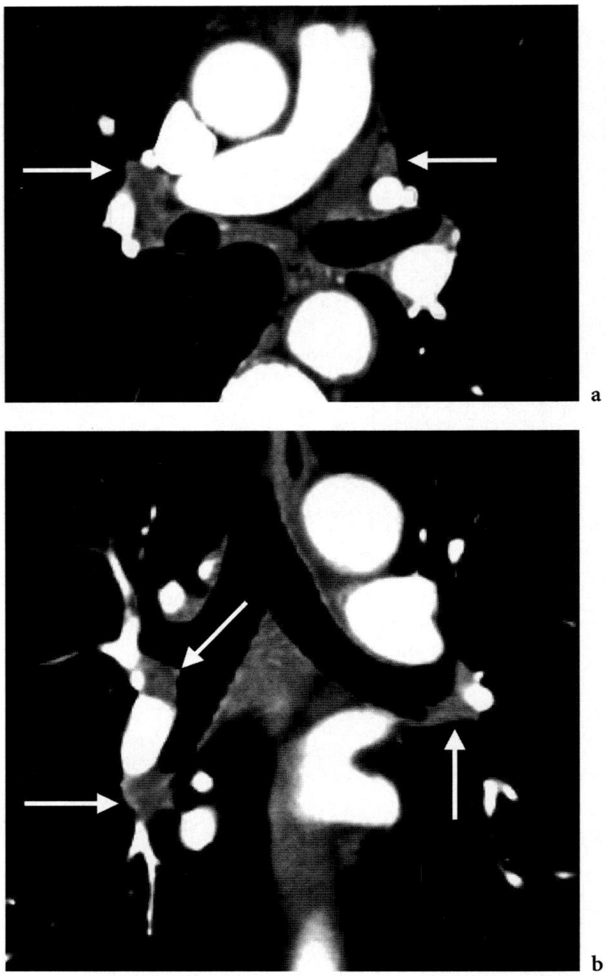

Fig. 17.4a, b. Contrast-enhanced CT pulmonary angiography in a patient with suspected acute PE. Lymphatic tissue in the mediastinum and in the pulmonary hilum (*arrows*) may be misinterpreted as embolic filling defects in central pulmonary vessels by less experienced observers if only axial sections (**a**) are used for diagnosis. Coronal multiplanar reformats of a high-resolution 4-slice multidetector-row CT acquisition (**b**) allow better differentiation of lymphatic tissue and vessels and may reduce sources of diagnostic error

itself to 2D and 3D visualization. This may in some instances improve PE diagnosis (Remy-Jardin et al. 1995). Potential pitfalls for PE diagnosis that have been cited relate to the incorrect interpretation of hilar lymphatic tissue as intraluminal filling defects; however, even for less experienced observers, diagnostic errors such as this are easy to avoid if familiarity with this potential pitfall is ensured. In the very few cases with residual diagnostic insecurity 3D visualization of multidetector-row CT data may be helpful in clarifying the relationship of hilar lymphatic tissue to the central pulmonary arteries, aid diagnosis in such instances, and help avoid diagnostic pitfalls (Fig. 17.4; Remy et al. 1998). The 3D visualization is generally of greater importance for conveying information on localization and extent of embolic disease to referring clinicians in an intuitive and palatable manner (Fig. 17.1).

Probably the most important advantage of high-resolution multidetector-row CT pulmonary angiography is the improved diagnosis of small peripheral emboli. Still with single-slice CT it could be shown that superior visualization of segmental and subsegmental pulmonary arteries can be achieved with thinner slice widths (e.g. 2 vs 3 mm; Remy-Jardin et al. 1997). however, with single-slice CT the range which can be covered with thin slice widths within one breath hold is limited (Remy-Jardin et al. 1997; Schoepf et al. 2000). The high spatial resolution of 1-mm or sub-millimeter-collimation data sets now allows evaluation of pulmonary vessels down to sixth-order branches (Ghaye et al. 2001) and significantly increases the detection rate of segmental and subsegmental pulmonary emboli (Fig. 17.5; Schoepf et al. 2002). This increase in the rate of detection is likely due to reduced volume averaging and the accurate analysis of progressively thinner vessels by use of thinner sections. Improved visualization with high-resolution multidetector-row CT is most striking in peripheral arteries with an anatomic course parallel to the scan plane. Such vessels tend to be most affected by volume averaging if thicker slices are used (Schoepf et al. 2002). The high spatial resolution along the scan axis of a thin-collimation multidetector-row CT data set, however, allows an accurate evaluation of the full course of such vessels. The inter-observer correlation for confident

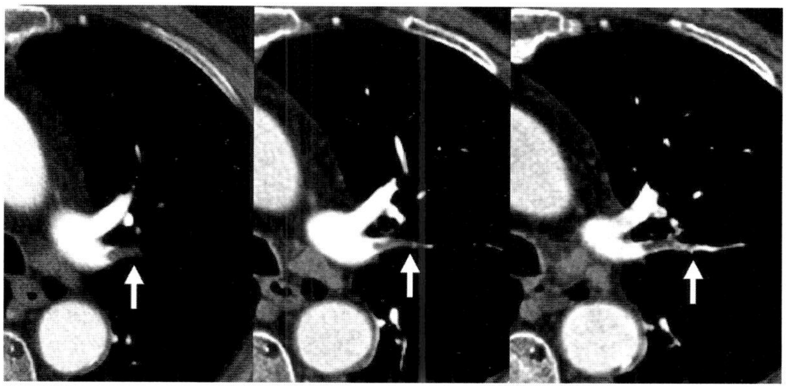

Fig. 17.5. Three-millimeter (*left*) and 2-mm (*middle*) axial reconstructions of a contrast-enhanced multislice CT data set suggest the presence of thrombus in a segmental artery supplying the posterior segment of the left upper lobe of the lung (*arrow*). Only 1-mm reconstruction (*right*) of the data set allows following the entire course of the segmental artery and unanimous visualization of the filling defect within the posterior subsegmental branch

detection of subsegmental emboli with high-resolution multidetector-row CT by far exceeds the reproducibility of other imaging modalities, i.e., invasive pulmonary angiography (Schoepf et al. 2002).

17.2.3 The Quandary of the Isolated Subsegmental Embolus

While traditional technical limitations of CT for the diagnosis of pulmonary emboli appear to have been successfully overcome with the advent of multidetector-row CT, we are now facing new challenges that are a direct product of our increased technical prowess. Small peripheral clots that might have gone unnoticed in the past are now frequently detected (Fig. 17.6).

While, based on a good-quality multidetector-row CT scan, there may be no doubt as to the presence of a small isolated clot, such findings will be increasingly difficult to prove in a correlative manner. Animal experiments that use artificial emboli as an independent gold standard indicate that high-resolution 4-slice multidetector-row CT is at least as accurate as invasive pulmonary angiography for the detection of small peripheral emboli (Baile et al. 2000); however, it appears highly unlikely that pulmonary angiography will be performed on a patient merely to prove the presence of an isolated embolus. Also, given the limited inter-observer correlation of pulmonary angiography which was pointed out previously (Diffin et al. 1998; Stein et al. 1999), it appears doubtful that this latter test, even if performed, would provide useful and adequate correlative proof for findings at high-resolution multidetector-row CT. Broad-based studies, such as PIOPED II, which set out to establish the efficacy of multidetector-row CT in suspected PE, account for this latter fact by using a composite reference test based on ventilation/perfusion scanning, ultrasound of the lower extremities, pulmonary angiography, and contrast venography to establish the PE status of the patient (Gottschalk et al. 2002).

Perhaps more importantly there is a growing sense of insecurity within the clinical community about how to manage patients in whom a diagnosis of isolated peripheral embolism has been established. It has been shown that 6 (PIOPED Investigators 1990) to 30% (Oser et al. 1996) of patients with documented PE present with clots only in subsegmental and smaller arteries, but the clinical significance of small peripheral emboli in subsegmental pulmonary arteries in the absence of central emboli is uncertain. It is assumed that one important function of the lung is to prevent small emboli from entering the arterial circulation (Gurney 1993). Such emboli are thought to form even in healthy individuals, although this notion has never been substantiated (Tetalman et al. 1973). Controversy also exists about whether the treatment of small emboli, once detected, may result in a better clinical outcome for patients (Remy-Jardin et al. 1996; Novelline et al. 1978; Goodman et al. 2000). There is little disagreement, however, that the presence of peripheral emboli may be an indicator for current deep vein thrombosis, thus potentially heralding more severe embolic events (Hull et al. 1994; Oser et al. 1996; Patriquin et al. 1998). A burden of small peripheral emboli may also have prognostic relevance in individuals with cardiopulmonary restrictions (Goodman et al. 2000; Oser et al. 1996; Gurney 1993) and for the development of chronic pulmonary hypertension in patients with thromboembolic disease (Oser et al. 1996).

Perhaps the most practical and realistic scenario for studying the efficacy of CT for the evaluation of patients with suspected PE is assessing patient outcome. There is a growing body of experience concerning the negative predictive value of a negative CT study and patient outcome if anticoagulation is subsequently withheld (Garg et al. 1999; Blachere et al. 2000;

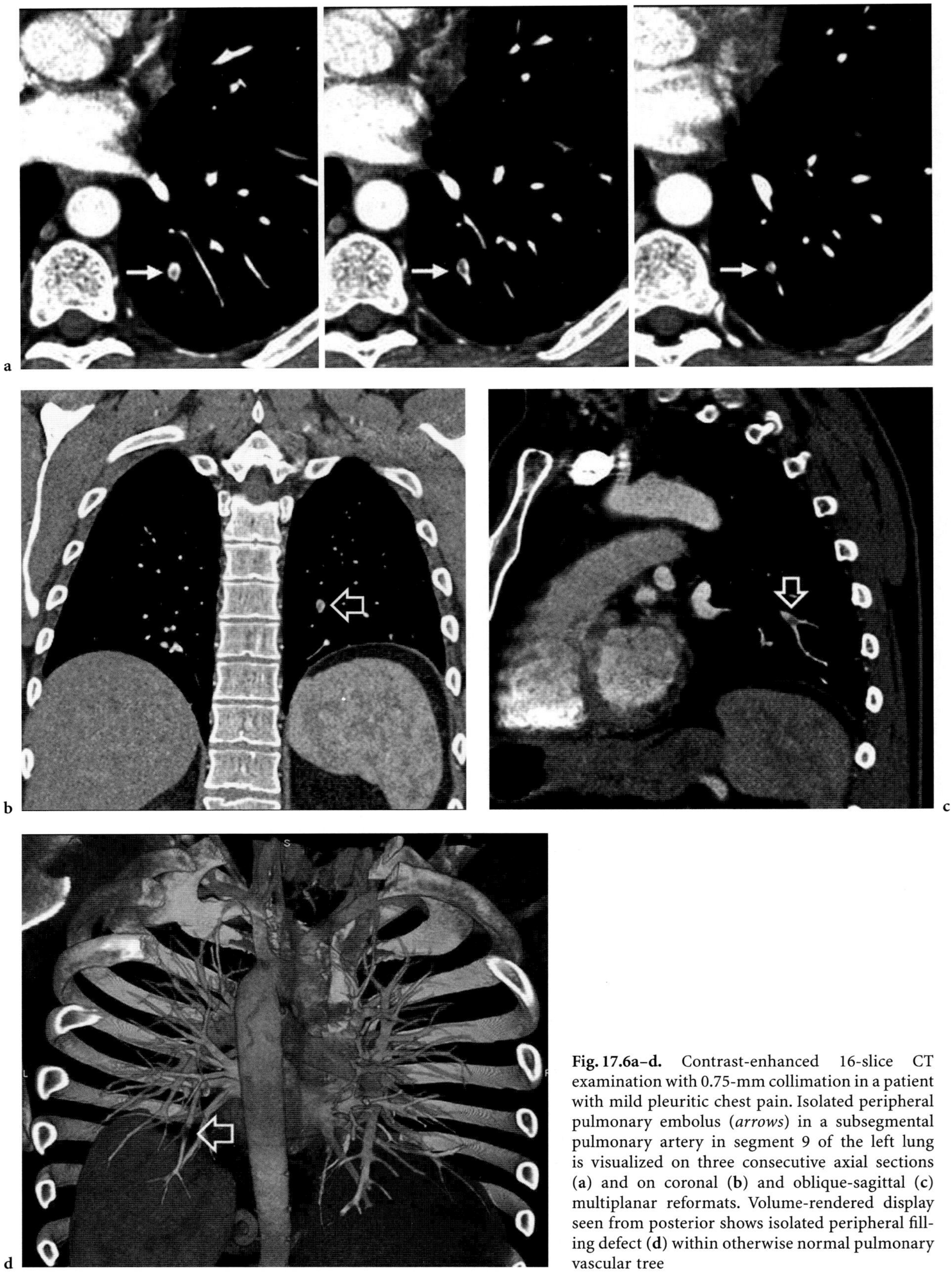

Fig. 17.6a–d. Contrast-enhanced 16-slice CT examination with 0.75-mm collimation in a patient with mild pleuritic chest pain. Isolated peripheral pulmonary embolus (*arrows*) in a subsegmental pulmonary artery in segment 9 of the left lung is visualized on three consecutive axial sections (**a**) and on coronal (**b**) and oblique-sagittal (**c**) multiplanar reformats. Volume-rendered display seen from posterior shows isolated peripheral filling defect (**d**) within otherwise normal pulmonary vascular tree

Goodman et al. 2000; Gottsater et al. 2001; Ost et al. 2001; Tillie-Leblond et al. 2002; Remy-Jardin et al. 2002; Swensen et al. 2002; Musset 2002). According to these studies the negative predictive value of a negative CT study is high, regardless of whether multidetector-row technology is used (Remy-Jardin et al. 2002) or whether underlying lung disease is present (Tillie-Leblond et al. 2002). The frequency of a subsequent clinical diagnosis of PE or DVT after a negative CT pulmonary angiogram is low and lower than that after a negative or low-probability V-Q scan (Goodman et al. 2000); thus, even single-slice CT is a reliable imaging tool for excluding clinically relevant PE so that it appears that anticoagulation can be safely withheld when the CT scan is normal and of good diagnostic quality (Goodman et al. 2000; Swensen et al. 2002).

With multidetector-row CT technology past limitations of CT for the diagnosis of PE should be effectively overcome, and for all practical purposes CT has become established as the first-line modality for imaging patients with suspected PE. Computed tomography has become an attractive means for a safe, highly accurate, and cost-effective diagnosis of pulmonary embolism. The lack of a clinically available gold standard for the diagnosis of PE suggests that the medical community should replace theoretical and academic discussions on the relative value of different imaging modalities with more realistic approaches based on patient outcome. Retrospective and prospective studies (Garg et al. 1999; Blachere et al. 2000; Goodman et al. 2000; Gottsater et al. 2001; Ost et al. 2001; Tillie-Leblond et al. 2002; Remy-Jardin et al. 2002; Swensen et al. 2002; Musset 2002) have demonstrated the high negative predictive value for a normal multidetector-row CT pulmonary angiography study. Once it is accepted by the medical community that a negative CT safely excludes the presence of pulmonary embolism, we believe use of CT for PE diagnosis will be unanimously embraced as the reference modality.

17.3 Multidetector-Row CT for Evaluating Pulmonary Hypertension

Pulmonary hypertension (PH) of the precapillary pulmonary circulation is a diagnostic challenge. The host of potential underlying disorders includes idiopathic disease, recurrent embolism, and structural lung changes among other more readily identifiable causes (Frazier et al. 2000). Computed tomography has traditionally been an important tool in the diagnostic algorithm of PH allowing for an accurate assessment of both, pathogenesis and extent of the disease. High-resolution CT (HRCT) is the gold standard to evaluate a patient with suspected PH for structural lung changes that may cause increased pre- or postcapillary pressure within the lung vessels. Mosaic attenuation on HRCT, combined with distal pruning of pulmonary arteries, is a sign of impaired pulmonary perfusion due to recurrent peripheral embolism as the underlying cause (Fig. 17.7). Contrast-enhanced CT allows for direct visualization of chronic thromboembolic changes and helps to determine if the disease is amenable to surgical thrombendarterectomy (Figs. 17.7, 17.8). If neither structural lung changes nor signs of thromboembolism are found in the absence of other identifiable etiologies for PH, such as congenital heart disease or tumor embolism, a diagnosis of primary pulmonary hypertension is usually considered. Since the differential diagnosis of PH includes diseases with both focal and diffuse character, the entire pathology frequently cannot be appreciated with a single CT technique. Thick-collimation single-slice CT may not suffice to assess interstitial changes. If only HRCT is performed, focal pathology, such as thromboembolism, is easily missed due to the high-frequency reconstruction algorithms and because scans are acquired at only every 10–20 mm. If single-slice CT is used for evaluation of patients with suspected PH, it is often necessary to perform both a contrast-enhanced spiral acquisition and HRCT for a comprehensive assessment of the underlying pathology. Now a single, breath-held, thin-collimation multidetector-row CT acquisition generates a set of raw data that provides all options for image reconstruction, addressing multiple diagnostic problems by performing a single contrast-enhanced scan (Figs. 17.7–17.9; Schoepf et al. 2001). In patients with suspected PH we routinely perform a thin-slice reconstruction of the entire chest, which can detect pulmonary emboli with high accuracy. In addition, from the same set of raw data 5-mm contiguous lung sections and HRCT sections at every 1 cm are routinely performed; thus, from a single set of raw data a comprehensive analysis of gross and diffuse lung changes and of thromboembolic disease becomes feasible.

17.4 Multidetector-Row CT Imaging of Systemic Arterial Supply to the Lung

Disorders of the systemic arterial supply to the lung are a not infrequent cause of massive hemoptysis and can

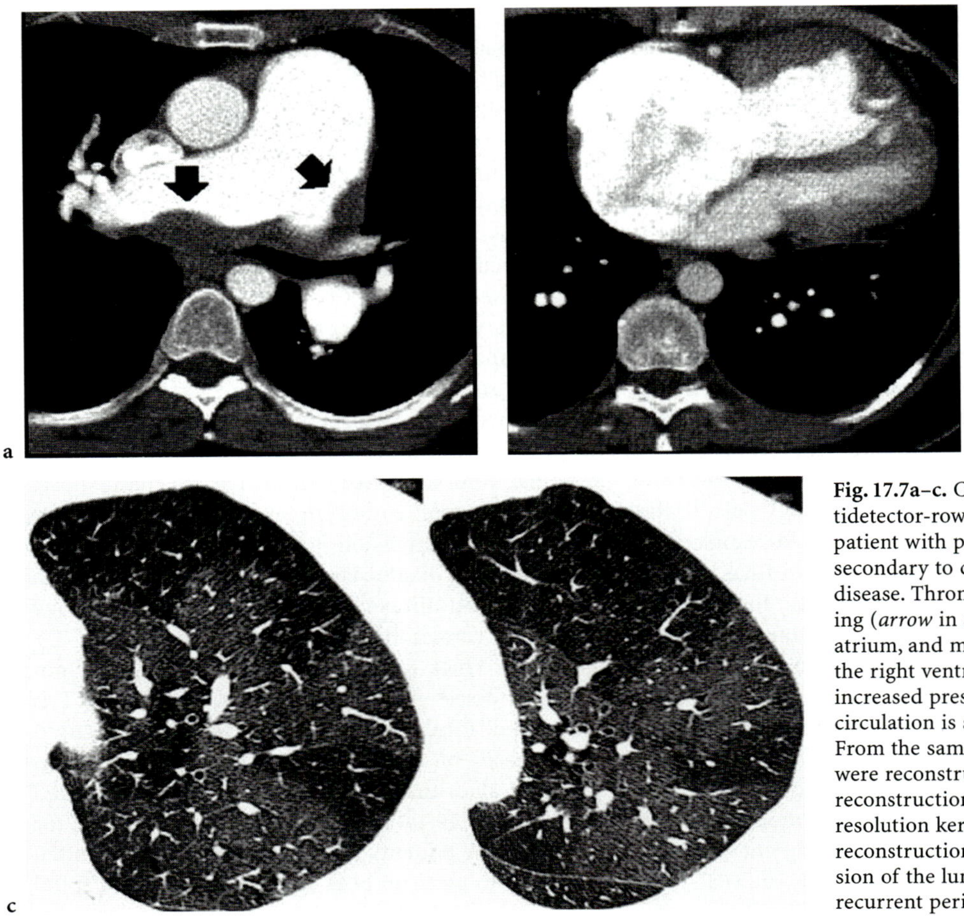

Fig. 17.7a–c. Contrast-enhanced multidetector-row CT angiography in a patient with pulmonary hypertension secondary to chronic thromboembolic disease. Thromboembolic wall thickening (*arrow* in **a**), dilatation of the right atrium, and muscular hypertrophy of the right ventricle (**b**) in response to increased pressure in the pulmonary circulation is seen on the axial images. From the same data set 1-mm sections were reconstructed with a 10-mm reconstruction increment and a high-resolution kernel. High-resolution reconstructions display mosaic perfusion of the lung parenchyma due to recurrent peripheral embolism (**c**)

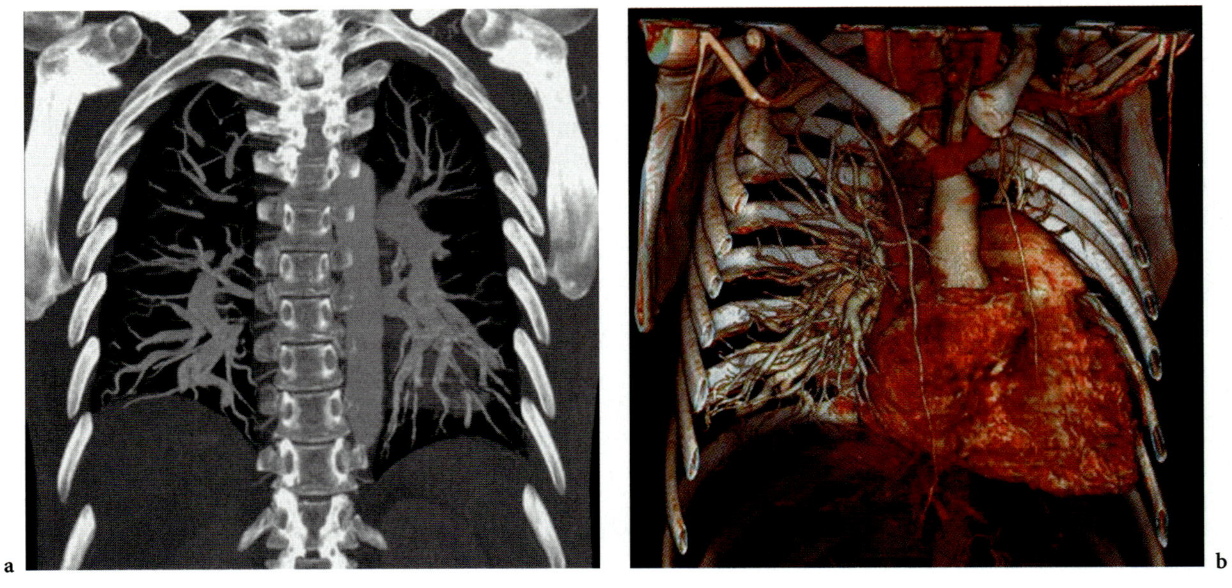

Fig. 17.8a, b. Patient with long-standing idiopathic pulmonary hypertension. Maximum intensity projection (**a**) and volume rendering (**b**) of a contrast-enhanced 16-slice CT data set, acquired in less than 10 s, demonstrates tortuous, cork-screw-like pulmonary arteries with distal pruning as hallmarks of the disease

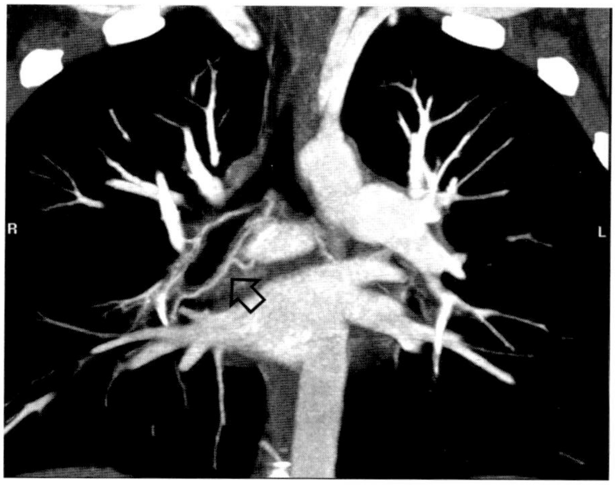

a

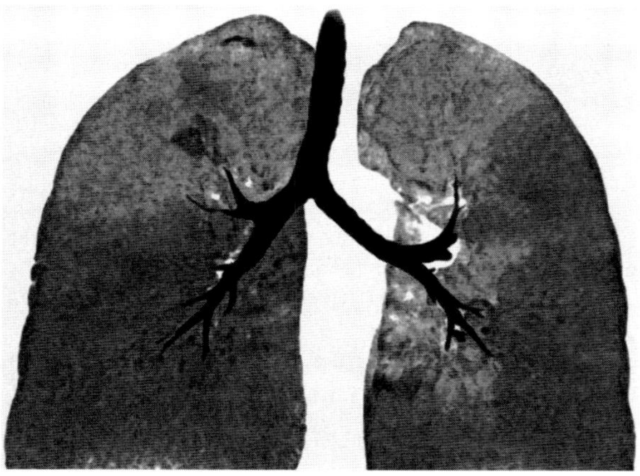

b

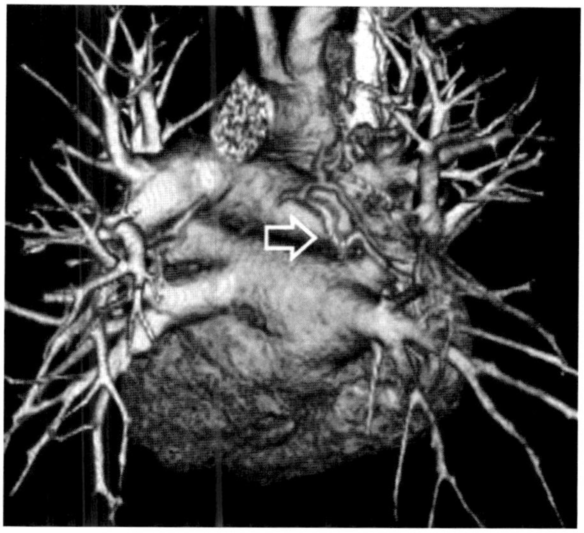

c

Fig. 17.9a–c. A 16-slice MDCT angiogram in a patient with long-standing thromboembolic disease. The pulmonary arteries in the right lower lobe are most affected by recurrent thromboembolism and appear obliterated on coronal maximum intensity projections (**a**). Diminished lung perfusion in the affected lower lobes of the lung with maintained perfusion in the upper lobes is demonstrated on coronal minimum intensity projections. (**b**) Blood flow to the right lower lobe is maintained via the bronchial arteries, which are hypertrophied (*arrow* in **a** and **c**) and have formed collaterals bypassing occluded and obliterated pulmonary arteries

lead to death, mainly by asphyxiation (Crocco et al. 1968). Systemic arterialization of the lung parenchyma is most often congenital in which case an aberrant systemic artery supplies the parenchyma involved in congenital pulmonary venolobar syndrome or bronchopulmonary sequestration (Fig. 17.10; Ellis 1991). Often these congenital conditions go unnoticed until hemoptysis occurs, leading to diagnostic work-up and detection of the disorder.

Bronchial arterial embolization, as a treatment for massive and recurrent hemoptysis, was first described in 1973 by Remy et al. (1974), and has since been established as a safe and effective procedure for treatment of this condition (Michelle et al. 2002). The planning and successful performance of this treatment depends on exact knowledge of the pulmonary vascular anatomy and the location of the hemorrhage. Computed tomography is readily available at most institutions, allowing for a fast diagnosis, even in patients with acute hemoptysis. Thin-section multidetector-row CT of the thorax is capable of providing high-resolution images and CT angiograms in a single session. This enables evaluation of structural changes of the lung parenchyma as well as of pulmonary vessels (Schoepf et al. 2001) which makes this technology very suitable for comprehensive imaging of disorders of the systemic arterial supply of the lung.

Chronic inflammatory disease can result in acquired systemic arterialization of the lungs, by causing anastomoses between pulmonary and systemic arteries. Most often the anastomoses develop between bronchial and pulmonary arteries within the lung parenchyma, but inflammatory processes in the lung may also cause transpleural anastomoses between pulmonary and systemic nonbronchial arteries. This can occur when an inflammatory process causes pleural adhesion resulting in neovascularization from regional systemic arteries (North et al. 1969; Webb and Jacobs 1977). Chronic vascular obstruction by inflammatory disorders (e.g., Takayasu's arteritis) or chronic thromboembolic changes of the pulmonary arteries can also cause anastomoses between the bronchial and pulmonary arterial systems, resulting in collateralization of the stenosed or obstructed pulmonary arterial

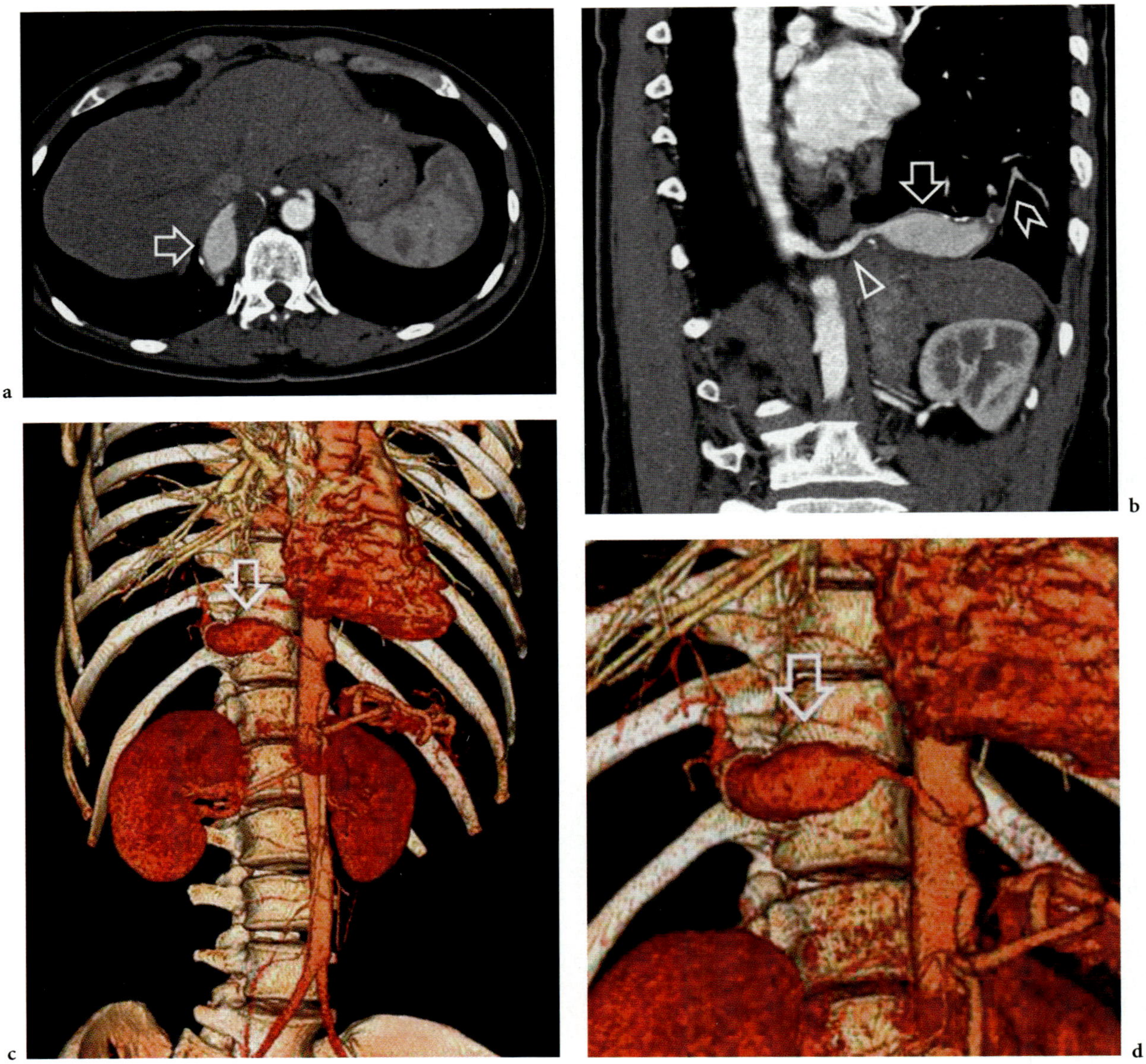

Fig. 17.10. High-resolution, contrast-enhanced 16-slice MDCT shows aneurismal dilatation (*large arrow* in **a–d**) of a systemic feeding artery, originating from the aorta cranial to the celiac trunk, supplying a bronchopulmonary sequestration. The feeding artery (*small arrow* in **b**) and the venous drainage (*double arrow* in **b**) are clearly displayed by high-resolution MDCT angiography, facilitating therapeutic planning, such as coil embolization of the vascular anomaly

bed by the systemic bronchial component of the dual pulmonary blood supply with subsequent hypertrophy of the bronchial arteries (Fig. 17.9; Boushy et al. 1969; Kauczor et al. 1994; Yarnada 1992).

17.5 Multidetector-Row CT Imaging of Malignancies of the Pulmonary Circulation

The role of multidetector-row CT for evaluation of thoracic malignancy is comprehensively covered by other contributions in this book. Specifically, CT angiography of the pulmonary circulation has its premier role in pre- and post-therapeutic evaluation of the vascular status of thoracic malignancies. The correct staging of tumors of the lung and of the mediastinum, foremost of bronchogenic carcinoma, is a cardinal prerequisite for appropriate tumor management. Multidetector-row CT imaging, with its high spatial resolution and its capability of scanning the entire thorax within a short breathhold in the most dyspneic of patients, has established itself as the modality of choice for this indication. Contrast-enhanced multidetector-row CT pulmonary angiography of the pulmonary circulation enables determining the exact location and extent of tumor mass with respect to pulmonary vessels, and tumor vascularity can be assessed. Over the course of therapy of bronchogenic carcinoma, therapeutic effects can be accurately monitored by follow-up volumetric multidetector-row CT scans. The major role of CT angiography is to determine the anatomical relation of tumor mass and pulmonary vasculature before and during therapy, that way also providing crucial information about the risk of hemorrhage, which is an apparent threat when tumor mass is located in the immediate proximity of vessels (Fig. 17.11) or when invasion of vessels has already occurred (Khanavkar et al. 1991). Visualization of the pulmonary vessels also plays a crucial role for surgical planning, since the appropriate surgical approach is determined by the relation of the tumor to vital anatomy such as the main bronchi and the central pulmonary vessels. This way, CT guides the decision of whether a more radical surgical approach becomes necessary, if tumor invasion of central structures is diagnosed. Centrally located tumors, that do not invade or surround adjacent vessels, are usually resected by a sleeve lobectomy and an end-to-end anastomosis of the main stem bronchus. If, however, tumor invasion of more centrally located pulmonary arteries is determined, angioplastic pulmonary artery reconstruction or pneumonectomy is indicated (Shields 1993). Post-surgical complications, such as arterial strictures and bronchoarterial fistulas following pulmonary artery reconstruction, or clot (Fig. 17.12) in the pulmonary artery stump after lobectomy, can be readily identified on follow-up CT angiography.

Autochthonous, however rare malignancies of the pulmonary vasculature, are neoplasms of the vessel wall, i.e., pulmonary artery sarcomas (Fig. 17.13; Parish et al.1996). The etiology of these tumors is obscure. Histopathologically, most pulmonary artery

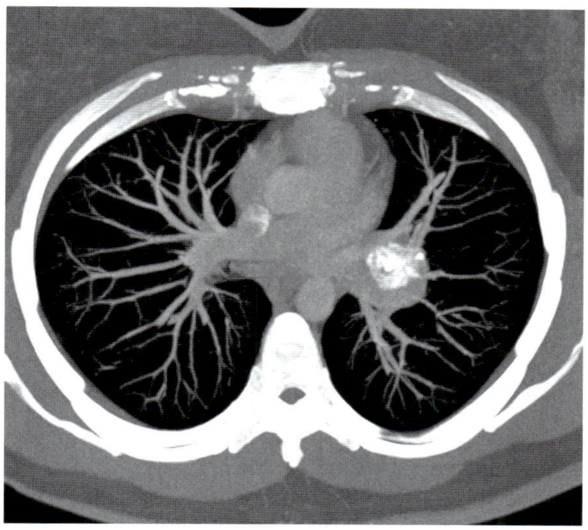
a

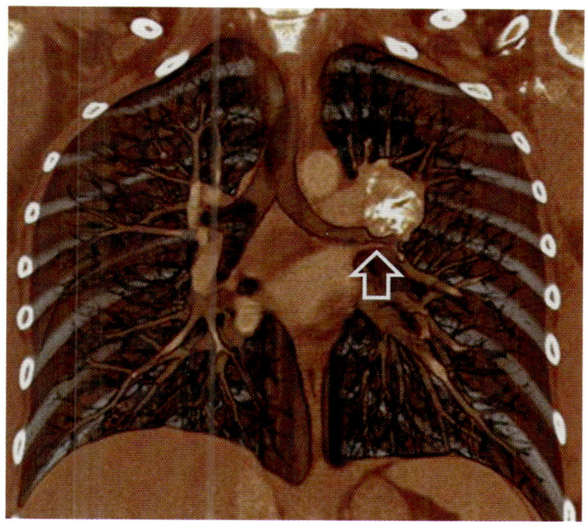
b

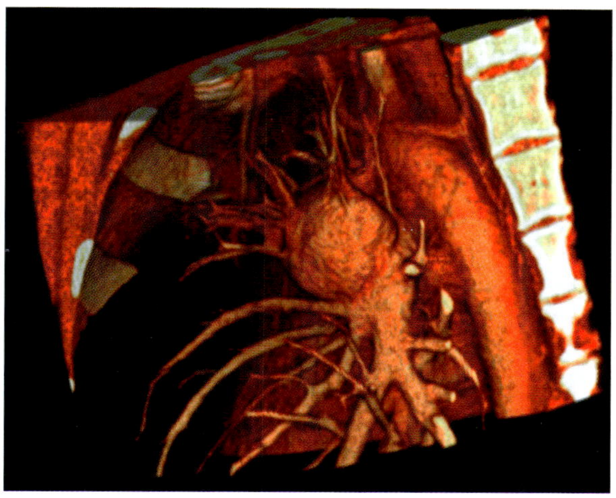
c

Fig. 17.11a–c. Metastasis from an abdominal neuroendocrine tumor to the left hilum assessed with contrast-enhanced multidetector-row CT. Axial maximum intensity projection (**a**) and volume-rendered displays seen from anterior (**b**) and oblique-posterior (**c**) perspectives. The heterogeneously calcified soft tissue mass is in immediate spatial relationship with the left main pulmonary artery. A focal polypoid lesion within the left upper lobe bronchus represents endobronchial extension of tumor (*arrow* in **b**)

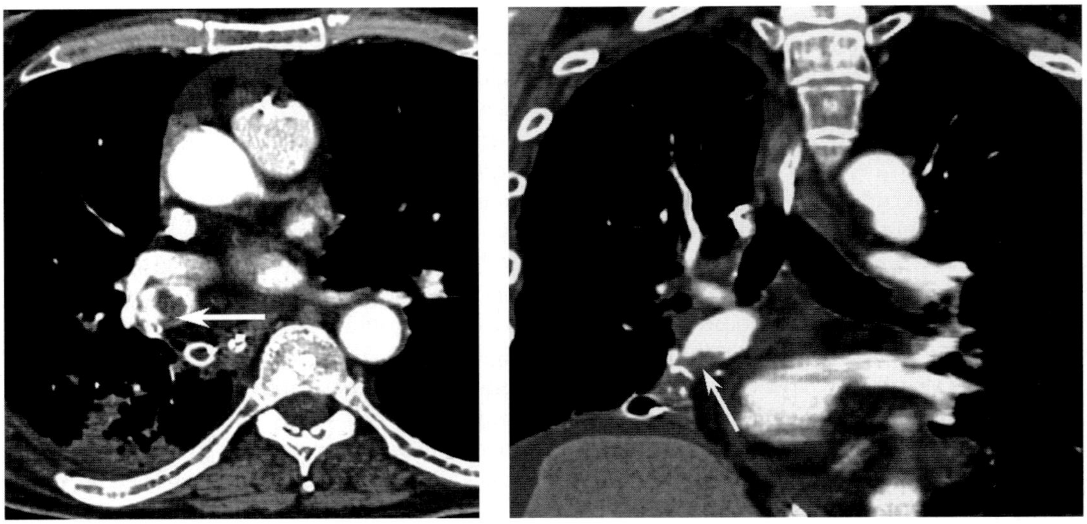

a b

Fig. 17.12a, b. Contrast-enhanced multidetector-row CT scan in a 54-year-old man 5 days after right middle and lower lobectomies. Axial sections (**a**) and coronal multiplanar reformats (**b**) show filling defects in the stump of the right pulmonary artery, representing thrombus formation arising from the suture line as opposed to PE

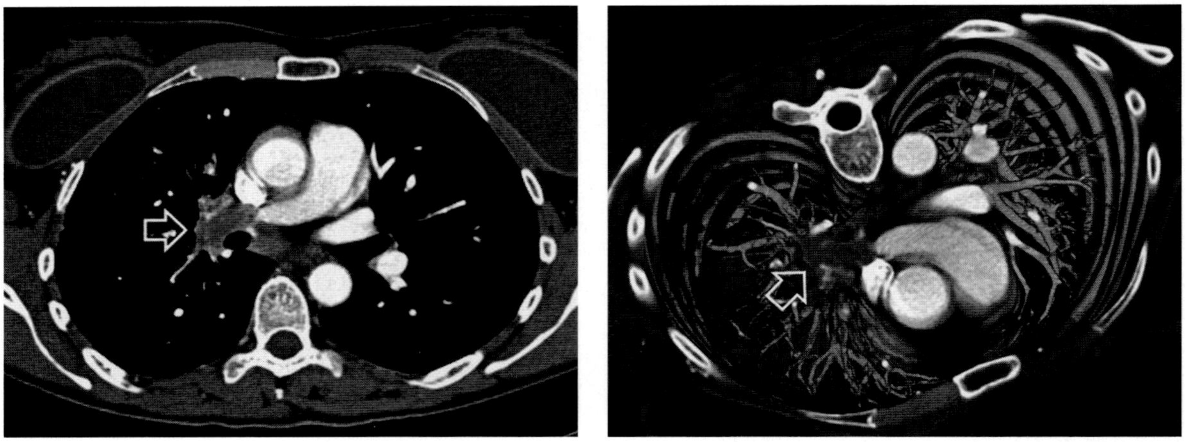

a b

Fig. 17.13a, b. Multidetector-row CT angiography performed in a 52-year-old woman with dyspnea. Axial sections obtained at the level of the main pulmonary artery (**a**) show an endoluminal filling defect in the right pulmonary artery which was initially felt to be consistent with chronic thromboembolic changes. Surgical exploration after failure of specific treatment established a diagnosis of pulmonary artery sarcoma. A 3D volume rendering of the MDCT data set (**b**) may be better suited for appreciating the mass-like nature of the right pulmonary artery lesion

sarcomas are leiomyosarcomas or "undifferentiated spindle cell sarcomas." Histopathologic classification, however, does not seem to be useful clinically or prognostically. Most pulmonary artery sarcomas arise from the dorsal area of the pulmonary trunk, although the tumors also may arise from the right (Fig. 17.13) and left pulmonary arteries, the pulmonary valve, and the right ventricular outflow tract. Because of its rarity and insidious growth characteristics, pulmonary artery sarcoma is often mistaken for pulmonary embolism, resulting in inappropriate therapy such as prolonged anticoagulation or thrombolysis. Symptoms and signs, such as weight loss, fever, anemia, and digital clubbing, may be subtle clues to diagnosis. Other characteristics, such as the absence of risk factors for deep vein thrombosis, high sedimentation rate, nodular parenchymal infiltrates on CT scans, and lack of response to anticoagulation, should raise the suspicion of a process other than pulmonary embolism. Computed tomographic angiography for a precise preoperative assessment is crucial for the appropriate exploration of the pulmonary artery to ensure complete resection and reconstruction.

17.6 Multidetector-Row CT Imaging of Congenital Abnormalities of the Pulmonary Circulation

17.6.1 Anomalous Origin of the Left Pulmonary Artery from the Right: "Pulmonary Artery Sling"

Anomalous origin of the left pulmonary artery is usually diagnosed in infancy because of the effect of the aberrant artery on the airway and often the associated tracheal or bronchial stenosis due to complete cartilage rings (Fig. 17.14; Lee et al. 2001). This can result in obstruction, feeding problems, and respiratory tract infections. Occasionally, the abnormality may be detected as an incidental finding in an asymptomatic adult or in the adult with respiratory complaints. The aberrant left pulmonary artery originates from the right pulmonary artery and travels across the midline posterior to the distal trachea or right main bronchus, where it turns abruptly to the left, passing between the esophagus and trachea to its destination in the left hilum. This anomalous artery has been called a sling (Fig. 17.14). Multidetector-row CT is well suited for imaging this and other congenital abnormalities. The high acquisition speed and high spatial resolution reduces the need for sedation in pediatric patients and facilitates 3D visualization of complicated vascular anatomy for surgical planning even if very low radia-

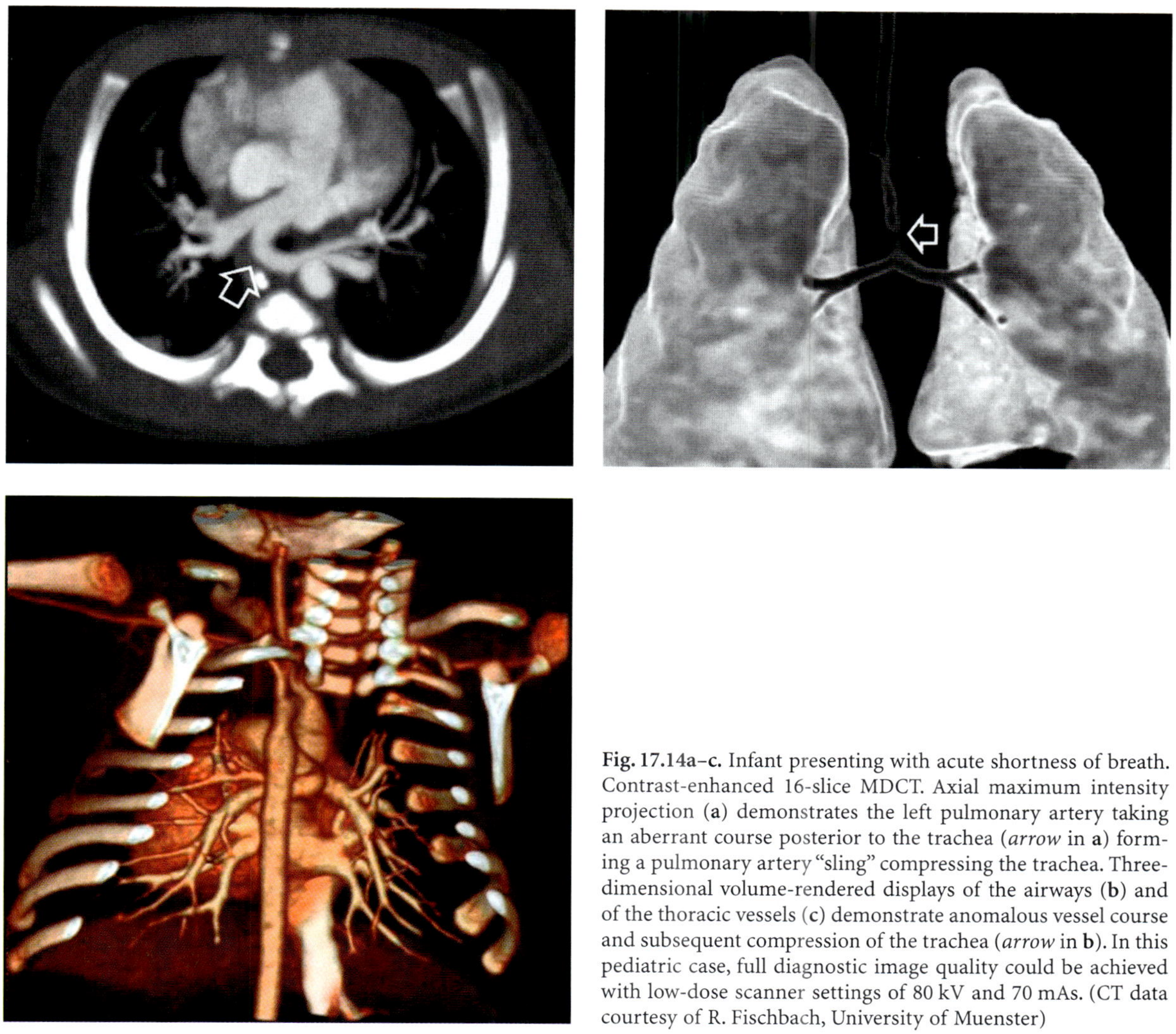

a b c

Fig. 17.14a–c. Infant presenting with acute shortness of breath. Contrast-enhanced 16-slice MDCT. Axial maximum intensity projection (**a**) demonstrates the left pulmonary artery taking an aberrant course posterior to the trachea (*arrow* in **a**) forming a pulmonary artery "sling" compressing the trachea. Three-dimensional volume-rendered displays of the airways (**b**) and of the thoracic vessels (**c**) demonstrate anomalous vessel course and subsequent compression of the trachea (*arrow* in **b**). In this pediatric case, full diagnostic image quality could be achieved with low-dose scanner settings of 80 kV and 70 mAs. (CT data courtesy of R. Fischbach, University of Muenster) tion dose settings, adapted to pediatric patients, are used (Fig. 17.14).

17.6.2 Pulmonary Arteriovenous Malformation

Pulmonary arteriovenous malformation can occur in isolation, be multiple, or be part of a systemic process where arteriovenous communications occur in the skin, mucous membranes, and other organs (hereditary hemorrhagic telangiectasia or Rendu-Osler-Weber disease; Swanson et al. 1999). Computed tomography has proved useful and highly sensitive for the detection of pulmonary arteriovenous malformation and is accepted as the method of choice for routine detection of this vascular abnormality. Apart from detection, CT angiography is also crucial for pretherapeutic evaluation of the angioarchitecture of pulmonary arteriovenous malformations, especially for assessing the number and configuration of feeding and draining vessels connected to the aneurysmal sac (Fig. 17.15). The therapy of choice consists of embolization of the vascular nidus and the number, course, and orientation of the feeding arteries are the most important factors that determine the technical difficulty and success rate of this procedure. With single-slice CT it often is necessary to obtain a thick collimation scan of the entire chest for detection of arteriovenous malformations and a high-resolution scan for dedicated evaluation of the angioarchitecture of detected lesions. With the introduction of MDCT technology acquisition of a single contrast-enhanced scan suffices for both lesion detection and accurate characterization for therapeutic planning (Fig. 17.15).

17.7. Limitations of Computed Tomography for Imaging of the Pulmonary Circulation

17.7.1 Contrast Media Injection

Despite of ever-advancing CT technology, there are still several factors that can render CT angiography of the pulmonary circulation inconclusive. The most common reasons for non-diagnostic CT studies comprise poor contrast opacification of pulmonary vessels, patient motion, and increased image noise due to excessive patient obesity.

Especially the advent of multidetector-row CT necessitates an extensive revision of contrast material injection protocols. Faster scan acquisition times allow scan acquisition during maximal contrast opacification of pulmonary vessels (Schoepf et al. 2000) but pose an increased challenge for correct timing of the contrast bolus. Strategies that have the potential to improve the delivery of contrast media for high and consistent vascular enhancement during CT pulmonary angiography include use of a test bolus or automated bolus-triggering techniques (Kirchner et al. 2000). Saline chasing (Hopper et al. 1997; Haage et al. 2000) has been used

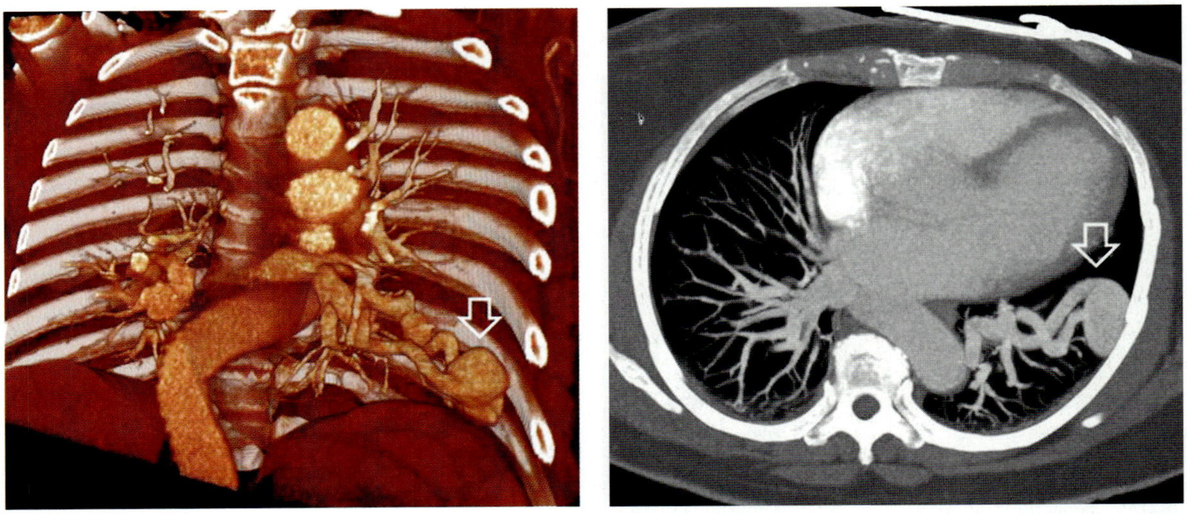

a b

Fig. 17.15. Volume rendering (**a**) and maximum intensity projection (**b**) of a left lower lobe pulmonary arteriovenous malformation evaluated with contrast-enhanced 16-slice multidetector-row CT angiography. The simple angioarchitecture of the arteriovenous malformation consists of a single feeding artery and a single draining vein, both connected to the aneurysmal sac for effective utilization of contrast media and reduction of streak artifacts arising from dense contrast material in the superior vena cava. Use of multi-phasic injection protocols has proved beneficial for general CT angiography (BAE et al. 1998; FLEISCHMANN et al. 2000) but has not been sufficiently evaluated for the pulmonary circulation.

17.7.2 Artifacts and Diagnostic Pitfalls

Another limitation that in some instances results in suboptimal diagnostic quality of CT pulmonary angiography is motion artifacts due to patient respiration or transmitted cardiac pulsation. The short breath-hold times that became feasible with multidetector-row CT should facilitate investigation of dyspneic patients (REMY-JARDIN et al. 2002) and reduce occurrence of respiratory motion artifacts. Similarly, artifacts arising from transmitted cardiac pulsation appear amenable to decreased temporal resolution with fast CT acquisition techniques (SCHOEPF et al. 2000). The ECG synchronization of CT scan acquisition allows for effective reduction of cardiac pulsation artifacts that might interfere with the unambiguous evaluation of cardiac structures, the thoracic aorta, and pulmonary structures (Fig. 17.16; SCHOEPF et al. 1999; FLOHR et al. 2002); however, the spatial resolution that could be achieved, e.g., with retrospectively ECG-gated technique using the previous generation of 4-slice multidetector-row CT scanners, was limited by the relatively long scan duration inherent to data oversampling (FLOHR et al. 2002); thus, high-resolution acquisition could only be achieved for relatively small volumes, e.g., the coronary arterial tree, but not for extended coverage of the entire chest. The advent of 16-slice scanners now effectively eliminates these previous tradeoffs. With 16-slice multidetector-row CT it is now possible to cover the entire thorax with sub-millimeter resolution in a single breath hold with retrospective ECG gating, effectively eliminating transmitted pulsation artifacts (Fig. 17.16). This way, potential sources of diagnostic pitfalls arising from cardiac motion can be effectively avoided.

17.7.3 Radiation Dose

Use of high-resolution multidetector-CT protocols was shown to improve visualization of pulmonary arteries (GHAYE et al. 2001) and the detection of small subsegmental emboli (SCHOEPF et al. 2002). In suspected PE, establishing an unequivocal diagnosis as to the presence or absence of emboli or other

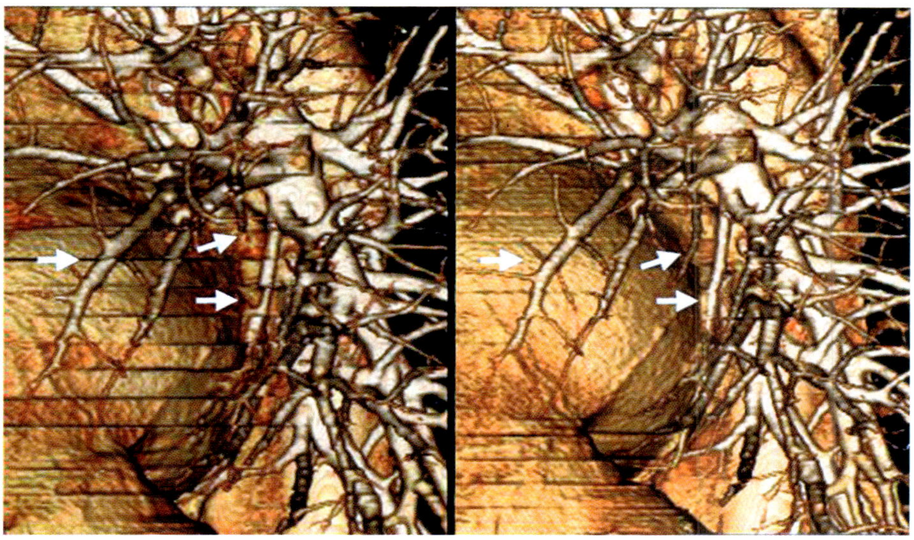

Fig. 17.16. Contrast-enhanced, retrospectively ECG-gated 16-clice CT pulmonary angiography study in a patient with suspected PE. Volume-rendered visualization of paracardiac pulmonary vessels in the left lower lobe. Image reconstruction during systole (*left panel*) results in severe stair-stepping artifacts along the course of the pulmonary vessels (*arrows in left panel*) due to transmitted cardiac motion. Image reconstruction of the same data set during the diastolic phase of the cardiac cycle (*right panel*) significantly reduces cardiac pulsation artifacts and enables almost motion-free analysis of paracardiac pulmonary vessels (*arrows in right panel*)

disease based on a high-quality multidetector-row CT examination may reduce the overall radiation burden of patients, since further work-up with other tests that involve ionizing radiation may be less frequently required; however, if a 4-slice multidetector-row CT protocol with 4×1-mm collimation is chosen to replace a single-detector CT protocol based on a 1×5-mm collimation, the increase is radiation dose ranges between 30% (Schoepf et al. 2001) and 100% (McCollough and Zink 1999). A similar increase in radiation dose, however, is not to be expected with the introduction of 16-slice multidetector CT technology with sub-millimeter resolution capabilities. The addition of detector elements should improve tube output utilization compared with current 4-slice CT scanners and reduce the ratio of excess radiation dose that does not contribute to actual image generation (Flohr et al. 2002). Also, sophisticated technical devices move into clinical practice, that modulate and adapt tube output relative to the geometry and X-ray attenuation of the scanned object, i.e., the patient (Kalender et al. 1999a,b; Gies et al. 1999). Substantial dose savings can thus be realized without compromising on diagnostic quality (Greess et al. 2002). The most important factor, however, for ensuring responsible utilization of multidetector-row CT's technical prowess is the increased radiation awareness that we currently observe among technologists and radiologists. It has been shown that diagnostic quality of chest CT is not compromised, if tube output is adjusted to the body type of the individual patient (Wildberger et al. 2001). Also, with multidetector-row CT radiologists are increasingly adapting to the concept of volume imaging and adjust their expectations with regard to the image quality in the individual axial slice that they require for establishing a diagnosis.

17.7.4 Data Management

Multidetector-row CT increases our diagnostic capabilities; however, the massive amount of data which is generated by this technique puts significant strain on any image analysis and archiving system. A high-resolution 16-slice multidetector-row CT study in a patient with suspected PE routinely results in 500–600 individual axial images; however, differently from focal lung disease, which can be accurately diagnosed by use of maximum intensity projection reconstructions that beneficially "condense" large-volume multidetector-row CT data sets (Gruden et al. 2002), a diagnosis of PE is usually most beneficially established based on individual axial sections. Interpretation of such a study is only feasible by use of digital workstations that allow viewing in "scroll-through" or "cine" mode. Development of dedicated computer-aided detection algorithms (Schoepf et al. 2002) may be helpful in the future for the identification of pulmonary emboli in large-volume multidetector-row CT data sets. Also, extensive storage capacities are an essential need for successful routine performance of multidetector-row CT in a busy clinical environment. Adapting this environment to the new demands which are generated by the introduction of ever-faster scanning techniques is not a trivial task. New modalities for data transfer, data archiving, and image interpretation will have to be devised in order to make full use of the vast potential of multidetector-row CT imaging.

References

Bae K, Heiken JP, Brink JA (1998) Aortic and hepatic peak enhancement at CT: effect of contrast medium injection rate – pharmacokinetic analysis and experimental porcine model. Radiology 206:455–464

Baile E, King GG, Muller NL, D'Yachkova Y, Coche EE, Pare PD, Mayo JR (2000) Spiral computed tomography is comparable to angiography for the diagnosis of pulmonary embolism. Am J Respir Crit Care Med 161:1010–1015

Bajc M, Bitzen U, Olsson B et al. (2002) Lung ventilation/perfusion SPECT in the artificially embolized pig. J Nucl Med 43:640–647

Blachere H, Latrabe V, Montaudon M et al. (2000) Pulmonary embolism revealed on helical CT angiography: comparison with ventilation-perfusion radionuclide lung scanning. Am J Roentgenol 174:1041–1047

Boushy SF, North LB, Trics JA (1969) The bronchial arteries in chronic obstructive pulmonary disease. Am J Med 46: 506–515

Brown MD, Rowe BH, Reeves MJ et al. (2002) The accuracy of the enzyme-linked immunosorbent assay D-dimer test in the diagnosis of pulmonary embolism: a meta-analysis. Ann Emerg Med 40:133–144

Crawford T, Yoon C, Wolfson K et al. (2001) The effect of imaging modality on patient management in the evaluation of pulmonary thromboembolism. J Thorac Imaging 16:163–169

Crocco JA, Rooney JJ, Fankushen DS, DiBenedetto RJ, Lyons HA (1968) Massive hemoptysis. Arch Intern Med 121: 495–498

Diffin D, Leyendecker JR, Johnson SP, Zucker RJ, Grebe PJ (1998) Effect of anatomic distribution of pulmonary emboli on interobserver agreement in the interpretation of pulmonary angiography. Am J Roentgenol 171:1085–1089

Dunn KL, Wolf JP, Dorfman DM et al. (2002) Normal D-dimer levels in emergency department patients suspected of acute pulmonary embolism. J Am Coll Cardiol 40:1475

Ellis K (1991) Developmental abnormalities in the systemic blood supply to the lungs. Am J Roentgenol 156:669–679
Fleischmann D, Rubin GD, Bankier AA, Hittmair K (2000) Improved uniformity of aortic enhancement with customized contrast medium injection protocols at CT angiography. Radiology 214:363–371
Flohr T, Prokop M, Becker C et al. (2002a) A retrospectively ECG-gated multislice spiral CT scan and reconstruction technique with suppression of heart pulsation artifacts for cardio-thoracic imaging with extended volume coverage. Eur Radiol 12:1497–1503
Flohr T, Stierstorfer K, Bruder H et al. (2002b) New technical developments in multislice CT. Part 1. Approaching isotropic resolution with sub-millimeter 16-slice scanning. Rofo Fortschr Geb Rontgenstr Neuen Bildgeb Verfahr 174: 839–845
Frazier AA, Galvin JR, Franks TJ, Rosado-De-Christenson ML (2000) From the archives of the AFIP: pulmonary vasculature: hypertension and infarction. Radiographics 20: 491–524; 530–531, 532
Garg K, Welsh CH, Feyerabend AJ et al. (1998) Pulmonary embolism: diagnosis with spiral CT and ventilation-perfusion scanning – correlation with pulmonary angiographic results or clinical outcome. Radiology 208:201–208
Garg K, Sieler H, Welsh CH et al. (1999) Clinical validity of helical CT being interpreted as negative for pulmonary embolism: implications for patient treatment. Am J Roentgenol 172:1627–1631
Ghaye B, Szapiro D, Mastora I et al. (2001) Peripheral pulmonary arteries: How far in the lung does multi-detector row spiral CT allow analysis? Radiology 219:629–636
Gies M, Kalender WA, Wolf H, Suess C (1999) Dose reduction in CT by anatomically adapted tube current modulation. I. Simulation studies. Med Phys 26:2235–2247
Goodman LR, Curtin JJ, Mewissen MW et al. (1995) Detection of pulmonary embolism in patients with unresolved clinical and scintigraphic diagnosis: helical CT versus angiography. Am J Roentgenol 164:1369–1374
Goodman LR, Lipchik RJ, Kuzo RS et al. (2000) Subsequent pulmonary embolism: risk after a negative helical CT pulmonary angiogram – prospective comparison with scintigraphy. Radiology 215:535–542
Gottsater A, Berg A, Centergard J et al. (2001) Clinically suspected pulmonary embolism: Is it safe to withhold anticoagulation after a negative spiral CT? Eur Radiol 11:65–72
Gottschalk A, Stein PD, Goodman LR, Sostman HD (2002) Overview of prospective investigation of pulmonary embolism diagnosis II. Semin Nucl Med 32:173–182
Greess H, Nomayr A, Wolf H et al. (2002) Dose reduction in CT examination of children by an attenuation-based online modulation of tube current (CARE Dose). Eur Radiol 12:1571–1576
Groell R, Peichel KH, Uggowitzer MM et al. (1999) Computed tomography densitometry of the lung: a method to assess perfusion defects in acute pulmonary embolism. Eur J Radiol 32:192–196
Gruden JF, Ouanounou S, Tigges S et al. (2002) Incremental benefit of maximum-intensity-projection images on observer detection of small pulmonary nodules revealed by multidetector CT. Am J Roentgenol 179:149–157
Gupta A, Frazer CK, Ferguson JM et al. (1999) Acute pulmonary embolism: diagnosis with MR angiography. Radiology 210:353–359
Gurney JW (1993) No fooling around: direct visualization of pulmonary embolism. Radiology 188:618–619
Haage P, Schmitz-Rode T, Hubner D et al. (2000) Reduction of contrast material dose and artifacts by a saline flush using a double power injector in helical CT of the thorax. Am J Roentgenol 174:1049–1053
Hopper KD, Mosher TJ, Kasales CJ et al. (1997) Thoracic spiral CT: delivery of contrast material pushed with injectable saline solution in a power injector. Radiology 205:269–271
Hu H, He HD, Foley WD, Fox SH (2000) Four multidetector-row helical CT: image quality and volume coverage speed (in process citation). Radiology 215:55–62
Hull R, Raskob GE, Ginsberg JS, Panju AA, Brill-Edwards P, Coates G, Pineo GF (1994) A noninvasive strategy for the treatment of patients with suspected pulmonary embolism. Arch Intern Med 154:289–297
Kalender WA, Wolf H, Suess C et al. (1999a) Dose reduction in CT by on-line tube current control: principles and validation on phantoms and cadavers. Eur Radiol 9:323–328
Kalender WA, Wolf H, Suess C (1999b) Dose reduction in CT by anatomically adapted tube current modulation. II. Phantom measurements. Med Phys 26:2248–2253
Kauczor HL, Schwickert HC, Mayer E, Schweden F, Schild HH, Thelen M (1994) Spiral CT of bronchial arteries in chronic thromboembolism. J Comput Assist Tomogr 18:855–861
Khanavker B, Stern P, Alberti W, Nakhosteen JA (1991) Complications associated with brachytherapy alone or with laser in lung cancer. Chest 99:1062–1065
Khorasani R, Gudas TF, Nikpoor N, Polak JF (1997) Treatment of patients with suspected pulmonary embolism and intermediate-probability lung scans: Is diagnostic imaging underused? Am J Roentgenol 169:1355–1357
Kirchner J, Kickuth R, Laufer U et al. (2000) Optimized enhancement in helical CT: experiences with a real-time bolus tracking system in 628 patients. Clin Radiol 55: 368–373
Kruip MJ, Slob MJ, Schijen JH et al. (2002) Use of a clinical decision rule in combination with D-dimer concentration in diagnostic workup of patients with suspected pulmonary embolism: a prospective management study. Arch Intern Med 162:1631–1635
Lee KH, Yoon CS, Choe KO et al. (2001) Use of imaging for assessing anatomical relationships of tracheobronchial anomalies associated with left pulmonary artery sling. Pediatr Radiol 31:269–278
Leveau P (2002) Diagnostic strategy in pulmonary embolism. National French survey. Presse Med 31:929–932
McCollough CH, Zink FE (1999) Performance evaluation of a multi-slice CT system. Med Phys 26:2223–2230
Meaney J, Weg JG, Chenevert TL, Stafford-Johnson D, Hamilton BH, Prince MR (1997) Diagnosis of pulmonary embolism with magnetic resonance angiography. N Engl J Med 336:1422–1427
Michelle LW, Peter S, Mark JH (2002) Percutaneous embolotherapy for life-threatening hemoptysis. Chest 121:95–102
North LB, Boushy SF, Houk VN (1969) Bronchial and intercostal arteriography in nonneoplastic pulmonary disease. Am J Roentgenol 107:328–342
Novelline R, Baltarowich O, Athanasoulis C, Greenfield A, McKusick K (1978) The clinical course of patients with suspected pulmonary embolism and a negative pulmonary angiogram. Radiology 126:561–567

Oser RF, Zuckerman DA, Gutierrez FR, Brink JA (1996) Anatomic distribution of pulmonary emboli at pulmonary angiography: implications for cross sectional imaging. Radiology 199:31–35

Ost D, Rozenshtein A, Saffran L, Snider A (2001) The negative predictive value of spiral computed tomography for the diagnosis of pulmonary embolism in patients with nondiagnostic ventilation-perfusion scans. Am J Med 110: 16–21

Oudkerk M, van Beek EJ, Wielopolski P et al. (2002) Comparison of contrast-enhanced magnetic resonance angiography and conventional pulmonary angiography for the diagnosis of pulmonary embolism: a prospective study. Lancet 359:1643–1647

Palmer J, Bitzen U, Jonson B, Bajc M (2001) Comprehensive ventilation/perfusion SPECT. J Nucl Med 42:1288–1294

Parish JM, Rosenow EC, 3rd, Swensen SJ, Crotty TB (1996) Pulmonary artery sarcoma. Clinical features. Chest 110: 1480–1488

Patriquin L, Khorasani R, Polak JF (1998) Correlation of diagnostic imaging and subsequent autopsy findings in patients with pulmonary embolism. Am J Roentgenol 171: 347–349

PIOPED Investigators (1990) Value of the ventilation/perfusion scan in acute pulmonary embolism. J Am Med Assoc 95:498–502

Prologo JD, Glauser J (2002) Variable diagnostic approach to suspected pulmonary embolism in the ED of a major academic tertiary care center. Am J Emerg Med 20:5–9

Qanadli SD, Hajjam ME, Mesurolle B et al. (2000) Pulmonary embolism detection: prospective evaluation of dual-section helical CT versus selective pulmonary arteriography in 157 patients. Radiology 217:447–455

Remy J, Voisin C, Dupuis C et al. (1974) Treatment of hemoptysis by embolization of the systemic circulation. Ann Radiol (Paris) 17:5–16 [in French]

Remy J, Remy-Jardin M, Artaud D, Fribourg M (1998) Multiplanar and three-dimensional reconstruction techniques in CT: impact on chest diseases. Eur Radiol 8:335–351

Remy-Jardin M, Remy J (1999) Spiral CT angiography of the pulmonary circulation. Radiology 212:615–636

Remy-Jardin M, Remy J, Wattinne L, Giraud F (1992) Central pulmonary thromboembolism: diagnosis with spiral volumetric CT with the single-breath-hold technique – comparison with pulmonary angiography. Radiology 185:381–387

Remy-Jardin M, Remy J, Cauvain O et al. (1995) Diagnosis of central pulmonary embolism with helical CT: role of two-dimensional multiplanar reformations. Am J Roentgenol 165:1131–1138

Remy-Jardin M, Remy J, Deschildre F et al. (1996) Diagnosis of pulmonary embolism with spiral CT: comparison with pulmonary angiography and scintigraphy. Radiology 200: 699–706

Remy-Jardin M, Remy J, Artaud D et al. (1997) Peripheral pulmonary arteries: optimization of the spiral CT acquisition protocol (see comments). Radiology 204:157–163

Remy-Jardin M, Tillie-Leblond I, Szapiro D et al. (2002) CT angiography of pulmonary embolism in patients with underlying respiratory disease: impact of multislice CT on image quality and negative predictive value. Eur Radiol 12: 1971–1978

Roberts DA, Gefter WB, Hirsch JA et al. (1999) Pulmonary perfusion: respiratory-triggered three-dimensional MR imaging with arterial spin tagging – preliminary results in healthy volunteers. Radiology 212:890–895

Schibany N, Fleischmann D, Thallinger C et al. (2001) Equipment availability and diagnostic strategies for suspected pulmonary embolism in Austria. Eur Radiol 11:2287–2294

Schluger N, Henschke C, King T et al. (1994) Diagnosis of pulmonary embolism at a large teaching hospital. J Thorac Imaging 9:180–184

Schoepf UJ, Becker CR, Bruening RD et al. (1999) Electrocardiographically gated thin-section CT of the lung. Radiology 212:649–654

Schoepf UJ, Helmberger T, Holzknecht N et al. (2000a) Segmental and subsegmental pulmonary arteries: evaluation with electron-beam versus spiral CT. Radiology 214: 433–439

Schoepf U, Bruening R, Konschitzky H, Becker CR, Knez A, Weber J, Muehling O, Herzog P, Huber A, Haberl R, Reiser M (2000b) Pulmonary embolism: comprehensive diagnosis using electron-beam computed tomography for detection of emboli and assessment of pulmonary blood flow. Radiology 217:693–700

Schoepf U, Bruening RD, Hong C, Eibel R, Aydemir S, Crispin A, Becker CR, Reiser MF (2001) Multislice helical CT imaging of focal and diffuse lung disease: comprehensive diagnosis with reconstruction of contiguous and high-resolution CT sections from a single thin-collimation scan. Am J Roentgenol 177:179–184

Schoepf U, Das M, Schneider AC, Anderson A, Wood SA, Costello P (2002a) Computer aided detection (CAD) of segmental and subsegmental pulmonary emboli on 1-mm multidetector-row CT (MDCT) studies. Radiology 225 (Suppl):384

Schoepf U, Holzknecht N, Helmberger TK, Crispin A, Hong C, Becker CR, Reiser MF (2002b) Subsegmental pulmonary emboli: improved detection with thin-collimation multidetector-row spiral CT. Radiology 222:483–490

Shields TW (1993) Surgical therapy for carcomoma of the lung. Clin Chest Med 14:121–147

Stein PD, Alavi A et al. (1992) Complications and validity of pulmonary angiography in acute pulmonary embolus. Circulation 85:462–468

Stein PD, Gottschalk A (2000) Review of criteria appropriate for a very low probability of pulmonary embolism on ventilation-perfusion lung scans: a position paper. Radiographics 20:99–105

Stein PD, Relyea B, Gottschalk A (1996) Evaluation of individual criteria for low probability interpretation of ventilation-perfusion lung scans. J Nucl Med 37:577–581

Stein PD, Henry JW, Gottschalk A (1999) Reassessment of pulmonary angiography for the diagnosis of pulmonary embolism: relation of interpreter agreement to the order of the involved pulmonary arterial branch. Radiology 210: 689–691

Swanson KL, Prakash UB, Stanson AW (1999) Pulmonary arteriovenous fistulas: Mayo Clinic experience 1982–1997. Mayo Clin Proc 74:671–680

Swensen SJ, Sheedy PF II, Ryu JH et al. (2002) Outcomes after withholding anticoagulation from patients with suspected acute pulmonary embolism and negative computed tomographic findings: a cohort study. Mayo Clin Proc 77: 130–138

Teigen CL, Maus TP, Sheedy PF II, Stanson AW, Johnson CM, Breen JF, McKusick MA (1995) Pulmonary embolism:

diagnosis with contrast-enhanced electron beam CT and comparison with pulmonary angiography. Radiology 194: 313–319

Tetalman MR, Hoffer PB, Heck LL, Kunzmann A, Gottschalk A (1973) Perfusion lung scan in normal volunteers. Radiology 106:593–594

Tillie-Leblond I, Mastora I, Radenne F et al. (2002) Risk of pulmonary embolism after a negative spiral CT angiogram in patients with pulmonary disease: 1-year clinical follow-up study. Radiology 223:461–467

Van Erkel AR, van Rossum AB, Bloem JL, Kievit J, Pattynama PNT (1996) Spiral CT angiography for suspected pulmonary embolism: a cost-effectiveness analysis. Radiology 201:29–36

Van Rossum AB, Pattynama PM, Mallens WM et al. (1998) Can helical CT replace scintigraphy in the diagnostic process in suspected pulmonary embolism? A retrolective–prolective cohort study focusing on total diagnostic yield. Eur Radiol 8:90–96

Van Rossum AB, van Erkel AR, van Persijn, van Meerten EL et al. (1998) Accuracy of helical CT for acute pulmonary embolism: ROC analysis of observer performance related to clinical experience. Eur Radiol 8:1160–1164

Webb WR, Jacobs RP (1977) Transpleural abdominal systemic artery – pulmonary artery anastomosis in patients with chronic pulmonary infection. Am J Roentgenol 129: 233–236

Wells PS, Anderson DR, Rodger M et al. (2001) Excluding pulmonary embolism at the bedside without diagnostic imaging: management of patients with suspected pulmonary embolism presenting to the emergency department by using a simple clinical model and d-dimer. Ann Intern Med 135:98–107

Wildberger JE, Mahnken AH, Schmitz-Rode T et al. (2001a) Individually adapted examination protocols for reduction of radiation exposure in chest CT. Invest Radiol 36:604–611

Wildberger JE, Niethammer MU, Klotz E et al. (2001b) Multislice CT for visualization of pulmonary embolism using perfusion weighted color maps. Rofo Fortschr Geb Rontgenstr Neuen Bildgeb Verfahr 173:289–294

Woodard PK (1997) Pulmonary arteries must be seen before they can be assessed. Radiology 204:11–12

Yamada I, Shibuya H, Matsubara O et al. (1992) Pulmonary artery disease in Takayasu's arteritis: angiographic findings. Am J Roentgenol 159:263–269

Zuckerman DA, Sterling KM, Oser RF (1996) Safety of pulmonary angiography in the 1990s. J Vasc Interv Radiol 7: 199–205

18 Thromboembolic Disease: Perfusion-Weighted Imaging of the Lung

J. E. Wildberger and M. U. Niethammer

CONTENTS

Standard computed tomography (CT) imaging in patients with suspected pulmonary embolism (PE) demonstrates mainly structural and morphological changes, e.g. the direct visualization of clot material following contrast enhancement. Compared to the gold standard – pulmonary arteriography – spiral CT has proven to be an efficient and sensitive imaging modality, especially for assessing central and segmental PE (Remy-Jardin et al. 1996; Harvey et al. 2000). Secondary changes, like air-trapping, dystelectasis and alternate diagnoses are safely depicted as well (Garg et al. 1999).

Using modern multi-slice CT (MSCT) scanners, further technical improvements have been readily achieved, as the whole lung volume can be covered within a single breathhold offering a dedicated analysis down to the subsegmental level (Ghaye et al. 2001; Schoepf et al. 2002).

Perfusion defects allow the direct parenchymal assessment of the extent of PE, especially for isolated subsegmental emboli. This information is reliably given by pulmonary angiography and perfusion-/ventilation scintigraphy (V/Q scans). Parenchymal density values and enhancement patterns after contrast media application are also linked to functional parameters, such as perfusion, ventilation and metabolic activity (Kazaroony 2001). Direct and indirect visualization of lung perfusion as an adjunct to CTA seems to be an attractive technique to improve the overall accuracy of PE diagnostics. Basis for this methodology is a high contrast bolus within the vessel lumen. Using high-concentrated, non-ionic contrast material followed by an additional chaser bolus, mean density values of approximately 300 Hounsfield units (HU) within the main pulmonary arteries are achievable in clinical routine (Wildberger et al. 2002). This guarantees a homogeneous filling of the lung microcirculation and peripheries as well.

Latter is mandatory, as density differences between normal lung tissue and areas with perfusion defects are quite small. Initial studies on matching pulmonary structure and perfusion have been performed using electron-beam tomography (EBT). Hoffman et al. (1995) stressed the importance of achieving near maximal enhancement for adaequate signal in the lung peripheries. The injection of contrast media (0.7 mL / kg body weight) directly into the right ventricular outflow tract using a sharp bolus geometry (2 s duration) led to (optimal) density values of approximately 800 HU in the vessel lumen. However, the authors also addressed the limitation between ideal technical performance under experimental conditions and the clinical reality in daily routine. A small patient study with a dedicated subtraction technique was published by Schoepf et al. (2000), performing a second thin-collimated, ECG-gated serio-scan on a 7.6 cm thick lung section after an initial standard EBT-examination for PE. Additional contrast media (40 mL) had to be administered with a high flow injection protocol (10 mL / s). A reduction in blood flow was depicted in case of vessel obstruction. The blood flow in the adjacent lung parenchyma was significantly reduced to 0.63 mL/min/mL, when compared to normal lung parenchyma with 2.27 mL/min/mL (P = .001) (Fig. 18.1).

A clinical approach was conducted on a single-slice scanner by performing region-of-interest

J. E. Wildberger, MD
Department of Diagnostic Radiology, University of Technology, Pauwelsstrasse 30, 52074 Aachen, Germany
M. U. Niethammer, MSc
Siemens Medical Solutions, Computed Tomography, Siemensstrasse 1, 91301 Forchheim, Germany

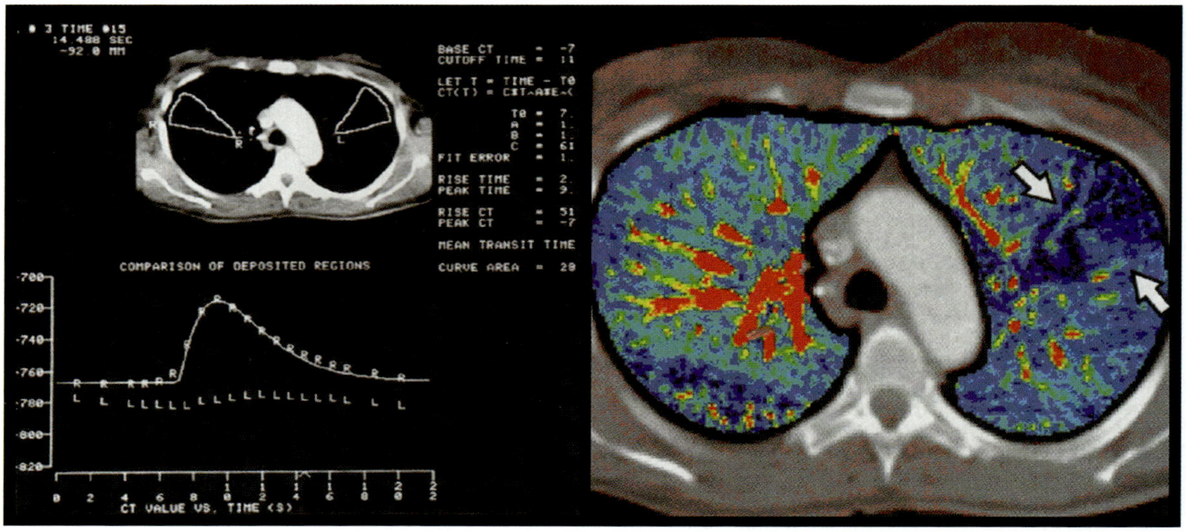

Fig. 18.1. Parenchymal time-attenuation curves in the occluded apicoposterior segment of the upper lobe of the left lung (L) and the nonoccluded corresponding segment in the upper lobe of the right lung (R). Parenchymal blood flow was 0.15 mL/min/mL in the occluded segment vs. 1.48 mL/min/mL in the nonoccluded segment. Cold spectrum colors delineate the perfusion deficit in the apicoposterior segment on the left side (arrows) (Figure 1 taken from Schoepf et al. 2000)

(ROI) measurements before and after intravenous contrast material had been administered (Groell et al. 1999). Initially, there was no density difference for all lung areas. In patients with scintigraphically proven perfusion defects, less enhancement was measured herein compared to non-affected lung segments (density before / after i.v. contrast: -826 ± 48 HU / -813 ± 57 HU, enhancement: 12 ± 18 HU in occluded segments vs. density before / after i.v. contrast: -825 ± 37 HU / -794 ± 45 HU, enhancement: 30 ± 17 HU in normal lung parenchyma; $p < 0.01$). However, this method was only feasible in patients with extensive central and segmental embolism. Another drawback of this method was the need for a second spiral scan, as these patients had to be examined twice, before and after intravenous contrast media application.

To the best of our knowlegde, a subtraction technique for the whole lung is technically not feasible with four-row MSCT, even with 0.5 s gantry rotation time. Our own animal investigations have been limited by the inability to correlate ventilation and perfusion parameters simultaneously with the in vivo assessment of related anatomic details such as diaphragm geometry, pulmonary vascular branching patterns and mediastinal anatomy including the beating heart (Fig. 18.2).

Therefore, we developed a new dedicated image post-processing technique from contrast-enhanced lung studies for the extraction of additional information related to parenchymal enhancement.

Image post-processing was performed on clinical data sets, acquired from MSCT chest examinations for clinical suspicion of PE. Non-ionic contrast media (Ultravist 370, Schering, Berlin, Germany) was applied intravenously using a double power injector (CT 9000 Digital Injection System; Liebel-Flarsheim, Cincinnatti, U.S.A.). Flow parameters were 3 mL / s, with a total amount of 120 mL, followed by a saline chaser bolus (3 mL / s, 30 mL). Start delay was 27 s in caudo-cranial direction. Imaging was performed on a commercially available MSCT (SOMATOM Volume Zoom; Siemens, Forchheim, Germany). Scan parameters were 120 kV / 140 kV and 100 mAs, using a rotation time of 0.5 s, a thin collimated spiral scan (4×1 mm) and a table speed of 7 mm / rotation (beam pitch: 1.75). Therefore, the entire chest was examined within approximately 21 s.

Radiological diagnoses regarding PE were established on thin collimated axial slices (slice thickness $_{eff.}$ 1.25 mm, reconstruction increment 0.8 mm, standard soft tissue kernel [B30]) in cine mode view on a workstation (Wizard, Siemens). Complete or incomplete occlusion of pulmonary arteries as well as direct visualization of emboli due to filling defects were considered as primary signs of PE.

The image post-processing algorithm for visualization of parenchymal density distribution was structured into 5 steps:

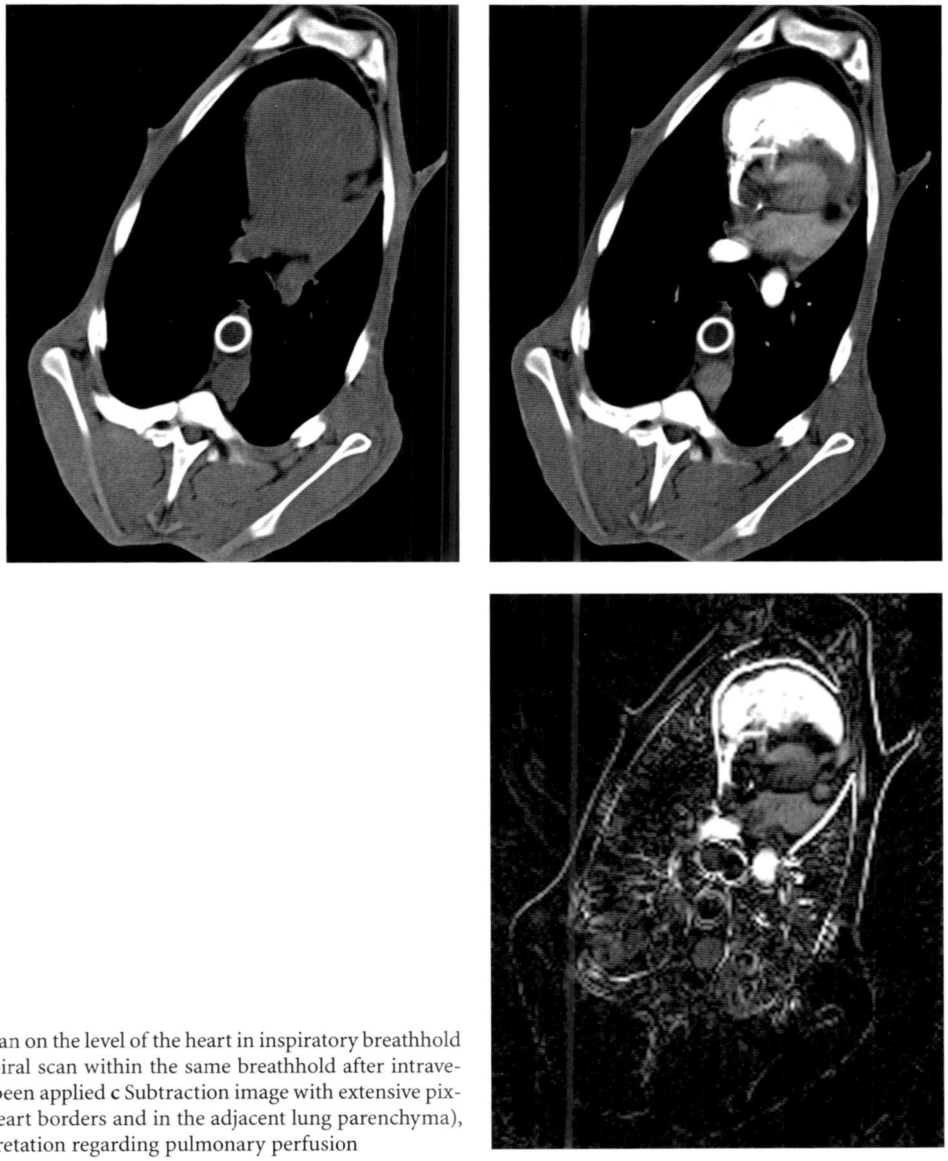

Fig. 18.2. **a** Native spiral scan on the level of the heart in inspiratory breathhold (pig study) **b** Repeated spiral scan within the same breathhold after intravenous contrast media had been applied **c** Subtraction image with extensive pixelshift (especially at the heart borders and in the adjacent lung parenchyma), obscuring detailed interpretation regarding pulmonary perfusion

18.1 Contour Definition by Identifying the Lung by Threshold Based Contour Finding/Segmentation Algorithm

In a first step, a binary mask of the image was derived by identifying lung areas and non-lung areas. A threshold based contour finder was used for segmentation, as lung tissue (low HU) is generally enclosed by high HU areas (pleura / chest wall). The threshold HU value separated both HU ranges and defined the contour of the lung.

To trace the lung contour, a standard algorithm has been adapted. The search proceeded counter-clockwise, starting from the detected starting point. The algorithm always considered the neighboring three pixels in the search direction and determined the first pixel with a value below the specified threshold as the next contour point.

To exclude pleural walls, 7 layers of pixels were removed at the border of segmented lung areas by applying the morphological operation of erosion five times to the binary segmentation mask, using the four connected neighbours as the structuring element (Fig. 18.3).

The centerpositions of each lung were derived from the segmentation mask and used as initial

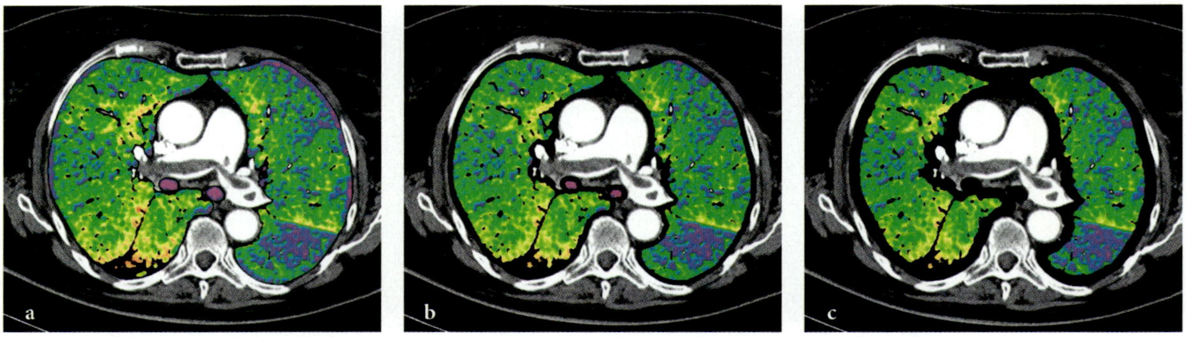

Fig. 18.3. Erosion of contour pixels: **a** No erosion **b** 7 layers of pixels eroded **c** 15 layers of pixels eroded

points for the segmentation of the next image. Segmentation proceeded automatically until the whole dataset was processed.

All following steps were performed on the extracted lung areas, exclusively.

18.2 Vessel Cutting

Major vascular structures and airways were removed by HU range selection to prepare images for subsequent filtering.

A lower threshold $HU_{B\ (B\ =\ Bronchi)}$ and an upper threshold $HU_{V\ (V\ =\ Vessel)}$ were specified, pixels below HU_B were identified as airways, pixels above HU_V as vessels. For optimal image visualization, vessel cutting had to be balanced between cutting all vessels and keeping as much lung pixels as possible. As there is an inter- and even intrapatient variability of the optimum HU_V, a percentage based definition of HU_V proved to be more general. Therefore, a combination of threshold and percentage based removal scheme was applied. The algorithm removed all pixels below HU_B. HU_B was fixed at a value of –990 HU. HU_V was individually adjusted to reach an arbitrary maximum share of 28% of removed pixels (Fig. 18.4).

18.3 Adaptive Filtering

The segmented dataset was reformated by linear interpolation to obtain a dataset with isotropic voxel spacing. An adaptive sliding mean value filter was applied, using an isotropic (spherical) 3D kernel with a diameter of 5 mm. In most datasets, this corresponded to 7 pixels (Fig. 18.5).

In this process, up to 7 adjacent slices were combined. Lost pixels due to vessel cutting were replaced to a specified extent, by the average of the pixel values from their 3D environment. When the filter was applied, the central pixel of each (kernel) volume was replaced by the mean value of all pixels in the volume. Pixels removed in preceding operations (segmentation, erosion, vessel cutting), were defined

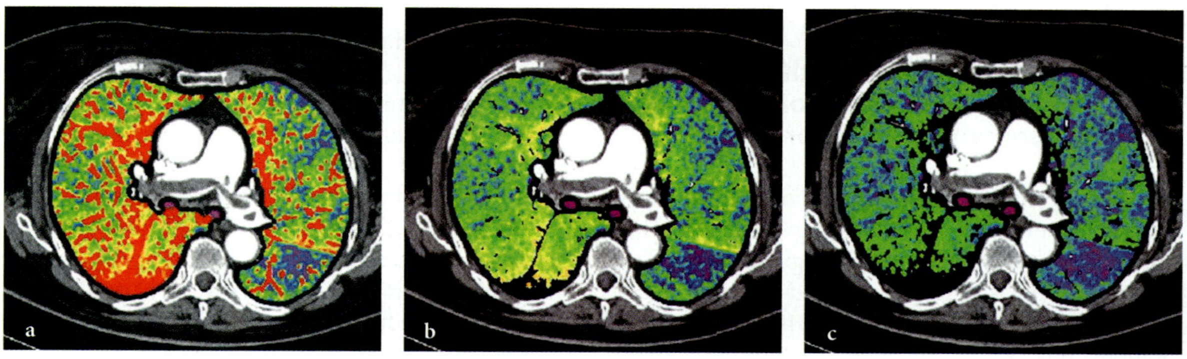

Fig. 18.4. Influence of vessel cutting settings (already color encoded): **a** Original image, no removal **b** HU_B = -990 HU, HU_V = -827 HU, 28% removed **c** HU_B = -990 HU, HU_V = -864 HU, 48% removed

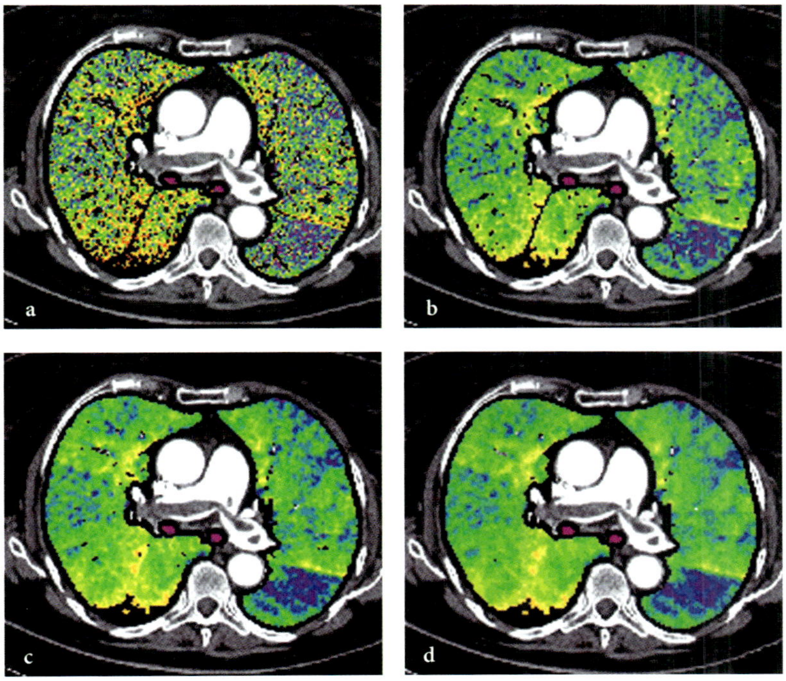

Fig. 18.5. Influence of kernel diameter: **a** No filter **b** 7 pixel, 4.9 mm **c** 9 pixel, 6.4 mm **d** 11 pixel, 7.8 mm

as invalid and did not contribute to the averaging density values. The user defined the minimum share of valid pixels in the volume, required for a valid averaging result. The limit was specified as a percentile value; in the following referred to as an "inclusion threshold". If the share was below the limit, the central pixel was set as invalid. As in the last processing step, all invalid pixels were replaced by the corresponding pixels of the original image. The inclusion threshold specified how many vascular structures and airways appeared in the processed parenchymal area. A heuristic approach with an inclusion threshold of 20% was utilized (Fig. 18.6).

The implementation of the adaptive filtering took advantage of a fast numerical convolution algorithm. In the following, it is described for a 2D filter, which can be easily generalized to 3D. In the image, all pixels that were invalid or outside the contour were set to zero. The image matrix and its binary mask were convoluted separately. The convolution of the binary mask yielded the number of valid pixels in the volume, corresponding to the position of the value in the matrix. The inclusion threshold was implemented by thresholding the matrix and setting all values below the computed limit to zero. To produce the filtered image, the convoluted image was divided by the convoluted mask, the division was carried out element-by-element. If an element of the convoluted mask array was zero, the result was set to invalid.

18.4 Color Encoding

To facilitate visualization of parenchymal enhancement, the resulting image was mapped onto a spectral color scale. Mapping was controlled by center and width, analogous to gray scale image mapping. As a subtraction technique from native data was not possible, no baseline was defined. A heuristic approach analyzed the parenchymal histogram and determined the window parameters automatically. The algorithm used the median of the processed parenchymal pixels as the center value, the width range was fixed to 100 HU (Fig. 18.7).

If requested, additional manual interactive windowing by the user was feasible.

18.5 Image Fusion with the Original Image

The resulting color encoded parenchymal images were overlayed onto the original CT images, as these CT source images were crucial for spatial orientation in the dataset. For overlay, all non-parenchymal pixels were replaced by the original pixels of the respective slice position and displayed in the usual CT gray scale presentation. In addition, the user was

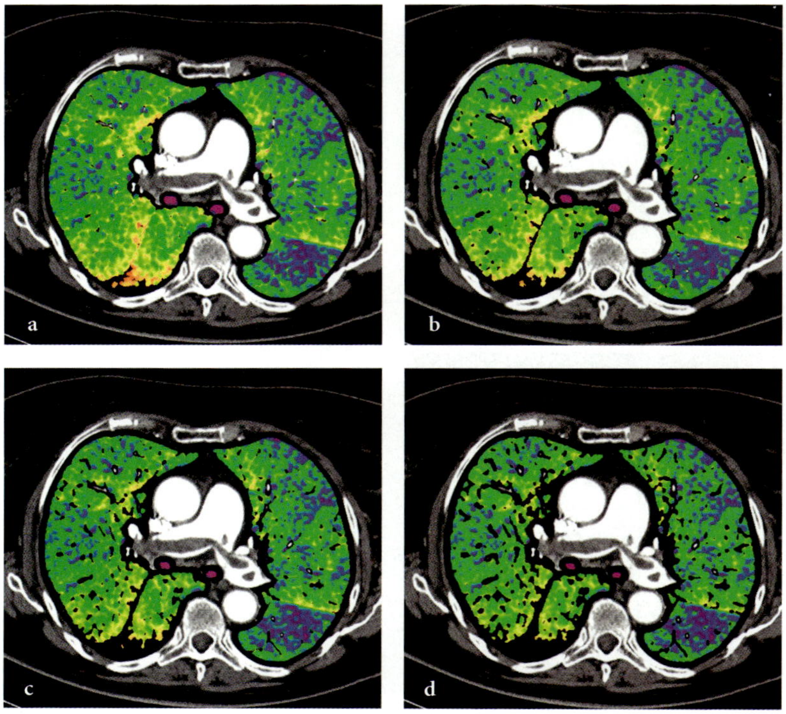

Fig. 18.6. Variation of inclusion threshold: **a** 5% **b** 20% **c** 35% **d** 50%

a

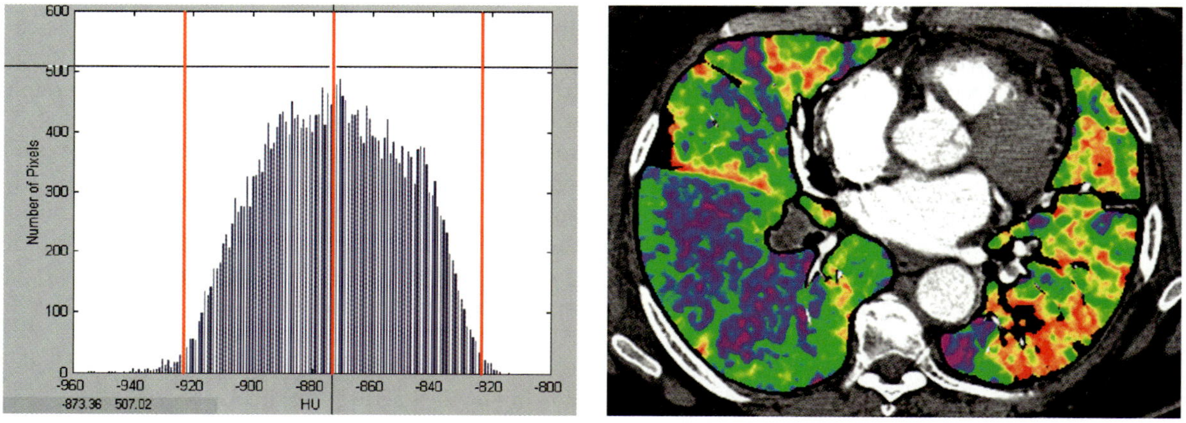

b

Fig. 18.7. a Histogram: Density distribution within the lung parenchma of the corresponding slice b. The second red line marks the median of the processed parenchymal pixels as the center value. The other red lines determine the width range, fixed to 100 HU **b** Resulting color encoded image

allowed to perform manual interactive windowing of the gray and the colored parts of the image.

These algorithms were implemented in a matlab based development environment (MatLab 5.3; The MathWorks Inc., Natick, U.S.A.) on a PC (Pentium III, 600 MHz). Modular software architecture allowed easy modifications and tests of new algorithms. The userinterface consisted of an image processing module and a viewing module for axial, sagittal and coronal display. All relevant parameters were accessible by the userinterface (Fig. 18.8).

These resulting color encoded images were evaluated for distribution of density values within the whole data set.

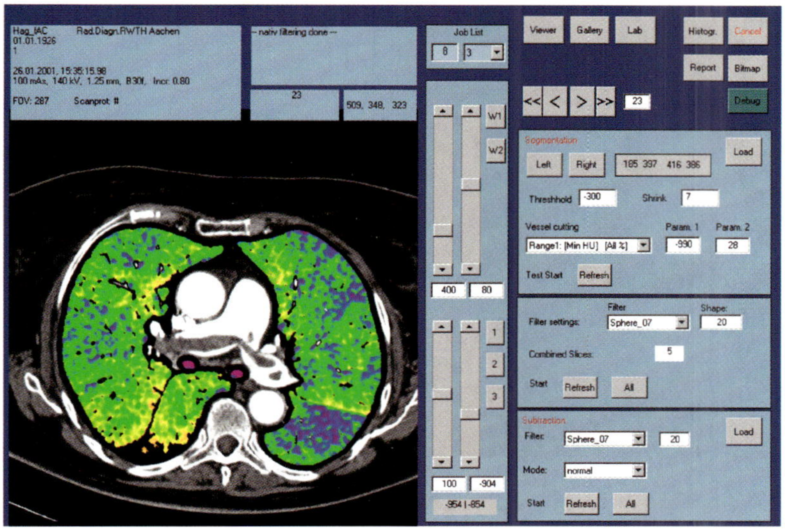

Fig. 18.8. Userinterface of the image processing module of the LungLab research environment

18.6 Clinical Examples

In patients with normal CT scans in axial scanning, color encoded display of lung parenchyma showed a quite homogeneous appearance of density values, displayed in bright green and partly yellow colors (Fig. 18.9). Anatomical details, such as lung fissures, were sharply delineated and allowed anatomical orientation, even on sagittal and coronal images. On axial and sagittal planes, a gravity dependent gradient was visible in ventro-dorsal direction in nearly every patient (green-blue encoded in the ventral lung areas).

In patients with acute PE, filling defects on CTA corresponded to areas of decreased densities, as arterial inflow into the lung parenchyma was impaired significantly in these lung segments. These areas were predominantly displayed in violet and dark blue colors (Fig. 18.10).

This methodology had limitations in patients with underlying lung disease, like emphysema,

a
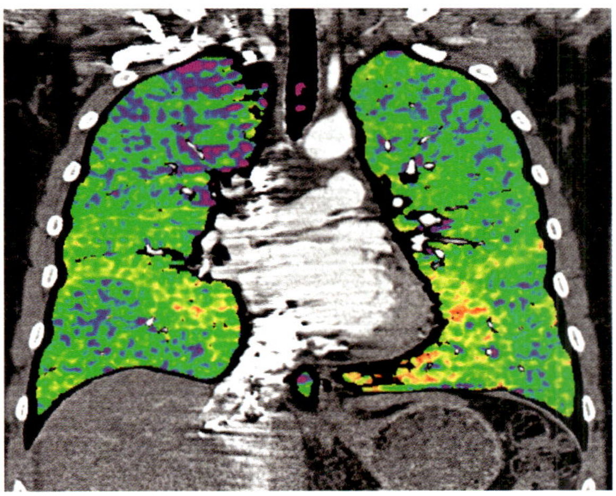

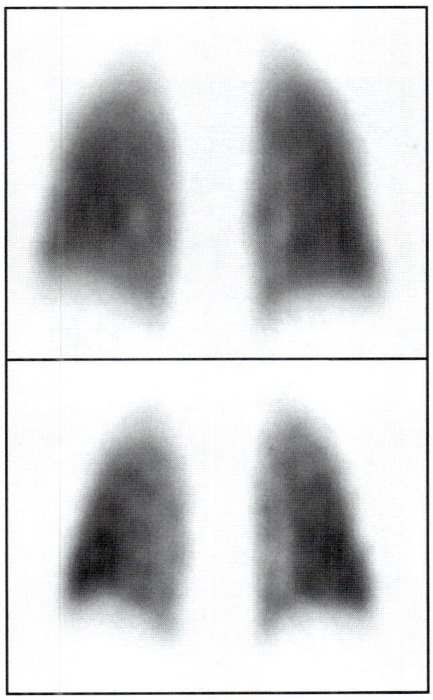
b

Fig. 18.9. Exclusion of pulmonary embolism. In coronary view, a homogeneous distribution of lung densities in green-yellow colors is depicted. Despite streaking artifacts in the right upper part of the thorax (due to contrast media application via the right arm veins), no circumscribed areas of de- or increased densities are delineated. Perfusion scintigraphy (upper right) and ventilation scintigraphy (lower right) are negative as well (Scintigraphy: Courtesy of Patrick Reinartz, MD, Department of Nuclear Medicine, University Hospital, RWTH Aachen, Germany)

a
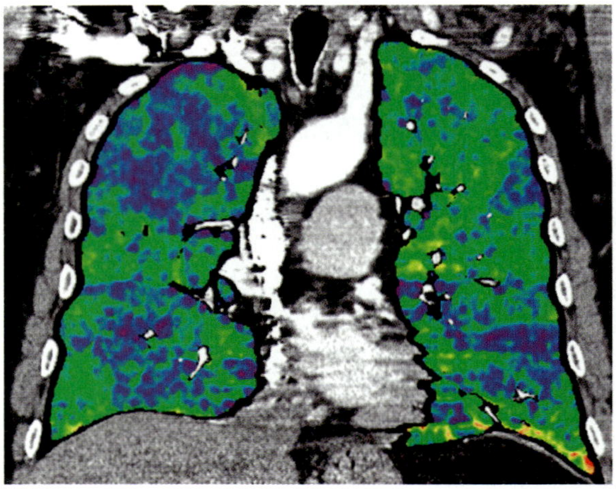

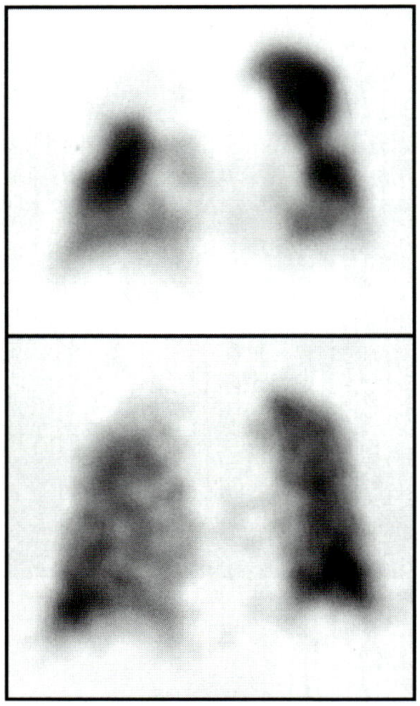
b

Fig. 18.10. Coronary view. Occluding emboli in the right upper lobe as well as in the right lower lobe and on the subsegmental and segmental level in the left lung. The downstream lung parenchyma shows decreased density distribution, corresponding to the mismatch on scintigraphy (perfusion scintigraphy (upper right) and ventilation scintigraphy (lower right); courtesy of Patrick Reinartz, MD, Department of Nuclear Medicine, University Hospital, RWTH Aachen, Germany)

pneumonia and lung fibrosis. Interpretation of areas with increased density values remain challenging, as several conditions may lead to this finding. In the patients with proven PE, dystelectatic areas led to an increase in lung density. Additional findings, such as pleural effusion, ground glass and mosaic attenuation pattern as well as atelectases for several reasons might had also effects on this methodology. Areas with increased density were displayed in red colors, and areas above the selected threshold were not color encoded at all, but were easily being assessed by adjusting the window settings for lung tissue. In these patients, interpretation of the perfusion weighted color maps together with the source images was mandatory for detailed analysis. Bullous emphysema could be delineated by circumscribed homogeneous violet areas, with lack of normal lung tissue (Fig. 18.11).

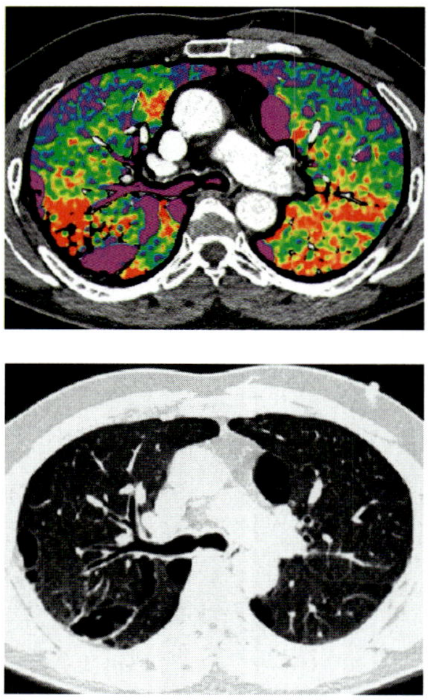

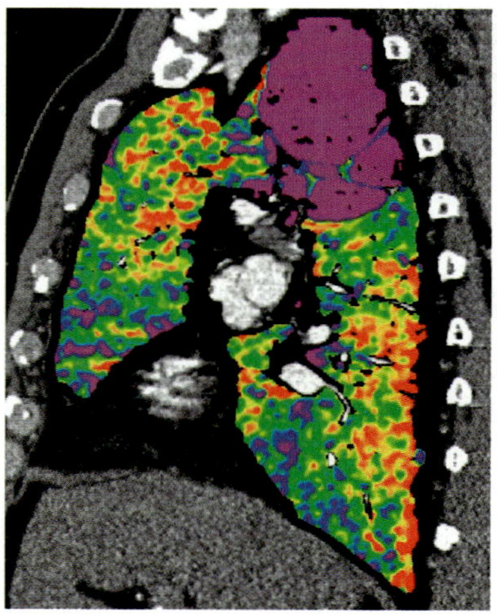

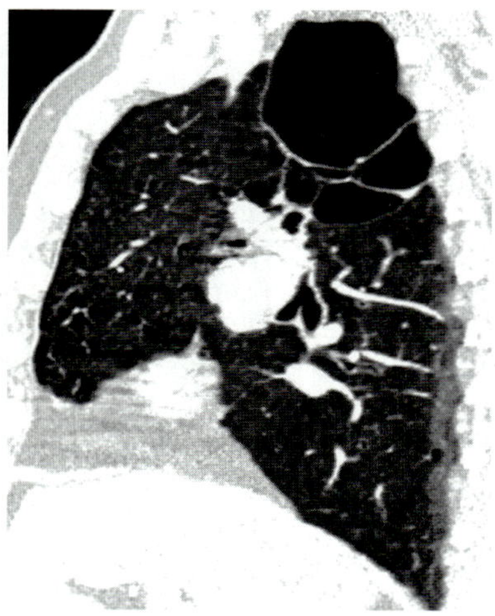

Fig. 18.11. Color encoded display of bullous emphysema. The bullae are displayed in homogeneous violet colors. Note that the absence of intrinsic structure herein allows the diagnosis. However, latter has to be confirmed on the corresponding source images in lung tissue settings [Width: 1200 HU, Center: -600 HU]

As the parenchymal histogram and the window parameters wee determined automatically, no further (subjective) windowing was needed. Informations of the lung perfusion were obtained by careful analysis of anatomic detail in all three directions.

Perfusion weighted color maps utilizing MSCT may serve as a additional imaging technique derived from data sets of the entire chest (Wildberger et al. 2001). Depiction of four slices within one gantry rotation allows a maximum volume coverage of 20 mm for dynamic MSCT studies at the moment. However, further advancement in CT-technique will form the basis for dynamic, multiphasic and real functional CT of the lungs, with eight-row and 16-row multislice CT-scanners at present or even flat-panel volume CT in the future. The post-processing method on parenchymal density distribution might serve as a basis for further developments in this field.

References

Garg K, Sieler H, Welsh CH, Johnston RJ, Russ PD (1999) Clinical validity of helical CT being interpreted as negative for pulmonary embolism: implications for patient treatment. Am J Roentgenol 172:1627–1631

Ghaye B, Szapiro D, Mastora I, Delannoy V, Duhamel A, Remy J, Remy-Jardin M (2001) Peripheral pulmonary arteries: how far in the lung does multi-detector row spiral CT allow analysis. Radiology 219:629–636

Groell R, Peichel KH, Uggowitzer MM, Schmid F, Hartwagner K (1999) Computed tomography densitometry of the lung: a method to assess perfusion defects in acute pulmonary embolism. Eur J Radiol 32:192–196

Harvey RT, Gefter WB, Hrung JM, Langlotz CP (2000) Accuracy of CT angiography versus pulmonary angiography in the diagnosis of acute pulmonary embolism: evaluation of the literature with summary ROC curve analysis. Acad Radiol 7:786–797

Hoffman EA, Tajik JK, Kugelmass SD (1995) Matching pulmonary structure and perfusion via combined dynamic multislice CT and thin-slice high-resolution CT. Comp Med Imaging Graph 19:101–112

Kazerooni EA (2001) Quantitative and functional CT of the chest. In: Müller NL, Grist TM (eds) Categorial course in diagnostic radiology: thoracic imaging – chest and cardiac. Syllabus, RSNA, pp 159 –167

Rémy-Jardin M, Rémy J, Deschildre F, Artaud D, Beregi JP, Hossein-Foucher C, Marchandise X, Duhamel A (1996) Diagnosis of pulmonary embolism with spiral CT: comparison with pulmonary angiography and scintigraphy. Radiology 200:699–706

Schoepf UJ, Bruening R, Konschitzky H, Becker CR, Knez A, Weber J, Muehling O, Herzog P, Huber A, Haberl R, Reiser MF (2000) Pulmonary embolism: comprehensive diagnosis by using electron-beam CT for detection of emboli and assessment of pulmonary blood flow. Radiology 217: 693–700

Schoepf UJ, Holzknecht N, Helmberger TK, Crispin A, Hong C, Becker CR, Reiser MF (2002) Subsegmental pulmonary emboli: improved detection with thin-collimation multidetector row spiral-CT. Radiology 222:483–490

Wildberger JE, Niethammer MU, Klotz E, Schaller S, Wein BB, Günther RW (2001) Multi-slice CT for visualization of pulmonary embolism using perfusion weighted color maps. Fortschr Roentgenstr 173:289–294

Wildberger JE, Mahnken AH, Sinha AM, Stargardt A, Haage P, Schaller S, Günther RW (2002) A differentiated approach to the diagnosis of pulmonary embolism and deep venous thrombosis using multi-slice CT. Fortschr Roentgenstr 174: 301–307

19 Multiple-Detector CT Venography

A. Nchimi and B. Ghaye

CONTENTS

19.1 Introduction

Deep venous thrombosis (DVT) and pulmonary embolism (PE) are two aspects of the same disease process termed venous thrombo-embolism (VTE). The VTE is a major health problem that is estimated to be associated with 300,000–900,000 hospitalisations and results in 50,000–150,000 deaths each year in the United States (National Institutes of Health 1986; Moser 1990; Ferris 1992). Early diagnosis and treatment significantly improve survival in patients with VTE (Dalen and Alpert 1975); however, the clinical diagnosis is difficult. Although ventilation–perfusion (V/Q) lung scan has been a common screening test of suspected PE, single-slice spiral CT angiography (SSCTA) was used increasingly in the 1990s, as it accurately defines emboli down to the level of the segmental pulmonary arteries, while revealing other non-embolic causes of thoracic symptoms (Remy-Jardin et al. 1996; Herold et al. 1999; Ghaye et al. 2002a). Drawbacks to the SSCTA as a screening test for PE included a rate of indeterminate examinations up to 13%, its relative inaccuracy for small clots located distal to the level of segmental arteries, and the duration of breath hold, up to 45 s, which may result into breathing artefacts (Ghaye et al. 2002a); thus, the role of SSCTA relative to V/Q scan remained a debate among clinicians during the past decade. Most of the limitations of SSCTA have been overcome with the use of multiple-detector CT angiography (MDCTA), who proved to be accurate down to the subsegmental arteries and requires a 10- to 20-s breathhold when using four rows (Ghaye et al. 2001). Regarding actual performances, if ever such refinement is required, there is little doubt that MDCTA will become the standard examination in patients suspected of PE, with the use of scanners with 16 or more rows.

Pulmonary emboli may represent the "tip of the iceberg", as a small PE may herald larger emboli to come, which imposes evaluation of venous clots (Goodman and Lipchik 1996; Goodman 2000). While clots in the lungs clearly influence the cardiopulmonary status of the patients, the major risk of death is from recurrent PE. In the PIOPED study, a recurrent embolic event was the cause of death in 90% of the patients dying of PE (Carson et al. 1992). The DVT is often asymptomatic and approximately 90% of PE arise from deep veins of the legs and pelvis (Moser 1990); therefore, it appears that opti-

A. Nchimi, MD
Department of Medical Imaging, University Hospital Sart Tilman B 35, 4000 Liège, Belgium
B. Ghaye, MD
Department of Medical Imaging, University Hospital Sart Tilman B 35, 4000 Liège, Belgium

misation of resolution of SCTA may be of less clinical importance than accurate assessment of residual DVT. Furthermore, dual assessment of both aspects of the disease is important with respect to therapeutic implications (Ferris 1992). Although the most common imaging strategy to rule out DVT in the extremities includes SCTA followed by ultrasound (US) (Goodman and Lipchik 1996; Fishman and Horton 2000), a single examination that accurately depicts both PE and DVT would be desirable to avoid delay in the diagnosis of VTE and limit cost.

19.2 Venous Imaging Techniques

Venous obstruction, among which DVT is the leading cause, and preoperative imaging of venous insufficiency, are the main indications for examination of the lower limb veins; for the latter, US is almost always sufficient (Reimer and Landwehr 1998). Ascending venography (VG) is still currently accepted as the most reliable test for the diagnosis of DVT and the gold standard against which all other diagnostic tests should be evaluated (Bauer and Flynn 1988; Bettmann 1997). The VG is considered the only technique available that accurately demonstrates all calf, muscular, deep and superficial veins. Uncertain initial results may require variations of the basic technique. Using proper technique in a cooperative patient, it is almost always possible to visualize the deep venous system and to determine whether venous occlusion is acute or chronic. This invasive test is limited by technical factors and complications, which may be minimized by a careful technique (Bettmann 1997). Inter- and intra-observer variability confirmed important operator dependence and the need for experience in performing and interpreting results (McLachlan et al. 1979; Picolet et al. 1990).

Ultrasound is an established and widely available technique for evaluation of the veins of both the lower and upper extremities. Advantages include non-invasive and inexpensive technique, and the ability to perform the examination at the patient's bedside, including dynamic manoeuvres. In the lower limbs US can be performed with the compression technique (Cogo et al. 1993), Doppler technique or both (Lensing et al. 1999). In a large meta-analysis, US showed sensitivities of 92–100% and specificities of 80–100%, when compared with VG for proximal veins in patients having symptoms of DVT. For distal or calf veins, sensitivity was 40–87% depending on technique. In asymptomatic patients, sensitivity was 38–100% for the proximal level, and 38–58% for the calf level, confirming that none of the US examination techniques had a sufficiently high sensitivity for calf veins (Lensing et al. 1999). In addition, US is operator dependent and has limitations above the inguinal ligament and below knee. Recently, Katz et al. found 30% of clots located below knee or above the inguinal ligament in 100 patients with positive CTV (Katz et al. 2002). Among 347 patients with VTE, we found DVT in 306 patients, bilateral in 55 patients. The distribution of clots in the 306 patients with DVT at CTV showed that 70% (837 of 1193) of the thrombosed veins were located below knee or above the inguinal ligament (Table 19.1). Furthermore, 24 of the 25 (96%) patients with isolated segmental DVT had involvement below knee or above the inguinal ligament (Table 19.2).

Similarly to CT, MR has the ability to allow for a combined evaluation of PE and venous thrombosis. Preliminary results of MR venography showed results similar to those of ascending VG (Carpenter et al. 1993; Ruehm et al. 2000). Widespread availability, lower cost, shorter examination time and higher accuracy for peripheral pulmonary arteries are currently the main advantages of CT over the emerging MR imaging. For both techniques, the risk of recurrent PE from missed DVT still needs assessment.

Table 19.1. Distribution of deep venous thrombosis at different venous levels in 306 patients with positive CT venography. *IVC* inferior vena cava

Venous level	No. of thrombosed venous segments
IVC	11
Iliac (common, internal and external iliac veins)	85
Femoral (common femoral, deep femoral and superficial femoral veins)	213
Popliteal level	143
Calf (anterior tibial, posterior tibial, peroneal, gastrocnemial, sural and tibioperoneal veins)	741

Table 19.2. Distribution of isolated DVT at different venous levels in 25 patients of 306 with positive CT venography

Venous level	No. of thrombosed venous segments
IVC	0
Iliac (common, internal and external iliac veins)	1
Femoral (common femoral, deep femoral and superficial femoral veins)	1
Popliteal	0
Calf (anterior tibial, posterior tibial, peroneal, gastrocnemial, sural and tibioperoneal veins)	23

In nuclear medicine imaging, radiolabelled thrombus-detecting agents are investigated, with the potential of screening the whole body for thrombo-embolic disease in a single examination, and differentiating between acute or chronic thrombosis (Blum and Handmaker 2000).

19.3 CT Venography

19.3.1 History

In 1978, Steele et al. first reported incidental detection of inferior vena cava (IVC) thrombosis with conventional CT in two patients (Steele et al. 1978). In 1980, Zerhouni et al. reported five cases demonstrating CT findings of ilio-femoral venous thrombosis (Zerhouni et al. 1980); thereafter, CT findings of DVT were refined in many papers published during the early 1980s (van Breda et al. 1979; Allgayer et al. 1981; Vujic et al. 1981; Hidalgo et al. 1982; Pagani et al. 1982; Pawar and Kay 1984). In 1987, Pillari et al. reported a series of 14 patients suspected of DVT who underwent CT of the legs after a negative venography. The CT was performed from the patella to the inferior third of the calves during infusion of 30% contrast medium in a foot vein. No further DVT was demonstrated, but abnormalities, such as muscular haemorrhage or occult knee-joint effusion, responsible of the clinical symptoms, were shown (Pillari et al. 1987). In 1988, Bauer and Flynn reported the clinical use of indirect CT venography (CTV) in patients with inconclusive VG, or when venous access in the foot was impossible. The CT scanning of the lower extremities and pelvis was obtained during a slow infusion of 150 ml of contrast medium in an arm vein for 10 min (Bauer and Flynn 1988). In 1991, Langer et al. reported a series of indirect CTV from the ankle to the pelvis in 15 patients. In the 6 patients suspected of having PE, the thorax was also scanned and concomitant pleuro-parenchymal changes were demonstrated. This report was the first to promote a combined incremental CT examination of the thorax, lower limbs, and pelvis in patients suspected of VTE (Langer et al. 1991). In 1994, Stehling et al. reported the first case of direct spiral CTV of the lower limbs following injection through a catheter inserted in a dorsal vein of the foot (Stehling et al. 1994); however, it was not until 1998 that Loud et al. reported the combination of spiral CT angiography of the pulmonary arteries and incremental CTV in 5 patients suspected of VTE. Veins were imaged from the lower calves to the diaphragm thanks to contrast medium recirculation that follows rapid infusion for SCTA (Loud et al. 1998).

19.3.2 Direct CT Venography

19.3.2.1 *Technique*

Stehling et al. reported the first case of direct spiral CTV in 1994 (Stehling et al. 1994). Diluted contrast medium was injected through a catheter placed in a dorsal foot vein. Tourniquets were used around the ankle to direct the contrast medium into the deep venous system. Axial, multiplanar and maximum intensity projection images allowed differentiation of acute DVT from chronic thrombus in a patient with ambiguous sonographic and venographic findings. Potential advantages over venography are the ability to perform 3D imaging, a tenfold reduction of contrast medium volume, increased patient comfort due to the low concentration of contrast medium, a supine position and a decreased risk of post-injection phlebitis. Layering of contrast medium in the vein may remain nevertheless a factor of suboptimal opacification (Stehling et al. 1994). With a 4-detector rows CT, a 5-mm collimation, 1.5–2.0 pitch, 100-mAs spiral covering both legs from the ankle to the diaphragm may be sufficient. For preoperative imaging of venous insufficiency, the contrast medium may be injected directly inside the varicose veins and the spiral length limited to the region of interest (Uhl et al. 2002).

19.3.2.2 *Indications and Results*

One study compared direct spiral CTV with conventional venography in 52 patients suspected of having DVT. Sensitivity of direct spiral CTV was 100%, specificity 96%, positive predictive 91% and negative predictive value 100%. The extension of DVT, particularly in pelvic veins and inferior vena cava (IVC), was better demonstrated with CTV. Interobserver agreement was 0.81–0.93 and 0.71–0.88 for direct CTV and conventional venography, respectively. Intra-observer agreement was 0.91–0.94 and 0.75–0.92, respectively. Global venous opacification was significantly better with direct CTV, despite a 80% reduction of volume of contrast medium (40 vs 200 ml). Major differences were found in the IVC, pelvic veins and deep femoral veins. Only 11% (compared with 25% with venography) of all deep veins were not opacified. The technique is less operator dependent than US or venography but remains susceptible to blood inflow that can mimic an intraluminal filling defect (Baldt et al. 1996). Direct CTV better demonstrates the relation between thrombus and vessel wall, confirming that conventional venography overestimated the prevalence of the so-called free-floating clots (Gartenschlager et al. 1996). The deep venous system is not always entirely opacified, and veno-puncture of both feet is required (Baldt et al. 1996, 1997). The technique can also be applied to evaluate venous thrombosis of the upper extremities (Zontsich et al. 1998). A combination with MDCTA of the pulmonary arteries is impossible, and any further imaging will require additional contrast medium injection; thus, direct CTV must be used either for DVT, with the same rationale as VG, or in selected patients with venous insufficiency requiring preoperative 3D diagnostic work-up.

19.3.3 Indirect CT Venography

19.3.3.1 Technique

The patient is positioned supine on the CT table with the feet directed towards the gantry. Feet are placed in the head holder or on a table extender and wrapped together with tape to limit leg motion. Such patient orientation allows for scanning from the ankle to the cervico-thoracic junction without repositioning. Legs are maintained slightly elevated on a folded blanket to avoid compression of the calf veins. In some centres, tourniquets are used, for preferential opacification of the deep venous system (Coche et al. 2001). Elastic stockings have recently been reported to increase venous enhancement between 30 and 34% ($p<0.0005$) at popliteal, femoral and iliac levels (Abdelmoumene et al. 2003). The arms are placed over the patient's head as with SCTA. Firstly, a scout view of the thorax is obtained. In some equipment allowing tube current modulation in spiral scanning for CTV, the scout view should include the whole trunk and lower limbs. Next, 120–150 ml of 240–300 mg iodine/ml contrast medium are injected at a flow rate of 3–5 ml/s through an antecubital vein for acquisition of MDCTA. After completion of examination of pulmonary arteries, the table may be either manually moved to place the reference laser at the level of the ankle or automatically positioned after prescription of CTV on the scout view. CTV starts approximately 210 s following the beginning of the injection using either sequential or spiral scanning.

1. With sequential technique, 5- to 10-mm-thick slices are acquired every 20–50 mm. Only 2.1% of the patients had DVT visible on one single slice when using a 20-mm slice interval. A slice interval >2 cm can potentially lead to either false-negative findings on CTV or an underestimation of the extent of DVT (Garg et al. 2001).
2. Using spiral technique, 3.75- to 10-mm-thick slices are usually obtained (El Hajjam et al. 1999; Cham et al. 2000; Duwe et al. 2000; Coche et al. 2001; Muller et al. 2001; Nicolas et al. 2001; Peterson et al. 2001). With 4-detector rows CT, a length of 100 cm can be scanned in approximately 20 s, using 4- to 5-mm collimation, 0.5-s rotation time and pitch of 1.8 (Schoepf et al. 2001; Wildberger et al. 2002).

Screening during the optimal time window of CTV is important for proper clot detection. Optimal vein analysis requires high level of luminal attenuation, homogeneous opacification and a sufficient vein to surrounding muscle gradient and vein-to-clot gradient. A gradient of 30 Hounsfield units (HU) is generally considered to be sufficient. Morphology and density of clots appear to vary with thrombus composition and age. Venous thrombus, generated in slow-flow conditions, are "red thrombus" predominantly composed of red blood cells. The relative concentration of protein, particularly globin, is responsible for high CT density values. Acute red thrombi have a higher haematocrit value than blood, due to increased concentration of globin. Recent clots (<8 days) appear homogeneous with average densities of 31±10 HU (Loud et al. 2000), 51 HU (Cham et al. 2000), 66±7 HU (Baldt et al. 1996), 76 HU (Lomas and Britton 1991) and 60–80 HU (Gmelin et al. 1992). With time, globin is broken down and removed by phagocytes, resulting in decreased attenuation values, which are sometimes at a lower level than normal blood (Lomas and Britton 1991). Subacute or chronic clots (>8 days) tend to become heterogeneous with areas of high attenuation and average densities of 28 HU (Lomas and Britton 1991), <50 HU (Gmelin et al. 1992) or 55±11 HU (Baldt et al. 1996).

Time-density curves of lower limb venous enhancement following SCTA of the pulmonary arteries have been studied using sequential, single or multiple-detector CT (Matar et al. 1999; Yankelevitz et al. 2000a; Szapiro et al. 2001). Curves at different levels of the lower limbs showed that all density values comprised in the time interval from venous enhancement mean peak (ranging from 93 to 137 HU) to mean densities at 420 s (ranging from 88 to 103 HU) were above reported attenuation values of recent clots. Time to reach maximum enhancement increased from IVC (93±9.5 s) to popliteal veins (141±57 s) and decreased for calf veins (124±32 s; Szapiro et al. 2001). Homogeneity of venous enhancement is another parameter that affects clot detection during CTV. Homogeneous enhancement is obtained after 150 s for above-knee veins, except for femoral vein (180 s), and 210 s for veins below the knees (Szapiro et al. 2001). When considering time-density curves, homogeneous venous opacification, vein-to-muscles and vein-to-clot gradients at different levels, an optimal time window for CTV was determined to be between 210 and 240 s for the calf level and 180–300 s for above-knee veins (Fig. 19.1). When using a sequential acquisition for CTV, a caudo-cranial acquisition is recommended, which starts at 210 s for the sural level (optimal time window). For faster CTV technique, such as multi-slice CT, the choice of direction of acquisition is irrelevant (Szapiro et al. 2001). Similar levels of enhancement (91–118 HU) were reported in clinical practice for above-knee veins, when starting CTV 180–210 s after contrast medium injection (Cham et al. 2000; Loud et al. 2000; Bruce et al. 2001; Wildberger et al. 2002).

19.3.3.2
Indication

Currently, the only stringent indication of indirect CTV is VTE. Combined SCTA of the pulmonary arteries and indirect CTV of the lower limbs allow for a complete one-session evaluation of VTE (Loud et al. 1998; Cham et al. 2000; Garg et al. 2000; Ghaye et al. 2000; Loud et al. 2000; Yankelevitz et al. 2000a).

19.4
Radiation Dose of CTV

Advantages of spiral scanning include faster acquisition, 3D imaging capability and absence of interslice gap. Drawbacks of the spiral technique include minimal increase in sensitivity for DVT, while resulting in a substantial increase in radiation dose and in number of images (Katz et al. 2002). Although their clinical significance is unknown, isolated short segmental DVT are not uncommon findings, especially in asymptomatic patients (Garg et al. 2000). Two small clots in the superficial and common femoral vein were missed, when using 40- to 50-mm interslice gap in 308 patients (0.6%; Loud et al. 2001); thus, as for the optimisation of MDCTA of the pulmonary arteries, the justification of spiral CTV will become in the near future an additional matter of debate. Technical parameters influencing the dose delivered to the patient have to be carefully selected. To the best of our knowledge, currently there is no published study comparing different irradiation parameters for CTV. Spiral technique requires careful selection of scanning parameters, in order to obtain acceptable radiation doses in comparison with sequential technique. For example, with sequential scanning (PQ 5000, Phillips, Eindhoven, The Netherlands), we used 100 mA, 1-s rotation speed and 130 kVp per slice (Szapiro et al. 2001). On a 4-row multislice scanner (HiSpeed QX/i, GE Medical systems, Milwaukee, Wis.), we performed scanning with a continuous spiral, 5-mm collimation, 30-mm/rotation table speed, 0.7-s rotation speed, 90 mA and 120 kVp, without significant degradation of the image quality. In comparison, Wildberger et al. used a 4×5-mm collimation, 30-mm/rotation table speed, 0.5-s rota-

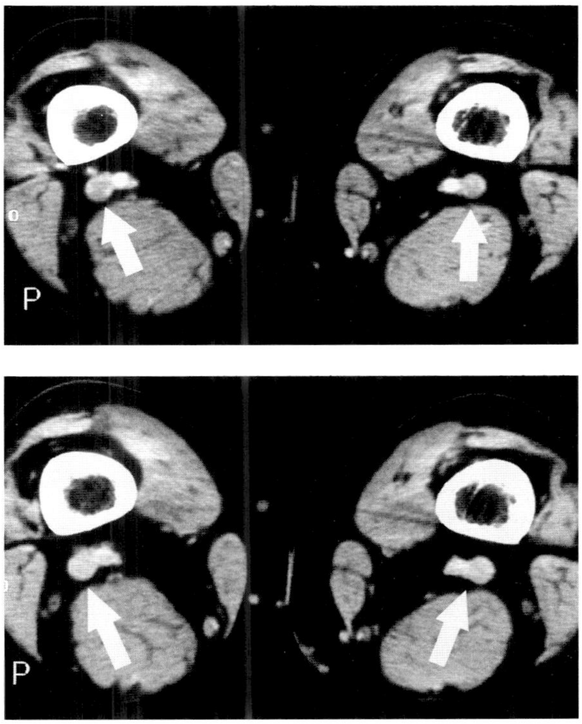

a

b

Fig. 19.1a, b. Heterogeneous venous enhancement. **a** Axial CT venogram at the popliteal level shows a pseudo-filling defect in both popliteal veins (*arrows*). Scanning was performed less than 180 s after start of contrast medium injection. **b** Axial CT venogram shows homogeneous enhancement after rescanning 30 s later tion speed, 120 kVp and 170 mAs and calculated the dose of CTV to be 9.3 mSv (Wildberger et al. 2002). Using 4×2.5 mm, 15 mm/s, 120 kVp and 130 mAs, a CTDI of 12.22 mGy and DLP of 1200 mGy.cm were reported. Using 16×1.5 mm, 24 mm/s, 120 kVp and 130 mAs, results were 10.50 mGy for CTDI and 1090 mGy.cm for DLP (Martin-Bouyer 2002). In other published clinical studies using spiral CT, parameters were variable (75–260 mA and 120–150 kVp and a pitch of 1–1.5) (El Hajjam et al. 1999; Cham et al. 2000; Coche et al. 2001; Muller et al. 2001). "Low-dose" technical parameters (75 mAs, 120 kVp) have been shown to be adequate when using dual-detector spiral CT, 6.5-mm slice thickness, 20-mm/s table feed and 1-s rotation speed (Coche et al. 2001). One study estimated the dose of CTV to be slightly less than that of a standard pelvic CT (Cham et al. 2000). In another study, the effective radiation dose of combined spiral SCTA–CTV was calculated to be approximately 57% of a dual-phase spiral CT of the liver (4.75 vs 8.3 mSv). Although such an evaluation depends on the specific technical parameters and type of scanner used, it was demonstrated that spiral CTV was responsible for 50% of the effective dose of the combined SCTA–CTV technique and of a significant increase in gonadal dose. Although the risk–benefit ratio remains limited in a mainly aged population, indications of CTV should be considered carefully in younger patients (Rademaker et al. 2001).

19.5 Image Interpretation

19.5.1 CT Signs of DVT

In clinical practice the differentiation between acute and chronic DVT is important for determination of the need for anticoagulation and duration of treatment (Bettmann 1997; Garg et al. 2001; Garg and Mao 2001).

19.5.1.1 Acute DVT

The CT signs of acute DVT have been described in case reports published in the 1980s (Steele et al. 1978; van Breda et al. 1979; Zerhouni et al. 1980; Allgayer et al. 1981; Vujic et al. 1981; Hidalgo et al. 1982; Pagani et al. 1982; Lien and Lund 1983; Pawar and Kay 1984; Seem et al. 1985; Vogelzang et al. 1988). The primary CT sign of DVT is the demonstration of intra-vascular clot, presenting as a complete, partial or juxta-mural filling defect, depending on the degree of venous occlusion. Recognition of clot with CT may be difficult in some cases, as fresh thrombus may exhibit attenuation values similar to contrast-enhanced blood (Zerhouni et al. 1980; Ghaye et al. 2000). Additional findings may contribute to establish the diagnosis: venous dilation compared with the normal contralateral side, obliteration of perivenous fat suggestive of oedema, high contrast ring-like rim of the venous wall due to contrast staining in the vasa vasorum or contrast accumulation around intraluminal clot, muscular swelling and opacification of collateral veins (Figs. 19.2–4; Loud et al. 1998; Ghaye et al. 2000). A non-opacified venous segment that is sandwiched by an opacified distal and proximal seg-

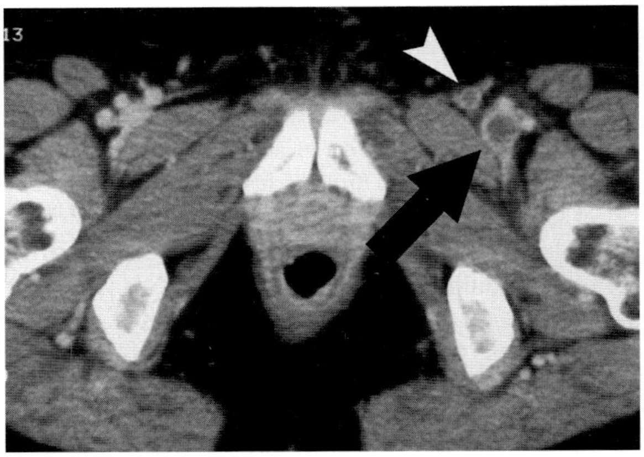

Fig. 19.2. Proximal acute deep venous thrombosis. Acute clots are demonstrated in the left common femoral vein (*arrow*) and left greater saphenous vein (*arrowhead*). Note dilation of the veins and infiltration of perivenous fat compared to the right side

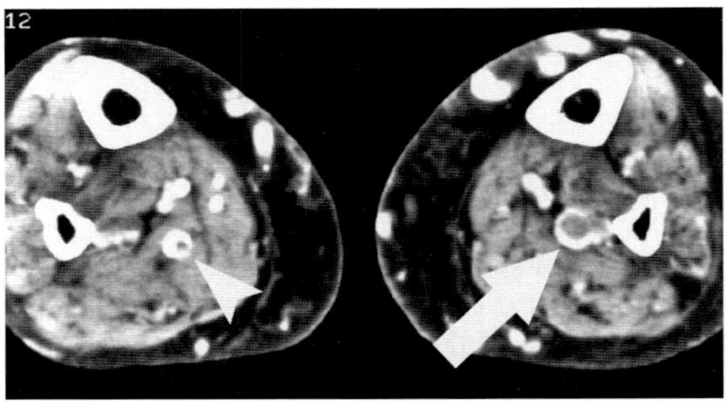

Fig. 19.3. Distal acute deep venous thrombosis. Acute clots are shown in the left internal peroneal vein (*arrow*) and in a right sural vein (*arrowhead*). Note dilation of thrombosed veins compared with normal and the presence of large subcutaneous collaterals

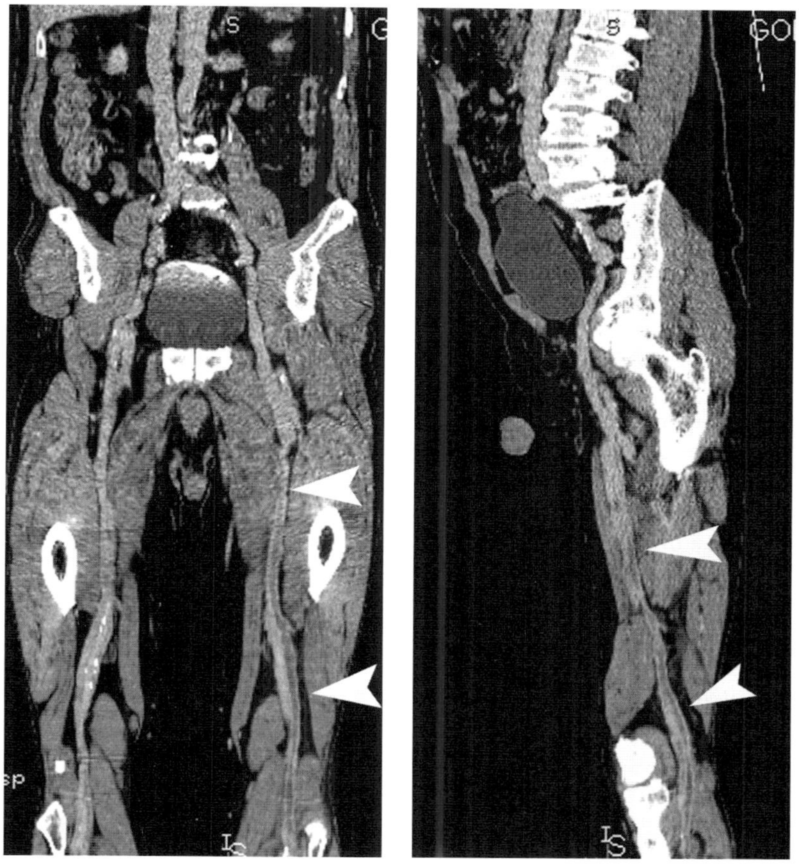

Fig. 19.4a, b. Acute deep venous thrombosis. Indirect MDCT venography was performed with a 4×5-mm collimation from the ankle to the diaphragm. A 2.5-mm-thick curved reformatting along the deep venous system of the left lower limb was performed. **a** Front and **b** lateral angles of rotation along the curve showed a continuous central filing defect involving the deep venous system, from the calf to the common femoral vein (*arrowheads*)

ment has to be interpreted with caution. Prolonged arterial phase of enhancement may occasionally be seen in patients with extensive bilateral DVT (Duwe et al. 2000).

19.5.1.2 Chronic DVT

Chronic DVT classically manifests as clots with an irregular margin, and occasionally containing calcifications. Thrombus is often eccentric with a large portion anchored to the vein wall. Thickening of the vein wall corresponds either to a hyperplastic response of the endothelium, or to residual thrombus incorporated in the vein wall. Partial clot recanalisation may result in a heterogeneous lumen and strands. Multiple deep or superficial collaterals are commonly encountered. Other signs include small retracted veins and ultimately a fibrous cord replacing the vein (Ghaye et al. 2002b); however, some chronic clots may show vein dilation, or perivascular and soft tissue oedema, which may mimic acute DVT (Gmelin et al. 1992; Garg and Mao 2001; Loud et al. 2001).

19.5.1.3 Recurrent DVT

Association of findings of acute and chronic DVT on CTV suggests the diagnosis of recurrent DVT (Garg and Mao 2001). Recurrent DVT is a major challenge in diagnostic imaging (Hull et al. 1983; Cronan and Leen 1989). Comparison with previous examinations improves confidence in diagnosis. Both CTV and US have been suggested to have a complementary role in unsolved cases (Garg and Mao 2001). The accuracy of CTV in predicting the age of the thrombus and recurrent DVT needs to be assessed.

19.5.2 Venous Anatomy

The CT venography enables recognition of DVT in veins which are difficult to assess with US or ascending venography, such as deep femoral vein, internal iliac vein, gonadal vein, renal vein and hepatic vein. Combination with SCTA may further demonstrate clots in the right heart, superior vena cava, right and left innominate veins and central part of the subclavian and jugular veins.

19.5.2.1
Normal Anatomy

Normal venous anatomy is displayed in Fig. 19.5. There is a wide variation in the distribution of calf veins, but they are mainly grouped into anterior tibial, posterior tibial and peroneal veins. Veins accompany the corresponding arteries and are duplicated in most cases. Posterior tibial and peroneal veins drain the sural veins and join to form the tibioperoneal trunk that joins the anterior tibial vein to form the popliteal vein, at the lower limit of the popliteus muscle. Gastrocnemial veins drain into the popliteal vein in most patients; however, they may drain at a lower level (i.e. the tibioperoneal trunk or the peroneal vein). The superficial femoral vein begins at the hiatus of the adductor magnus muscle and accompanies the corresponding artery through the crus. It joins the deep femoral vein to form the common femoral vein that drains the superficial circumflex, pudendal and the greater saphenous vein, at the level of the inguinal ligament, to form the external iliac vein. The veins that are located below the inguinal ligament have numerous valves. Deep veins may communicate with the superficial veins via trans-fascial (perforating) veins. A corresponding artery does not accompany greater and lesser saphenous veins, as other superficial veins. Above the inguinal ligament, both the internal and external iliac vein join on each side to form common iliac vein. Both common iliac vein have an upper, anterior and internal oblique course, with the vertical orientation of the left-sided vein being less marked. Both veins join to form the inferior vena cava that has a vertical course in the retroperitoneum, right to the abdominal aorta, ending immediately above the diaphragmatic hiatus, in the inferior posterior aspect of the right atrium, after having received the following veins: lumbar, right testicular/ovarian, renal, right adrenal, inferior phrenic and hepatic. The diameter of the veins reflects their capacious role. The venous calibre is similar to that of the corresponding artery for popliteal vein, superficial and common femoral veins, external and common iliac veins and IVC. Veins below the popliteal level, deep femoral vein and internal iliac vein have a calibre superior to the corresponding artery.

19.5.2.2
Anatomic Variants

Anatomic variants should be recognized to avoid false-negative results of CTV. Duplication is usual for posterior tibial, anterior tibial and peroneal veins. Partial duplication of popliteal and/or superficial femoral veins may be frequently encountered, particularly in patients with DVT. The IVC may be occasionally duplicated or left sided (Wagner and Mark 1969; Kouroukis and LeClerc 1996). Duplication represents a classic pitfall in US (Loud et al. 2001; Ghaye et al. 2002b). Embryological remnants of the sciatic vein may rarely be seen with popliteal vein draining either in deep femoral or in internal iliac veins. Unusual venous pathways may be associated with absence of usual normal venous segment.

19.5.3
Interpretative Pitfalls

19.5.3.1
Pitfalls Related to Technique

Theoretical advantages of the sequential technique are reduction of number of slices and of total irradiation; however, short segmental DVTs have unknown clinical significance and are likely to be overlooked with sequential scanning. Obviously, the risk increases as the interslice gap is larger. With spiral scanning, the risk of missing a short clot is almost completely minimised (Fig. 19.6). Furthermore, spiral technique offers orthogonal reformatting capability that may be useful in equivocal cases. Inhomogeneous opacification of the veins may cause pseudo-filling defects, which may simulate DVT (Garg and Mao 2001; Ghaye et al. 2002b). Such artefacts may be flow related or due to improper selection of scanning time (Fig. 1; Glazer et al. 1981; Barnes et al. 1982; Vogelzang et al. 1985; Garg et al. 2000; Peterson et al. 2001; Ghaye et al. 2002b). The time-to-peak venous enhancement is highly variable among patients (Yankelevitz et al. 2000a). The influence of individual physiological parameters on venous enhancement, such as age, body weight and height, cardiac output, hydration and renal function, has to be evaluated. In patients with heart failure, severe distal arterial obstruction or impaired flow dynamics, such as abdominal vein compression, adding a further delay of 60 s is recommended before CTV acquisition (Garg et al. 2000). A contrast-blood interface is occasionally observed in dilated varicose veins, due to reduced local flow

Fig. 19.5a–i. Normal venous anatomy. An MDCT venography was performed with a 4×5-mm collimation from the ankle to the diaphragm. **a** The three paired calf veins, adjacent to the corresponding arteries (*arrowheads*). **b** Tibioperoneal trunk (*arrows*) and gastrocnemial veins (*arrowheads*). **c** Popliteal vein (*arrows*). **d** Deep (*arrowheads*) and superficial femoral veins (*arrows*). **e** Smaller veins joining the common femoral vein (*arrows*), such as the circumflex veins, are seen (*arrowheads*). **f** External iliac (*arrows*) and gluteal veins (*arrowheads*). **g** The latter at an upper level joins the other pelvic veins, to form the internal iliac vein (*arrowheads*). **h** The left ovarian vein (*arrowheads*) and **i** both renal veins (*arrowheads*) joining the inferior vena cava (*arrows*)

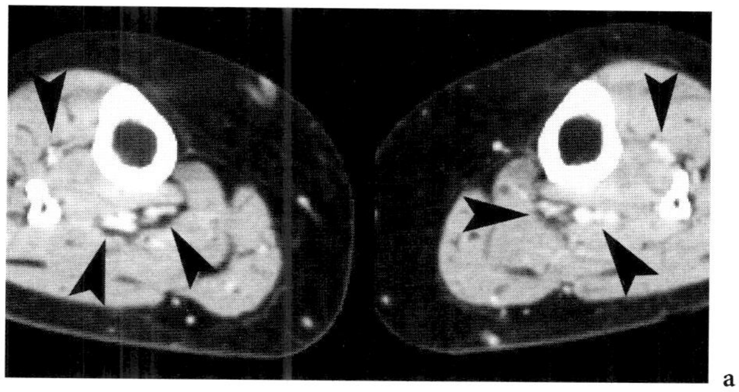

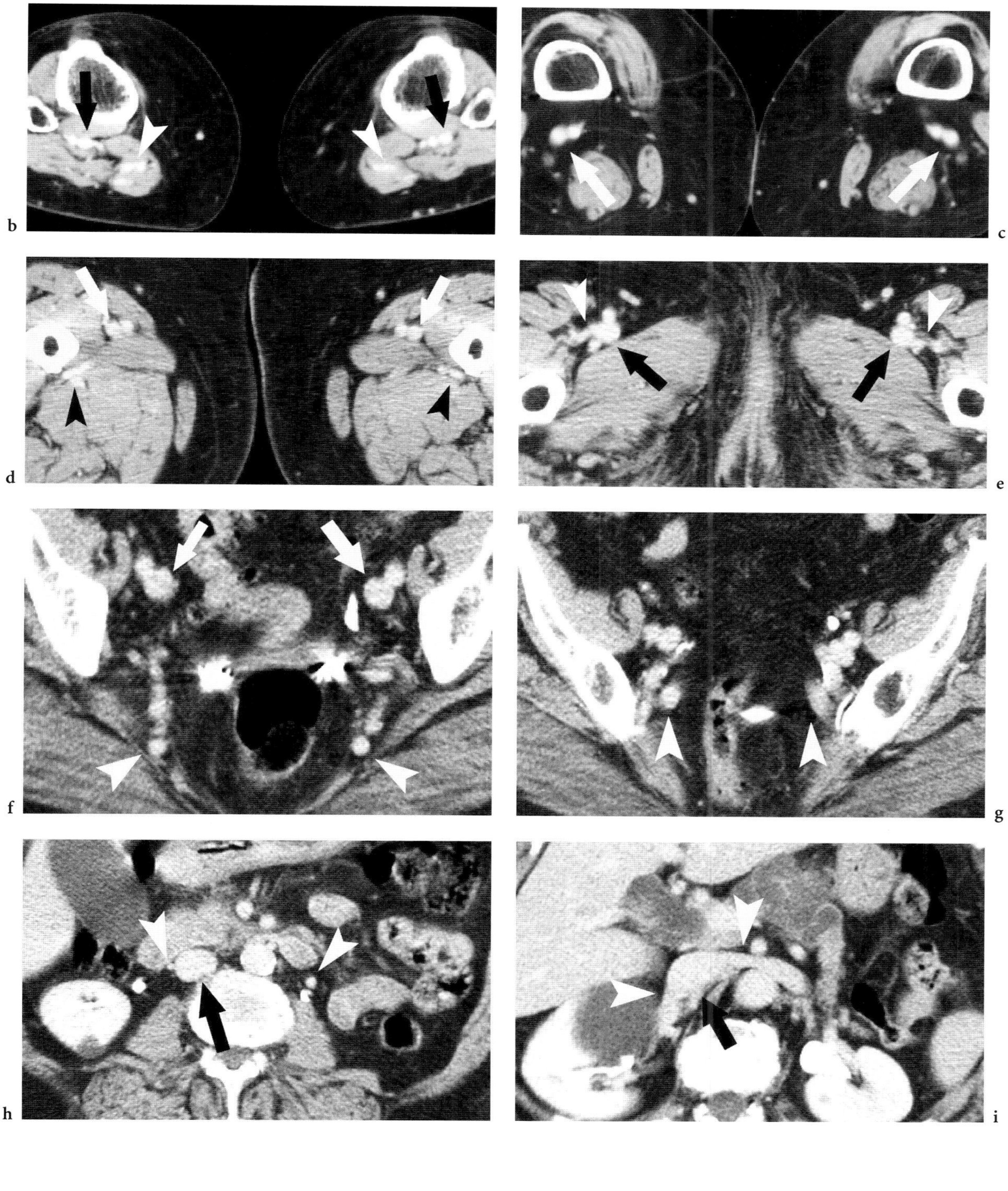

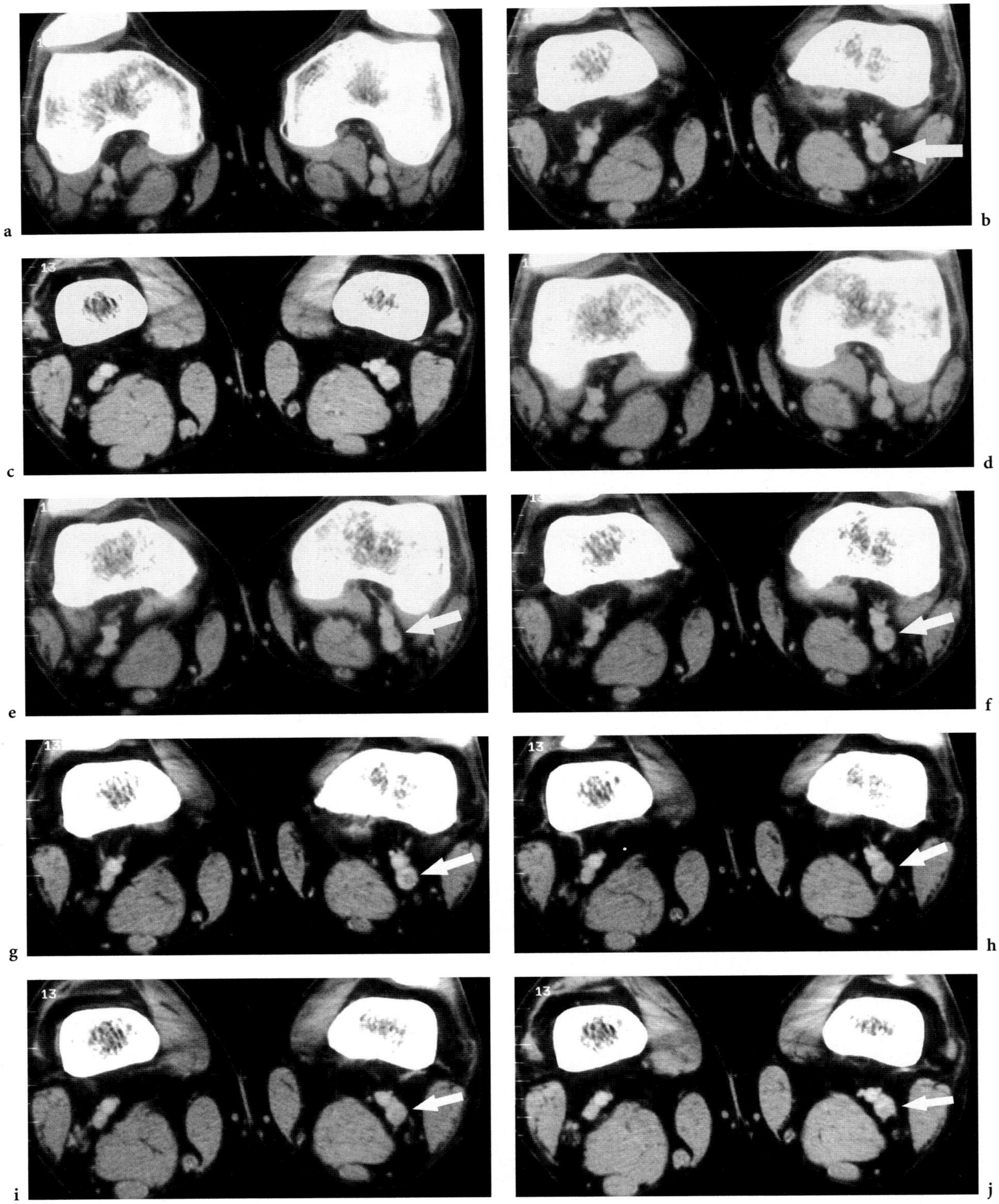

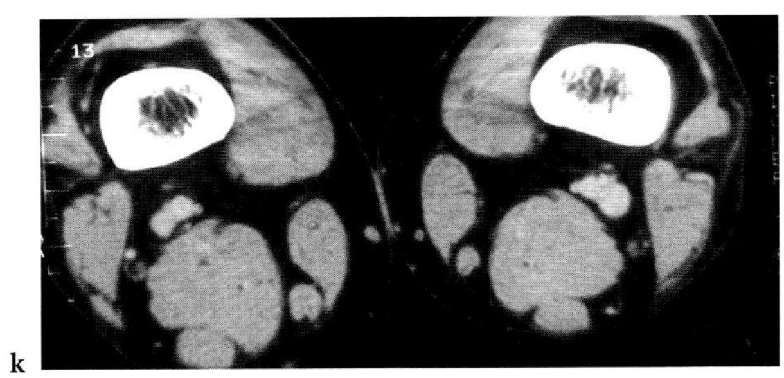

Fig. 19.6a–k. Comparison of sequential scanning and spiral scanning at the popliteal level. **a–c** Five-millimetre-thick axial CT venograms were acquired sequentially 20 mm apart. Suspicion of DVT in the left popliteal vein (*arrow*). **d–k** Five millimetre-thick axial CT venograms were acquired using spiral technique on the same area without reinjection of contrast medium. The DVT was confirmed in the right popliteal vein

(YOUSSEFZADEH et al. 1998; GHAYE et al. 2002b). Rescanning the area 1–2 min later shows homogeneous filling in varicosities with patent lumen; however, insufficient venous opacification can occur in an unpredictable manner, which may limit CTV in some patients (MATAR et al. 1999). In clinical practice, sufficiently homogeneous enhancement is obtained in 84–99% of the patients depending on the anatomic level. Poor opacification leading to indeterminate results of CTV has been reported in 1–5% of the patients (CHAM et al. 2000; DUWE et al. 2000; GARG et al. 2000, 2001; LOUD et al. 2000; BRUCE et al. 2001). In one study, patients with fair- to poor-quality SCTA (5%; 27 of 541) were more likely to have fair- to poor-quality CTV (52%; 14 of 27; CHAM et al. 2000); otherwise, CTVs acquired with "low-dose" or thin slices can produce noisy images with lumen of the vessels difficult to interpret, particularly in obese patients (YANKELEVITZ et al. 2000b).

19.5.3.2 Normal or Pathological Structures

Some normal structures may present with a hypervascular rim and a central hypodensity mimicking DVT: volume averaging integrating a venous valve; lymph node; sciatic nerve; aponeurosis or tendon; obstructed and dilated ureter or bowel loop with non-opacified lumen (ZERHOUNI et al. 1980; ALLGAYER et al. 1981; DUWE et al. 2000; CICCOTOSTO et al. 2002a; GHAYE et al. 2002b). Abnormal or pathological structures may also wrongly suggest DVT: thrombosed arteries or bypass; haematoma; abscess; popliteal cyst; and acute compartment syndrome (GHAYE et al. 2002b).

19.5.3.3 Streak Artefacts

Orthopaedic material, bone, calcification and opacified bladder or ureter can produce streak or beam-hardening artefacts, which may be responsible of endovascular hypodensities when crossing a normally opacified vessel. The sharp and straight appearance of these artefacts that extend in the surrounding tissue may help to establish the correct diagnosis (CHAM et al. 2000; GHAYE et al. 2002b). Such artefacts seem to be reduced by the use of multiple-detector CT compared with single-slice CT.

19.6 Potential Benefits of Combined Spiral CT Angiography and CTV

The potential benefits of combining spiral CT angiography (SCTA) and CTV are multiple. It is a rapid one-stop-shop examination of both aspects of VTE, which allows for immediate treatment of patients who have isolated DVT, without further delay by other types of diagnostic examinations. Neither separate venipuncture nor additional contrast medium injection are necessary, as only the contrast medium already in circulation from SCTA is used. Little time (30–240 s) is added to the overall examination duration, depending on the technique used, with negligible additional cost, although this may vary from country to country (PETERSON et al. 2001). Total room transit time of the patient is between 15 and 25 min. Preliminary results have suggested that combined SCTA–CTV is more cost-effective in selected patients than a combination of other tests (CENSULLO et al. 1999). The technical quality of CTV is not dependent on patient collaboration or mobility; therefore, it may be useful in ICU patients who are intubated, or who are unable to hold their breath, or in whom leg symptoms cannot be assessed (GARG et al. 2000). CTV is not limited by leg cast or painful compression, dressing, oedema, open wounds, severe burns or trophic changes of lower limbs or obesity (BALAKRISHNAN and GHEILER 1993; GARG et al. 2000; COCHE et al. 2001). Patient comfort is preserved, as no further mobilisation is required. CTV provides adequate visualisation of veins that are difficult to image with US, such as iliac veins and IVC, which is advantageous to guide further interventions, such as catheter placement for thrombolysis or IVC filter introduction (Figs. 19.7, 19.8; LOUD et al. 1998). CTV demonstrates anomalies compressing the venous system (BAUER and FLYNN 1988; GHAYE et al. 2000). These findings may be responsible for the patient's symptoms and may have an impact on management. Examples are given by gastrointestinal tract perforation, abdominal tumour, haematoma or other fluid collections, ascites, portal vein thrombosis and arterial embolism (EL HAJJAM et al. 1999; GHAYE et al. 2000; COCHE et al. 2001; NICOLAS et al. 2001); thus, combined SCTA–CTV results in a complete evaluation of potential sources of clots by screening the lower limbs veins, IVC, superior vena cava and the heart chambers.

CTV may also decrease multiple referrals to CT for suspected malignancy as an underlying cause for VTE (SCHOEPF et al. 2001). It is a valuable baseline

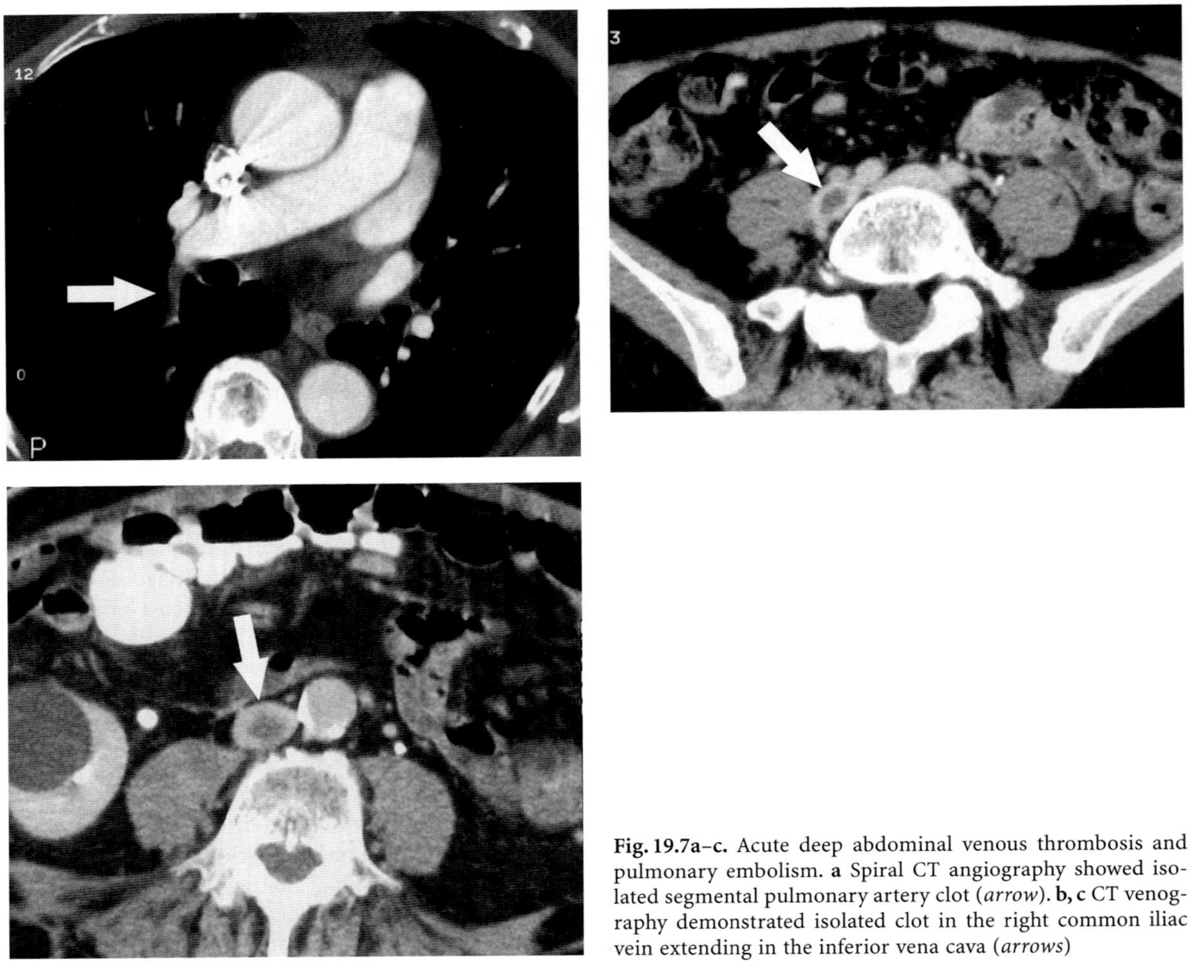

Fig. 19.7a–c. Acute deep abdominal venous thrombosis and pulmonary embolism. **a** Spiral CT angiography showed isolated segmental pulmonary artery clot (*arrow*). **b, c** CT venography demonstrated isolated clot in the right common iliac vein extending in the inferior vena cava (*arrows*)

for follow-up of VTE or against which any further development should be evaluated (Loud et al. 1998). The technique is less operator dependent than US or venography. A potential role in the workup of paradoxical embolism has been suggested (Fig. 19.9; Delalu et al. 2000).

19.7 Clinical Results

CTV has been performed using sequential (Garg et al. 2000; Ghaye et al. 2000; Katz et al. 2000; Loud et al. 2000, 2001; Garg et al. 2001; Ciccotosto et al. 2002b), spiral (El Hajjam et al. 1999; Cham et al. 2000; Duwe et al. 2000; Muller et al. 2001; Peterson et al. 2001; Ciccotosto et al. 2002b; Wildberger et al. 2002) or mixed technique (Coche et al. 2001; Nicolas et al. 2001). Results are most often compared with US, which is known to be a weak standard of reference. In such comparisons, results of CTV were 71–100% sensitivity, 92–100% specificity, 53–100% positive predictive value and 97–100% negative predictive value. Global inter-technique agreement was 0.84 to 1.00 between CTV and US (El Hajjam et al. 1999; Ghaye et al. 2000). Agreement was lower for infrapopliteal veins (kappa=0.57) than for popliteal and supra-popliteal veins (kappa=0.78–0.87; El Hajjam et al. 1999). Inter-observer agreement was 0.59–0.95 (Coche et al. 2001; Garg et al. 2001; Ciccotosto et al. 2002b). A moderate correlation (kappa=0.53) between CTV or US and venography in one study may be partially explained by the fact that venography was mainly applied in patients with discordant results of CTV and US (Ghaye et al. 2000). Preliminary results did not show any difference whether sequential or spiral technique was used. The overall

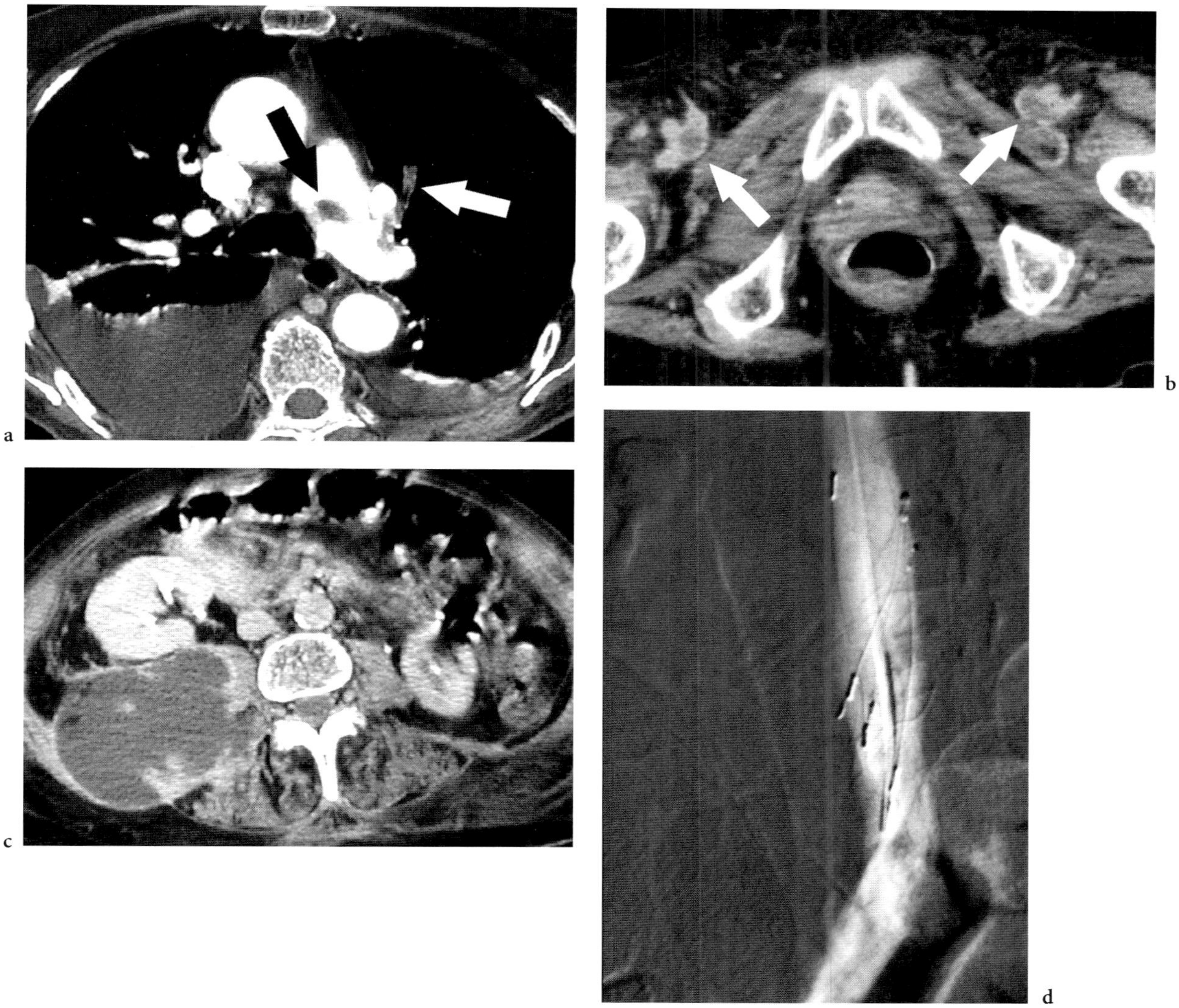

Fig. 19.8a–d. Acute DVT and pulmonary embolism. A 82-year-old woman, under prophylactic dose of low molecular weight heparin, presented with isolated dyspnoea syndrome. **a** Spiral CT angiography of the thorax showed massive pulmonary embolism (*arrows*). **b** CT venography demonstrated non-symptomatic bilateral thrombosis of the common femoral veins (*arrows*). **c** CT venography at the level of the abdomen showed an asymptomatic large retroperitoneal haematoma. **d** Following findings of the combined SCTA–CTV, she was treated by percutaneous insertion of a bird's-nest-type inferior vena cava filter introduced via right jugular route

detection rate of DVT in CTV in patients with PE was 32–89% (mean 59%). Except in one series, CTV increased the percentage of positive results for VTE by 11–36% (mean 23%; Cham et al. 2000; Garg et al. 2000; Katz et al. 2000; Coche et al. 2001; Loud et al. 2001; Nicolas et al. 2001; Jonetz-Menzel et al. 2001). In one study the addition of CTV to STCA increased the accuracy of detection of VTE from 69 to 88% (Censullo et al. 1999). Other advantages were more accurate demonstration of extension of DVT, particularly in pelvic and abdominal veins (Figs. 19.7, 19.10; Garg et al. 2000; Ghaye et al. 2000; Loud et al. 2001; Nicolas et al. 2001). Additional findings and alternative diagnoses of the clinical symptoms were also provided by CTV (Ghaye et al. 2000; Katz et al. 2000; Coche et al. 2001; El Hajjam et al. 1999). Other authors have suggested performing limited CTV of the pelvis only or of pelvis and abdomen, in combination with SCTA, when a previous US was negative. In this condition, additional DVT was demonstrated in 2–8% of the patients suspected of PE (Ferretti et al. 1998; Au et al. 2001; Walsh and Redmond 2002).

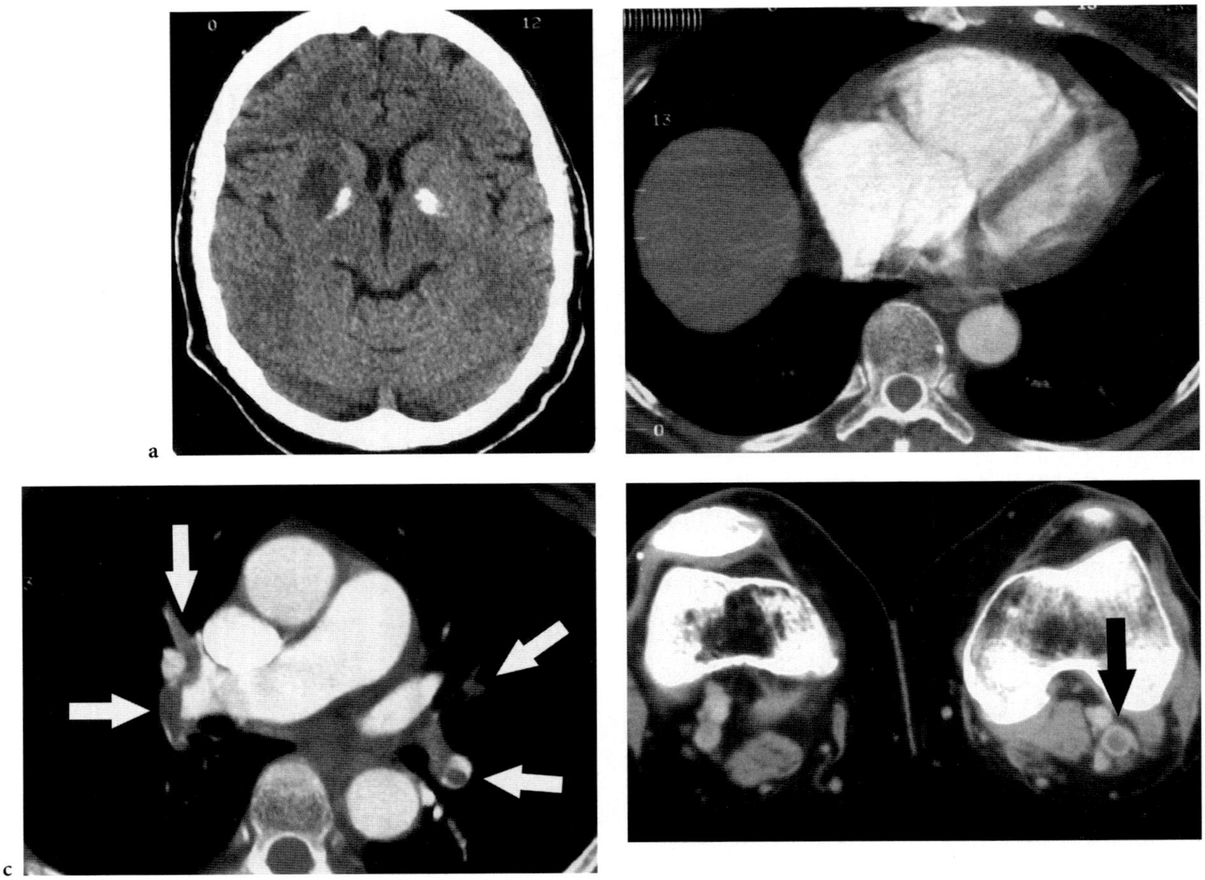

Fig. 19.9a–d. Paradoxical embolism. A 66-year-old woman presented with left hemiparesis. Echocardiography revealed right-to-left intracardiac shunt. **a** A CT of the brain demonstrated an ischaemic area in the right putamen. **b, c** Spiral CT of the thorax showed severe dilation of the right heart cavities. Multiple asymptomatic emboli were demonstrated in central and segmental pulmonary arteries (*arrows*). **d** CT venography showed segmental asymptomatic thrombosis of the left popliteal vein (*arrow*)

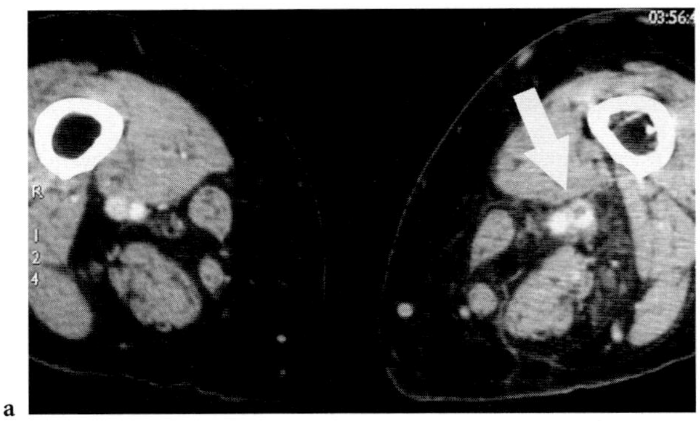

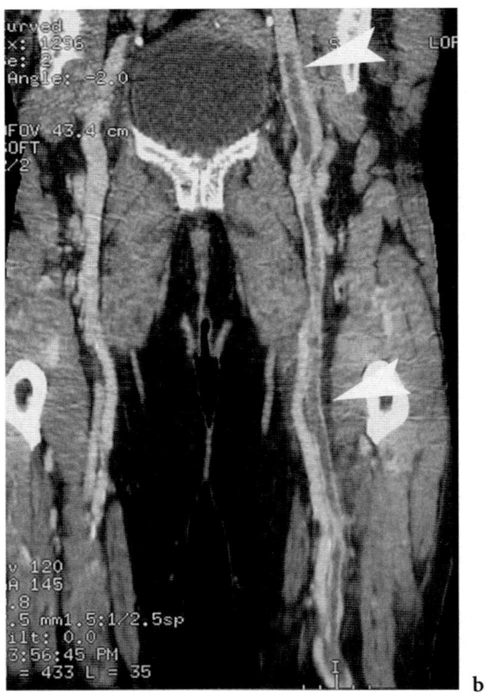

Fig. 19.10. Acute DVT. Indirect MDCTV was performed with a 4×5-mm collimation from the ankle to the diaphragm. **a** Five-millimetre-thick axial slice at the level of the popliteal vein showed venous clot and perivenous fat infiltration (*arrow*). **b** Frontal 2.5-mm-thick curved reformation of the deep venous system of the left lower limb showed a continuous central filling defect involving the deep venous system, from the knee to the external iliac vein (*arrowheads*)

19.8 Conclusion

Regarding all advantages, combined SCTA–CTV appears as an outstanding imaging technique for patients suspected having VTE which will challenge the current standards in diagnostic workup in the near future. The technique is time- and cost-effective and allows an "all in one" accurate visualisation of the pulmonary arteries, cardiac chambers, limb, pelvic, retroperitoneal and mediastinal veins. Correct choice of imaging parameters and reasonable use of the spiral mode while imaging the veins decreases the irradiation dose to an acceptable level. Clinical results suggest that CTV should be performed in combination with SCTA in patients suspected having PE, except in young patients, unless US has recently been performed.

References

Abdelmoumene Y, Chevallier P, Barghouth G et al. (2003) Technical innovation. Optimization of multidetector CT venography performed with elastic stockings on patients' lower extremities: A preliminary study of nonthrombosed veins. Am J Roentgenol 180: 1093-1094

Allgayer B, Reiser M, Ries G, Feuerbach S (1981) Computed tomographic demonstration of venous thrombosis of different etiologies. Eur J Radiol 1:204–206

Au VW, Walsh G, Fon G (2001) Computed tomography pulmonary angiography with pelvic venography in the evaluation of thrombo-embolic disease. Australas Radiol 45:141–145

Balakrishnan C, Gheiler EL (1993) Computed tomography for diagnosis of deep venous thrombosis in burn patients. Plast Reconstr Surg 91:1174–1175

Baldt MM, Zontsich T, Stumpflen A et al. (1996) Deep venous thrombosis of the lower extremity: efficacy of spiral CT venography compared with conventional venography in diagnosis. Radiology 200:423–428

Baldt MM, Zontsich T, Kainberger F, Fleischmann G, Mostbeck G (1997) Spiral CT evaluation of deep venous thrombosis. Semin Ultrasound CT MR 18:369–375

Barnes PA, Bernardino ME, Thomas JL (1982) Flow phenomenon mimicking thrombus: a possible pitfall of the pedal infusion technique. J Comput Assist Tomogr 6:304–306

Bauer AR, Flynn RR (1988) Computed tomography diagnosis of venous thrombosis of the lower extremities and pelvis with contrast material. Surg Gynecol Obstet 167:12–15

Bettmann MA (1997) Venography. In: Baum S (ed) Abrams' angiography, vol 2. Little, Brown, Boston, pp 1743–1754

Blum JE, Handmaker H (2000) Role of small-peptide radiopharmaceuticals in the evaluation of deep venous thrombosis. Radiographics 20:1187–1193

Bruce D, Loud PA, Klippenstein DL, Grossman ZD, Katz DS (2001) Combined CT venography and pulmonary angiography: How much venous enhancement is routinely obtained? Am J Roentgenol 176:1281–1285

Carpenter JP, Holland GA, Baum RA, Owen RS, Carpenter JT, Cope C (1993) Magnetic resonance venography for the detection of deep venous thrombosis: comparison with contrast venography and duplex Doppler ultrasonography. J Vasc Surg 18:734–741

Carson JL, Kelley MA, Duff A et al. (1992) The clinical course of pulmonary embolism. N Engl J Med 326:1240–1245

Censullo ML, Ernst RD, Kawashima A, Caskey CI, Sandler CM (1999) CT venography as an adjunct to CT pulmonary angiography for the detection of pulmonary thromboembolic disease. Radiology 213 (Suppl):558

Cham MD, Yankelevitz DF, Shaham D et al. (2000) Deep venous thrombosis: detection by using indirect CT venography. Radiology 216:744–751

Ciccotosto C, Goodman LR, Washington L, Quiroz FA (2002a) Indirect CT venography following CT pulmonary angiography: spectrum of findings. J Thorac Imaging 17:18–27

Ciccotosto C, Filippone A, Storto ML, Ricciardi M, Salcuni M, Bonomo L (2002b) Accuracy of multislice CT for acute deep venous thrombosis: variability of observer performance related to clinical experience. Eur Radiol 12 (Suppl):150

Coche EE, Hamoir XL, Hammer FD, Hainaut P, Goffette PP (2001) Using dual-detector helical CT angiography to detect deep venous thrombosis in patients with suspicion of pulmonary embolism: diagnostic value and additional findings. Am J Roentgenol 176:1035–1039

Cogo A, Lensing WA, Prandoni P, Hirsh J (1993) Distribution of thrombosis in patients with symptomatic deep vein thrombosis: implications for simplifying the diagnostic process with compression ultrasound. Arch Intern Med 153:2777–2780

Cronan JJ, Leen V (1989) Recurrent deep venous thrombosis: limitations of US. Radiology 170:739–742

Dalen JE, Alpert JS (1975) Natural history of pulmonary embolism. Prog Cardiovasc Dis 17:259–270

Delalu P, Ferretti GR, Bricault I, Ayanian D, Coulomb M (2000) Paradoxical emboli: demonstration using helical computed tomography of the pulmonary artery associated with abdominal computed tomography. Eur Radiol 10:384–386

Duwe KM, Shiau M, Budorick NE, Austin JH, Berkmen YM (2000) Evaluation of the lower extremity veins in patients with suspected pulmonary embolism: a retrospective comparison of helical CT venography and sonography. Am J Roentgenol 175:1525–1531

El Hajjam M, Qanadli SD, Mignon F, Sissakian J, Chagnon S, Lacombe P (1999) Combined double helical CT phlebography of the lower extremities and CT pulmonary angiography: new approach for thromboembolic disease diagnosis. Radiology 213 (Suppl):126

Ferretti GR, Ayanian D, Ranchoup Y, Thony F, Bosson JL, Coulomb M (1998) CT assessment of abdominal and pelvic veins in patients suspected of acute pulmonary embolism and presenting with normal sonography of the lower limbs. J Radiol 79:327–330

Ferris EJ (1992) George W. Holmes Lecture. Deep venous thrombosis and pulmonary embolism: correlative evaluation and therapeutic implications. Am J Roentgenol 159:1149–1155

Fishman EK, Horton KM (2000) CT of suspected pulmonary embolism: study design optimization. Am J Roentgenol 175:1002–1003

Garg K, Mao J (2001) Deep venous thrombosis: spectrum of findings and pitfalls in interpretation on CT venography. Am J Roentgenol 177:319–23

Garg K, Kemp JL, Wojcik D et al. (2000) Thromboembolic

disease: comparison of combined CT pulmonary angiography and venography with bilateral leg sonography in 70 patients. Am J Roentgenol 175:997–1001
Garg K, Kemp JL, Russ PD, Baron AE (2001) Thromboembolic disease: variability of interobserver agreement in the interpretation of CT venography with CT pulmonary angiography. Am J Roentgenol 176:1043–1047
Gartenschlager M, Klose KJ, Schmidt JA (1996) Floating venous thrombi: diagnosis with spiral-CT-phlebography. Rofo Fortschr Geb Rontgenstr Neuen Bildgeb Verfahr 164:376–381
Ghaye B, Szapiro D, Willems V, Dondelinger RF (2000) Combined CT venography of the lower limbs and spiral CT angiography of pulmonary arteries in acute pulmonary embolism: preliminary results of a prospective study. JBR-BTR 83:271–278
Ghaye B, Szapiro D, Mastora I et al. (2001) Peripheral pulmonary arteries: How far in the lung does multi-detector row spiral CT allow analysis? Radiology 219:629–636
Ghaye B, Remy J, Remy-Jardin M (2002a) Non-traumatic thoracic emergencies: CT diagnosis of acute pulmonary embolism : the first 10 years. Eur Radiol 12:1886–1905
Ghaye B, Szapiro D, Willems V, Dondelinger RF (2002b) Pitfalls in CT venography of the lower limbs and abdominal veins. Am J Roentgenol 178:1465–1471
Glazer GM, Callen PW, Parker JJ (1981) CT diagnosis of tumor thrombus in the inferior vena cava: avoiding the false-positive diagnosis. Am J Roentgenol 137:1265–1267
Gmelin E, Link J, Judaschke S, Marienhoff N (1992) Nonenhanced CT of thrombosed calf veins. Rofo Fortschr Geb Rontgenstr Neuen Bildgeb Verfahr 156:338–341
Goodman LR (2000) CT diagnosis of pulmonary embolism and deep venous thrombosis. Radiographics 20:1201–1205
Goodman LR, Lipchik RJ (1996) Diagnosis of acute pulmonary embolism: time for a new approach. Radiology 199:25–27
Herold CJ, Hahne J, Ghaye B et al. (1999) Prospective evaluation of pulmonary embolism: diagnostic performance of spiral CT angiography in the ESTIPEP trial. Radiology 213:126–127
Hidalgo H, Korobkin M, Breiman RS, Heaston DK, Moore AV, Ram PC (1982) CT demonstration of subcutaneous venous collaterals. J Comput Assist Tomogr 6:514–518
Hull RD, Carter CJ, Jay RM et al. (1983) The diagnosis of acute, recurrent, deep-vein thrombosis: a diagnostic challenge. Circulation 67:901–906
Jonetz-Mentzel L, Basche S, Eger C (2001) CT phlebography and CT angiography of the pulmonary arteries in the diagnosis of acute lung embolism. Eur Radiol 11 (Suppl):137
Katz DS, Loud PA, Klippenstein DL, Shah RA, Grossman ZD (2000) Extra-thoracic findings on the venous phase of combined computed tomographic venography and pulmonary angiography. Clin Radiol 55:177–181
Katz DS, Loud PA, Bruce D et al. (2002) Combined CT venography and pulmonary angiography: a comprehensive review. Radiographics S22:3-19
Kouroukis C, LeClerc JR (1996) Pulmonary embolism with duplicated inferior vena cava. Chest 109:1111–1113
Langer B, Kauffman P, Bechara M, Aguiar ET, Aun R (1991) Diagnosis of deep venous thrombosis of the lower limbs by computed tomography. Rev Paul Med 109:149–152
Lensing AW, Kraaijenhagen R, van Beek EJR, Buller HR (1999) Diagnosis of venous thrombosis. In: Oudkerk M, van Beek EJR, ten Cate (Eds) pp 44-70, Blackwell, London
Lien HH, Lund G (1983) Collateral veins in inferior caval vein occlusion demonstrated via CT. Eur J Radiol 3:319–323
Lomas DJ, Britton PD (1991) CT demonstration of acute and chronic iliofemoral thrombosis. J Comput Assist Tomogr 15:861–862
Loud PA, Grossman ZD, Klippenstein DL, Ray CE (1998) Combined CT venography and pulmonary angiography: a new diagnostic technique for suspected thromboembolic disease. Am J Roentgenol 170:951–954
Loud PA, Katz DS, Klippenstein DL, Shah RD, Grossman ZD (2000) Combined CT venography and pulmonary angiography in suspected thromboembolic disease: diagnostic accuracy for deep venous evaluation. Am J Roentgenol 174:61–65
Loud PA, Katz DS, Bruce DA, Klippenstein DL, Grossman ZD (2001) Deep venous thrombosis with suspected pulmonary embolism: detection with combined CT venography and pulmonary angiography. Radiology 219:498–502
Martin-Bouyer Y (2002) Phleboscanner. Presented at the 2nd symposium on volumetric multislice CT, A. Blum Organization, Nancy, 7–8 October
Matar LD, Ramirez JA, McAdams HP, Farrell MA, Herndon JE (1999) Optimal timing of CT venography following CT pulmonary angiography using a multidetector row helical scanner: work in progress. Radiology 213 (Suppl):472–473
McLachlan MS, Thomson JG, Taylor DW, Kelly ME, Sackett DL (1979) Observer variation in the interpretation of lower limb venograms. Am J Roentgenol 132:227–229
Moser KM (1990) Venous thromboembolism. Am Rev Respir Dis 141:235–249
Muller C, Kopka L, Funke M, Funke C, Grabbe E (2001) Diagnosis of lung embolism and underlying venous thrombosis in multi-slice spiral CT. Rofo Fortschr Geb Rontgenstr Neuen Bildgeb Verfahr 173:528–535
National Institutes of Health (1986) Prevention of venous thrombosis and pulmonary embolism. J Am Med Assoc 256:744–749
Nicolas M, Debelle L, Laurent V et al. (2001) Incremental lower extremity CT venography, a simplified approach for the diagnosis of deep venous thrombosis in patients with pulmonary embolism. J Radiol 82:251–256
Pagani JJ, Thomas JL, Bernardino ME (1982) Computed tomographic manifestations of abdominal and pelvic venous collaterals. Radiology 142:415–419
Pawar SV, Kay CJ (1984) Soft-tissue CT changes in pelvic venous thrombosis. Am J Roentgenol 143:605–607
Peterson DA, Kazerooni EA, Wakefield TW et al. (2001) Computed tomographic venography is specific but not sensitive for diagnosis of acute lower-extremity deep venous thrombosis in patients with suspected pulmonary embolus. J Vasc Surg 34:798–804
Picolet H, Leizorovicz A, Revel D, Chirossel P, Amiel M, Boissel JP (1990) Reliability of phlebography in the assessment of venous thrombosis in a clinical trial. Haemostasis 20: 362–367
Pillari G, Zito J, Chang JB et al. (1987) Lower extremity swelling: computerized tomography following negative venography. Cardiovasc Intervent Radiol 10:261–263
Rademaker J, Griesshaber V, Hidajat N, Oestmann JW, Felix R (2001) Combined CT pulmonary angiography and venography for diagnosis of pulmonary embolism and deep vein thrombosis: radiation dose. J Thorac Imaging 16:297–299
Reimer P, Landwehr P (1998) Non-invasive vascular imaging of peripheral vessels. Eur Radiol 8:858–872

Remy-Jardin M, Remy J, Deschildre F et al (1996) Diagnosis of pulmonary embolism with spiral CT: comparison with pulmonary angiography and scintigraphy. Radiology 200: 699–706

Ruehm SG, Wiesner W, Debatin JF (2000) Pelvic and lower extremity veins: contrast-enhanced three-dimensional MR venography with a dedicated vascular coil: initial experience. Radiology 215:421–427

Schoepf UJ, Kessler MA, Rieger CT et al. (2001) Multislice CT imaging of pulmonary embolism. Eur Radiol 11: 2278–2286

Seem E, Stranden E, Stiris MG (1985) Computed tomography in deep venous thrombosis with limb oedema. Acta Radiol Diagn 26:727–730

Steele JR, Sones PJ, Heffner LT (1978) The detection of inferior vena caval thrombosis with computed tomography. Radiology 128:385–386

Stehling MK, Rosen MP, Weintraub J, Kim D, Raptopoulos V (1994) Spiral CT venography of the lower extremity. Am J Roentgenol 163:451–453

Szapiro D, Ghaye B, Willems V, Zhang L, Albert A, Dondelinger RF (2001) Evaluation of CT time-density curves of lower-limb veins. Invest Radiol 36:164–169

Uhl JF, Lemasle P, Gillot C, Verdeille S, Bouyer YM, Mugel T (2002) 3D Imaging of the venous system by CT venography (interactive CD-Rom), presented at the 88th scientific assembly and annual meeting of the RSNA, 1–6 December, Chicago

Van Breda A, Rubin BE, Druy EM (1979) Detection of inferior vena cava abnormalities by computed tomography. J Comput Assist Tomogr 3:164–169

Vogelzang RL, Gore RM, Neiman HL, Smith SJ, Deschler TW, Vrla RF (1985) Inferior vena cava CT pseudothrombus produced by rapid arm-vein contrast infusion. Am J Roentgenol 144:843–846

Vogelzang RL, Gore RM, Anschuetz SL, Blei AT (1988) Thrombosis of the splanchnic veins: CT diagnosis. Am J Roentgenol 150:93–96

Vujic I, Stanley J, Tyminski LJ (1981) Computed tomography of suspected caval thrombosis secondary to proximal extension of phlebitis from the leg. Radiology 140: 437–441

Walsh G, Redmond S (2002) Does addition of CT pelvic venography to CT pulmonary angiography protocols contribute to the diagnosis of thromboembolic disease? Clin Radiol 57:462-465

Wagner M, Mark L (1969) Duplication of the inferior vena cava and its role in recurrent pulmonary emboli. J Am Med Assoc 209:108–109

Wildberger JE, Mahnken AH, Sinha AM et al. (2002) A differentiated approach to the diagnosis of pulmonary embolism and deep venous thrombosis using multi-slice CT. Rofo Fortschr Geb Rontgenstr Neuen Bildgeb Verfahr 174:301–307

Yankelevitz DF, Gamsu G, Shah A et al. (2000a) Optimization of combined CT pulmonary angiography with lower extremity CT venography. Am J Roentgenol 174:67–69

Yankelevitz DF, Cham MD, Shaham D, Henschke CI (2000b) Common diagnostic pitfalls of indirect CT venography. Radiology 217 (Suppl):127

Youssefzadeh S, Liskutin J, Dorffner R, Bankier A, Hubsch P (1998) Venous contrast fluid level in computed tomography. Clin Radiol 53:528–531

Zerhouni EA, Barth KH, Siegelman SS (1980) Demonstration of venous thrombosis by computed tomography. Am J Roentgenol 134:753–758

Zontsich T, Turetschek K, Baldt M (1998) CT-phlebography. A new method for the diagnosis of venous thrombosis of the upper and lower extremities. Radiologe 38:586–590

20 CT Angiography of the Thoracic Aorta

G. D. Rubin

CONTENTS

Introduction

Although aortography has long been considered the standard for aortic imaging, there are several reasons why spiral or helical CT may be superior to conventional arteriography for assessing the thoracic aorta. Firstly, the volumetric acquisition of spiral CT enables clear delineation of the aortic arch, tortuous brachiocephalic arterial branches, and adjacent aneurysms and pseudoaneurysms. Because aortography is a projectional technique, the commonly occurring overlap of these structures can confound their visualization and delineation of anatomic relationships. Secondly, blood-pool imaging provided by the intravenous administration of iodinated contrast media allows simultaneous visualization of true and false luminal flow channels, intramural hematomas communicating with the aortic lumen, and slow perigraft flow around thoracic aortic stent grafts. Finally, the aortic wall and non-communicating intramural collections are directly visualized. These advantages together with the rapid, non-invasive means with which CT angiography (CTA) is acquired has resulted in CTA challenging conventional arteriography for the assessment of many thoracic aortic abnormalities. The purpose of this chapter is to review the technical factors that must be considered when acquiring and interpreting thoracic aortic CT angiograms as well as the range of disease states for which CTA can be valuable.

G. D. Rubin, MD
Department of Radiology, S-072, Stanford University School of Medicine, Stanford, California 94305-5105, USA

20.1 Imaging Techniques

The first step in performing thoracic aortic CTA is to determine the anatomic coverage required to assess the clinical question. At a minimum, the initiation point of the CT scan should be at the base of the neck so that the proximal aspect of the common carotid and vertebral arteries are included within the CT scan. Inferiorly, coverage should extend to include the origin of the celiac axis. The inclusion of the supra-aortic branches is important when lesions involving the aortic arch extend into these brachiocephalic branches, which commonly occurs in the setting of both aneurysmal disease and aortic dissection. The purpose of including the celiac origin is that lesions of the distal thoracic aorta can be accurately localized relative to this anatomic landmark, which can greatly facilitate planning of endovascular and open repair. There may be some instances when additional anatomic coverage is necessary. For example, in the setting of acute aortic dissection, frequently imaging through the abdomen and pelvis is necessary due to signs and symptoms of diminished blood flow to the abdominal viscera or lower extremity. Similarly, some disease processes may warrant inclusion of portions of the upper extremities particularly when assessing for sources of embolization to the hands.

Finally, occasionally, a greater degree of anatomic coverage to include the entirety of the carotid arterial circulation may be warranted, particularly in the setting of assessment of large vessel arteritis and aortic dissection associated with symptoms of cerebral ischemia.

To ensure that all relevant anatomy is included in the CT angiograms, thoracic aortic CT angiography begins with a relatively thick section unenhanced localizing scan prescribed from a frontal scout view of the chest and upper abdomen. Usually, 5-mm nominal section thickness associated with a high pitch (2.0 for SDCT and 1.3–1.7 for MDCT) is sufficient to localize the relevant landmarks; however, there are several clinical scenarios where thinner sections should be acquired for these unenhanced views. Specifically, when the assessment is for acute chest pain and intramural hematoma is a diagnostic consideration, unenhanced views can be very valuable for identifying a hyperattenuative mural crescent corresponding to the intramural hematoma. Because 10-mm-thick sections can result in substantial volume averaging, 5-mm nominal thick sections are advised for the unenhanced portion of the scan in this setting. Additionally, when assessing stent grafts, 5-mm-thick unenhanced sections can be useful for mapping the location of calcifications around the stent graft, which can subsequently mimic an endoleak following contrast administration. Because these initial unenhanced scans are thick, a relatively low tube current and potential is satisfactory for this acquisition. We typically use 120 kV and 100 mA. Not only does this dose save radiation exposure to the patient, it also minimizes tube heating that can subsequently limit the current at which the X-ray tube is operated for single-detector-row CT when acquiring the CTA.

Based on these localizing sections, the initiation point and terminus of the CT angiograms, as well as the field of view for reconstruction, is determined.

20.2 Contrast Medium

Prior to performing the CT angiogram, the iodinated contrast administration protocol must be determined. As a general rule, we do not perform CT angiography at a flow rate less than 4 ml/s and for thoracic aortic CT angiograms with durations less than 20 s we prefer at least 5 ml/s injection rate. The duration of the bolus should be equivalent to the duration of the CT scan, and therefore the volume of contrast required is determined by multiplying the CT scan duration by the flow rate. We have found that a volume of at least 80 ml of iodinated contrast medium (350 mg of iodine/ml) is necessary for reliable opacification. This volume of contrast medium at the recommended flow rate is readily delivered through a 20- or 22-G antecubital intravenous catheter. Because highly attenuative undiluted contrast medium within the in-flowing veins can obscure adjacent structures, we always perform thoracic aortic CT angiography through a right antecubital venous source to avoid opacification of the left brachiocephalic vein which can substantially obscure the origins of the brachiocephalic, left, common carotid, and left subclavian arteries. Because of the high flow rates employed in CTA, iodinated contrast medium should always be non-ionic.

The final and critical step for optimizing contrast medium delivery is the determination of the scan delay time following initiation of the contrast medium bolus. In the past we relied upon a preliminary injection of 15 ml of iodinated contrast medium coupled with serial CT sections acquired within the proximal descending aorta to obtain a time-attenuation curve. We selected the time from the initiation of the injection to the peak of this curve as the scan delay for the CT angiogram. The availability of automated scan-triggering capabilities on the CT scanner has led us to abandon this approach. On our CT scanners equipped with this feature, approximately 8 s is required from the time that contrast medium arrives in the descending aorta until the enhancement is recognized and the CTA acquisition is initiated; therefore, we determine the injection duration to be equal to the scan duration plus 8 s. We have found this direct method of visualizing aortic enhancement to be the most reliable method for achieving consistently high-quality CT angiograms.

20.3 CTA Acquisition

Thoracic aortic CT angiography should be performed with a nominal section thickness of 3 mm or less coupled with a relatively high pitch value of 2.0 for SDCT and 1.3–1.7 for MDCT. A 1.25-mm section thickness is not required for the majority of thoracic aortic applications; however, it can be of particular value when a detailed assessment of the supra-aortic branches is indicated. The gantry rotation period should be minimized to the lowest value available in order to minimize the duration of the acquisition and the dosage of contrast medium. Occasionally, larger patients may benefit from the use of a slower gantry rotation period to overcome excessive image noise, thus enabling a higher mA•S product. Recently introduced techniques for cardiac gating of CT data may prove valuable in the assessment of the ascending aorta and in particular the coronary arteries; however, these techniques are not widespread and therefore are not discussed further in this chapter.

The CT angiogram should be performed within a single breath hold. If breath holding is not possible due to mechanical ventilation of the patient or extreme dyspnea, attempts should be made to avoid sudden gasps for air by allowing the patient to breathe quietly throughout the acquisition rather than attempting a breath hold that cannot be completed.

For the vast majority of CT angiograms, an arterial phase acquisition is sufficient; however, for the assessment of stent-graft repair of aortic aneurysm, delayed views can be very important to assess for endoleak. We typically acquire these views 70 s after the initiation of the arterial phase acquisition and use 2.5- to 5-mm nominal section thickness through the stent graft.

20.4 Reconstruction

The CT angiogram and delayed views when acquired should be reconstructed with an interval that is equivalent to 50% of the effective section thickness. For most acquisitions, a 1.5-mm reconstruction interval is appropriate. The reconstruction field of view should be minimized to only include the relevant arterial anatomy and typically ranges between 25 and 30 cm. We usually use a soft or standard reconstruction algorithm for CT angiograms as these reconstruction algorithms minimize noise in the data which greatly facilitate the creation of 3D views.

A detailed description of 3D rendering is beyond the scope of this chapter. In general, we find the use of curved planar reformations, volume renderings, and shaded-surface displays (SSD) most useful for assessing the thoracic aorta. Furthermore, thin-slab maximum intensity projections (MIP) may be useful; however, full-volume MIPs are rarely useful in the thoracic aorta. A more detailed discussion of these techniques is given below.

20.5 SDCT vs MDCT

For imaging of the thoracic aorta, single-detector-row CT (SDCT) scanners are adequate for the majority of applications; however, MDCT typically results in superior image quality. This is because MDCT scans are usually acquired with narrower effective section thickness, and a shorter period of time, and with less contrast medium. In particular, the shorter scan duration allows for substantially shorter breath-hold periods and more consistent enhancement across the scan acquisition. Furthermore, diminished pulsation-related artifacts through the heart and great vessels have been observed with MDCT (Fig. 20.1). A final consequence of the use of MDCT is that the shorter scan time results in a substantial reduction in contrast medium utilization (Rubin et al. 2000).

Imaging of extended vascular territories beyond the thorax and in particular through the abdomen and pelvis require the use of MDCT to image the entire volume within a single breath hold. The use of SDCT limits the application of thoracic CT aortography to the thoracic aorta alone (Fig. 20.2).

20.6 Technical Considerations for Interpretation

The interpretation of thoracic aortic CT angiograms is greatly facilitated by the use of a workstation to perform soft-copy reading. Scrolling through a stack of transverse sections allows easy integration of the longitudinal dimension in these large three-dimensional data sets. Moreover, substantial variations in the degree of aortic enhancement requires customization of window width and level settings. It is important to adjust the display setting to ensure that the aortic lumen does not appear to be white to facilitate discrimination of luminal enhancement from mural calcifications. Additionally, when assessing delayed images for endoleaks following stent-graft repair, very narrow windows are frequently required for the detection of subtle endoleaks.

20.6.1 Common Artifacts in Thoracic CTA

Two artifacts result in the majority of interpretative limitations of thoracic aortic CTA: perivenous streaks

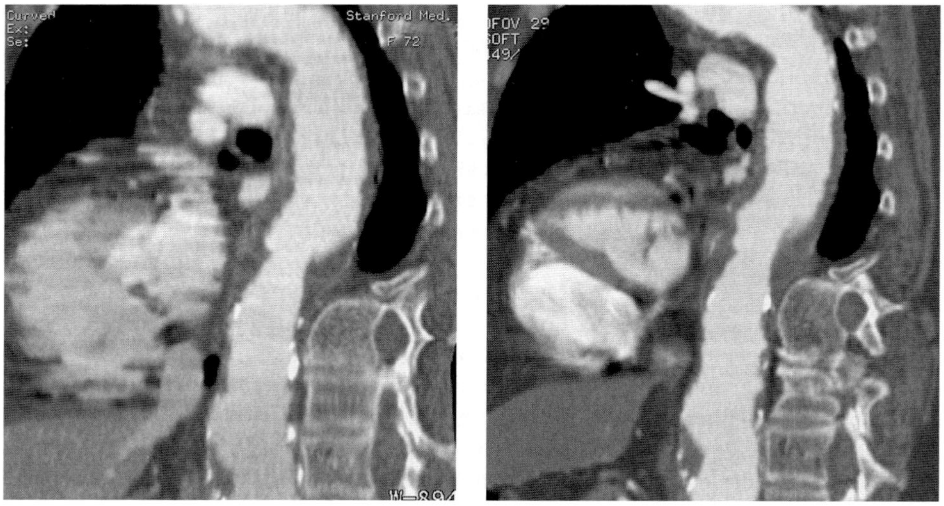

a b

Fig. 20.1. **a** Single-detector CT (SDCT) and **b** multidetector-row CT (MDCT) curved planar reformations through the thoracic aorta in a patient with extensive descending aortic atherosclerotic plaque. These two scans illustrate important differences between SDCT and MDCT acquisitions. The SDCT acquisition (3-mm collimation, pitch 2) demonstrates substantial pulsation-related misregistration artifacts throughout the heart as well as in the left pulmonary artery. These artifacts are reduced on the MDCT scan, particularly in the left pulmonary artery and the left and right ventricles. This is due to the substantially greater table speed of the 2.5 mm, pitch 6.0, acquisition resulting in the heart being imaged in substantially fewer heartbeats

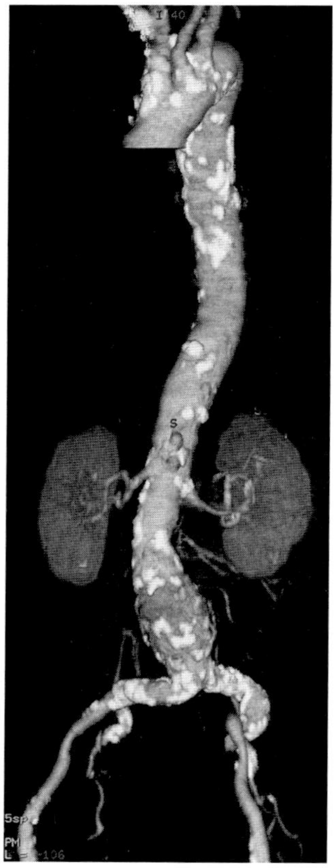

Fig. 20.2. Volume rendering of MDCT angiogram from the thoracic inlet through the common femoral arteries. These emanations required 28 s to image 510 mm with 2.5-mm-thick sections

and arterial pulsation. Both of these artifacts tend to have their greatest influence on the visualization of the ascending aorta and therefore are particularly important to bear in mind when assessing patients suspected of aortic dissection.

Perivenous streaks are likely caused by a combination of beam hardening and motion caused by transmitted pulsation in veins carrying undiluted contrast medium to the heart. Strategies designed to minimize this artifact include the use of dilute contrast medium solutions (Remy-Jardin et al. 1992; Rubin et al. 1996b), caudal to cranial scan direction, and femoral venous access (Prokop et al. 1993). In practice, perivenous streaks are rarely confused with intimal dissection in the ascending aorta as their orientation typically varies from section to section and they typically extend beyond the confines of the aortic wall. The most problematic region for perivenous artifacts is the origin of the supra-aortic branches adjacent to an opacified left brachiocephalic vein. Perivenous streaks in this region can mask extension of intimal flaps into these branches as well as occlusive disease caused by atherosclerotic plaque at their origins. If detected at the time of initial section reconstruction (within 2 min of bolus initiation), then delayed sections can be rapidly prescribed to enable reimaging during a second pass of arterial contrast prior to the equilibrium phase. Other than this rapid intervention and reinjection at another site, there are no techniques to adequately overcome obscured brachiocephalic arterial origins once the equilibrium phase has begun. The best prevention of this limitation is ensuring that peripheral venous access is from the right upper extremity.

Arterial pulsation has been recognized as a cause of false-positive aortic dissection on conventional and helical CT scans. The increasing acquisition speed of helical CT scanners may ultimately result in the elimination of this artifact; however, in the meantime there is an intervention that can be retrospectively applied to the raw scan data to minimize these artifacts. "Segmented" or "weighted half-scan" reconstruction is an alternative interpolation technique that minimizes the amount of projection data required to generate a cross section. As implemented by General Electric, this results in a reduction of projection data required to reconstruct a cross section from the standard 360 to 225°. For a 1-s gantry rotation period, segmented reconstruction effectively increases the temporal resolution of the CT scan from 1 to 0.6 s. This has been demonstrated to eliminate artifacts that might be misconstrued as intimal flaps on conventional CT scans (Posniak et al. 1993). It is available for helical scans as well. Its use is typically required if an equivocal finding is present on a single image and should not be considered necessary when linear filling defects are visualized entirely within the confines of the aortic wall on sequential reconstructions – an indication of a true intimal flap (Fig. 20.3).

Arterial pulsation and perivenous streaks can also create distractions on SSDs and MIPs, even after the superior vena cava has been edited from the data. Aortic pulsation, which tends to be more pronounced in thinner individuals, results in a serrated appearance to arteries, which can mimic fibromuscular dysplasia in blood vessels such as renal arteries, but is rarely a limitation in the chest. It is useful to always bear in mind the discordance between gantry rotation and cardiac pulsation, which can explain some unusual CT images.

Because the cardiac period is spread over a longer distance longitudinally as the table speed of the CT scanner increases, pulsation artifacts are less frequent with the higher table speeds found with MDCT (Rubin et al. 2000). As gantry rotation period diminishes from 2 to 1 to 0.8 to 0.5 s, the temporal resolution of the scan improves and variations in aortic position appear more discrete, thus accentuating pulsation artifacts. Longer gantry rotation will smooth these artifacts due to smearing of the information over a longer period of time. An extreme example of this condition occurs during gadolinium-enhanced 3D MRA, where data are acquired for each anatomic location across the entire acquisition. The result is a very smooth appearing aortic surface, the

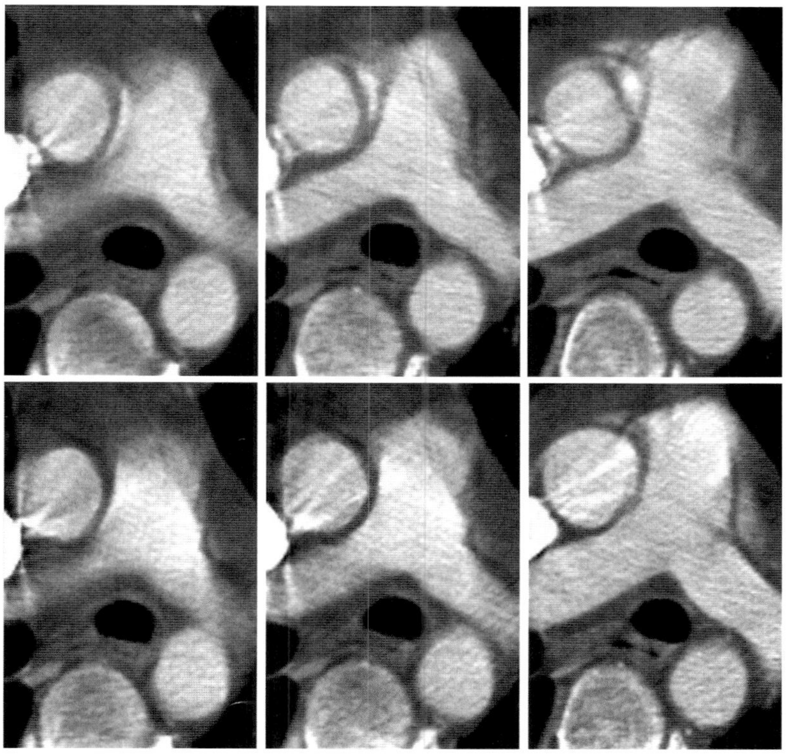

Fig. 20.3. *Top row:* Contiguous 3.75-mm transverse section MDCT sections obtained through the ascending aorta in a patient who had been run over by a tractor. Acquisition parameters are 3.75-mm detector width, pitch 6.0, table speed of 22.5 mm per rotation, and 0.8 s per rotation. An apparent linear filling defect is present within the ascending aorta on all three sections. This filling defect persisted even with the reconstruction of overlapping sections (not shown). *Bottom row:* Identical image locations from the same CT acquisition reconstructed with a half scan or segmented reconstruction algorithm. The segmented reconstruction requires approximately 220° of data resulting in an effective temporal resolution of 0.5 mm. By reconstructing the sections using this algorithm, the apparent linear filling defects are revealed to be motion-related artifacts, and thus there is no suspicion for ascending aortic injury

position of which represents the average position of the aorta across the entire acquisition.

20.7 Alternative Visualization: Reformation and Rendering

Although primary reconstructed transverse sections remain the mainstay of CTA interpretation, alternative visualization techniques can substantially augment diagnosis and provide an efficient means of communicating critical anatomic relationships to referring clinicians. The four most popular means of alternative visualization for CTA data: multiplanar reformation (MPR); SSD; MIP; and volume rendering (VR).

The MPR, which includes curved planar reformations (CPR) as well as traditional sagittal, coronal, and oblique tomograms, are typically a single voxel thick, but all MPRs can be broadened by combining information from adjacent voxels to obtain a thickened tomogram, referred to as a thin-slab or multi-planar volume rendered (MPVR) view (Napel et al. 1993). The thickness of the slab and method with which the slab is computed are user specified. The advantage of displaying anatomy with thin slabs is that pre-rendering segmentation or editing is not required, and some of the difficulties inherent in demonstrating vessel origins that originate in different but nearby planes, such as occurs with the branches of the aortic arch, are overcome. Despite these advantages, however, the single-voxel thick tomogram, particularly the CPR, is the most useful of the MPR techniques (Rubin et al. 1995). Its advantage is best appreciated when visualization of the luminal contents of the aorta or its branches is critical, such as in cases of aortic dissection or aortic stent-graft deployment. The relationship of intimal flaps to branch ostia can be well depicted, mural thrombus, atheroma, or hematoma to the flow lumen and branch ostia, and the interior of stents or stent grafts can be assessed for stenosis from neointima or for branch origin stenosis due to overlying graft material.

As commonly implemented, SSDs (Cline et al. 1991; Magnusson et al. 1991) are relatively simple three-dimensional views that render the entire volume or an edited subvolume to display complex three-dimensional relationships, particularly in regions of vessel overlap. The typical implementation on imaging workstations begins with the application of a single threshold value which converts the 12-bit deep CT data into a binary or 1-bit data set – above or below the threshold value. While this approach may result in artifacts and misrepresentation of the anatomy, the arbitrary selection of a threshold value or the necessity to select only a single threshold value is most limiting clinically when assessing vascular occlusive disease for stenosis grading, differentiating calcified plaque from luminal enhancement, and visualizing mural thrombus (Rubin et al. 1994, 1995). For the most part, thoracic aortic disease is not occlusive, but rather aneurysmal (true or false), aberrant branching (congenital), and intimal dissection or intramural hematoma. For all of these applications with the exception of intramural hematomas and some thrombosed false lumina, SSD provides the best simulation of lesion anatomy for surgical planning.

Maximum intensity projections (Rubin et al. 1994; Keller et al. 1989; Napel et al. 1992), while of value for CTA of other vascular territories, has limited applicability when assessing the thoracic aorta outside of thick-slab or MPVR applications. Calcified atheroma by itself is rarely of clinical significance, and the configuration of the aortic arch and its adjacency to other opacified structures, such as pulmonary arteries and veins, results in substantial vessel overlap; therefore, when assessing the thoracic aorta, the advantage that MIP–CTA allows simultaneous visualization and differentiation of the opacified flow lumen and mural calcium does not offer substantial clinical utility, and the inability of MIP to allow overlapping structures to be discerned is a substantial limitation (Fig. 20.3).

The final and most complex rendering technique is VR (Drebin et al. 1988; Levoy 1991; Rusinek et al. 1989; Fishman et al. 1987; Rubin et al. 1996a). There are many different versions and interfaces for VR, but the general approach is that all voxel values are assigned an opacity level that varies from total transparency to total opacity. This opacity function can be applied to the histogram of voxel values as a whole or to regions of the histogram that are classified as specific tissue types. With the latter approach, rectangular or trapezoidal regions are selected that correspond to the range of attenuation values for a structure (Johnson et al. 1996; Kuszyk et al. 1996). The "walls" of the trapezoid slope from an opacity plateau to the baseline of complete transparency in an attempt to account for partial-volume effects at the edges of structures. Regions at the walls of the trapezoidal regions or in positions where the opacity curve has a steep slope are referred to as transition zones in the ensuing protocols and are analogous to threshold levels with SSDs. Lighting effects may be simulated in a similar fashion as with SSD. Because there is no surface definition with VR, lighting effects are applied based on the spatial gradient (i.e., variability of attenuation within a local neighborhood of voxels). Near the edges of structures, the spatial variation in attenuation changes more rapidly (a high gradient) than in the center of structures (a low gradient). Lighting effects are most pronounced in regions of high spatial gradients. Because lighting effects and variations in transparency are simultaneously displayed, it is frequently useful to view VRs in color. The color is applied to the attenuation histogram to allow differentiation of pixel values and to avoid ambiguity with lighting effects, which are encoded in gray scale. Other variables, such as specular reflectivity, which models the "shininess" of a surface, may be available but should be used with caution to avoid confounding the visualization.

20.8 Clinical Applications

20.8.1 Thoracic Aortic Aneurysm

The CTA is a useful tool for diagnosing thoracic aortic aneurysms, determining their extent, and predicting appropriate management (Quint et al. 1996). While the diagnosis of aortic aneurysms is readily made from transverse sections, an assessment of the extent of the lesion, particularly when the brachiocephalic branches are involved, is facilitated by an assessment of CPRs and SSDs (Fig. 20.4).

In general, thoracic aortic aneurysms greater than 5 cm are at an increased risk for rupture. Although thoracic aortic aneurysm expand at a slower rate than abdominal aortic aneurysms, surgical repair is contemplated when thoracic aneurysms reach a diameter of 5–6 cm (Masuda et al. 1992; Dapunt et al. 1994). Helical CT can facilitate surgical planning by delineating the extent of the aneurysm and the involvement of aortic branches. In fact, Quint and colleagues (1996) found that an analysis of transverse sections and multiplanar reformations was 94% accurate with a positive predicative value of 95% and negative predictive value of 93% for successfully predicting the need for hypothermic circulatory arrest. With the exception of the elimination of one false-negative result, the addition of MPRs did not alter the predictions made from the transverse sections alone. Three-dimensional renderings were not evaluated in this study (Quint et al. 1996).

Because of the tortuosity and curvature of the thoracic aorta, aneurysm sizing is performed most accurately when double-oblique tomograms are generated perpendicular to the aortic flow lumen. The challenge of such an approach is that data concerning the risk of aneurysm rupture and expansion rate are based on measurements made from transverse sections, where true diameters can be overestimated. Furthermore, the measurement technique must be reproducible to assess the rate of aneurysm expansion on sequential studies.

The most complete measure of aneurysm size, however, is not the determination of true aortic diameters or even cross-sectional area, but aneurysm volume. Currently, this approach has substantial drawbacks. While the volumetric data of helical CT should be excellent for determining aneurysm volume, the accurate segmentation of both patent, thrombosed, and atheromatous elements of the aorta must be segmented from the adjacent structures to make this determination. The only technique available to perform this is painstaking manual segmentation performed by drawing regions of interest around the aorta on each cross section. Furthermore, to date aneurysm expansion has been studied primarily in terms of radial expansion of the aorta. While aneurysm volume determination is an attractive measure of aneurysm growth based on theoretical considerations, data concerning the risk of aneurysm rupture and guidelines for intervention are based on traditional transverse diameter measurements (Masuda et al. 1992; Dapunt et al. 1994).

20.8.2 Thoracic Aortic Dissection

The critical clinical issue required of any imaging test applied to a patient suspected of having an aortic dissection is the identification of an intimal flap and its localization to the ascending (type A) or descending (type B) aorta. This fundamental diagnostic feature that determines the need for emergent repair can be addressed by at least four imaging modalities: angiography; CT; magnetic resonance imaging (MR); and transesophageal echocardiography (TEE).

The relative accuracy of these modalities has been debated in the medical literature and is confounded by the fact that technical improvements in CT, MR, and TEE have outpaced our ability to compare them in appropriately designed prospective trials. Recent opinion has shifted toward MRI or TEE as the most sensitive tests for aortic dissection (Cigarroa et al. 1993).

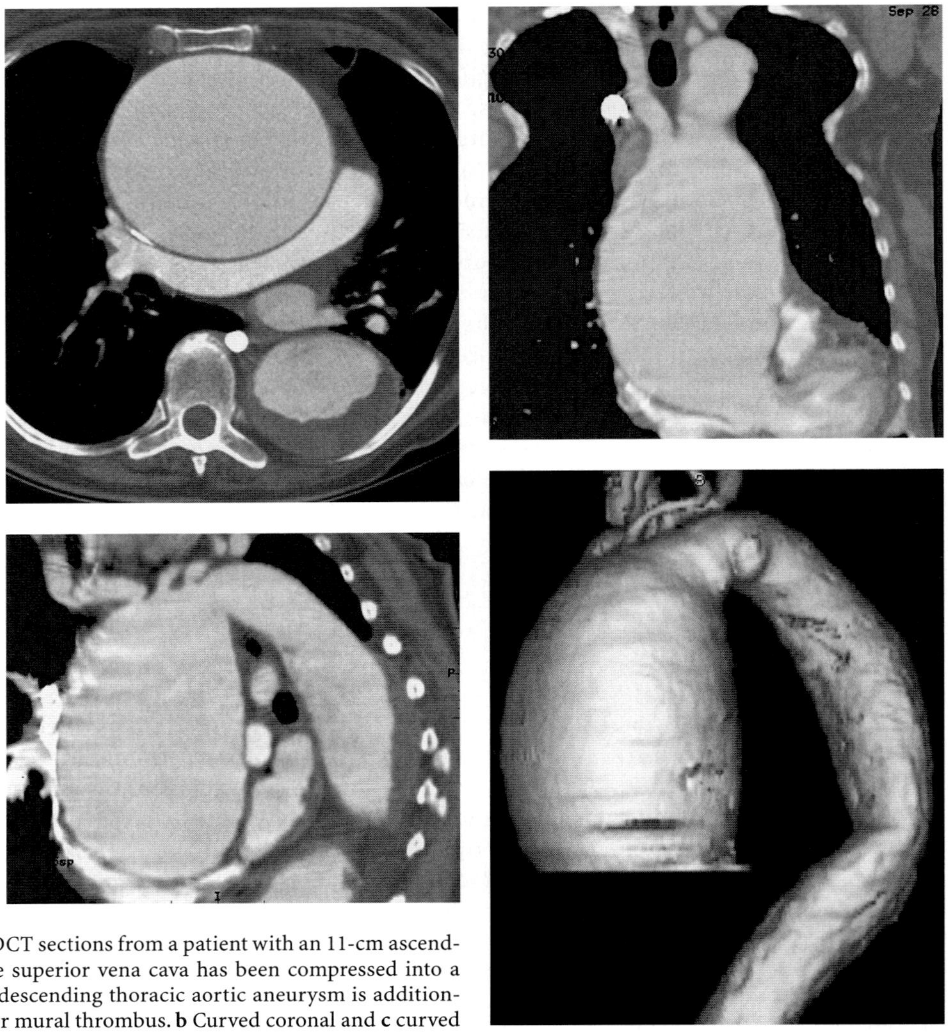

Fig. 20.4. **a** Transverse MDCT sections from a patient with an 11-cm ascending aortic aneurysm. The superior vena cava has been compressed into a slit-like configuration. A descending thoracic aortic aneurysm is additionally present with posterior mural thrombus. **b** Curved coronal and **c** curved sagittal reformations demonstrate origins of all supra-aortic branches from the ascending aortic aneurysm. The curved coronal reformation (**b**) demonstrates the marked displacement of the left ventricle resulting from this large aneurysm. **d** Shaded-surface display further improves depiction of the full extent of the aneurysm particularly at its distal neck

Unfortunately, much of this opinion is based on comparative studies where state-of-the-art MR or TEE is compared with relatively primitive conventional CT technique (Erbel et al. 1989; Nienaber et al. 1993). In 1989, Erbel and colleagues studied 164 consecutive patients with suspected aortic dissection. All patients were studied with transthoracic echocardiography and TEE, 85 patients were studied with CT, and 96 patients were studied with aortography. The technique for CT scanning was 10-mm-thick sections acquired at 20- to 40-mm intervals through the chest. Details of how iodinated contrast was administered are not given. Not surprisingly, CT was found to be less sensitive (77%) than echocardiography (98%) and aortography (89%) in those patients with surgical proof (Erbel et al. 1989). In 1993 Nienaber and co-workers compared 110 patients with suspected aortic dissection who underwent at least two of three imaging tests: TEE; CT; or MR. The CT was found to have lower sensitivity (93.8%) than TEE (97.7%) and MR (98.3%) and lower specificity (87.1%) than MR (97.8%). For this study, 80–100 ml of contrast were administered during the course of 5- to 15-min scans that were performed with section intervals of 20 mm (Nienaber et al. 1993). To date, there have been no comparisons of helical CT to either MR or TEE, and while it is tempting to discount these prior studies because of the substantial advances that have occurred in CT imaging, TEE and MR have undergone further improvements as well.

The TEE has progressively improved with the introduction of biplane and multiplane probes that substantially reduce the blind spots and ambiguous reverberation artifacts that can limit the accuracy of monoplane devices (Cigarroa et al. 1993). Newer MR techniques, employing a dynamic intravenous injection of gadolinium coupled with a rapid breath-held gradient-echo acquisition, have also yielded impressive images that should improve the diagnostic accuracy of MR over that of spin-echo and cine techniques (Prince et al. 1996; Krinsky et al. 1997). The one modality that has not been substantially improved has been conventional angiography. Currently, the primary indication for diagnostic arteriography of acute aortic dissection is in the setting of arrhythmia or ECG abnormalities suggestive of coronary artery involvement and myocardial ischemia. It is likely that in appropriately skilled hands, the accuracy of TEE, CT, and MR will be nearly identical for the diagnosis of aortic dissection. Access to these three modalities is another issue, however.

Because patients suffering from acute aortic dissection are typically critically ill and potentially in need of an emergent operation, expediency of diagnosis is important. In a center where experienced cardiologists are available to perform state-of-the-art TEE in the emergency room to identify the presence of an intimal flap in the ascending aorta, this will likely be the preferred first-line imaging test. An additional advantage of TEE over CT acutely is its ability to identify aortic valvular insufficiency, which in the setting of acute aortic dissection will indicate the need for emergent valve replacement in addition to aortic repair. When high-quality TEE is unavailable, however, in most institutions CT will be the modality that is most accessible and staffed to handle potentially hemodynamically unstable patients (Fig. 20.5).

When considering the clinical utility of a diagnostic test, it is useful to consider the likelihood that a test will suggest an alternative diagnosis when the primary diagnosis is not present. Figure 20.6 illustrates a case where the combination of acute chest pain and diminished right brachial and radial pulses were highly suggestive of aortic dissection. No dissection was identified; however, a high-grade stenosis of the brachiocephalic artery origin and an occluded bypass graft originating on the anterior surface of the ascending aorta and inserting onto a proximally stenosed left anterior descending coronary artery was found on CTA. It is unlikely that either of these abnormalities would have been detected with TEE.

In the setting of chronic aortic dissection or acute dissection that does not necessitate emergent operation, other imaging issues emerge that cannot be addressed by TEE. These include the extension of the intimal flap into aortic branches, true luminal compression by the false lumen limiting blood flow into the abdomen, and the presence of fenestrations that allow communication between the true and false lumen. Clinically relevant aortic branch involvement typically is intraabdominal where mesenteric ischemia, renal insufficiency, and lower extremity claudication indicate extension into mesenteric, renal, and iliac arteries, respectively. Intervention, either surgically or using catheter-based techniques, may be required. The CT appears to be excellent for establishing extension of intimal flaps into aortic branches; however, its accuracy has not been established. When considering catheter-based interventions, preprocedural CT can be very useful. The simultaneous visualization of all aortic lumina can help to avoid confusion in the angiography suite that results from opacification of only one of three or more lumina in a complex dissection. The CT scan can also help identify the best route for achieving access to aortic branches.

While the superior spatial resolution and improved aortic enhancement provided by helical CT results in substantially better images than conventional CT, some pitfalls persist. Pulsation in the ascending aorta can mimic an intimal flap. This artifact tends to be less of a problem with helical CT as the generation of closely overlapping sections in the region of the suspected artifact or intimal flap, displayed sequentially as a cine loop, usually establishes the artifact as rotating or moving relative to the aorta. Examination of wide windows may document extension of artifacts beyond the aortic wall. The use of segmented reconstruction of the helical scan data may eliminate motion artifacts observed on standard reconstructions (Posniak et al. 1993). Finally, differential flow in the true and false lumina can result in the spurious appearance of a thrombosed false lumen when scan delay is based upon a timing study directed to the true lumen of the aorta. In the setting of suspected aortic dissection, bolus timing should be performed just below the aortic arch, where transverse cross sections of the distal ascending and proximal descending aorta can be evaluated. A region of interest is placed in both the true and false lumens of and two curves are generated. A delay time that assures some false luminal opacification is selected and the bolus duration then extended by the number of seconds between the true luminal peak and the selected delay

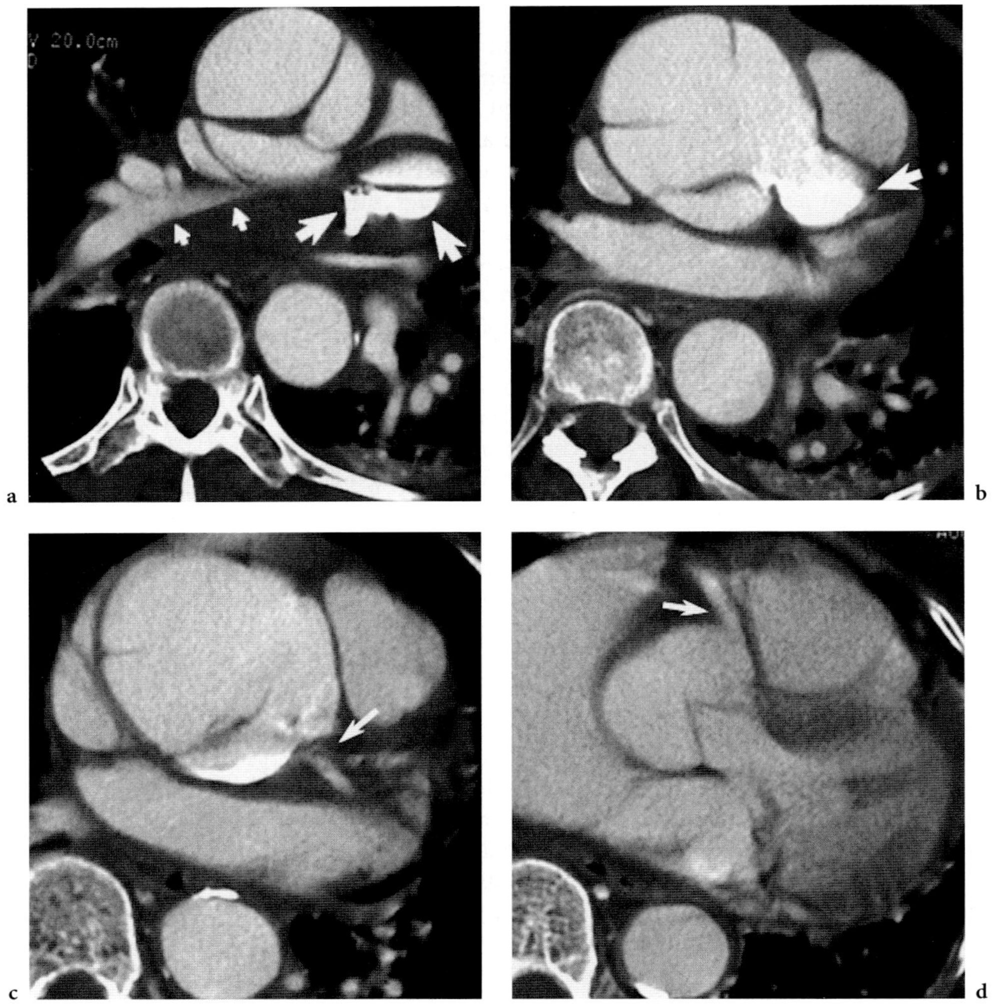

Fig. 20.5. a, b Transverse CT sections in a patient with acute chest pain demonstrates a type-A aortic dissection with posteromedial rupture of the proximal ascending aorta and active extravasation of arterial contrast medium into the mediastinum through a pseudoaneurysm (*large arrows*). A mediastinal hematoma is resulting in substantial right pulmonary arterial compression (*small arrows*). **c** The original left main coronary artery could be visualized one section below this image, which demonstrates the proximal left, centered, and circumflex coronary arteries (*arrow*) originated immediately below the pseudoaneurysm from the left sinus of Valsalva. **d** The right coronary artery origin is clearly uninvolved (*arrow*), as is the aortic valve

time. This assures true and false luminal opacification for the duration of the helical acquisition.

When considering alternative visualization techniques in the setting of aortic dissection, it should not be surprising that MIPs are limited as they do not demonstrate the intimal flap unless it is oriented perpendicular to the MIP. Curved planar reconstructions can be very useful for displaying the flap within the center of the vessel, whereas SSDs depict the interface of the intimal flap with the aortic wall.

20.8.3 Intramural Hematoma

Although initially recognized pathologically in 1920, intramural hematoma has only recently been recognized as a distinct clinical entity from aortic dissection. Several mechanisms have been proposed, including spontaneous rupture of vasa vasorum, intimal fracture at an atherosclerotic plaque, and intramural propagation of hemorrhage adjacent to a penetrating

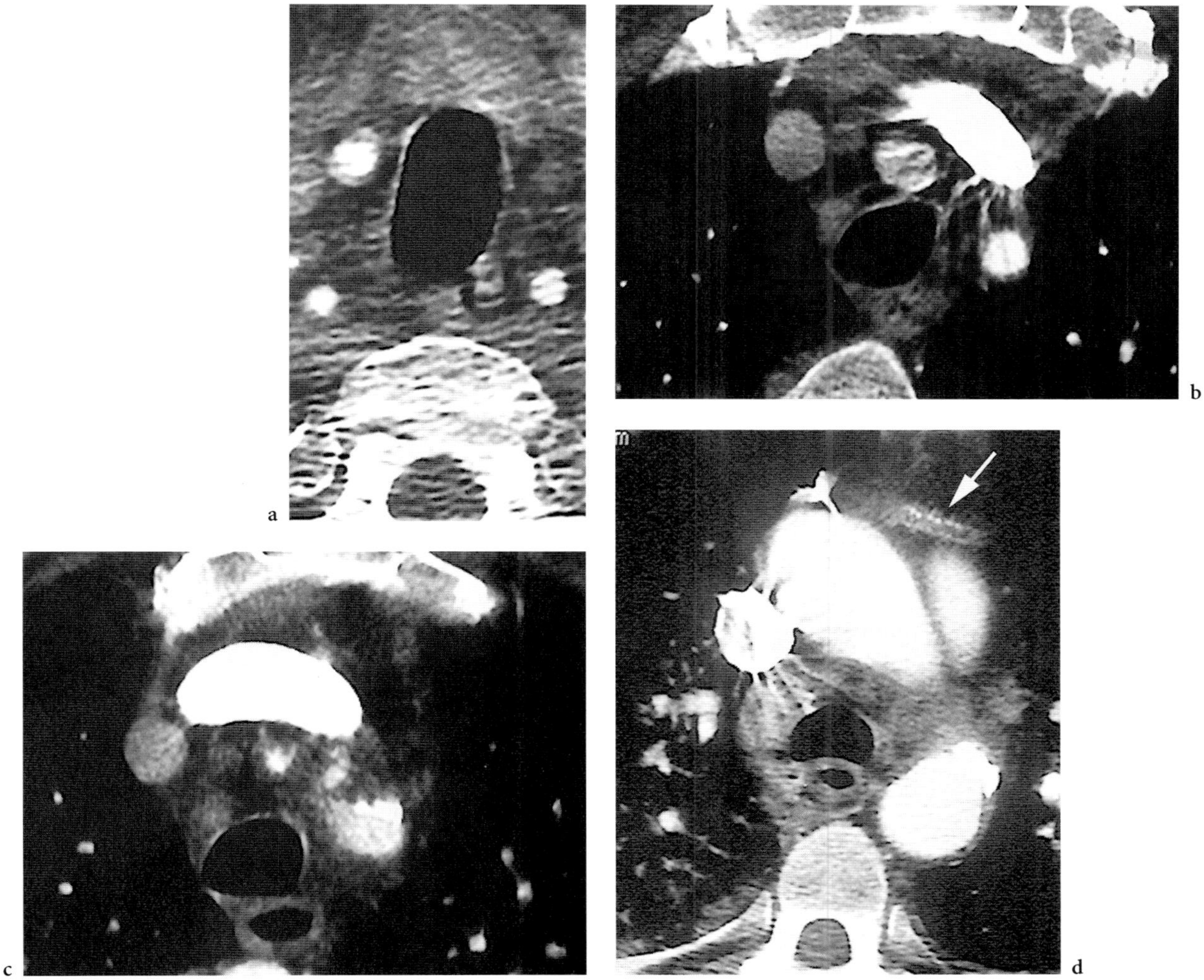

Fig. 20.6. a–c Transverse sections acquired with 3-mm collimation and 2.0 pitch in a patient with acute chest pain and diminished right brachial and radial pulses. One centimeter above the aortic arch (**c**), there is a high-grade stenosis of the brachiocephalic artery origin and a narrow left common carotid artery origin. One centimeter cephalad (**b**) the brachiocephalic artery is normal caliber but the left common carotid artery is nearly occluded. At the thoracic inlet (**a**) the left common carotid artery is completely occluded. Note that both vertebral arteries are large in this patient with unsuspected, although substantial, flow limitation into both carotid arteries. Below the aortic arch (**c, d**) a thrombosed coronary artery bypass graft (*arrow*) from the ascending aorta to the left anterior descending coronary artery is demonstrated. The findings were confirmed arteriographically and serial enzymes established the diagnosis of acute myocardial infarction

atherosclerotic ulcer. Regardless of the cause, patients with intramural hematomas exhibit signs and symptoms as well as risk profiles that are virtually identical to classic aortic dissection (Nienaber et al. 1995).

Kazerooni and co-workers, based on an analysis of conventional CTs in 16 patients, described the CT appearance of intramural hematomas caused by penetrating atherosclerotic ulcers. In addition to the visualization of at least one ulcer in 15 of 16, the intramural hematoma was visualized in all 16, and its subintimal location was confirmed by the observation of displaced intimal calcifications in 13 patients (Fig. 20.7; Kazerooni et al. 1992). While intramural hematomas associated with ulceration tend to predominate in the descending aorta (Kazerooni et al. 1992), the distribution of all intramural hematomas was 48% ascending aortic, 8% aortic arch, and 44% descending aortic in one series (Nienaber et al. 1995).

In Quint's series two patients in whom intramural hematomas were identified, but an associated

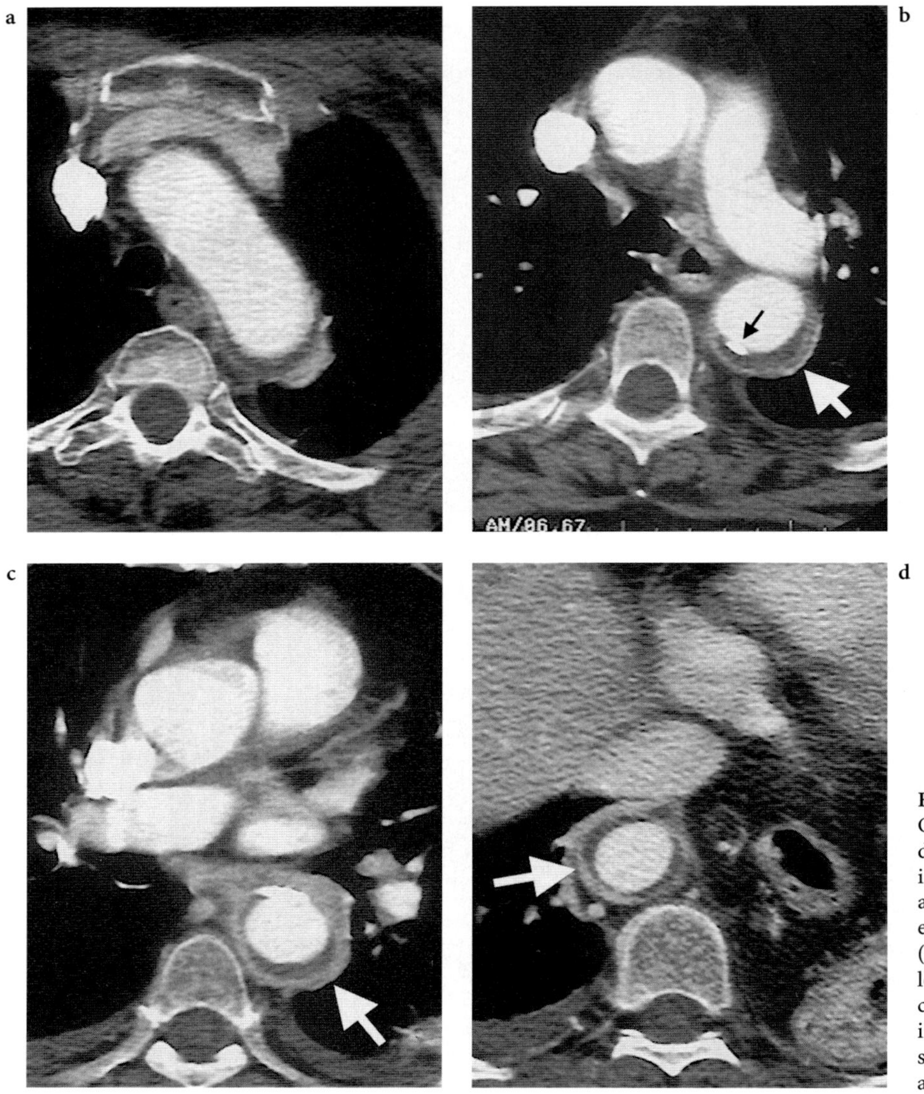

Fig. 20.7a–d. Transverse CTA sections demonstrate a descending thoracic aortic intramural hematoma associated with marked aortic wall enhancement and thickening (*white arrow*). The subintimal location of the hematoma is confirmed by the presence of intimal calcium on its internal surface (*black arrow*). Ulceration was not identified

ulceration could not be identified, were scored as false-negative examinations (Quint et al. 1996). Recognizing that intramural hematoma formation has two proposed mechanisms: (a) extension of a penetrating ulcer into the media with subsequent bleeding into the aortic wall; and (b) primary disruption of vasa vasorum without penetrating ulcer formation (Kazerooni et al. 1992; Gore 1952). The diagnoses in these cases may have been correct given a primary intramural bleed as the mechanism for intramural hematoma formation, which need not be associated with ulceration.

Unenhanced sections typically reveal a high-attenuation crescent within the wall of the aorta (Fig. 20.8). Another finding that is seen in the setting of intramural hematoma is intense enhancement and thickening of the aortic wall external to the hematoma, which may represent adventitial inflammation.

20.8.4 Thoracic Aortic Trauma

Prior to the introduction of helical CT, unenhanced conventional CT scanning was used to detect mediastinal hemorrhage as an indirect sign of aortic injury. In a meta-analysis of 18 previously published series of post-traumatic thoracic CT revealed that mediastinal hemorrhage had a specificity of 87.1% and a sensitivity of 99.3% for predicting aortic

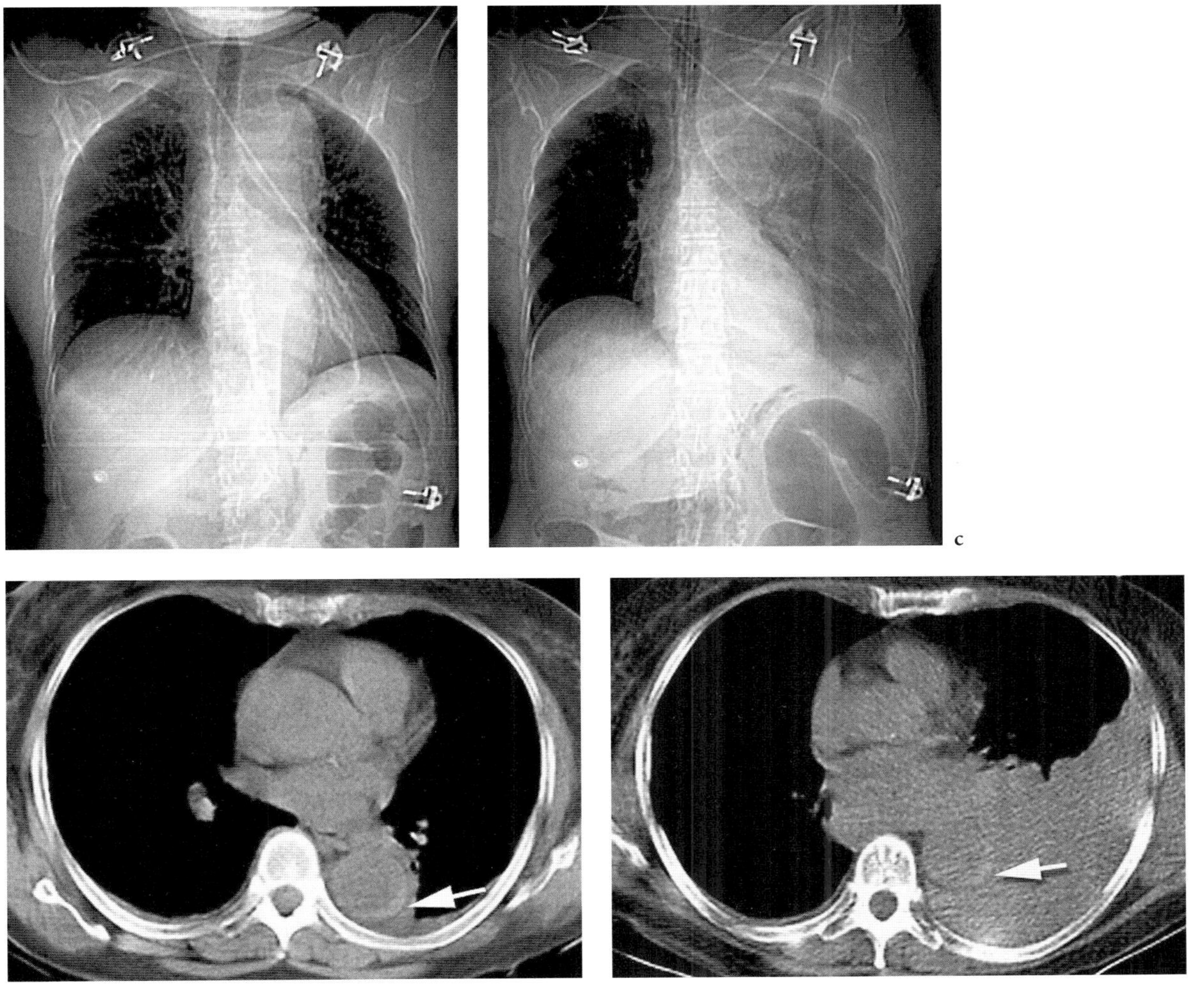

Fig. 20.8. **a** Frontal projectional radiograph of the chest demonstrates a widened aortic arch in a patient with acute chest pain. **b** Unenhanced transverse CT section obtained in anticipation of performing a CT angiogram demonstrates a high-attenuation crescent within the posterior wall of the descending aorta (*arrow*). A small left pleural effusion is present. This high-attenuation crescent is pathognomonic for an intramural hematoma. Prior to performing the ensuing CT angiogram, the patient became acutely hemodynamically unstable on the CT table necessitating cardiopulmonary resuscitation. **c** Forty-five minutes after the initial acquisition, **a, b** the patient was stabilized hemodynamically. A repeat frontal projectional radiograph demonstrates that the left hemothorax is now filled with fluid. **d** Transverse CT section at this time demonstrates a large left pleural effusion (*arrow*), which was subsequently demonstrated to represent blood due to acute rupture of the aorta at the site of the intramural hematoma. The high-attenuation crescent within the aortic wall, which is now displaced anteriorly, compared with the earlier cross section, is still visible

injury (Mirvis et al. 1996). Reliance on CT for triaging patients to angiography only when CT was suspicious resulted in an overall cost savings of over $365,000.00 in their own series of 677 trauma patients with chest radiographic abnormalities warranting aortic imaging (Mirvis et al. 1996). While these results are impressive, many have argued that the confident identification of mediastinal hematoma, particularly on unenhanced CT, is extremely difficult (Raptopoulos 1994), and that the presence of mediastinum hematoma is insufficiently sensitive and specific for thoracic aortic injury.

The application of helical CTA to suspected aortic trauma offers the critical advantage of direct visualization of the aortic tear (Fig. 20.9). Although initial reports did not rely on the use of high-resolution helical acquisitions coupled with high-flow iodinated contrast injections, the results were encouraging. Gavant and colleagues published the first helical CTA series of aortic injury. Using 7-mm collimation

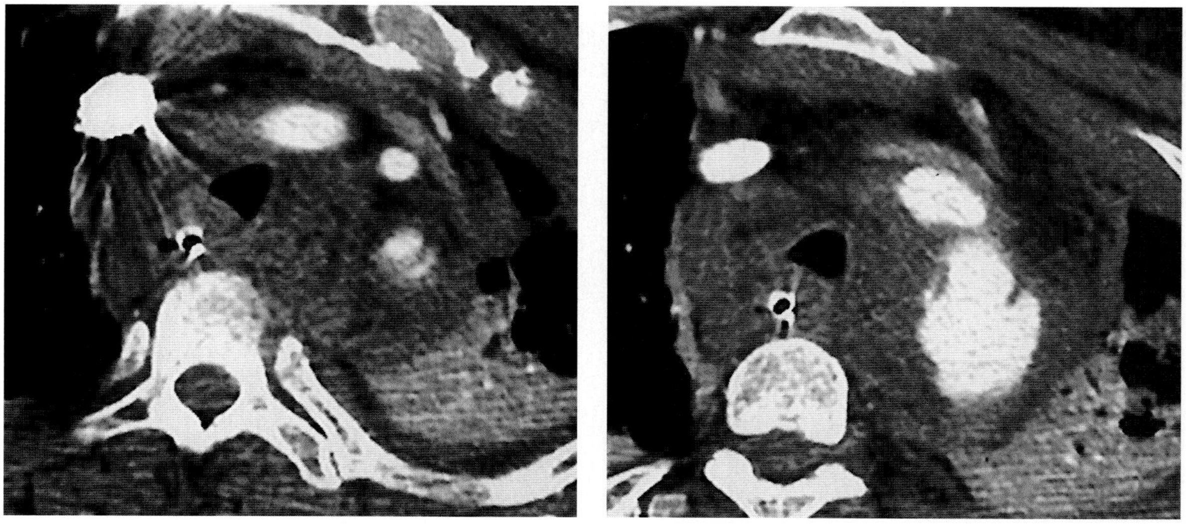

a b

Fig. 20.9a, b. Status after high-speed motor vehicle accident: gross aortic injury. Transverse helical CTA sections demonstrate aortic injury with pseudoaneurysm formation at the aortic isthmus. An intimal injury extends into the left subclavian artery. There is extensive mediastinal hematoma. The findings were confirmed in the operating room

and a contrast medium flow rate of 1.5–2.0 ml/s, they found that the sensitivity of CT was greater than that of conventional arteriography (100 vs 94.4%), but the specificity and positive predictive values were less than those of conventional arteriography (81.7 and 47.4%, respectively, for CT vs 96.3 and 81% for aortography) in a subset of 127 of 1518 patients with nontrivial blunt thoracic trauma who under went both CT and aortography. Perhaps the most encouraging result of this study was that no false-negative results occurred in the 21 patients with aortic injury (Gavant et al. 1995).

Gavant subsequently described the CT appearance of 38 thoracic aortic or great vessel injuries in 36 patients identified with helical CT and confirmed with aortography or surgery. Six (17%) of these cases were found to have either no or "difficult-to-detect" para-aortic or mediastinal hematoma. Transverse sections showed either an intimal flap or thrombus protruding into the aortic lumen in all cases. Of 28 injuries to the descending aorta, 23 (82%) were associated with a pseudoaneurysm. In subjectively comparing the value of the reconstructed transverse sections to multiplanar reformations and 3D renderings, the authors felt that the transverse sections were best for depicting the proximal and distal extent of the lesion, and aside from the fact that multiplanar reformations and 3D renderings "portray the thoracic aortic lumen in a familiar light" did not contribute substantially to the identification and characterization of aortic injury (Gavant et al. 1996).

A recent publication by Parker and colleagues (2001) reported on an investigation of 142 patients with abnormal chest radiographs following trauma that were suggestive of aortic injury. All patients had CTA and conventional thoracic aortography. The sensitivity and negative predictive value of CT were 100%. Fourteen false-positive CT results occurred and were attributed to a conservative approach where ductus bumps, bronchial artery infundibula, and hemomediastinum (Parker et al. 2001). Similar results have been reported by Dyer and colleagues (1999).

20.8.5 Congenital Anomalies

Congenital anomalies of the thoracic aorta and aberrant branches of the descending aorta such as CT, vascular rings, aberrant supra-aortic branching, coarctation (Fig. 20.10), and enlarged bronchial arteries or major arteriopulmonary communicating arteries are easily diagnosed and characterized (Katz et al.1995; Hopkins et al. 1996) with helical CT. The use of conventional angiography for the diagnosis and characterization of lesions such as pulmonary sequestration should no longer be necessary if a thin-section volumetric acquisition is appropriately acquired with adequate contrast enhancement. The simultaneous visualization of the airways complements vascular visualization by allowing a direct determination of the specific structures responsible

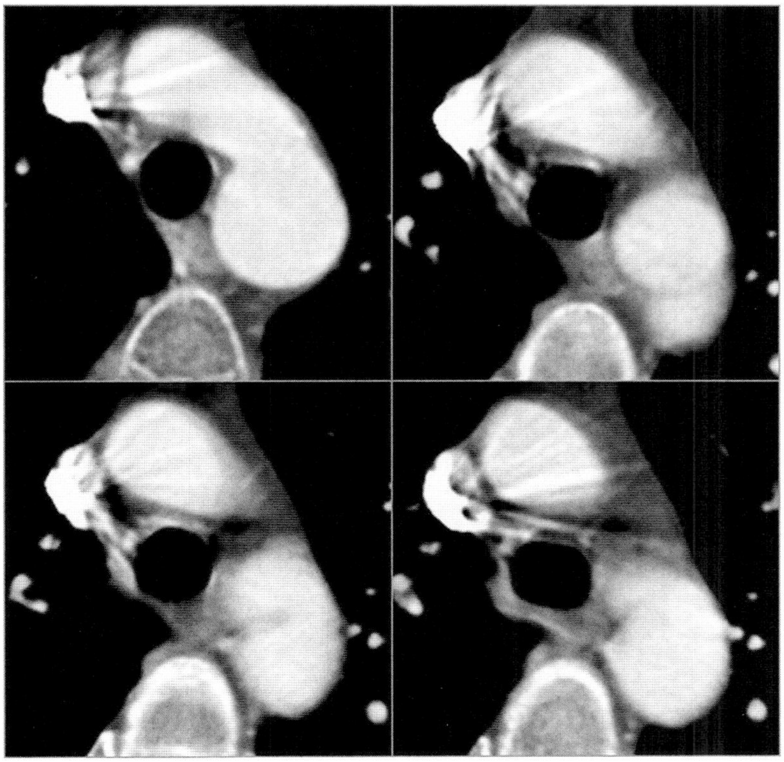
a

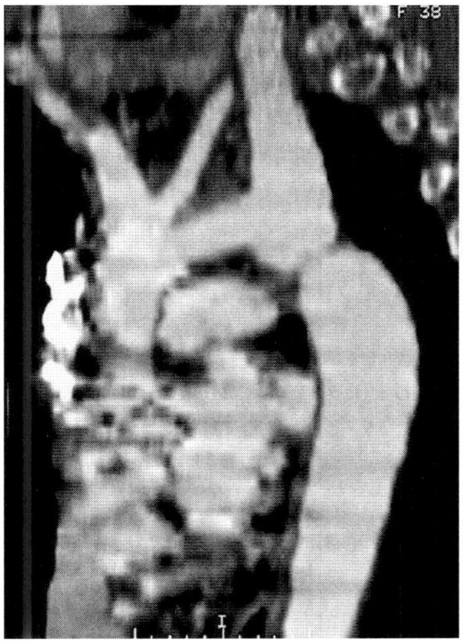
b

Fig. 20.10. **a** Consecutive transverse sections acquired with 3 mm collimation, 2.0 pitch demonstrate a linear filling defect in the proximal descending aorta. The lesion is difficult to characterize from the transverse sections alone. **b** Curved planar reformation demonstrates a very short region of aortic coarctation, and a hypoplastic aortic arch with bovine branching pattern and enlarged left subclavian artery

for tracheobronchial narrowing and the presence of aberrant airways. While aortic stenosis secondary to coarctation is clearly demonstrated and enlarged intercostal arteries can be visualized as well, further study must be performed to determine the extent with which the thin webs that often are present in these lesions can be identified and the degree of aortic stenosis determined.

20.8.6 Assessment of Open and Endovascular Interventions

Vascular clips, sternal wires, and graft materials typically result in relatively little artifact on helical CT scans (Fig. 20.11). As a result, helical CTA is an excellent means for assessing the thoracic aorta for perianastomotic complications following aortic or coronary artery bypass graft placement (Fig. 20.12) and complications relating to placement of access cannulas for cardiopulmonary bypass. In fact, the patency of coronary artery bypass grafts often can be determined on helical CT scans and should be routinely examined, particularly in the setting of acute chest pain and the exclusion of aortic dissection as the indication for thoracic CTA.

The CTA is also very useful for the assessment of endoluminal stent grafts (Armerding et al. 2000). The success of aneurysm treatment by stent-graft deployment is dependent upon ensuring that the aneurysm has been completely excluded. Perigraft flow can be very slow and thus during flush aortography may be undetected (Fig. 20.13). Because helical CTA relies upon generalized arterial opacification from an intravenous injection rather than a local aortic injection, opacification of perigraft channels are frequently detected on postdeployment CT angiograms, when aortography suggested complete exclusion. Furthermore, because the origins of the brachiocephalic branches are typically tortuous in the setting of thoracic aortic aneurysm, it can be challenging to demonstrate the relationship of the stent graft and the brachiocephalic arterial origins arteriographically. Other complications, such

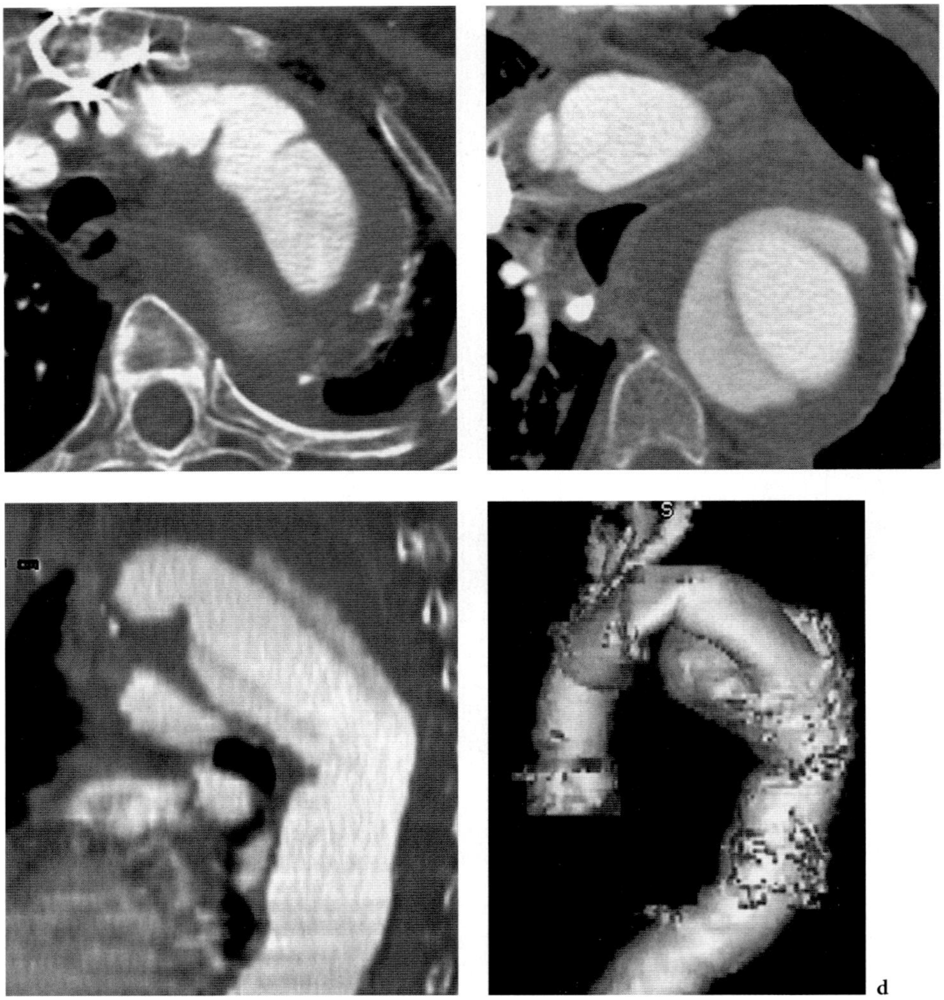

Fig. 20.11. a, b Transverse CT sections to the aortic arch and proximal descending aorta demonstrates the appearance of an elephant-trunk graft which can simulate a primary aortic dissection. Folds in the **a** proximal aspect of the graft mimic intimal flaps, whereas **b** dual-lumen appearance within the descending aorta mimics the true and false lumen of the aortic dissection. **c** Curved planar reformation of the descending aorta demonstrates the characteristic appearance of the elephant-trunk graft extending into the descending aorta. The proximal descending aorta is sutured around the mid graft and a substantial tail of the graft is left within the aortic lumen for subsequent recovery at thoracotomy and placement of an extended descending thoracic aortic graft. **d** Shaded-surface displays facilitate visualization of the complex relationships present in the aortic distal arch. An interposition graft is additionally present in the proximal ascending aorta

as aortic branch occlusions (Fig. 20.14), retroperitoneal hematoma, and iliac arterial dissection or occlusion, are also demonstrable (Fig. 20.15).

20.9 Conclusion

Nine years after its introduction (Napel et al. 1992; Rubin et al. 1993), spiral or helical CTA is being embraced as an important noninvasive tool for imaging the thoracic aorta and its branches. The high degree of accessibility and ease with which the studies are performed make it a viable alternative to aortography. Once familiar with the principles of CTA, the acquisition phase of the examination can be completed in as little as 15 min.

Nevertheless, important challenges remain for CTA. The capabilities of MDCT to acquire thinner sections in shorter scan times have resulted in a veritable explosion of imaging data for radiologists to analyze. In this environment, efficient image processing workstations and software is critical to improving

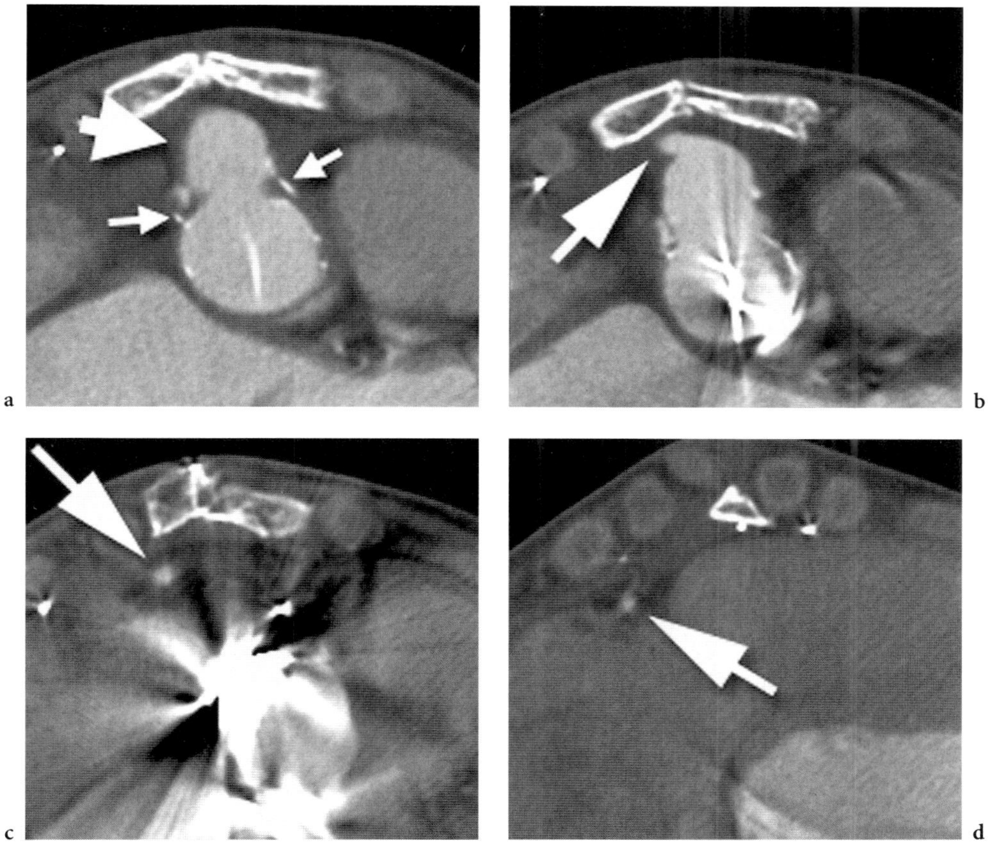

Fig. 20.12. **a** Transverse CT sections obtained with 2.5-mm thickness and displayed at 10-mm increments demonstrate a dehisced coronary artery implantation button. The rings of the button are visualized as punctate high-attenuation structures in the *upper left image* (*small arrows*). A 1.5-cm pseudo-aneurysm had formed at the implantation site (*large arrow*). **b–d** Despite the presence of the anastomotic dehiscence in associated pseudo-aneurysm, patency within the right coronary artery is demonstrated (*arrows*)

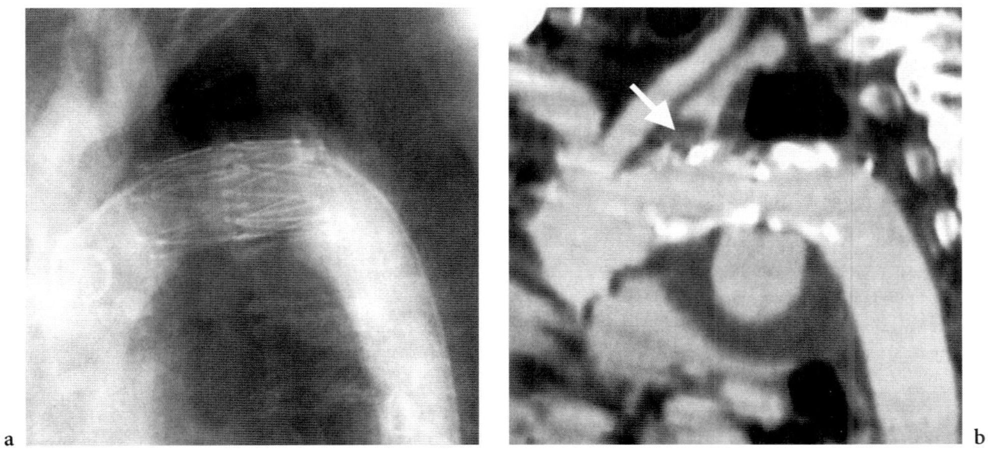

Fig. 20.13. **a** Aortogram status after deployment of a stent-graft (Dacron covered modified Z stent) over a pseudoaneurysm of at the aortic isthmus. The pseudoaneurysm appears to be completely thrombosed. **b** CPR CTA obtained 4 h after stent-graft deployment demonstrates that the pseudoaneurysm is still patent. Additionally, the stent graft covers the origin of the left subclavian artery, and a thrombus (*arrow*) has formed in the proximal left subclavian artery. The patient underwent transection of the left subclavian artery approximately 5 cm from its origin through a limited incision in the neck. The distal left subclavian artery was transplanted onto the left common carotid artery

our ability to efficiently interpret these volumetric CT data (Rubin et al. 1996a).

Finally, helical CT technology is far from static. Every year new advances in engineering bring better image quality, improved resolution, and faster scan times. As medical imagers, we must not become complacent, but rather constantly challenge ourselves to consider how we might further improve upon our utilization of CT equipment to maximize the collection of information relevant to diagnosis and therapy.

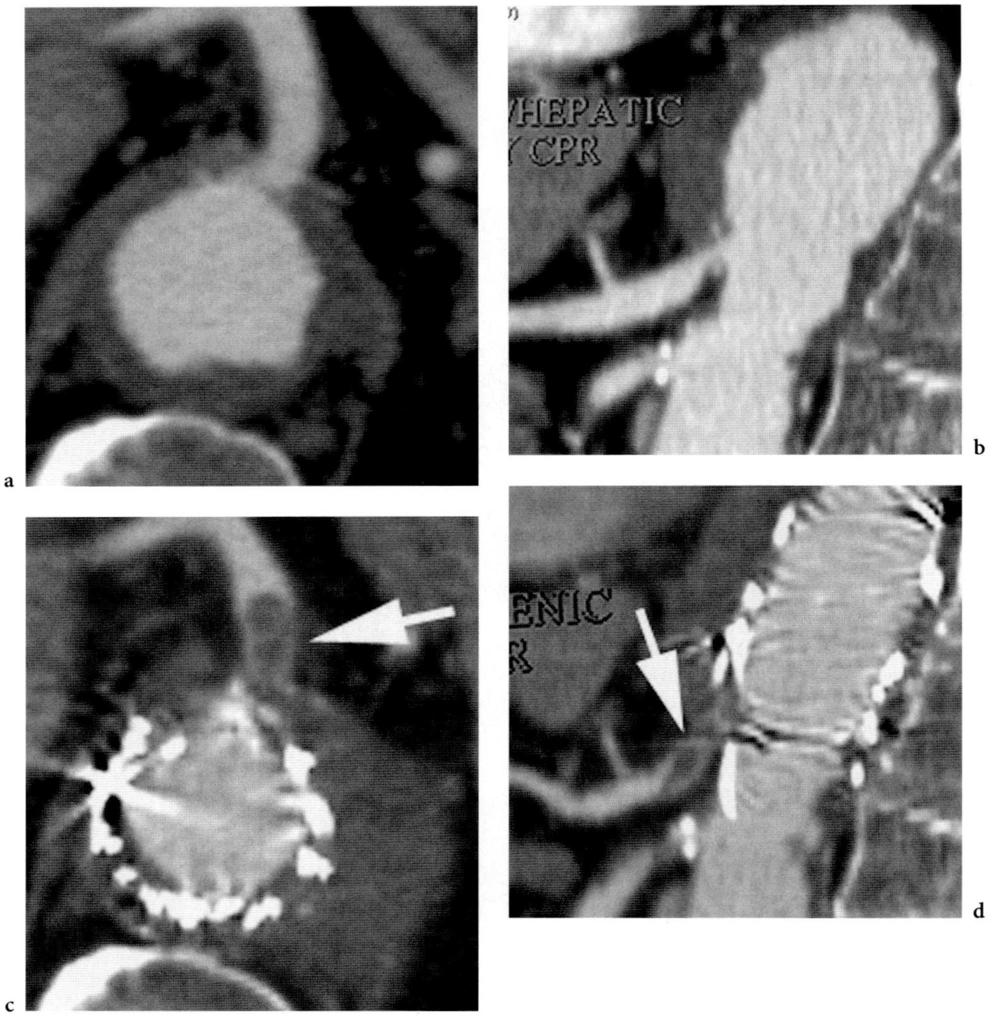

Fig. 20.14. a Transverse sections and **b** curved sagittal reformation through the celiac origin demonstrates a celiac origin stenosis at the distal extent of a thoracoabdominal aortic aneurysm. **c** Transverse CT section and **d** curved sagittal reformation following treatment of the thoracoabdominal aortic aneurysm with a stent graft demonstrates inadvertent occlusion of the celiac origin with thrombus (*arrows*) present in the proximal centimeter of the celiac axis

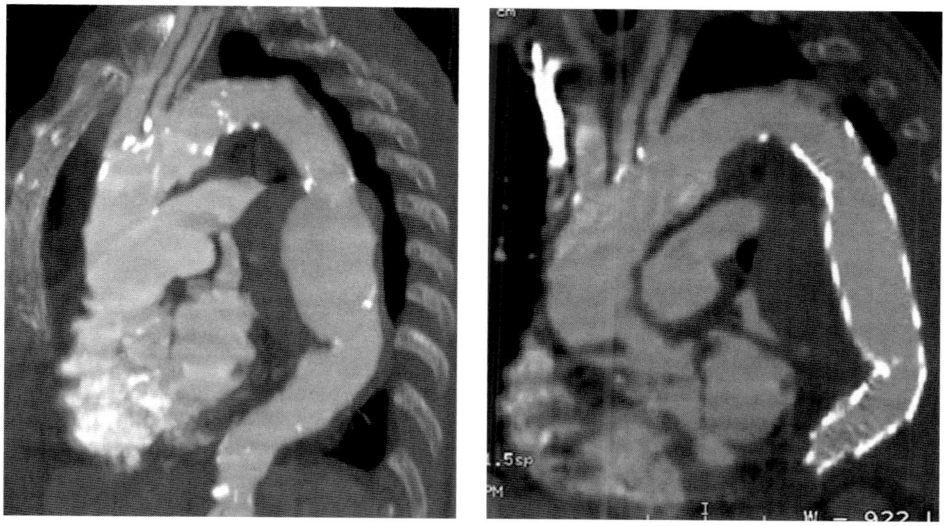

a b

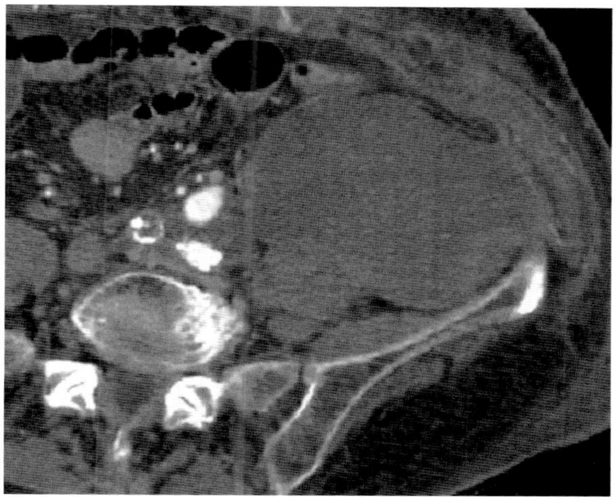

c

Fig. 20.15. **a** Curved thin-slab para-sagittal maximum intensity projection demonstrates a large descending thoracic aortic aneurysm with mural thrombus. **b** Curved planar reformation following deployment of a descending aortic stent graft demonstrates successful isolation of the aneurysm. **c** Transverse sections through the pelvis demonstrate a large retroperitoneal hematoma as well as a complete thrombosis of the right common iliac artery that occurred following deployment of the stent graft. An oval enhancing structure anterior to the common iliac arteries represents a small graft conduit sutured to the distal aorta into which the stent graft was introduced for primary deployment

References

Armerding MD, Rubin GD, Beaulieu CF et al. (2000) Aortic aneurysmal disease: assessment of stent-graft treatment-CT versus conventional angiography. Radiology 215: 138–146

Cigarroa JE, Isselbacher EM, DeSanctis RW, Eagle KA (1993) Medical progress. Diagnostic imaging in the evaluation of suspected aortic dissection: old standards and new directions. AJR 161:485–493

Cline HE, Lorensen WE, Souza SP et al. (1991) 3D Surface rendered MR images of the brain and its vasculature. J Comput Assist Tomogr 15:344–351

Dapunt L, Galla JD, Sadeghi AM et al. (1994) The natural history of thoracic aortic aneurysms. J Thorac Cardiovasc Surg 107:1323–1333

Drebin RA, Carpenter L, Hanrahan P (1988) Volume rendering. Comput Graph 22:65–74

Dyer DS, Moore EE, Mestek MF et al. (1999) Can chest CT be used to exclude aortic injury? Radiology 213:195–202

Erbel R, Daniel W, Visser C, Engberding R, Roelandt J, Rennollet H (1989) Echocardiography in diagnosis of aortic dissection. Lancet 4:457–461

Fishman EK, Drebin B, Magid D et al. (1987) Volumetric rendering techniques: applications for three-dimensional imaging of the hip. Radiology 163:737–738

Gavant ML, Manke PG, Fabian T, Flick PA, Graney MJ, Gold RE (1995) Blunt traumatic aortic rupture: detection with helical CT of the chest. Radiology 197:125–133

Gavant ML, Flick P, Manke P, Gold RE (1996) CT aortography of thoracic aortic rupture. AJR 166:955–961

Gore I (1952) Pathogenesis of dissecting aneurysm of the aorta. Arch Pathol Lab Med 53:142–153

Hopkins KL, Patrick LE, Simoneaux SF, Bank ER, Parks WJ, Smith SS (1996) Pediatric great vessel anomalies: initial clinical experience with spiral CT angiography. Radiology 200:811–815

Johnson PT, Heath DG, Bliss DF, Cabral B, Fishman EK (1996) Three-dimensional CT: real-time interactive volume rendering. Am J Roentgenol 167:581–583

Katz M, Konen E, Rozsenman J, Szeinberg A, Itzchak Y (1995) Spiral CT and 3D image reconstruction of vascular ring and associated tracheobronchial anomalies. J Comput Assist Tomogr 19:564–568

Kazerooni EA, Bree RL, Williams DM (1992) Penetrating atherosclerotic ulcers of the descending thoracic aorta: evaluation with CT and distinction from aortic dissection. Radiology 183:759–765

Keller PJ, Drayer BP, Fram EK, Williams KD, Dumoulin CL, Souza SP (1989) MR angiography with two-dimensional acquisition and three-dimensional display. Radiology 173: 527–532

Krinsky GA, Rofsky NM, DeCorato DR et al. (1997) Thoracic aorta: comparison of gadolinium-enhanced three-dimensional MR angiography with conventional MR imaging. Radiology 202:183–193

Kuszyk BS, Heath DG, Bliss DF, Fishman EK (1996) Skeletal 3-D CT: advantages of volume rendering over surface rendering. Skeletal Radiol 25:207–214

Levoy M (1991) Methods for improving the efficiency and versatility of volume rendering. Prog Clin Biol Res 363: 473–488

Magnusson M, Lenz R, Danielsson PE (1991) Evaluation of methods for shaded surface display of CT volumes. Comput Med Imaging Graph 15:247–256

Masuda Y, Takanashi K, Takasu J, Morooka Y, Inagaki Y (1992) Expansion rate of thoracic aortic aneurysms and influencing factors. Chest 102:461–466

Mirvis SE, Shanmuganathan K, Miller BH, White CS, Turney SZ (1996) Traumatic aortic injury: diagnosis with contrast-enhanced thoracic CT: five year experience at a major trauma center. Radiology 200:413–422

Napel S, Marks MP, Rubin GD et al. (1992) CT angiography with spiral CT and maximum intensity projection. Radiology 185:607–610

Napel S, Rubin GD, Jeffrey RB Jr (1993) STS-MIP: a new reconstruction technique for CT of the chest. J Comput Assist Tomogr 17:832–838

Nienaber CA, Kodolitsch Y, Nicolas V et al. (1993) The diagnosis of thoracic aortic dissection by noninvasive imaging procedures. N Engl J Med 328:1–9

Nienaber CA, Kodolitsch Y von, Petersen B et al. (1995) Intramural hemorrhage of the thoracic aorta: diagnostic and therapeutic implications. Circulation 92:1465–1472

Parker MS, Matheson TL, Rao AV et al. (2001) Making the transition: the role of helical CT in the evaluation of potentially acute thoracic aortic injuries. Am J Roentgenol 176:1267–1272

Posniak HV, Olson MC, Demos TC (1993) Aortic motion artifact simulating dissection on CT scans: elimination with reconstructive segmented images. AJR 161:557–558

Prince MR, Narasimham DL, Jacoby WT et al. (1996) Three-dimensional gadolinium-enhanced MR angiography of the thoracic aorta. AJR 166:1387–1397

Prokop M, Schaefer CM, Leppert AGA, Galanski M (1993) Spiral CT angiography of thoracic aorta: femoral or antecubital injection site for intravenous administration of contrast material? Radiology 189:111

Quint LE, Francis IR, Williams DM et al. (1996) Evaluation of thoracic aortic disease with the use of helical CT and multiplanar reconstructions: comparison with surgical findings. Radiology 201:37–41

Raptopoulos V (1994) Chest CT for aortic injury: maybe not for everyone. AJR 162:1053–1055

Remy-Jardin M, Remy J, Wattinne L, Giraud F (1992) Central pulmonary thromboembolism: diagnosis with spiral volumetric CT with the single-breath-hold technique – comparison with pulmonary angiography. Radiology 185:381–387

Rubin GD, Dake MD, Napel SA, McDonnell CH, Jeffrey RBJ (1993) Abdominal spiral CT angiography: initial clinical experience. Radiology 186:147–152

Rubin GD, Dake MD, Napel S et al. (1994) Spiral CT of renal artery stenosis: comparison of three-dimensional rendering techniques. Radiology 190:181–189

Rubin GD, Dake MD, Semba CB (1995) Current status of three-dimensional spiral CT scanning for imaging the vasculature. Radiol Clin North Am 33:51–70

Rubin GD, Lane MJ, Bloch DA, Leung AN, Stark P (1996a) Optimization of contrast enhanced thoracic spiral CT. Radiology 201:785–791

Rubin GD, Beaulieu CF, Argiro V et al. (1996b) Perspective volume rendering of CT and MR images: applications for endoscopic imaging. Radiology 199:321–330

Rubin GD, Shiau MC, Leung AN, Kee ST, Logan LJ, Sofilos MC (2000) Aorta and iliac arteries: single versus multiple detector-row helical CT angiography. Radiology 215:670–676

Rusinek H, Mourino MR, Firooznia H, Weinreb JC, Chase NE (1989) Volumetric rendering of MR images. Radiology 171: 269–272

MDCT of the Heart

21 Detection and Quantification of Coronary Calcium with MDCT

R. FISCHBACH

CONTENTS

R. FISCHBACH, MD
Department of Clinical Radiology, University of Muenster, Albert-Schweitzer-Strasse 33, 48149 Muenster, Germany

21.1 Introduction

Coronary heart disease (CHD) is the leading cause of death, illness, and disability in populations worldwide. Strategies to reduce the risk of CHD include the early initiation of primary preventive measures including lifestyle changes and/or medical therapy in patients with subclinical disease. The reliable identification of presymptomatic patients, however, it remains problematic by conventional risk assessment based on traditional risk factors. Direct visualization and quantification of the coronary atherosclerotic plaque burden would be desirable to more precisely determine a patient's coronary heart risk. In recent years there has been an important increase of interest in the use of noninvasive measurement of coronary arterial calcification as a screening test for coronary atherosclerosis. Since coronary artery calcification is conceived as a manifestation of atherosclerosis in the arterial wall, the detection of coronary calcifications may serve as a marker for the presence of coronary artery disease. The most frequent application of coronary calcium scoring has thus become the assessment of an individual's future risk for a myocardial event. This indication and the predictive value of coronary artery calcium measurement and its role in the assessment of myocardial event risk has always been a matter of debate.

Until the introduction of subsecond mechanical CT scanners, coronary calcium measurement remained a domain of electron beam computed tomography (EBCT). Due to the limited number of EBCT scanners available in dedicated imaging centers, access to coronary CT scanning has long been restricted. On the other hand, the scan protocol and the quantification method remained quite uniform for a decade. Many of the whole-body multidetector row CT systems installed currently are equipped with the necessary hard- and software to perform examinations of the heart using either prospective triggering of sequential scans or retrospective gating of spiral CT scans. This development opens CT scanning of the heart for a larger patient population. Parallel to the introduction of a growing range of MDCT systems capable of performing ECG-synchronized cardiac scans, different scan protocols have been suggested and new approaches for the quantification of coronary artery calcifications have been introduced. Presently, no accepted standards exist for performing MDCT studies for quantification of coronary artery calcifications.

This chapter gives an overview of the basic concepts of imaging of coronary artery calcification and reviews current techniques and indications for the so-called calcium scoring examination with special regard to MDCT technique.

21.2 Coronary Heart Disease

Cardiovascular disease has been the leading cause of death in the United States ever since 1900, with the exception of the influenza epidemic in 1918. Although remarkable advances have been made in prevention and treatment of CHD, it remains the major cause of mortality and morbidity in the industrialized nations and accounts for 54% of all cardiovascular deaths and 22% of all deaths in the United States (American Heart Association 2002). From 1990 to 2000, the death rate from CHD declined 25%, but the absolute number of deaths decreased only 7.6%. The CHD typically manifests in middle-aged and older, predominantly male, individuals. The average age of a person having a first myocardial infarction is 65 years in men and 70 years in women. In up to 50% of CHD victims, sudden coronary death or nonfatal myocardial infarction is the first manifestation of disease, and approximately 50% of patients with acute myocardial infarction die within the first month of the event (Chambless et al. 1997a; Thaulow et al. 1993). The identification of asymptomatic persons with subclinical disease who are at high risk of developing a future coronary event and who could potentially benefit from preventive efforts thus is of major economical and clinical importance. CHD is the product and manifestation (myocardial infarction, stable and unstable angina, and myocardial dysfunction) of coronary artery disease (CAD) in the form of coronary atherosclerosis.

Traditionally, CHD risk stratification has been based on well-known clinical and biochemical factors. Moderately effective preventive treatment is available: lipid lowering with HMG-CoA reductase inhibitors (statins) or antiplatelet therapy (aspirin) have both resulted in decreased incidence rates of coronary events (Antiplatelet Trialists' Collaboration 1994; Shepherd et al. 1995). The CHD thus seems to be a suitable target for screening efforts. However, many myocardial events are not accounted for by these risk factors alone; therefore, efforts have been made to develop new diagnostic modalities that may provide an improved approach to CHD risk assessment.

21.3 Coronary Artery Calcification

Autopsy studies have shown that coronary artery calcification is an excellent marker of coronary artery disease (McCarthy and Palmer 1974; Rifkin et al. 1979). Histomorphological evaluation of coronary arteries at autopsy has produced good correlation between coronary artery calcification and overall plaque burden (Rumberger et al. 1995; Sangiori et al. 1998; Schmermund et al. 2001), but it is not known whether the amount of calcium reflects the amount of total plaque over time or after therapeutic intervention. Calcification seems to be a better marker for overall coronary plaque burden than individual stenosis based on residual lumen size (Sangiori et al. 1998). Calcifications are frequently present long before clinical manifestation of atherosclerotic disease. Although coronary artery calcification is found more frequently in advanced lesions, it may be histologically identified early in the disease process and has been detected in lesions that are seen as early as the second decade of life. On the other hand, atherosclerotic plaque can be present when coronary calcium is either absent or not detectable by CT, even though histopathological studies confirmed an intimate relation between coronary atherosclerotic plaque area and coronary calcium area.

21.3.1 Pathophysiology of Coronary Artery Calcification

The development of coronary atherosclerosis can be described as a sequence of changes in the arterial wall. An in-depth description of the pathophysiology would be beyond the scope of this chapter and the interested reader is referred to the literature (Stary et al. 1994, 1995; VIRMANI et al. 2000). Initial lesions seem to occur secondary to an injury of the coronary artery endothelium. Circulating histiocytes traverse the injured vascular endothelium and gather in the arterial wall. These histiocytes transform into macrophages and can accumulate lipid. Lipid accumulation can be identified as fatty streaks, the initial and intermediate lesions in atherosclerotic plaque formation. Histologically, different types of atherosclerotic lesions can be distinguished, which has led to a classification system suggested by the American Heart Association. Lesions are designated by Roman numerals I through VI (see Fig. 21.1).

Initial and intermediate lesions are types I–III. The advanced atherosclerotic lesions are subdivided into lesions types IV–VI. The type-IV lesion (atheroma) is characterized by extracellular intimal lipid accumulation, the lipid core. The type-V lesion contains fibrous connective tissue formation. If parts of the lesion are calcified, it becomes a type-Vb lesion. If the lipid core is absent, the type-Va or type-Vb lesion is classified as type Vc. Type-IV and type-V lesions may develop fissures, hematoma, and/or thrombus (type-VI lesion). Although this classification system suggests a linear sequence of events, plaque development seems to be more complex (VIRMANI et al. 2000). This is suggested by angiographic studies, which have shown that rapid progression of minor lesions to high-grade stenosis may occur in only a few months (AMBROSE et al. 1988; MANCINI and PITT 2002).

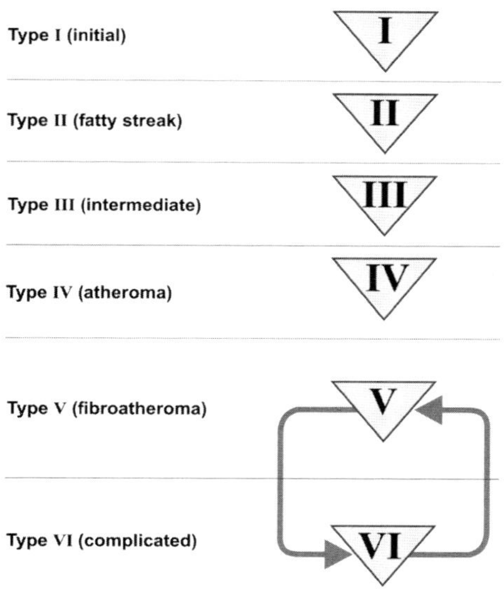

Fig. 21.1. Sequence of atherosclerotic lesions according to the classification system by the American Heart Association and the American College of Cardiology. The early lesion is characterized by isolated macrophage foam cells (type-I lesion) or mainly intracellular lipid accumulation (type II). Type-II changes and early extracellular lipid pools characterize the intermediate lesion. The more advanced lesions contain a core of extracellular lipids (atheroma, type IV), or multiple lipid cores and fibrotic layers or calcifications (type V). A lesion with a surface defect and associated thrombus or hematoma is the "complicated" type-VI lesion. (Modified according to STARY et al. 1995)

21.3.2 Plaque Morphology and Degree of Calcification

Apatite in the form of hydroxyapatite $\{[Ca\ (Ca_3(PO_4)_2)_3]^{2+}\ 2\ OH^-\}$ and carbonate apatite is the predominant mineral form in calcified lesions. Atherosclerotic calcification is an organized, regulated process similar to bone formation that occurs only when other aspects of atherosclerosis are also present. Nonhepatic Gla-containing proteins, such as osteocalcin, which are actively involved in the transport of calcium out of vessel walls, are suspected to have key roles in the pathogenesis of coronary calcification. Osteopontin and its mRNA, known to be involved in bone mineralization, and mRNA for bone morphogenetic protein-2a, a potent factor for osteoblastic differentiation, have been identified in calcified atherosclerotic lesions. Although the process of calcium accumulation in atherosclerotic lesions is not fully understood, it seems to be an active process, which involves mechanisms similar to bone formation and resorption (DOHERTY and DETRANO 1994; JEZIORSKA et al. 1998; WEXLER et al. 1996). Regardless of the mechanisms involved, it is evident that calcium is very common in advanced atherosclerotic lesions.

Histologically, coronary artery plaque can be also classified as plaque rupture, plaque erosion, vulnerable plaque, fibroatheroma, fibrous plaque, plaque hemorrhage, and healed plaque rupture. Rupture is characterized by an acute luminal thrombus with connection to a plaque with a lipid-rich core. Plaque erosion represents a plaque with an intact fibrous cap and acute luminal thrombus. The "vulnerable plaque" or thinned-cap fibroatheroma shows a plaque with a thin fibrous cap and infiltration of macrophages. The pattern of calcification was correlated with the plaque morphology in a histomorphologic study of patients dying suddenly with severe coronary disease (BURKE et al. 2001). The greatest amount of calcium was found in healed ruptures followed by fibroatheroma. Acute plaque ruptures were most frequently seen in segments with speckled or no calcification, but did also occur in areas with diffuse calcifications. From these observations it can be assumed that calcification reflects healing of plaque rupture and intraplaque hemorrhage as well as a response to inflammation in the plaque. Calcification may thus be seen as an attempt of the arterial wall to stabilize itself, since calcified and fibrotic plaques are much stiffer than lipid-rich lesion. The previous concepts suggesting that calcification is associated with plaque instability are not be supported by recent data.

In a study of 40 patients with acute coronary syndromes and no or moderate angiographic coronary disease, 36% of culprit lesions were not calcified (Schmermund et al. 1998). Since most acute ruptures seem to occur in areas with only little calcification, it is questionable whether coronary calcification could be a marker for plaque instability. Furthermore, we will have to accept that calcification pattern is not helpful in localizing potentially vulnerable lesions as it has been shown that unstable plaque can be present in vessels with a wide range of calcification patterns as well as in vascular segments without detectable calcium deposits.

Even if the individual calcification or calcified plaque does not equal a possible future culprit lesion, the presence and extent of coronary artery calcifications reflect the total plaque burden and as such the likelihood of the presence of potentially vulnerable lesions. Using this concept, the demonstration of coronary artery calcium accumulation identifies the patient with coronary artery disease and the degree of calcification can be considered a potential risk factor (Schmermund and Erbel 2001).

21.3.3 Prevalence of Coronary Artery Calcification

The prevalence of coronary artery calcification in asymptomatic as well as symptomatic persons is well studied. Table 21.1 shows data from an early study investigating the prevalence of coronary artery calcification in asymptomatic men and women of various ages (Janowitz et al. 1993). The prevalence in men is evidently higher than the prevalence in women well into the postmenopausal period and it is obvious that the prevalence is age dependent. Several investigators have since reported coronary calcium scores in large asymptomatic populations (see Fig. 21.2). The calcium score distributions published for these asymptomatic mainly white American populations can be used to classify patients compared with the expected norm. All investigators (Hoff et al. 2001; Raggi et al. 2000; Wong et al. 2002) report a steep increase in coronary calcium score with age: the

Table 21.1. Prevalence of coronary artery calcification detected by CT in asymptomatic men and women. Adapted from (Janowitz et al. 1993)

Age (years)	Asymptomatic	
	Men (%)	Women (%)
<29	11	6
30–39	21	11
40–49	44	23
50–59	72	35
60–69	85	67
70–79	94	89
80–89	100	100

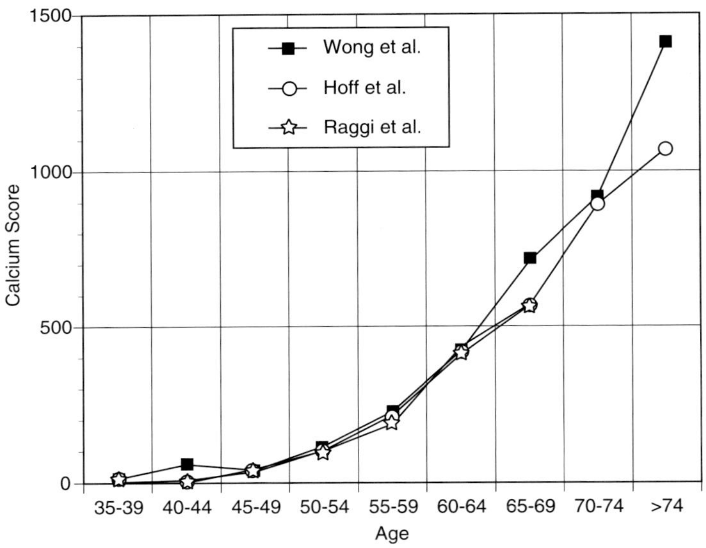

Fig. 21.2. Coronary artery calcium score in asymptomatic populations. Age- and gender-adjusted 75th percentile of coronary artery calcium in asymptomatic male patient populations reported by Raggi et al. (2000), Hoff et al. (2001), and Wong et al. (2002). All investigators found a remarkable increase of calcium scores with age. The reported 75th percentile calcium score is quite similar in the different groups

75th percentile ranges between 36 and 44 for men between 45 and 50 years; between 101 and 116 for men between 50 and 55 years; and 410 and 434 for men between 60 and 65 years. Interestingly, the absolute calcium scores are quite similar in the different North American populations studied.

Even though there is a positive association of the amount of coronary artery calcium and age, coronary artery calcification is not an inevitable aspect of aging. In older adults with minimal clinical cardiovascular disease, 16% of the individuals examined had no detectable coronary artery calcifications (Newman et al. 2000).

21.4 Imaging of Coronary Artery Calcification

Calcium strongly attenuates X-rays due to its relatively high atomic number; therefore, a variety of radiological imaging techniques, including chest X-ray, fluoroscopy, EBCT, as well as conventional, spiral, and MDCT, are suitable methods for detecting coronary calcifications.

21.4.1 Conventional X-ray Techniques

Chest film has the least sensitivity and only extensive calcifications can be identified (Souza et al. 1978). Fluoroscopy has a much higher sensitivity compared with plain chest radiography, but characterization, quantification, and documentation are problematic using a projection technique. Furthermore, fluoroscopy requires a skilled and experienced examiner. Nevertheless, fluoroscopically detected calcifications were shown to carry significant prognostic information. A prospective study using fluoroscopy in high-risk asymptomatic population found that individuals with detectable coronary calcifications were three times as likely to develop angina or to experience myocardial infarction or death than persons without coronary calcifications (Detrano et al. 1994). Margolis et al. (1980) assessed the significance of coronary artery calcification in 800 symptomatic patients who underwent cardiac fluoroscopy. Calcification was shown by fluoroscopy in 250, of whom 236 (94%) had ≥75% stenosis of one or more major coronary arteries at angiography. The 5-year survival for patients with coronary artery calcifications was 58%, compared with 87% in patients without coronary artery calcifications. The prognostic significance of coronary artery calcification was independent of gender, status of the coronary vessels at angiography, left ventricular function, or results of exercise tests.

21.4.2 CT Imaging Techniques

Due to the high attenuation of calcium, CT is extremely sensitive in depicting vascular calcifications (Fig. 21.3). Conventional single-section imaging with acquisition times in the range of 2–5 s allowed identification of coronary artery calcifications, but calcifications are blurred because of cardiac motion and small lesions may not be detected. Despite these drawbacks, conventional CT seems to be more sensitive in detecting calcifications than fluoroscopy (Rienmüller and Lipton 1987). Still, motion artifacts and resulting volume averaging and breathing misregistration due to different inspiration depth precluded exact calcium quantification.

21.4.2.1 Electron Beam CT

The introduction of EBCT in the mid-1980s made quantification of coronary artery calcifications fea-

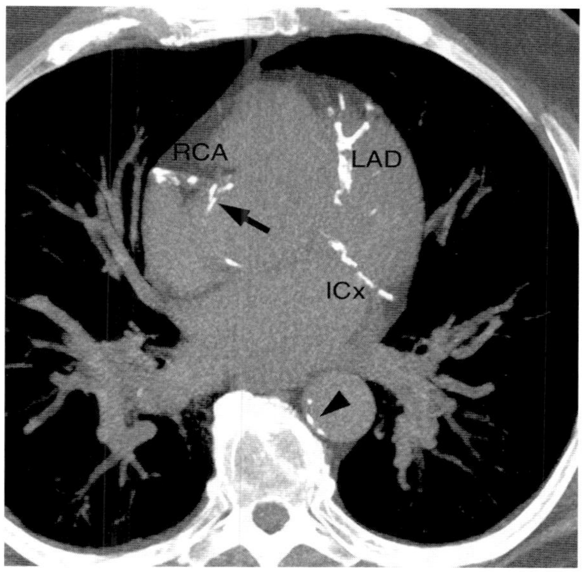

Fig. 21.3. Maximum intensity projection image of an MDCT coronary scan depicting severely calcified coronary arteries. The right coronary artery (*RCA*), the left anterior descending artery (*LAD*), and the left circumflex (*ICx*) show diffuse calcifications. Small calcium accumulations are seen in the wall of the ascending (*arrow*) and descending aorta (*arrowhead*)

sible. The first reports on EBCT to quantify coronary artery calcifications were published in the late 1980s (Agatston et al. 1990; Tannenbaum et al. 1989). The EBCT was shown to be much more sensitive than fluoroscopy in detecting small and less densely calcified plaque. Only 52% of calcifications detected by EBCT had been detected by fluoroscopy in the study by Agatston and coworkers (1990).

The EBCT uses an electron beam to sweep stationary tungsten target rings to generate images. A typical scan protocol for coronary calcium detection consists of contiguous 3-mm sections covering the heart with 100-ms exposure time per slice. The scans are prospectively triggered from the electrocardiogram (ECG) of the patient, usually at 80% of the R–R interval. The examination is performed during one or two breath holds. Using EBCT with ECG triggering allowed for the first time to obtain cross-sectional images of the heart with high spatial and temporal resolution. The current is presently limited to 630 mAs, which results in image noise, especially in obese patients. Signal-to-noise ratio, however, is critical for distinguishing small calcifications from image noise.

The EBCT-based calcium quantification has been criticized for its high variability in measurement results. Interscan variability may hamper accurate serial measurements in follow-up studies. The reported mean percentage variability for the calcium score in repeat examinations ranges between 15 and 49% (see Table 21.2). This variability is well within the reported annual calcium progression rate, rendering interpretation of yearly follow-up examinations difficult.

The major reasons for this variability are artifacts due to either cardiac motion in scan misregistration or patient motion occurring during the long breath-hold times. The most important factor, however, seems to be the quantification method (see below) and the thick section thickness, which renders the measurement susceptible to partial-volume effects.

21.4.2.2 Multidetector CT

The development of subsecond rotation speeds in mechanical scanners in conjunction with the development of partial scan reconstruction algorithms provided a significant improvement in temporal resolution. Limited volume coverage and slow scan speed were major drawbacks of single-section CT. In comparisons of EBCT and ECG controlled sequential CT scanning (Becker et al. 1999; Budoff et al. 2001) the variability between the two modalities was poor (42–84%). In combination with electrocardiogram-based synchronization of image reconstruction from subsecond single-section spiral CT, agreement in the classification of subjects as "healthy" or "diseased" based on calcium score categories was above 90% (Carr et al. 2000).

The now widely available MDCT scanners offer the possibility of cardiac imaging with similar or even better image quality than EBCT. This is due mainly to advantages of acquisition geometry, adjustable tube current, and the possibility of continuous spiral scanning. Four-slice CT systems were introduced in 1998. These systems achieved rotation times as fast as 500 ms, resulting in a temporal resolution of a partial scan of 250 ms for a prospective triggering technique. Latest-generation systems offer rotation times of down to 420 ms and can acquire up to 16 slices with nearly isotropic resolution. Despite the fast technological development in MDCT systems, these systems still have a potential disadvantage of inferior temporal resolution compared with a 100-ms exposure time by EBCT. Motion artifacts, especially in the rapidly moving right coronary artery, become increasingly problematic with higher heart rates or cardiac contractility; however, the tube current can

Table 21.2. Results of reproducibility measurements using electron beam CT

Reference	No. of patients	Calcium score variability (%)	Volume score variability (%)
Kajinami et al. (1993)	25	34	-
Shields et al. (1995)	50	38	-
Wang et al. (1996)	72	29	-
Yoon et al. (1997)	50	37	28.2
Callister et al. (1998)	52	19	18
Devries et al. (1995)	91	49	-
Achenbach et al. (2001)	120	19.9	16.2
Mao et al. (2001)	60	24	-
	57	15[a]	-

[a]Triggering of the scan at 40% R–R interval

be adjusted to improve the signal-to-noise ratio considerably, which helps to distinguish small calcifications from image noise (BIELAK et al. 1994).

Extensive validation studies to determine the equivalence of EBCT and MDCT have not been performed. Initial experiences show good correlation of EBCT measurement and prospectively triggered MDCT. A recent study compared different quantification methods and found volume and mass indexes to be superior to the traditional calcium score for comparing the results of EBCT and MDCT and for determining significant coronary artery disease (BECKER et al. 2001).

21.5 Quantification of Coronary Artery Calcification

Computed tomography allows for reliable measurements of lesion area and lesion attenuation. On the basis of these measurements quantification of coronary artery calcifications can be performed using calcium area, calcium score based on area and plaque density or volume, as well as mass measurement.

21.5.1 Traditional Calcium Score

The initial quantification method introduced by AGATSTON et al. (1990) uses EBCT for the quantification of coronary calcification and introduced a method for coronary artery calcification quantification, which has since been referred to as "Agatston score" or calcium score. The Agatston score in its original form is assessed from 20 contiguous 3-mm sections of the heart. A threshold of 130 Hounsfield units (HU) is empirically set to identify calcifications. This threshold was introduced to exclude noise from the evaluation, since it was more than two standard deviations of the average attenuation of the aorta. In its original form, only plaques related to the coronary arteries with a minimum lesion size of 1 mm^2 or two adjacent pixels are included in the calculation to exclude random image noise. The analysis software highlights any lesion that contains the minimum number of pixels with more than 130 HU. The observer has to identify scoreable coronary artery lesions and assigns each lesion to the left main coronary artery, the left anterior descending artery, the left circumflex artery, or the right coronary artery. A region of interest is placed around each lesion and area and maximum CT number of each lesion is determined. The calcium score is then calculated by multiplying the individual lesion area with a weighting factor. The maximum CT number per lesion determines this weighting factor. The factor is 1 for a peak lesion attenuation of 130–199 HU, 2 for 200–299 HU, 3 for 300–399 HU, and 4 for a lesion with a density ≥400 HU. The sum of all lesion scores is the vessel score and all vessel scores are summed to calculate the total calcium score.

The use of a density-dependent weighting factor makes the area-based Agatston score nonlinear and can mean a dramatic change in the lesion and overall score based on just a single pixel. Only slight changes in the position of a lesion in the measured section, as in repeat examinations, can induce significant changes in the number of registered pixels and the calcium score of a given lesion. Figure 21.4 uses an example to illustrate how differences in pixel attenuation of the same lesion from partial-volume effect can influence score results.

21.5.1.1 Problems Using the Calcium Score in MDCT

When applying the Agatston method to coronary calcium scanning based on MDCT technology, it has to be kept in mind that the Agatston score was initially designed for a special protocol and modality (EBCT). Any changes in image acquisition parameters such as scan volume, section thickness, image increment, image reconstruction kernels, and X-ray spectrum will influence the quantification result.

For example, calcium scans with a four-channel MDCT using a 4 2.5-mm detector configuration and prospective triggering will produce 2.5-mm sections instead of 3-mm sections, thus giving more images per volume. Consequently, the resulting score would be falsely high and mathematical operations need to be introduced to correct for this. If MDCT calcium scanning is performed using spiral data acquisition with overlapping image reconstruction, as suggested by some groups, the number of sections per volume will further increase. Since the absolute CT number of a calcium deposit will differ with different CT systems and image protocols, not only the measured area but also the maximum CT number and thus the weighting function for the Agatston score will be affected.

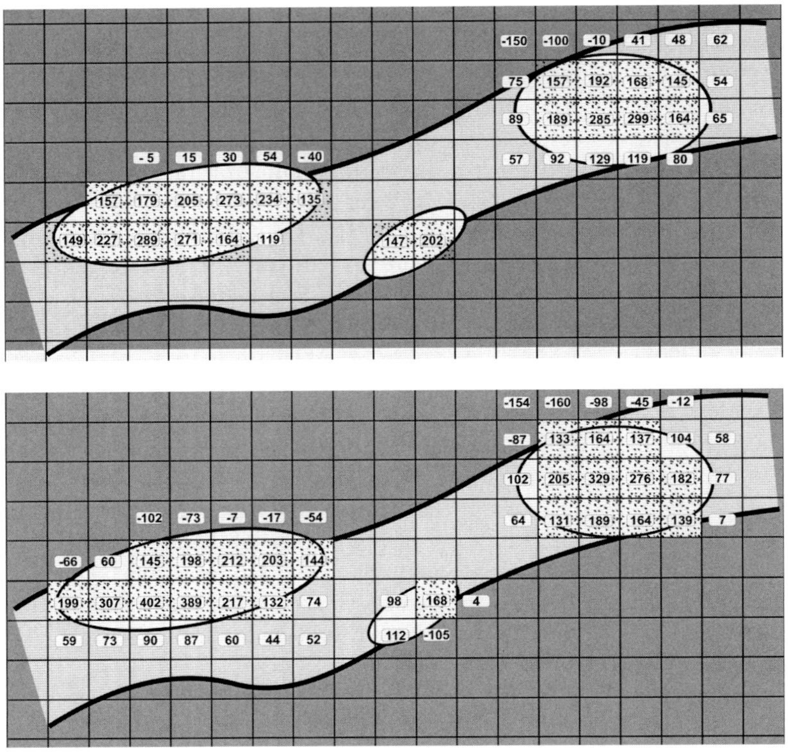

a, b

Fig. 21.4a, b. Calculation of the calcium score and effect of partial volumes. This figure illustrates the calcium quantification using the calcium score. The *grid* represents the pixel matrix. A vessel is depicted containing three oval calcified lesions (*white*). The perivascular fat (*dark gray*) has negative CT numbers. The CT number for pixels representing the calcified lesions is given. Every pixel with a CT number above 130 is registered as calcified. The measured CT number in pixels that contain calcified plaque and perivascular fat or vascular structures are an average of the underlying tissues and are only scored as calcium-containing plaque (*speckled pattern*) if the CT number exceeds the threshold of 130 HU. In **a** the left lesion contains 11 pixels with CT numbers greater 130. The greatest CT number is 289, the lesion score is 2 11. The small lesion is scored as 2 2, and the plaque on the right contains eight registered pixels with a peak density of 299 HU, resulting in a lesion score of 2 8. The vessel score in this case would be 22+4+16=42. In **b** the same vessel is depicted with a slight change in the position of vessel regarding to the pixel matrix. This change in position results in important changes in registered CT numbers. The first lesion now scores as 4 11, the small lesion has only one registered pixel, and the right lesion is counted as 3 11. The vessel score in this case would be 44+1+33=78

21.5.2 Calcium Volume Score

The poor reproducibility of calcium quantification results with the use of the Agatston score has been realized when calcium scoring was employed to follow the progression or possible regression of coronary atherosclerotic plaque. The Calcium Volume Score (CVS) has been introduced to improve the reproducibility of calcium measurements (Callister et al. 1998a, 1998b). The CVS for each lesion are calculated as the number of voxels in the volume data set that belong to the calcification multiplied by the volume of one voxel. The determination of calcified plaque volume is independent from the section thickness or image overlap used. An increase in the number of sections scored when overlapping image reconstruction is chosen or when smaller slice thickness is generated is automatically accounted for; therefore, the comparability between different modalities is improved over the traditional calcium score. The lack of a density-dependent weighting factor further reduces the influence of partial-volume effects.

Since the measured volume of a calcification depends on the attenuation of the lesion as well as the threshold used, the CVS does not represent the true volume of the calcification (Ulzheimer and Kalender 2003). If the traditional threshold 130 HU is employed, the CVS overestimates the volume of very dense calcifications and underestimates the volume of less dense calcifications. Since the tube current used also affects the attenuation of a calcified lesion, and attenuation influences the lesion volume, a measurement which is standardized, reproducible, and independent of scanner hardware as well as image acquisition parameters is desirable, especially in view of the rapidly increasing diversity of the MDCT systems available.

21.5.3 Calcium Mass

It has been suggested that the most reliable calcium quantification method would be an absolute hydroxyapatite (Ca–HA) mass measurement, which can be performed similar to bone mineral density assessment (Ulzheimer and Kalender 2003). The Ca–HA mass is proportional to the mean CT number of a calcification multiplied with the lesion volume. Since objects that are smaller than the section thickness are displayed with decreased mean CT numbers, Ca–HA mass automatically corrects for linear partial-volume effects. Furthermore, Ca–HA mass has the advantage to represent a real physical measure, which can be reliably obtained regardless of differences in CT systems and scanning protocols when using appropriate calibration. To obtain absolute values for the calcium mass, a calibration measurement of a sufficiently large calcification with known Ca–HA density has to be performed (Hong et al. 2002; Ulzheimer and Kalender 2003). The specific calibration factor needs to be determined for all scanners and protocols. Several commercial analysis software packages allow for mass quantification. It can be expected that the need for reproducible quantification results will result in the replacement of the Agatston score with mass measurements. Large-size studies supporting this assumption are still lacking.

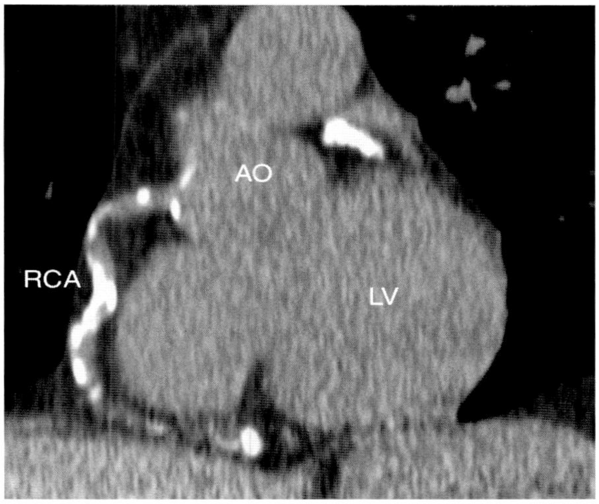

Fig. 21.5. Retrospective ECG gating and overlapping image reconstruction yields motion-free high-resolution images, which allow multiplanar reformation showing the heavily calcified right coronary artery (*RCA*). High-attenuation calcification, intermediate attenuation vascular and cardiac structures, and the dark perivascular fat are well differentiated

21.6 MDCT Examination Technique

Imaging of coronary calcifications is typically performed using a low-dose technique without contrast enhancement. The scan time should be as short as possible to avoid patient motion and breathing artifacts. Synchronization of the image acquisition or image calculation with the cardiac motion is mandatory to scan the heart at reproducible positions to avoid gaps or overlaps, which would result in image misregistration; therefore, continuous ECG recording is necessary to either trigger image acquisition in sequential scanning or to synchronize the image generation in spiral scans. The best possible temporal resolution is required for motion-free image acquisition.

The coronary arteries are easily recognized in their epimyocardial course surrounded by the low-attenuation periarterial fat. Due to the high density of vascular calcifications, even small calcium deposits are detected with high sensitivity (Fig. 21.5).

The patient is positioned like in any other examination of the thorax. The scan extends form the midlevel of the left pulmonary artery down to the diaphragm and is planned on a scout image. All MDCT scanners are able to cover this 10- to 15-cm range in one breath hold. Continuous table feed as in spiral technique allows for somewhat faster volume coverage than sequential, stepwise scanning. In order to keep the scan protocols comparable with the increasing number of scanners and possible image acquisition parameters, standard parameters for MDCT scanning should be developed. So far, no official recommendations exist. A recommendation of image and acquisition and evaluation parameters is given in Table 21.3.

21.6.1 Sequential Scanning

In prospectively triggered sequential scanning, each scan is started at a predefined position in the cardiac cycle. In this approach the next R–R interval is estimated from the previous R–R intervals. As long as the heart rate and rhythm remain constant, a prospective estimation of the duration of the next R–R interval can be used to reliably position the scan in the mid- to late diastole. In patients with change in heart rate during the necessary breath hold or with arrhythmia motion artifacts can impose a major problem for reliable calcium quantification (Mao et al. 1996). In EBCT scanning most groups use a 80% delay of the R–R interval for the scan. Recently, a 40% delay has been recommended to increase the scan reproducibility (Mao et al. 2001). For sequential MDCT scan-

Table 21.3. Recommendations for image acquisition and evaluation parameters for coronary calcium quantification with MDCT scanners

Data acquisition	
Scan mode	Spiral
Tube voltage (kV)	120
Tube current (mA)	100
ECG gating	Retrospective gating in mid- to late diastole, usually 50–60% R–R interval; individual selection of reconstruction window with least motion artifacts is suggested
Breath hold	Inspiration
Field of view (cm)	22
Matrix	512
Scan range	Entire heart from 1 cm below tracheal bifurcation to diaphragm
Image reconstruction	
Section thickness (mm)	3
Reconstruction increment	1.5
Filter kernel	Medium smooth
Data evaluation	
Threshold (HU)	130
Minimal lesion size	1 pixel
Motion artifacts	Include in region of interest
Reporting	No. of calcified vessels, calcium mass, and calcium volume score. The Agatston score cannot be recommended

ning, no systematic evaluations have been performed to determine the optimal timing of scan triggering. Due to the longer image exposure in MDCT an earlier trigger time in the R–R interval than the commonly used 80% as in EBCT seems to be preferential. In coronary MDCT angiography initial investigations based on spiral scanning and retrospectively gated image reconstruction have shown a wide variation of optimal reconstruction windows. A reconstruction window of 50–60% yielded best results in terms of motion-free images (Hong et al. 2001; Kopp et al. 2001). Since motion-free images are crucial for reliable calcium quantification a similar timing can be expected to yield favorable results in prospectively triggered MDCT scanning. In our experience individual test scans at the mid-cardiac level with 50, 60, or 70% R–R interval can be used to check for the optimal timing (Fig. 21.6). The best result can then be used for the entire cardiac scan.

21.6.2 Spiral Scanning

Spiral image acquisition has several advantages over sequential scanning. The continuous data acquisition speeds up the scanning process and images can be reconstructed at any position in the scanned volume. A slow table motion during the spiral data acquisition is necessary to allow for oversampling of spiral scan projections (Ohnesorge et al. 2000). This is necessary to allow consistent retrospective ECG-synchronized selection of data for image reconstruction

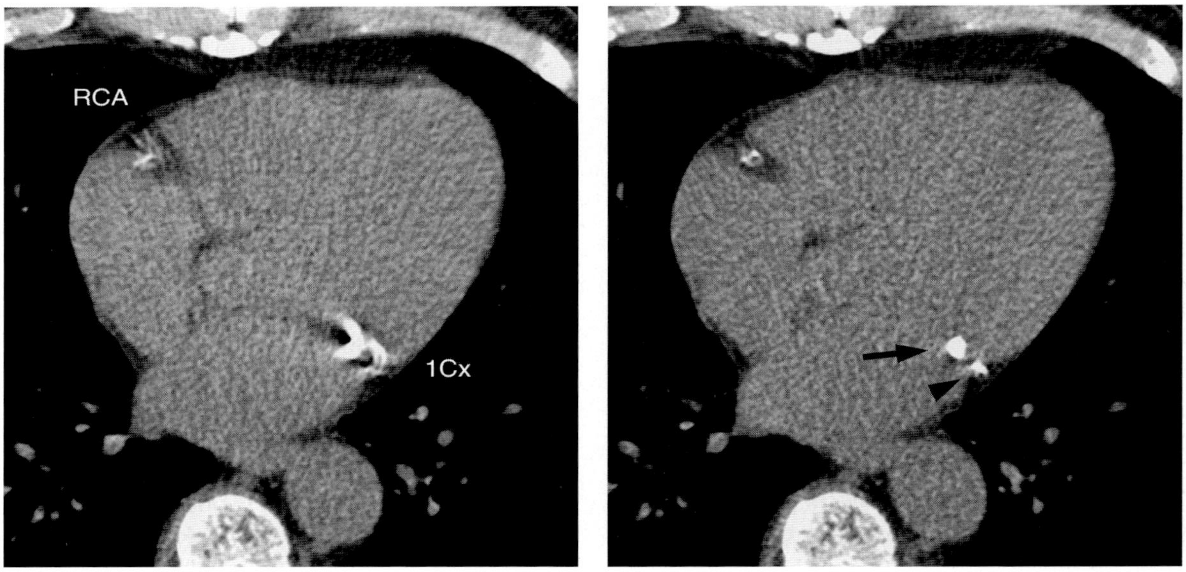

Fig. 21.6a, b. Scan in the mid-cardiac level at **a** 50% R–R interval and **b** 60% R–R interval. Motion artifacts affect the depiction of the right coronary artery (*RCA*) and the left circumflex (*lCx*). The lCx is not well delineated from calcifications of the mitral valve, which is better appreciated on the motion-free image obtained at 60% R–R interval

in a predefined phase of the cardiac cycle. As with prospectively ECG-triggered scan a specific position of the reconstruction window in relation to the R-peaks of the recorded ECG trace is chosen. Since image reconstruction is performed retrospectively after the data acquisition, an optimal agreement with the desired phase of cardiac cycle is assured. The user can perform additional reconstructions, if motion artifacts should occur; thus, misregistration due to changes in heart rate is kept minimal and spiral scanning can improve the robustness of image reconstruction in arrhythmia assuring a direct relation of the positions of the reconstructed images and heart rate. This renders spiral MDCT more stable in terms of image quality and probably measurement reproducibility than competing sequential scanning techniques.

Another important factor is overlapping image reconstruction, which is possible with any desired image increment. The use of overlapping image acquisition had already resulted in improved reproducibility of sequential coronary scans (Achenbach et al. 2001). The same effect was shown in an initial study using spiral MDCT and overlapping image increment (Ohnesorge et al. 2002). Overlapping image generation decreases the influence of partial-volume effects and increases the sensitivity for small lesions.

The obvious disadvantage of spiral scan technique with highly overlapping pitch is the continuous irradiation of the patient even in cardiac phases that are not used for image reconstruction; thus, the radiation exposure is higher than in sequential scanning. The use of a prospective tube current modulation can compensate for this disadvantage. In phases of the cardiac cycle that are not important for image reconstruction the tube current can be drastically reduced, and the nominal tube current is only used during the desired mid-diastolic phase (Fig. 21.7).

21.6.3 Radiation Exposure

Calcium measurement is applied mainly to apparently healthy individuals; therefore, radiation exposure has been a concern all along. The radiation exposure should be kept as low as reasonably achievable. Since image noise is a major concern in differentiating small calcifications from noise, a lower level is defined. If prospective triggering is used for MDCT scanning, the effective dose is approximately 1 mSv, which is similar to EBCT (McCollough 2003). The MDCT with constant tube output during spiral

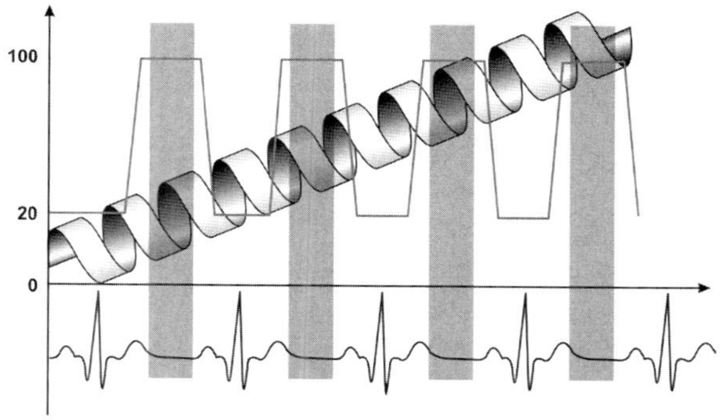

Fig. 21.7. Spiral scanning with tube-output modulation. The tube current is reduced to 20% of the nominal value during the systole and is increased to 100% during mid-diastole. The image reconstruction window is placed within the normal tube output

scanning will almost double the radiation exposure. The ECG-controlled tube output modulation can achieve a mean dose reduction of 48% for men and 45% for women (Jakobs et al. 2002). Considering the advantages of MDCT spiral scanning regarding reproducibility of calcium measurements, this slightly higher effective dose for spiral data acquisition should be acceptable.

21.7 Clinical Applications of Coronary Calcium Measurement

Reports on the potential for CT imaging of coronary calcifications to identify patients with CHD began early with the papers of Tannenbaum et al. (1989) and Agatston et al. (1990). In their study, Agatston et al. (1990) demonstrated that EBCT was much more sensitive than fluoroscopy in detecting coronary calcifications and that patients with symptomatic CHD displayed higher mean calcium scores than asymptomatic subjects (Fig. 21.8).

21.7.1 Coronary Artery Calcification and Angiographic Stenosis

In subsequent years studies have been conducted to confirm these initial results and to assess the ability of CT to identify patients with significant coronary artery obstruction. Accuracies for predicting angiographic stenoses were reported by several investigators. Table 21.4 lists the reported sensitivities and

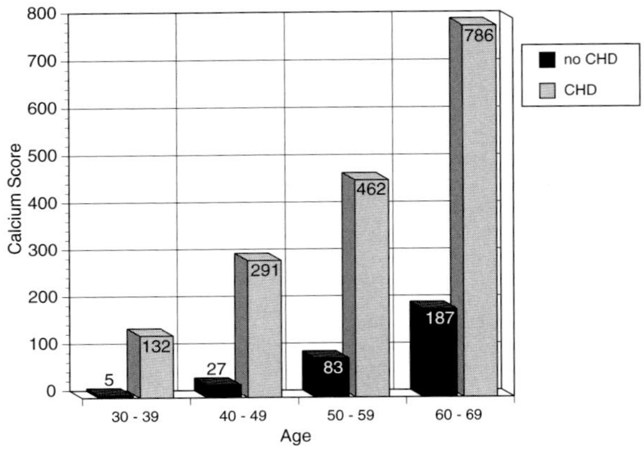

Fig. 21.8. Comparison of mean absolute calcium scores in 475 symptomatic patients without and 109 patients with a diagnosis of coronary heart disease. The calcium score increases with patient age and there is a significant difference between patients with and without coronary heart disease (AGATSTON et al. 1990)

specificities of CT coronary calcium scanning for predicting angiographic stenoses. There is only a moderate correlation between calcification score, as demonstrated by CT, and coronary narrowing, as shown by catheter angiography (DETRANO et al. 1996). Positive arterial remodeling may be an explanation for the relative lack of correlation between the degree of calcification and luminal narrowing (GLAGOV et al. 1987; SANGIORI et al. 1998). In patients under 50 years, the sensitivity of calcification detected by CT is approximately 85%, with a specificity of approximately 45% as compared with coronary angiography for the detection of significant coronary artery stenosis. In older individuals, the sensitivity of coronary calcification in predicting obstructive CAD is close to 100%, whereas the specificity remains low due to the high prevalence of coronary calcium deposits in elderly individuals.

The pattern of calcification may be useful in predicting luminal narrowing. The pattern of calcification can be classified as absent, speckled, fragmented, or diffuse (FRIEDRICH et al. 1994). Fragmented calcifications represent single linear or wide calcification >2 mm, whereas diffuse calcifications represent segments of continuous calcification >5 mm. Diffuse calcification is more strongly associated with luminal narrowing than speckled calcification (KAJINAMI et al. 1995; TUZCU et al. 1996).

21.7.2 Coronary Artery Calcification and Differential Diagnosis of Chest Pain

A positive coronary calcium scan has only a low predictive value for identifying stenoses but a concomitant high negative predictive value for ruling out obstructive CAD in the absence of detectable calcifications. It has therefore been suggested to apply calcium scanning to patients with a low to intermediate likelihood of coronary heart disease presenting with chest pain. Even though CT scanning does not allow for assessment of presence and severity of coronary stenoses, the knowledge of the presence or absence of coronary artery calcification can be helpful in making further decisions regarding diagnostic or therapeutic measures.

A negative predictive value of 98% has been reported for coronary chest pain or myocardial infarction in subjects with acute symptoms and nonspecific ECG (MCLAUGHLIN et al. 1999). A negative CT Calcium scan was furthermore shown to carry prognostic information. In 192 patients observed for a mean of 50 months, after undergoing an EBCT when presenting to the emergency room because of chest pain, subjects without coronary calcium accumulations had a significantly lower coronary event rate than subjects with a positive CT scan (GEORGIOU et al. 2001).

It has to be kept in mind, however, that even though a negative CT scan result for calcium does imply a low likelihood of significant luminal obstruction, the presence of atherosclerotic plaque cannot

Table 21.4. Relationship of coronary calcium and obstructive coronary artery disease in coronary angiography

Reference	No. of patients	Age (years)	Sensitivity (%)	Specificity (%)	Positive predictive value (%)	Negative predictive value (%)
BREEN et al. (1992)	100	47	100	47	62	100
FALLAVOLLITA et al. (1994)	106	44	85	45	66	70
DEVRIES et al. (1995)	140	58	97	41	55	94
RUMBERGER et al. (1995)	139	51	99	62	57	97
BUDOFF et al. (1996)	710	56	95	44	72	84
HABERL et al. (2001)	1764	56	99	39	57	97

be excluded. In this context, it has to be stressed that culprit plaque in sudden coronary death may contain only little calcium and consequently is not reliably identified by CT.

21.7.3 Coronary Artery Calcification and Disease Progression

Coronary artery calcification constitutes a surrogate of total plaque burden and plaque burden is closely related to the risk of future myocardial events. The possibility to observe changes in coronary atherosclerotic involvement non-invasively is an appealing concept for assessment of disease progression and efficacy of primary or secondary preventive measures in CAD.

Several studies have tracked changes of coronary calcium by EBCT. Score progression seems to be accelerated in patients with obstructive CAD compared with patients who have no clinically manifest disease (27 vs 18%; Janowitz et al. 1991). A mean annual rate of calcium score increase for untreated patients between 24 and 36% has been found. Recent studies have shown the ability of calcium quantification to monitor the progression of coronary calcification and to document the effect of risk factor modification and medical treatment (Achenbach et al. 2002; Budoff et al. 2000; Callister et al. 1998a; Maher et al. 1999). In 66 patients with coronary calcifications the observed increase in coronary calcium volume score was 25% without treatment and decreased to 8.8% under treatment with statins (Achenbach et al. 2002). It has not been shown whether a decrease in calcium progression also represents a decrease in future event risks. Since multiple trials on lowering cholesterol levels have shown a decrease in mortality, it is plausible that decrease in calcium score progression may be a valuable tool in monitoring and comparing such therapies.

If progression is to be assessed in an individual person, a high reliability of the calcium quantification is mandatory. Reported variability from many EBCT studies, however, precludes a meaningful interpretation of calcium measurements in the individual patient. The MDCT with spiral scanning, overlapping image reconstruction, and use of calcium mass measurement has resulted in a variability of 5% in a first study (Ohnesorge et al. 2002). This study will need confirmation, but a significant improvement for follow-up or therapy control studies may be expected.

21.7.4 Coronary Artery Calcification and Screening for CAD

21.7.4.1 Conventional Identification of Subjects at Risk of CAD

According to the Air Force/Texas Coronary Atherosclerosis Prevention Study (AFCAPS/TexCAPS), only 37% of acute events can potentially be prevented using lipid-lowering therapy as primary prevention in individuals with average cholesterol levels (Downs et al. 1998); therefore, risk assessment tools or screening tests are required that will reliably identify asymptomatic individuals at high risk of hard coronary events to efficiently target therapy.

The risk of developing CAD depends on a wide range of environmental and biochemical factors, many of which have been identified in prospective epidemiological studies. Among these well-recognized risk factors are tobacco smoking, high LDL cholesterol levels, low HDL cholesterol, diabetes mellitus, arterial hypertension, and family history of premature myocardial infarction (Table 21.5). These and other risk factors interact in a complex way, making a simple risk assessment in the individual patient complicated; however, algorithms derived from large prospective epidemiological studies, such as the Framingham Study (Anderson et al. 1991; Wilson et al. 1998) in the United States and the Prospective Cardiovascular Münster (PROCAM) Study (Assmann et al. 2002) in Germany, can be used to calculate a person's risk of CAD. A person is said to be at increased risk if his or her absolute risk of suffering a future myocardial event within the next ten years exceeds 20%. Calculation of an individual's CAD risk is possible either by using scoring systems and risk charts or computer assisted algorithms. (The Framingham

Table 21.5. Risk factors for developing coronary heart disease. *BMI* body mass index

Causal risk factors	Predisposing risk factors	Conditional risk factors
Hypercholesterolemia	BMI >30 kg/m^2	Triglycerides
Arterial hypertension	Sedentary lifestyle	Lipoprotein (a)
Cigarette smoking	Family history of premature myocardial infarction	Homocystein
Diabetes mellitus	Male gender	Fibrinogen
	Metabolic syndrome	Plasminogen activator inhibitor
	Social factors	C-reactive protein

risk score is available at http://www.nhlbi.nih.gov/guidelines/cholesterol/atglance.pdf. The PROCAM risk algorithm can be accessed interactively on the Internet at: http://www.chd-taskforce.com)

Subpopulations at a significantly increased global risk of CAD can be identified with a high level of exactness using scores or algorithms for risk assessment. Epidemiological studies have shown that in many individuals without clinically apparent symptoms the risk of developing a future myocardial infarction may equal or even exceed that of persons with a history of coronary heart disease (Assmann et al. 2002); however, it remains questionable whether the presence of subclinical manifestations of atherosclerosis in these presymptomatic patients can be diagnosed with sufficient certainty based on traditional risk factors alone.

Even if standard or traditional risk factor analysis is quite accurate in identifying populations at risk, exercise stress testing, which is also commonly used to screen for CAD, is characterized by a low accuracy in predicting events. The sensitivity of stress testing for identification of asymptomatic middle-aged men at risk for a future myocardial event is less than 40% (Detrano and Froelicher 1988). This is not surprising, since more than two-thirds of acute coronary events in previously asymptomatic individuals are due to rupture or erosion of non-obstructive coronary plaque (Petursson et al. 1995; Virmani et al. 2000). Non-obstructive CAD seldom causes stress-induced myocardial ischemia and thus perfusion imaging does not improve the detection rate of subclinical CAD.

21.7.4.2 Coronary Artery Calcification and Predicting Events

The use of noninvasive measurement of coronary artery calcification as a screening test for coronary atherosclerosis has received remarkable interest in recent years and has generated much controversy. Coronary calcium detection by CT makes the assumption that direct demonstration of atherosclerotic vessel wall involvement in asymptomatic populations with increased CHD risk is helpful to identify as well as to stratify individuals at risk.

To evaluate a possible benefit from CT calcium screening, we first should realize that the main purpose of CAD screening is classification of asymptomatic persons as likely or not likely to have CAD. Early diagnosis of cases with subclinical CAD should reduce morbidity and mortality from the specific disease among the population screened, because screening leads to a course of action proven to save lives. If coronary CT screening cannot achieve a significant reduction of morbidity and mortality, it cannot be deemed effective; therefore, we need to prove that calcium screening of the entire adult population, or even a subpopulation, leads to effective preventive therapy with a substantial benefit, before we can recommend this diagnostic test to healthy individuals and accept the involved expenditure of health care resources. Furthermore, calcium screening should identify high-risk individuals better than traditional risk factor analysis.

In a comparison of persons dying of CHD and age- and gender-matched individuals dying of other causes, three times as much calcium was found in the CHD group (Eggen et al. 1965). Coronary calcium was even nine times as abundant in persons under 50 years of age dying suddenly, when compared with matched controls dying from accidents (Schmermund et al. 2001).

Four prospective studies have addressed the prognostic information of coronary calcium scanning in asymptomatic individuals for predicting coronary events (Arad et al. 2000; Detrano et al. 1999; Raggi et al. 2000; Wong et al. 2000). Results of these studies are not conclusive, since most of the studies report on a limited number of hard coronary events, the majority of end points being revascularizations (possibly triggered by the scan results). Furthermore, some of the studies enrolled self-referred subjects or subjects referred for scanning because of cardiovascular risk factors.

Arad et al. (2000) reported an odds ratio of 22 for the prediction of myocardial infarction or death in 1173 self-referred men and women, when comparing event rates in the group with calcium scores greater than 160 vs event rates among subjects with calcium scores less than 160 (see Table 21.6). The subjects were followed for 3.6 years and 18 myocardial infarctions and coronary deaths were registered. The positive predictive value increased as a function of the calcium score, indicating that calcium quantification may be a valid test for vulnerable atherosclerotic plaque.

Raggi et al. (2000) gave a relative risk of 21 for myocardial infarction or cardiovascular death in subjects with a calcium score greater than the 75th percentile when compared with individuals with a calcium score lower than the 25th percentile. While the absolute calcium score had a wide variation in the asymptomatic individuals studied, a calcium score in the upper age and gender-adjusted quartile seemed to identify subjects at risk better (see Table 21.7) than an increased absolute calcium score. Twenty-seven

Table 21.6. Coronary calcium thresholds and test performance for identifying subjects with future myocardial infarction or coronary death. (Adapted from GUERCI and ARAD 2001)

Score	Sensitivity	Specificity	Positive predictive value	Negative predictive value	Overall accuracy	Odds ratio (95% CI)
>80	0.89	0.74	0.05	0.99	0.74	22.3 (5.1–97.4)
>160	0.83	0.82	0.07	0.99	0.82	22.2 6.4–77.4)
>600	0.55	0.94	0.13	0.98	0.94	20.3 (7.8–53.1)

events were registered in the 632 subjects during a mean observation of 32 months. Approximately two-thirds of the observed events occurred in patients with mild to moderate amounts of coronary artery calcium (calcium scores <400). Subjects with massive calcifications (calcium scores >400) represented only 7% of the population scanned and accounted for 22% of all events. On the other hand, 70% of the events observed (19 of 27) occurred in 181 subjects with a calcium score above the 75th percentile adjusted for gender and age.

In a study of 926 subjects, who were either referred because of risk factors or self-referred, the highest calcium score quartile was associated with a relative risk of cardiovascular events of 9 compared with subjects without coronary calcification (WONG et al. 2000). A limitation of this investigation is the high number of revascularizations (23 of 28 reported events) during a mean follow-up of 3.3 years after scanning.

In the South Bay Heart Watch Study, 29 myocardial infarctions and 17 coronary deaths were reported during 44 months of follow-up in 1196 asymptomatic high-risk subjects (DETRANO et al. 1999). Calcium detection by CT failed to improve the identification of patients at risk compared with traditional risk factor assessment in this study, which was carried out in a population originally screened by fluoroscopy.

O'MALLEY et al. (2000) performed a meta-analysis regarding the literature on using CT calcium to predict future events in asymptomatic adults. Their results show that the relative risk of calcification for a myocardial infarct or CAD-related death varies from 1 to 22 with a weighted mean of 4.2; thus, there is a strong indication that coronary calcium scanning may predict myocardial infarction in asymptomatic populations. The question remains as to whether calcium scanning performs better than conventional risk factor analysis.

On the basis of the investigations in asymptomatic persons, some authors would argue that the demonstration of coronary artery calcium, which means the presence of subclinical CAD, should shift an asymptomatic patient from a primary to a secondary prevention category (HECHT 2001). Even though this seems logical, it has not been proven that a positive or increased calcium score is equivalent to a prior myocardial infarction. Even if an increased calcium score puts a person at increased risk, as several investigations imply, one cannot be sure that any benefit would be reached by therapeutic intervention. It has been suggested that the coronary plaque burden should provide a better indicator of the probability of developing an acute coronary syndrome than a person's age and could replace age as a risk factor in the Framingham risk scores to improve risk assessment (GRUNDY 2001).

Table 21.7. Coronary calcium scores and risk of myocardial events according to RAGGI et al. (2000). In 632 asymptomatic persons 8 fatal and 19 nonfatal myocardial infarcts were observed. Use of adjusted calcium quartiles discriminates better between risk statuses than use of an absolute calcium score

	Absolute calcium scores			
	0	1–99	100–400	>400
No. of patients	292	219	74	47
Annual event rate	0.11	2.1	4.1	4.8
	Age- and gender-adjusted calcium score quartile			
	First	Second	Third	Fourth
No. of patients		351	100	181
Annual event rate	0.2	0.2	1.4	4.5

21.7.4.3 Ongoing Trials

Three prospective epidemiological trials under way will examine this issue. One part of the Prospective Army Coronary Calcium (PACC) study (O'MALLEY et al. 1999) is a prospective cohort study of 2000 participants followed for at least 5 years to establish the relation between coronary calcification and cardiovascular events in an unselected, "low-risk" army population. The Multi-Ethnic Study of Atherosclerosis (MESA) will use a cohort of 6500 American adults who will undergo CT scanning and will be followed for coronary events for 7 years.

Another population-based, prospective cohort study was begun in Germany in 2000. The RECALL (Risk Factors, Evaluation of Coronary Calcium and Lifestyle) study is designed to define the relative risk associated with EBCT-derived coronary calcium score for myocardial infarction and cardiac death in 4200 men and women aged 45–75 years in an unselected urban population from the large, heavily industrialized Ruhr area (Schmermund et al. 2002).

21.7.5 Conclusion

Risk factor assessment and non-invasive imaging of atherosclerosis by CT calcium scanning aim at selecting subjects at a high risk for a future coronary event. While cardiovascular risk factors have been shown to increase CAD risk 1.5 to 5 times (Chambless et al. 1997b; Wilson et al. 1998), odds ratios for increased coronary calcium detected by CT of 22 are reported. This indicates a strong association between coronary calcification and CAD risk, even though formal proof in prospective population-based studies is still lacking.

Since atherogenesis is a dynamic process, which represents the result of a life-long exposure of an individual to a variety of predisposing factors, manifestations of subclinical CAD, as indicated by a positive CT calcium scan, may point to individuals with an increased future cardiac risk. In this respect, coronary calcium may outperform clinical risk factor analysis in asymptomatic subjects, since the simple presence of even a combination of risk factors does not mean presence of subclinical CAD. Coronary plaque burden has been shown to be a good predictor for future coronary events in angiographic follow-up studies. Since coronary calcium is a reliable marker for CAD and since the amount of coronary calcium reflects total coronary plaque burden, demonstration of coronary artery calcification may thus be of value in improving risk stratification of asymptomatic populations with moderate to increased global coronary heart risk or in assessing disease progression.

There is no formal proof that CHD risk can be reduced in patients with elevated coronary calcium scores. Neither is there a consensus in the professional societies on how to use the results of calcium scoring for risk factor management or therapeutic decisions and who should undergo CT scanning at all. In groups with intermediate or increased risk, calcium scanning may be of value, but long-term prospective studies will have to decide this issue.

The MDCT scanning, especially using spiral technique with overlapping slice reconstruction and calcium quantification based on calibrated system and calcium mass measurement, holds promise to be developed as the reference technique in the future.

References

Achenbach S, Meissner F, Ropers D et al. (2001) Overlapping cross-sections significantly improve the reproducibility of coronary calcium measurements by electron beam tomography: a phantom study. J Comput Assist Tomogr 25:569–573

Achenbach S, Ropers D, Pohle K et al. (2002) Influence of lipid-lowering therapy on the progression of coronary artery calcification: a prospective evaluation. Circulation 106:1077–1082

Agatston A, Janowitz W, Hildner F et al. (1990) Quantification of coronary artery calcium using ultrafast computed tomography. J Am Coll Cardiol 15:827–832

Ambrose JA, Tannenbaum MA, Alexopoulos D et al. (1988) Angiographic progression of coronary artery disease and the development of myocardial infarction. J Am Coll Cardiol 12:56–62

American Heart Association (2002) Heart disease and stroke statistics: 2003 update. American Heart Association, Dallas, Texas

Anderson K, Wilson P, Odell P et al. (1991) An updated coronary risk profile: a statement for health professionals. Circulation 83:356–362

Antiplatelet Trialists' Collaboration (1994) Collaborative overview of randomized trials of antiplatelet therapy. I: Prevention of death, myocardial infarction, and stroke by prolonged antiplatelet therapy in various categories of patients. Br Med J 308:81–106

Arad Y, Spadaro LA, Goodman K et al. (2000) Prediction of coronary events with electron beam computed tomography. J Am Coll Cardiol 36:1253–1260

Assmann G, Cullen P, Schulte H (2002) Simple scoring scheme for calculating the risk of acute coronary events based on the 10-year follow-up of the prospective cardiovascular Munster (PROCAM) study. Circulation 105:310–315

Becker CR, Knez A, Jakobs TF et al. (1999) Detection and quantification of coronary artery calcification with electron-beam and conventional CT. Eur Radiol 9:620–624

Becker CR, Kleffel T, Crispin A et al. (2001) Coronary artery calcium measurement: agreement of multirow detector and electron beam CT. Am J Roentgenol 176:1295–1298

Bielak LF, Kaufmann RB, Moll PP et al. (1994) Small lesions in the heart identified at electron beam CT: calcification or noise? Radiology 192:631–636

Budoff M, Lane K, Bakhsheshi H et al. (2000) Rates of progression of coronary calcium by electron beam tomography. Am J Cardiol 86:8–11

Budoff MJ, Mao S, Zalace CP et al. (2001) Comparison of spiral and electron beam tomography in the evaluation of coronary calcification in asymptomatic persons. Int J Cardiol 77:181–188

Burke AP, Weber D, Kolodgie F et al. (2001) Pathophysiology of calcium deposition in coronary arteries. Herz 26:239–244

Callister T, Raggi P, Lippolis N et al. (1998a) Effect of HMG-CoA reductase inhibitors on coronary disease as assessed by electron-beam computed tomography. N Engl J Med 339:1972–1978

Callister TQ, Cooil B, Raya SP et al. (1998b) Coronary artery disease: improved reproducibility of calcium scoring with an electron-beam CT volumetric method. Radiology 208: 807–814

Carr JJ, Crouse JR III, Goff DC Jr et al. (2000) Evaluation of subsecond gated helical CT for quantification of coronary artery calcium and comparison with electron beam CT. Am J Roentgenol 174:915–921

Chambless L, Keil U, Dobson A et al. (1997a) Population versus clinical view of case fatality from acute coronary heart disease: results from the WHO MONICA Project 1985–1990. Multinational MONItoring of Trends and Determinants in CArdiovascular Disease. Circulation 96:3849–3859

Chambless LE, Heiss G, Folsom AR et al. (1997b) Association of coronary heart disease incidence with carotid arterial wall thickness and major risk factors: the Atherosclerosis Risk in Communities (ARIC) Study, 1987–1993. Am J Epidemiol 146:483–494

Detrano RC, Froelicher VF (1988) Exercise testing: uses and limitations considering recent studies. Prog Cardiovasc Dis 31:837–845

Detrano R, Wong N, Tang W (1994) Prognostic significance of cardiac cinefluoroscopy for coronary calcific deposits in asymptomatic high risk subjects. J Am Coll Cardiol 24: 354–358

Detrano R, Hsiai T, Wang S et al. (1996) Prognostic value of coronary calcification and angiographic stenoses in patients undergoing coronary angiography. J Am Coll Cardiol 27:285–290

Detrano RC, Wong ND, Doherty TM et al. (1999) Coronary calcium does not accurately predict near-term future coronary events in high-risk adults. Circulation 99:2633–2638

Doherty T, Detrano R (1994) Coronary arterial calcification as an active process: a new perspective on an old problem. Calcif Tissue Int 54:224–230

Downs J, Clearfield M, Weis S et al. (1998) Primary prevention of acute coronary events with lovastatin in men and women with average cholesterol levels: results of the AFCAPS/TexCAPS research. J Am Med Assoc 279:1615–1622

Eggen DA, Strong JP, McGill HC (1965) Coronary calcification: relationship to clinically significant coronary lesions and race, sex and topographic distribution. Circulation 32: 948–955

Friedrich G, Moes N, Muhlberger V et al. (1994) Detection of intralesional calcium by intracoronary ultrasound depends on the histologic pattern. Am Heart J 128:435–441

Georgiou D, Budoff MJ, Kaufer E et al. (2001) Screening patients with chest pain in the emergency department using electron beam tomography: a follow-up study. J Am Coll Cardiol 38:105–110

Glagov S, Weisenberg E, Zarins CK et al. (1987) Compensatory enlargement of human atherosclerotic coronary arteries. N Engl J Med 316:1371–1375

Grundy SM (2001) Coronary plaque as a replacement for age as a risk factor in global risk assessment. Am J Cardiol 88: 8E–11E

Guerci AD, Arad Y (2001) Potential use of Ca++ scanning to determine the need for and intensity of lipid-lowering therapy in asymptomatic adults. Curr Cardiol Rep 3: 408–415.

Hecht HS (2001) Impact of plaque imaging by electron beam tomography on the treatment of dyslipidemias. Am J Cardiol 88:406–408

Hoff JA, Chomka EV, Krainik AJ et al. (2001) Age and gender distributions of coronary artery calcium detected by electron beam tomography in 35,246 adults. Am J Cardiol 87: 1335–1339

Hong C, Becker CR, Huber A et al. (2001) ECG-gated reconstructed multi-detector row CT coronary angiography: effect of varying trigger delay on image quality. Radiology 220:712–717

Hong C, Becker CR, Schoepf UJ et al. (2002) Coronary artery calcium: absolute quantification in nonenhanced and contrast-enhanced multi-detector row CT studies. Radiology 223:474–480

Jakobs TF, Becker CR, Ohnesorge B et al. (2002) Multislice helical CT of the heart with retrospective ECG gating: reduction of radiation exposure by ECG-controlled tube current modulation. Eur Radiol 12:1081–1086

Janowitz WR, Agatston AS, Viamonte M Jr (1991) Comparison of serial quantitative evaluation of calcified coronary artery plaque by ultrafast computed tomography in persons with and without obstructive coronary artery disease. Am J Cardiol 68:1–6

Janowitz WR, Agatston AS, Kaplan G et al. (1993) Differences in prevalence and extent of coronary artery calcium detected by ultrafast computed tomography in asymptomatic men and women. Am J Cardiol 72:247–254

Jeziorska M, McCollum C, Wooley D (1998) Observations on bone formation and remodelling in advanced atherosclerotic lesions of human carotid arteries. Virchows Arch 433: 559–565

Kajinami K, Seki H, Takekoshi N et al. (1995) Noninvasive prediction of coronary atherosclerosis by quantification of coronary atery calcification using electron comuted tomography: comparison with electrocardiographic and thallium exerxise stress results. J Am Coll Cardiol 26: 1209–1221

Kopp AF, Schroeder S, Kuettner A et al. (2001) Coronary arteries: retrospectively ECG-gated multi-detector row CT angiography with selective optimization of the image reconstruction window. Radiology 221:683–688

Maher JE, Bielak LF, Raz JA et al. (1999) Progression of coronary artery calcification: a pilot study. Mayo Clin Proc 74: 347–355

Mancini GB, Pitt B (2002) Coronary angiographic changes in patients with cardiac events in the Prospective Randomized Evaluation of the Vascular Effects of Norvasc Trial (PREVENT). Am J Cardiol 90:776–778

Mao SS, Oudiz RJ, Bakhsheshi H et al. (1996) Variation of heart rate and electrocardiograph trigger interval during ultrafast computed tomography. Am J Card Imaging 10: 239–243

Mao S, Bakhsheshi H, Lu B et al. (2001) Effect of electrocardiogram triggering on reproducibility of coronary artery calcium scoring. Radiology 220:707–711

Margolis JR, Chen JT, Kong Y et al. (1980) The diagnostic and prognostic significance of coronary artery calcification. A report of 800 cases. Radiology 137:609–616

McCarthy J, Palmer F (1974) Incidence and significance of coronary artery calcification. Br Heart J 36:499–506

McCollough CH (2003) Patient dose in cardiac computed tomography. Herz 28:1–6

McLaughlin VV, Balogh T, Rich S (1999) Utility of electron beam computed tomography to stratify patients presenting to the emergency room with chest pain. Am J Cardiol 84:327–328, A328

Newman A, Naydeck B, Sutton-Tyrell K et al. (2000) Coronary artery calcification in older adults with minimal clinical or subclinical cardiovascular disease. J Am Geriatr Soc 48: 256–263

O'Malley PG, Taylor AJ, Gibbons RV et al. (1999) Rationale and design of the Prospective Army Coronary Calcium (PACC) Study: utility of electron beam computed tomography as a screening test for coronary artery disease and as an intervention for risk factor modification among young, asymptomatic, active-duty United States Army Personnel. Am Heart J 137:932–941

O'Malley PG, Taylor AJ, Jackson JL et al. (2000) Prognostic value of coronary electron-beam computed tomography for coronary heart disease events in asymptomatic populations. Am J Cardiol 85:945–948

Ohnesorge B, Flohr T, Becker C et al. (2000) Cardiac imaging by means of electrocardiographically gated multisection spiral CT: initial experience. Radiology 217:564–571

Ohnesorge B, Flohr T, Fischbach R et al. (2002) Reproducibility of coronary calcium quantification in repeat examinations with retrospectively ECG-gated multisection spiral CT. Eur Radiol 12:1532–1540

Petursson M, Jonmundsson E, Brekkan A et al. (1995) Angiographic predictors of new coronary occlusions. Am Heart J 129:515–520

Raggi P, Callister TQ, Cooil B et al. (2000) Identification of patients at increased risk of first unheralded acute myocardial infarction by electron-beam computed tomography. Circulation 101:850–855

Rienmüller R, Lipton M (1987) Detection of coronary artery calcification by computed tomography. Dynam Cardiovasc Imaging 1:139–145

Rifkin R, Parisi A, Folland E (1979) Coronary calcification in the diagnosis of coronary artery disease. Am J Cardiol 44: 141–147

Rumberger JA, Simons DB, Fitzpatrick LA et al. (1995) Coronary artery calcium area by electron-beam computed tomography and coronary atherosclerotic plaque area. A histopathologic correlative study. Circulation 92:2157–2162

Sangiori G, Rumberger J, Severson A et al. (1998) Arterial calcification and not lumen stenosis is correlated with atherosclerotic plaque burden in humans: a histologic study of 723 coronary artery segments using nondecalcifying methodology. J Am Coll Cardiol 31:126–133

Schmermund A, Erbel R (2001) Unstable coronary plaque and its relation to coronary calcium. Circulation 104: 1682–1687

Schmermund A, Baumgart D, Adamzik M et al. (1998) Comparison of electron-beam computed tomography and intracoronary ultrasound in detecting calcified and noncalcified plaques in patients with acute coronary syndromes and no or minimal to moderate angiographic coronary artery disease. Am J Cardiol 81:141–146

Schmermund A, Schwartz RS, Adamzik M et al. (2001) Coronary atherosclerosis in unheralded sudden coronary death under age 50: histo-pathologic comparison with "healthy" subjects dying out of hospital. Atherosclerosis 155:499–508

Schmermund A, Möhlenkamp S, Stang A et al. (2002) Assessment of clinically silent atherosclerotic disease and established and novel risk factors for predicting myocardial infarction and cardiac death in healthy middle-aged subjects: rationale and design of the Heinz Nixdorf RECALL Study. Risk factors, evaluation of coronary calcium and lifestyle. Am Heart J 144:212–218

Shepherd J, Cobbe S, Ford I et al. (1995) West of Scotland Coronary Prevention Study Group. Prevention of coronary heart diesease with pravastatin in men with hypercholesterolemia. N Engl J Med 333:1301–1307

Souza A, Bream P, Elliott L (1978) Chest film detection of coronary artery calcification: the value of CAC triangle. Radiology 129:7–10

Stary HC, Chandler AB, Glagov S et al. (1994) A definition of initial, fatty streak, and intermediate lesions of atherosclerosis. A report from the Committee on Vascular Lesions of the Council on Arteriosclerosis, American Heart Association. Arterioscler Thromb 14:840–856

Stary HC, Chandler AB, Dinsmore RE et al. (1995) A definition of advanced types of atherosclerotic lesions and a histological classification of atherosclerosis. A report from the Committee on Vascular Lesions of the Council on Arteriosclerosis, American Heart Association. Circulation 92:1355–1374

Tannenbaum S, Kondos G, Veselik K et al. (1989) Detection of calcific deposits in coronary arteries by ultrafast computed tomography. J Am Coll Cardiol 15:827–832

Thaulow E, Erikssen J, Sandvik L et al. (1993) Initial clinical presentation of cardiac disease in asymptomatic men with silent myocardial ischemia and angiographically documented coronary artery disease (the Oslo Ischemia Study). Am J Cardiol 72:629–633

Tuzcu E, Berkalp B, Franco A de et al. (1996) The dilemma of diagnosing coronary calcification: angiography versus intravascular ultrasound. J Am Coll Cardiol 27:832–838

Ulzheimer S, Kalender WA (2003) Assessment of calcium scoring performance in cardiac computed tomography. Eur Radiol 13:484–497

Virmani R, Kolodgie FD, Burke AP et al. (2000) Lessons from sudden coronary death: a comprehensive morphological classification scheme for atherosclerotic lesions. Arterioscler Thromb Vasc Biol 20:1262–1275.

Wexler L, Brundage B, Crouse J et al. (1996) Coronary artery calcification: pathophysiology, epidemiology, imaging methods, and clinical implications. A statement for health professionals from the American Heart Association. Circulation 94:1175–1192

Wilson PW, D'Agostino RB, Levy D et al. (1998) Prediction of coronary heart disease using risk factor categories. Circulation 97:1837–1847

Wong ND, Hsu JC, Detrano RC et al. (2000) Coronary artery calcium evaluation by electron beam computed tomography and its relation to new cardiovascular events. Am J Cardiol 86:495–498

Wong ND, Budoff MJ, Pio J et al. (2002) Coronary calcium and cardiovascular event risk: evaluation by age- and sex-specific quartiles. Am Heart J 143:456–459

22 MDCT Angiography of the Coronary Arteries

C. R. Becker

CONTENTS

22.1 Introduction

Contrast-enhanced CT studies of the coronary arteries were performed first to visualize the vessel lumen and to achieve an angiographic-like presentation of the coronary arteries in combination with 3D post-processing methods (Moshage et al. 1995). Because short exposure times are essential for coronary CT angiography, investigations initially were performed with electron-beam CT scanners. These dedicated cardiac CT scanners were originally designed to measure myocardial perfusion (Boyd 1983). For morphological assessment of cardiac structures a restrictive scan protocol allows for 100 ms exposure time, 3-mm slice thickness, and 130-kVp and 630-mA electron-gun power. The acquisition of every single slice is triggered prospectively by the ECG signal at the end-systole phase of the cardiac cycle. A recent technical update of this scanner type will allow for shorter exposure times, thinner slices, and higher electron-gun power; however, the feasibility to image the contrast-enhanced coronary arteries has not yet been demonstrated clinically.

C. R. Becker, MD
Department of Radiology, University Hospital Grosshadern, University of Munich, Marchioninistrasse 15, 81377 Munich, Germany

Multidetector-row helical CT scanners are operated with a different acquisition mode called retrospective ECG gating. The combination of fast gantry rotation, slow table movement and multislice-helical acquisition allows for acquisition of a high number of X-ray projection data. The ECG trace is recorded simultaneously during the helical scan acquisition. The X-ray projections of the mid-diastolic phase are selected to reconstruct images from the slow-motion diastole phase of the heart. In MDCT the exposure time (>210 ms) is longer and the radiation exposure (~10 mSv) is higher than in electron-beam CT. On the other hand, image quality is superior in MDCT compared with electron-beam CT because of higher spatial resolution and lower image noise.

In MDCT an attempt has been made to improve temporal resolution by multisector reconstruction. For this technique X-ray projections of more than one heart beat are used to reconstruct an image. This technique requires absolutely consistent data from at least two consecutive heart beats for successful image reconstruction. Unfortunately, the rhythm of the human heart may change rapidly, in particular under special conditions such as breath holding and Valsalva maneuver. For this reason, this technique is of limited practical use under clinical conditions.

The redundant radiation occurring during the radiation exposure in the systole can substantially be reduced by a technique called prospective ECG tube-current modulation. On the basis of the ECG signal the X-ray tube current is switched to its nominal value during the diastole phase and is reduced significantly during the systole phase of the heart, respectively. This technique is most effective in patients with low heart rates. If the heart rate is lower that 60 beats per minute, the radiation exposure will be reduced by approximately 50% (Jakobs et al. 2002).

In addition, retrospective ECG gating allows for reconstruction of images at any time within the cardiac cycle; however, with the currently available exposure time in MDCT the image quality is only poor if the images are reconstructed in the systole. The accuracy of the functional assessment by MDCT may be influenced if motion artifacts are present or if beta-blockers have been administered.

22.2 Patient Preparation

In 16-row-detector CT scanner with 420-ms gantry rotation an optimized partial view scan lasts approximately 210 ms. Reasonably good image quality with this exposure time can only be achieved in patients with low heart rates (40–60 beats per minute; HONG et al. 2001). Therefore, caffeine or any drug that increases the heart rate, such as atropine or nitroglycerin, should be avoided prior to a cardiac CTA investigation. Instead, the use of beta-blocker may become necessary for patient preparation aiming at a heart rate of 60 beats per minute or less.

To consider beta-blocker for patient preparation contraindications (bronchial asthma, AV block, severe congestive heart failure, aortic stenosis, etc.; RYAN et al. 1996) have to be ruled out and informed consent must be obtained from the patient. In case the heart rate of a patient is significantly above 60 beats/min, 50–200 mg of Metoprolol tartrat can be administered orally 30–90 min prior to the investigation. Alternatively, 5–20 mg of Metoprolol tartrat divided into four doses can be administered intravenously (RYAN et al. 1996) immediately prior scanning. Monitoring of vital functions, heart rate, and blood pressure is essential during this approach. The positive effect of beta-blocker on MDCT scanning is fourfold: better patient compliance; less radiation exposure and cardiac motion artifacts; and higher vascular enhancement.

22.3 Contrast Admininistration

Timely accurate and homogeneous vascular lumen enhancement is essential for full diagnostic capability of coronary MDCT angiography studies. Higher contrast enhancement is superior to identify small vessels in MDCT; however, dense contrast material in the right atrium may result in streak artifacts arising from the right atrium and interfering with the right coronary artery. On the other hand, coronary atherosclerosis is commonly associated with calcifications that may interfere with dense contrast material and hinders the assessment of the residual lumen. A contrast medium flow rate of 1 g/s iodine by peripheral venous injection in an antecubital vein will result in an enhancement of approximately 250–300 HU, which allows for delineation of intermediate (91±21 HU) as well as high dense plaques (419±194 HU; SCHROEDER et al. 2001).

The final vessel enhancement will also depend on the cardiac output. In patients with low cardiac output, e.g., under beta-blocker medication, the contrast media will accumulate in the cardiac chambers and lead to a higher enhancement than in patients with high cardiac output where the contrast agent will be diluted by non-enhanced blood faster.

The circulation time can be determined by a test bolus of 5 g iodine injected with a flow rate of 1 g/s iodine and followed by a saline chaser bolus. A series of scans is acquired at the level of the ascending aorta every other second. The arrival time of the test bolus can be determined by taking the delay time between start of the contrast injection and peak enhancement of the ascending aorta into account.

In a 4-detector-row CT scanning may start directly at the time of the pre-determined peak enhancement of the test bolus. Scanning with a 16-detector-row CT requires an additional delay time to allow the contrast media to reach the left ventricular system and the coronary arteries. In our current experience, another 6 s should be added to the peak enhancement of the test bolus to allow for complete enhancement of the left ventricular system in a 16-detector-row CT. The contrast media has to be injected for the duration of the scan and the delay time and therefore has to be maintained for 40 and 26 s in a 4- and 16-detector-row CT, respectively. In a 16-detector-row CT the sequential injection of contrast media and saline allows for selective enhancement the left ventricular system with a washout of contrast in the right ventricular system (Fig. 22.1). In general, the use of a dual high-power injector has been found to be mandatory in MDCT to keep the contrast bolus compact (HOPPER et al. 1997), to reduce the total amount of contrast media (HAAGE et al. 2000) and to allow for a central venous enhancement profile by a peripheral venous injection (HITTMAIR et al. 2001).

Alternatively, beginning of the CT scan can be triggered automatically by the arrival of the contrast bolus. A pre-scan is taken at the level of the aortic root and a region of interest is placed into the ascending aorta. When contrast injection starts repeated scanning at the same level is performed every second. If the density in the ascending aorta reaches 100 HU, a countdown begins until the acquisition starts. Right in front of the CT scan acquisition the patient is instructed to hold his breath. A delay time of 4 and 10 s has to be

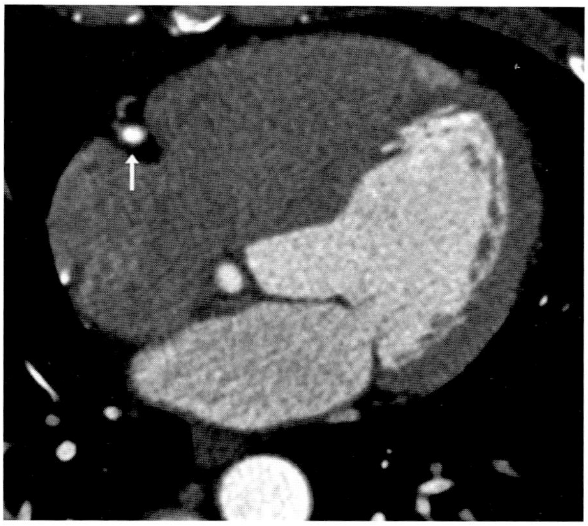

Fig. 22.1. In a 16-row-detector CT complete and homogenous enhancement of the left ventricle and the coronary arteries can be achieved by a dedicated contrast protocol. The contrast medium has passed the right ventricle and the flush with saline results in a washout of the contrast medium from the right ventricle (*arrow*)

added in a 4- and 16-detector-row CT, respectively, to allow for timely adequate contrast enhancement.

22.4 MDCT Scanning

For retrospective ECG gating with MDCT the pitch factor (detector collimation/table feed per gantry rotation) must not exceed 0.3 to allow for scanning the heart at any heart rate higher than 40 beats per minute. In a 4-detector-row CT with 1-mm slice collimation and 500-ms gantry rotation a typical scan range of 12 cm lasts approximately 40 s. In a 16-detector-row CT with 0.75-mm slice collimation currently 12 channels are used at a gantry rotation time of 420 ms. Tube current is set to 400 and 500 effective mAs in a 4- and 16-detector-row CT, respectively, with an acquisition time of 40 and 20 s, respectively.

The patients should be instructed not to press when taking a deep breath in order to avoid the Valsalva maneuver. The Valsalva maneuver increases the intra-thoracic pressure preventing the influx of contrast media through the superior vena cava into the right atrium. Non-enhanced blood from the inferior vena cava entering the right atrium leads to an inhomogeneous enhancement of the cardiac volume during the CTA scan.

Retrospective ECG gating always begins with a careful analysis of the ECG trace recorded with the helical scan. The image reconstruction interval is best been placed in between the T- and the P-wave of the ECG corresponding to the mid-diastole interval. The point of time for the least coronary motion may be different for every coronary artery. Least motion artifacts may result for reconstructing the RCA, LAD, and LCX at 50, 55, and 60% of the RR-interval, retrospectively. Individual adaptation of the point of time for reconstruction seems to further improve image quality (Hong et al. 2001); however, the lower the heart rate, the easier it is to find the best interval for all tree major branches of the coronary artery tree. Images are reconstructed with spatial in-plane resolution of 0.6 by 0.6 mm. The slice thickness and reconstruction increment is 1.3 with 0.7 mm and 1 with 0.5 mm in 4- and 16-detector-row CT, respectively.

The patient room time is approximately 15 minutes and image reconstruction and post-processing can be performed within approximately 10 min. Because coronary CT angiography (CTA) is performed with thin slices and low image noise, the radiation dose with tube current modulation is significantly higher (~5 mSv) than that for calcium screening (~1 mSv) however, the radiation of a CTA investigation is comparable to what is applied during a diagnostic coronary catheter procedure.

22.5 Image Post-Processing

Detection of coronary artery stenoses in axial CT images is problematic since every slice displays only a small fragment of the entire coronary artery. Multiplanar reformatting, volume rendering, virtual coronary endoscopy, and shaded-surface display does not seem to be suited to reconstruct CT images of the coronary arteries to detect coronary artery stenosis (Vogl et al. 2002). Maximum intensity projection (MIP) post-processing of CT images was found to be helpful in following the course of the coronary arteries and in creating angiographic-like projections that allow for better detection of coronary artery stenoses.

For that purpose, standardized thin (5 mm) MIP slabs with 2.5-mm increment between the slabs are reconstructed in three different planes similar to standard cardiac catheter projections (Johnson 1996). The MIP along the inter- and atria-ventricular groove creates images in similar planes as the right anterior oblique (RAO; Fig. 22.2a) and left anterior

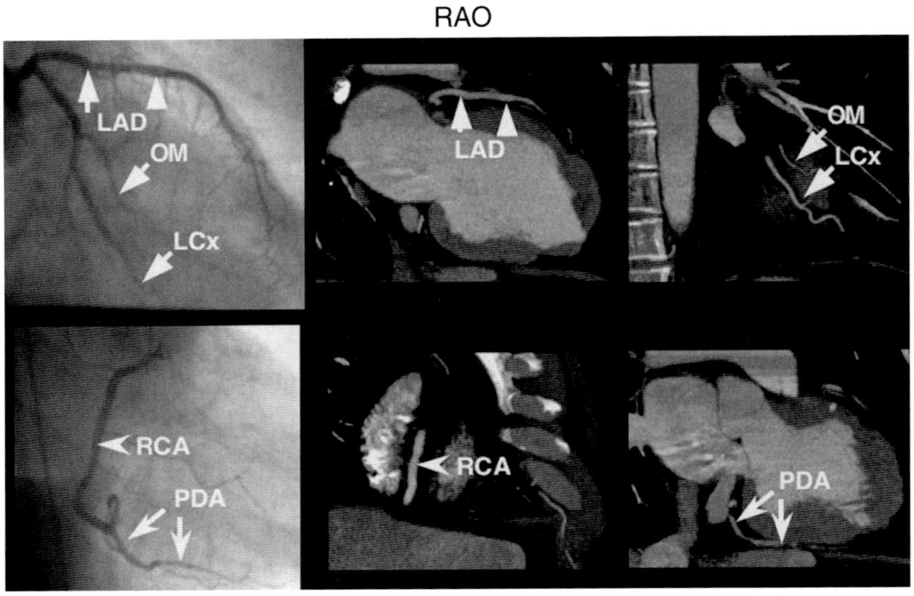

Fig. 22.2. **a** For the right anterior oblique (RAO) maximum intensity projection (MIP) images are reconstructed in a plane connecting the right and circumflex coronary artery in the atrium-ventricular grove. **b** The MIP images are best suited to display the course of the right and circumflex coronary artery. *RCA* right coronary artery, *OM* obtuse marginal branch, *LCx* left circumflex coronary artery, *PDA* posterior descending coronary artery, *RCA* right coronary artery, *LAD* left anterior descending, *AV* arteriovenous

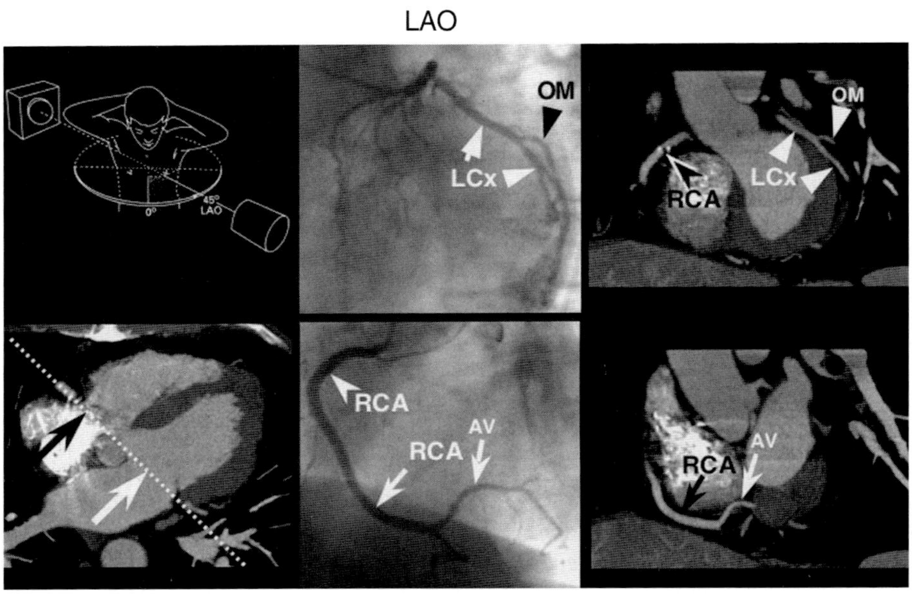

Fig. 22.3. **a** For the left anterior oblique (LAO) MIP images are reconstructed along the interventricular grove. **b** The reformatted images allow following the course of the left anterior descending coronary artery. *RCA* right coronary artery, *OM* obtuse marginal branch, *LCx* left circumflex coronary artery, *AV* arteriovenous

oblique (LAO; Fig. 22.3a) angiographic projections, respectively. The RAO–MIP slabs demonstrate best the course of the left anterior descending coronary artery (Fig. 22.2b). The LAO–MIP slabs display the course of the RCA and LCX (Fig. 22.3b). In addition, similar to coronary angiography, an oblique projection (LAO/OBL–MIP; Fig. 22.4a) can be reconstructed following the long axis of the heart. This projection plane spreads the branches of the LAD and is therefore called the "spider view." The "spider view" is well suited to demonstrate the proximal part of all three major coronary arteries (Fig. 22.4b).

22.6 Detection of Coronary Artery Stenoses

Every finding from post-processed MIP images has to be confirmed in the original axial CT slices. The primary axial slices are superior to any post-processing method to rule out CAD. Image analysis begins with identification of the coronary artery segments in the axial CT slices. Coronary segments can be numbered (Table 22.1) according to the model suggested by the American Heart Association (Fig. 22.5; Austen et al. 1975).

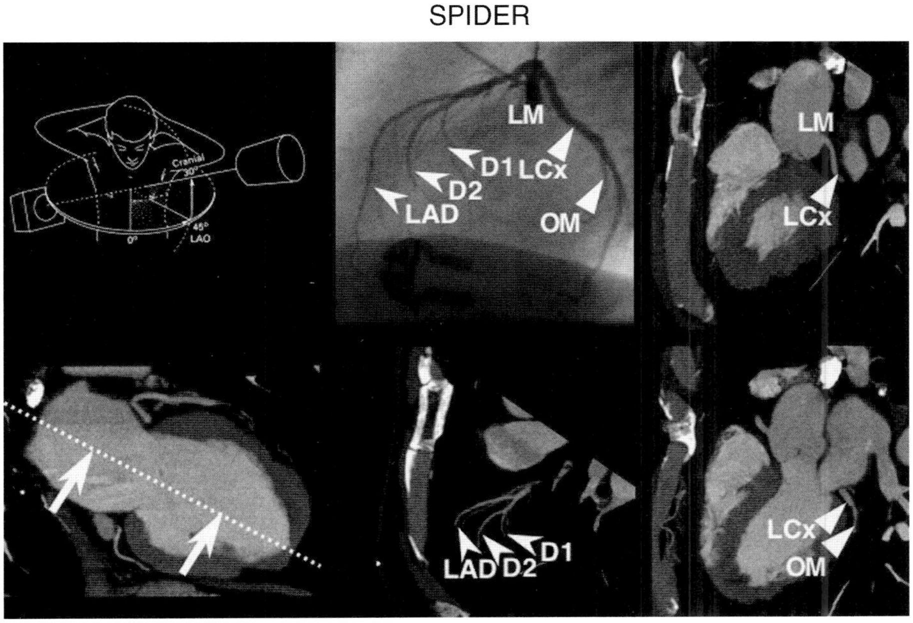

Fig. 22.4. a The plane of the "spider" (LAO oblique) view is positioned along the long axis of the heart and **b** displays the course of the left anterior coronary artery and the diagonal branches. *OM* obtuse marginal branch, *LCx* left circumflex coronary artery, *LAD* left anterior descending, *D1* first diagonal branch, *D2* second diagonal branch

Table 22.1. Segment numbering according to the American Heart Association scheme (Austen. 1975)

Segment no.	Name	Abbreviation	Segment	Begin	End
1	Right coronary artery	RCA	Proximal	Ostium	RV
2	Right coronary artery	RCA	Middle	RMD	AM
3	Right coronary artery	RCA	Distal	AM	Crux cordis
4	Posterior descending coronary artery	PDA		Crux cordis	Apex
5	Left main coronary artery	LCA		Ostium	Bifurcation
6	Left anterior descending	LAD	Proximal	Bifurcation	D1
7	Left anterior descending	LAD	Middle	D1	D2
8	Left anterior descending	LAD	Distal	D2	Apex
9	First diagonal branch	D1			
10	Second diagonal branch	D2			
11	Left circumflex coronary artery	LCX	Proximal	Bifurcation	OM
12	Obtuse marginal branch	OM			
13	Left circumflex coronary artery	LCX	Distal	OM	PD
14	Posterolateral branch	PL			
15	Posterior descending branch	PD			

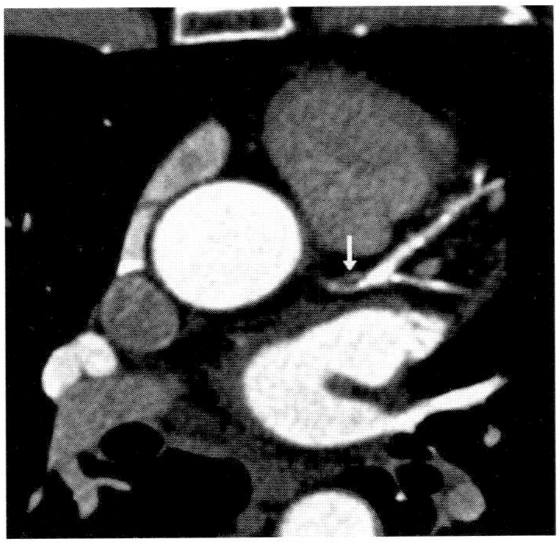

Fig. 22.5. Hemodynamically significant stenosis of the left main coronary artery (*arrow*) caused by a noncalcified coronary artery wall lesion

The morphology of calcifications may give a first hint for the presence or absence of significant stenoses in the coronary arteries. From electron-beam CT studies Kajinami et al. (1997) reported that the positive predictive value for significant stenosis (75%) was 0.04 in none, 0.18 in spotty (Fig. 22.6), 0.32 in long, 0.40 in wide, and 0.56 in diffuse (Fig. 22.7) coronary calcifications, respectively. Significant coronary stenosis may lead to a hemodynamically relevant blood flow reduction that may lead to myocardial ischemia with clinical symptoms such as angina pectoris. A lumen-narrowing scoring system according to Schmermund et al. (1998) may be used to describe different grades of coronary artery stenosis: A=angiographically normal segment (0% stenosis); B=non-obstructive disease (1–49% lumen diameter stenosis); C=significant (50–74%) stenosis; D=high-

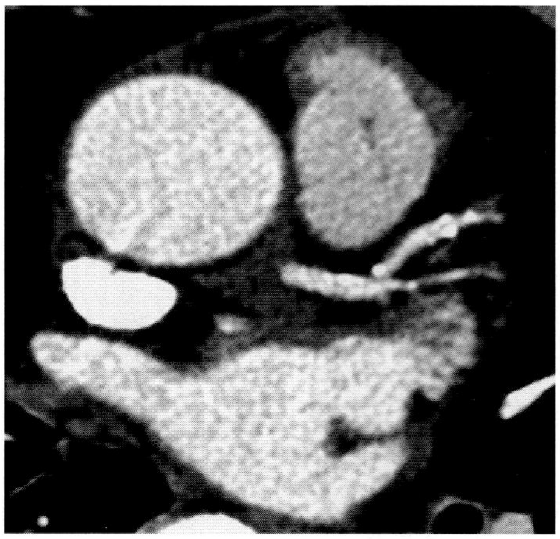

Fig. 22.6. The positive predictive value of spotty coronary calcifications is only 18%

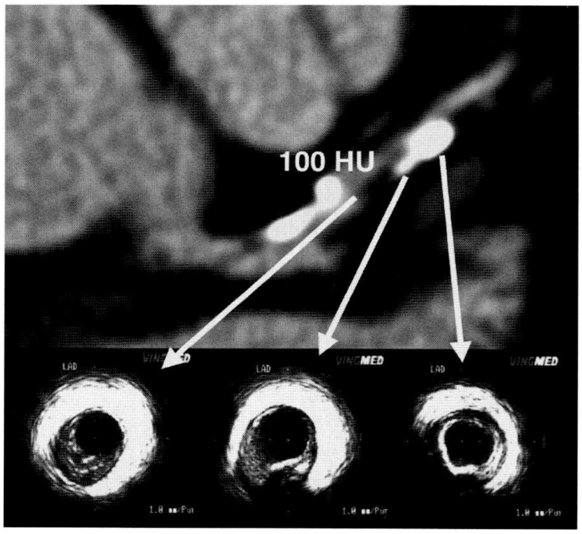

Fig. 22.7. The positive predictive value of diffuse coronary calcifications is 56%. Figure shows different types of coronary artery wall lesions in comparison with intravascular ultrasound. All lesions cause stenosis of the vessel. Diffuse calcification (*right*), mixed lesion with calcified components (*middle*), and non-calcified lesion component with soft tissue attenuation of 100 HU (*left*)

grade (75–99%) stenosis; and E=total occlusion (100% stenosis).

In comparison with cardiac catheter, several studies (Table 22.2) have shown that MDCT angiography has a mean sensitivity, specificity, and positive and negative predictive value for detecting significant coronary artery stenoses is 85, 88, 76, and 97%, respectively (Fig. 22.8; Achenbach et al. 2001; Nieman et al. 2001, 2002; Knez et al. 2000); however, the findings of a significant stenosis detected by MDCT are neither specific for the site nor the degree of the stenosis in cardiac catheter. On the other hand, with the high negative predictive value coronary artery disease (CAD) can reliably be ruled out by coronary MDCT angiography. In particular, patients with a low to moderate pretest probability (50%; Table 22.3; Gibbons et al. 1999) may be good candidates for a coronary CTA investigation.

22.7 Limitations for Detecting Coronary Stenosis

Initial experiences revealed a number of limitations already known from coronary CTA studies performed with electron-beam CT. Schmermund et al. (1998) reported that small vessel diameter may lead to false-positive findings. They also reported that extensive calcifications might interfere with the detection of coronary artery stenoses, resulting in false-negative results compared with selective coronary angiography. A reason for this observation may be that standard CT soft tissue reconstruction kernels are leading to a "blooming" of dense material such as coronary stents or calcifications that obscure the vessel lumen and wall changes.

Because of the limited spatial resolution in CTA and the "blooming" of calcifications, the definite assessment of the degree of coronary artery stenoses

Table 22.2. Comparison between MDCT angiography and cardiac catheter for detection significant coronary artery stenosis

Reference	No. of patients	Sensitivity (%)	Specificity (%)	Positive predictive value (%)	Negative predictive value (%)	Not assessible
Nieman . (2001)]	35	83	90	81	97	30
Achenbach . (2001)	64	85	76	59	98	32
Knez . (2001)	44	78	98	85	96	6
Nieman . (2002)	58	95	86	80	97	0
Mean	–	85	88	76	97	17

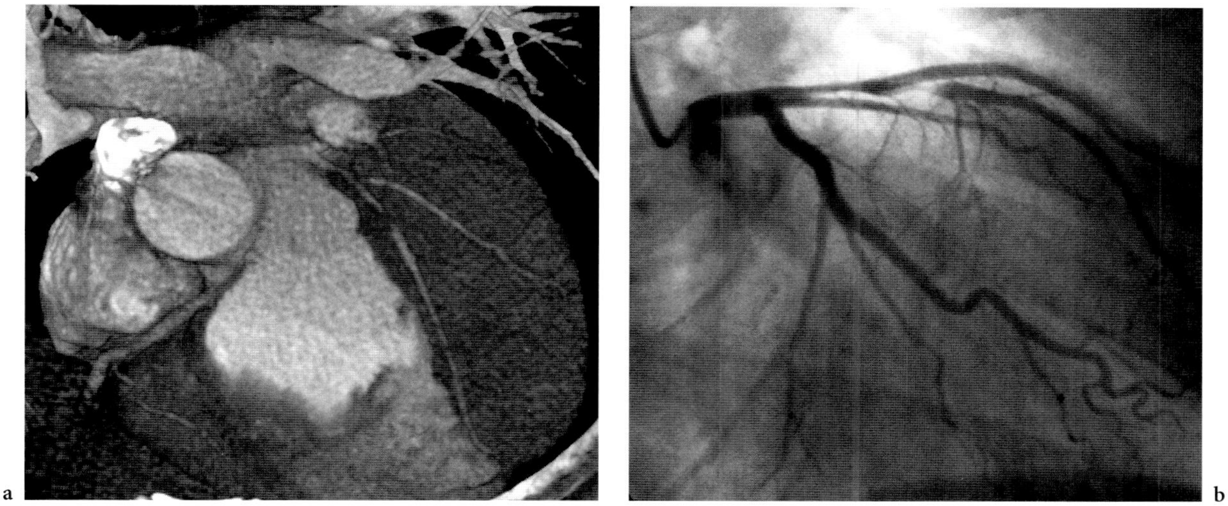

Fig. 22.8a, b. Hemodynamically significant stenosis of the left anterior descending coronary artery. **a** Contrast-enhanced CT vs **b** catheter angiogram

Table 22.3. Pre-test likelihood (in percent) of CAD in symptomatic patients according to age and gender (Gibbons 1999)

	Non-angina chest pain		Atypical angina		Typical angina	
Age (years)	Men	Women	Men	Women	Men	Women
30–39	4	2	34	12	76	26
40–49	13	3	51	22	87	55
50–59	20	7	65	31	93	73
60–69	27	14	72	51	94	86

still remains problematic; therefore, coronary CTA is currently not suited to determine the progression in patients with known CAD, typical angina, or obvious myocardial ischemia on exercise testing. These patients are better approached by cardiac catheter examination with the option to perform percutaneous coronary interventions in the same session (Nakanishi et al. 1997).

It should be considered when interpreting coronary CTA that details like collateral vessels, contrast runoff, and direction of filling of coronary arteries are not visualized by CTA. Finally, the hemodynamic relevance of coronary artery stenoses may not reliably be determined without wall motion or perfusion information about the myocardium under rest and exercise.

Further limitations have been seen in patients with a body mass index above 30 (Vogl et al. 2002) and absolute arrhythmia (Herzog et al. 2002) leading to a degradation of image quality in CTA by severe image noise and cardiac motion artifacts.

22.8 Coronary Atherosclerosis

More than displaying the coronary artery lumen only, MDCT as a cross-sectional modality is able to display the coronary artery wall. Coronary calcifications can easily be assessed, even without contrast media, and represent an advanced stage of atherosclerosis; however, as different stages of coronary atherosclerosis may be present simultaneously, calcifications may also be associated with more early stages of coronary atherosclerosis. The entire extent of coronary atherosclerosis, however, will be underestimated by assessing coronary calcifications alone (Wexler et al. 1996). With contrast enhancement calcified as well as non-calcified lesions can completely be assessed by MDCT simultaneously.

Cardiac catheter seems to be not suited to assess the entire extent of coronary atherosclerosis completely. Histological and intravascular ultrasound (IVUS) studies have shown that high atherosclerotic plaque burden can be found even in the absence of high-grade coronary stenoses on conventional coronary angiography. From the clinical standpoint the correlation between acute cardiac events and high-grade coronary artery stenoses is only poor. Recently, it has been reported that 68% of the patients who received coronary angiography by incidence prior to their acute cardiac event did not show any significant coronary artery stenoses (Ziada et al. 1999). In early stages of CAD, the coronary arteries may undergo a process of positive remodeling that compensates for the coronary wall thickening and keeps the inner lumen of the vessel unchanged (Glagov et al. 1987). The pathomechanism of this phenomenon is still unknown, but the underlying type of coronary artery disease may be a fibrous cap atheroma with accumulation of cholesterol. In cases of inflammatory processes the fibrous cap of an atheroma may become thinned, putting the plaque at risk for rupture and consecutive thrombosis (Virmani et al. 2000).

The current gold standard to assess coronary atherosclerosis in vivo is IVUS ultrasound. Comparing IVUS with MDCT, Schroeder et al. (2001) reported that coronary lesions classified as soft, intermediate, and dense, as determined by IVUS, correspond to plaque with a density of 14±26, 91±21, and 419±194 HU in MDCT, respectively.

It seems to be that different histological stages of atherosclerosis are present with different morphological patterns in MDCT. In heart specimen studies it turned out that Hounsfield densities of non-calcified plaques seem to depend on the ratio between lipid and fibrous tissue and may increase from atheroma (~50-HU) and fibroatheroma to fibrotic (~90-HU) lesions. As we have observed in coronary arteries of symptomatic patients, coronary thrombi (Fig. 22.9) present as very low dense (~20-HU) and inhomogeneous plaques (Table 22.3; Becker et al. 2000).

Commonly spotty calcified lesions may be found in MDCT angiography studies that may be associated with minor wall changes in conventional coronary angiography only (Kajinami et al. 1997); however, it is known that such calcified nodules may also be the source of unheralded plaque rupture and consecutive thrombosis (Fig. 22.10), and may lead to sudden coronary death in very rare cases (Virmani et al. 2000).

Even in contrast-enhanced studies coronary calcifications can easily be detected and quantified because the density of calcium (>350 HU) is beyond the density of the contrast media in the coronary artery lumen (250–300 HU; Hong et al. 2002); however, because of partial-volume effects, it is much more difficult to quantify non-calcified plaques. The optimal quantification algorithm for atherosclerosis determined by MDCT is still under development.

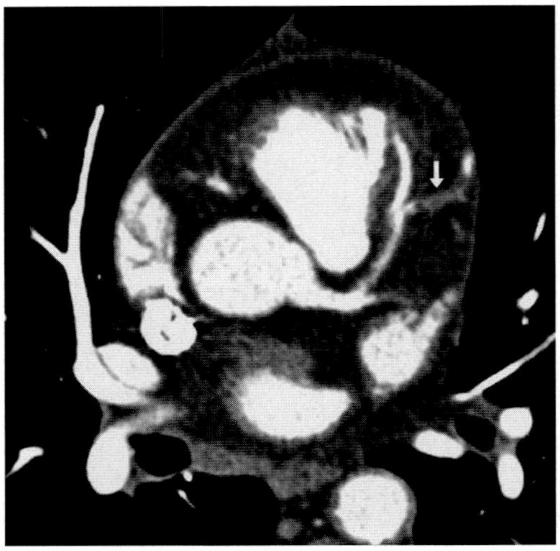

Fig. 22.9. Irregular, inhomogeneous and low dense plaque in the left anterior descending coronary artery in a patient with acute coronary syndrome. The lesion most likely reflects a thrombus in the coronary artery

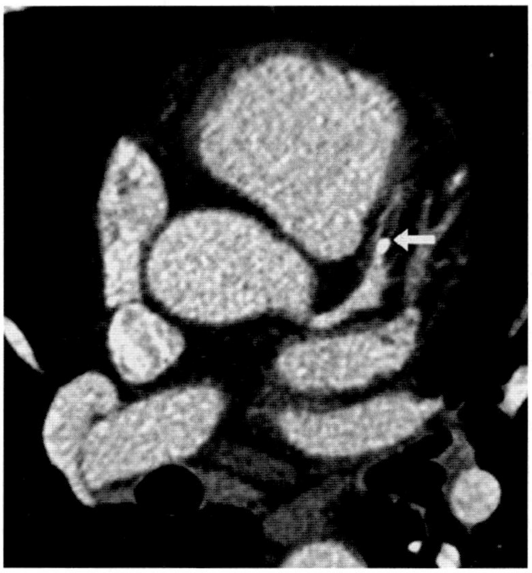

Fig. 22.10. Calcified nodule (*arrow*) with consecutive thrombus formation in a patient with unstable angina

In patients with extensive coronary calcifications, non-calcified plaques are uncommon most likely because the previously described "blooming" artifact prevents assessment. Therefore, and because the coronary artery stenosis cannot be reliably assessed (Kajinami et al. 1997), contrast-enhanced MDCT is currently not recommended in patients presenting with diffuse calcifications (>100 mg CaHA or Agatston Score >500).

22.9 Additional Findings

A late uptake of contrast media after first pass in the myocardium of patients after infarction was observed in CT approximately 17 years ago (Masuda et al. 1984). It is likely that this kind of myocardial enhancement may correspond to interstitial uptake of contrast media within necrotic myocytes, 6 weeks to 3 months after onset. To allow for superior detection of the late myocardial enhancement with the new-generation MDCT scanners, images should be acquired with thick slices, high signal-to-noise ratio, and reconstructed with a very soft tissue kernel at 80 kVp tube voltage. The optimal point of time for scanning may be between 10 and 40 min after first pass (Huber et al. 1981).

Frequently in patients with known history of CAD subendocardial or transmural myocardial infarction scars can been identified as dark zones commonly detected in the region. Every region of the myocardium can be assigned to the territory of the coronary vessel supplying it. The LAD supplies the anterior left ventricular wall with the roof of the left ventricle, the apex, the superior part of the septum, and the anterior papillary muscle. The posterior left ventricular wall and the posterior papillary muscle then are supplied by the LCX (Fig. 22.11). The inferior left ventricular wall and the inferior part of the septum finally is supplied by the RCA. Below the mitral valve all three territories can be identified in one axial slice.

Later development of a subendocardial or transmural myocardial infarction may lead to a thinning of the myocardial wall or myocardial aneurysm, respectively. Due to hypokinesia in the aneurysm, thrombus formation is likely to develop in the cardiac chamber and can be detected by CTA (Fig. 22.12) even more so than by transthoracic ultrasound (Masuda et al. 1984).

In addition, paracardial findings are frequently observed in CTA studies and should be reported. These findings include lymph node enlargement, pulmonary nodules, and tumors (Horton et al. 2002), or even quite commonly esophageal hernias. These incidental findings should trigger an additional reconstruction with a larger field of view or a more dedicated (CT) investigation should then be recommended.

22.10 Conclusion

The newest generation of MDCT now allows for consistently good image quality when regular sinus rhythm is present and the heart rate is in the range between 40 and 60 beats per minute. Extensive calcifications may hinder the detection of coronary stenosis; however, the high negative predictive value of CTA may justify the investigation of symptomatic patients with low to moderate pre-test probability of CAD (Nieman et al. 2002) to exclude a coronary macroangiopathy and to avoid unnecessary cardiac catheter procedures. The predictive value of atherosclerotic lesions detected by MDCT for cardiac events

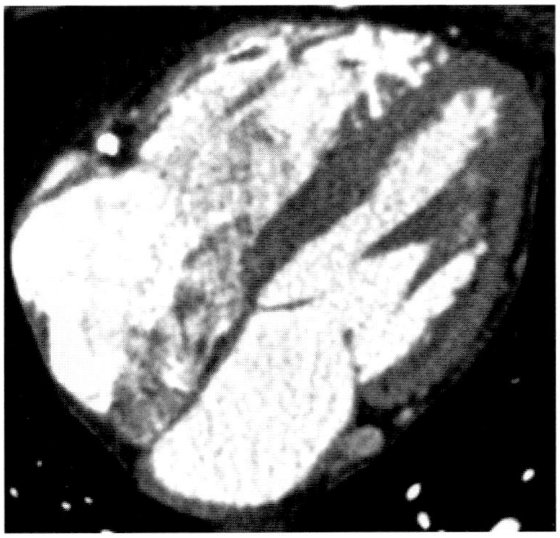

Fig. 22.11. Subendocardial myocardial infarction scar in the posterior wall including the posterior papillary muscle. This area is supplied by the circumflex coronary artery

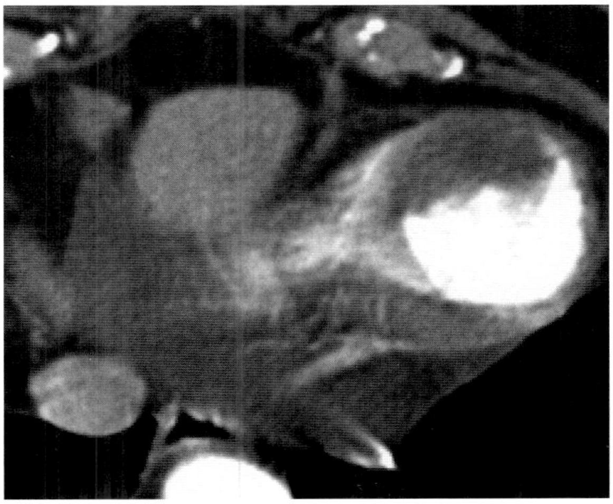

Fig. 22.12. Thrombus in the apex of the left ventricle as a result of hypokinesia after myocardial infarction

Table 22.4. Coronary artery plaque entities and morphological appearance in MDCT

Plaque entity type	AHA	Calcification (HU)	Density	Shape	Remodeling	Possible symptoms
Atheroma	IV	No	~50	Smooth	Positive	No
Fibroatheroma	Va	No	~70	Smooth	Positive/negative	No
Fibrotic lesion	Vc	No	~90	Smooth	Positive/negative	No
Fibrocalcified plaque	Vb	Yes	~90 or absent	Smooth	Negative	Chronic stable angina
Thrombus	VI	No	~20	Irregular	High-grade stenosis or occlusion	Acute unstable angina

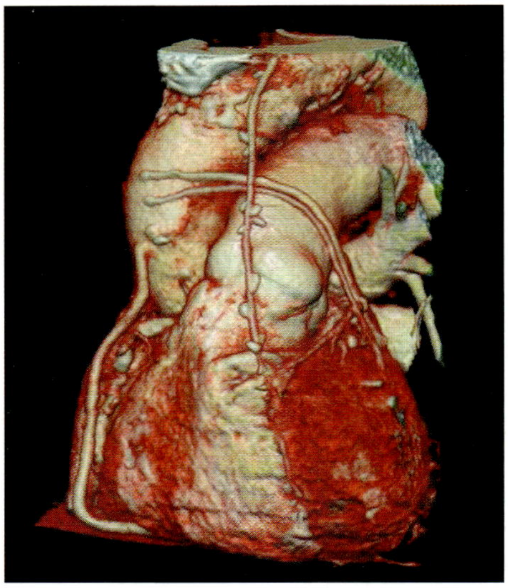

Fig. 22.13. Volume-rendered multidetector-row CT study of a patient with a left internal mammary artery bypass graft to the LAD territory and two venous grafts to the LAD and circumflex CA territories

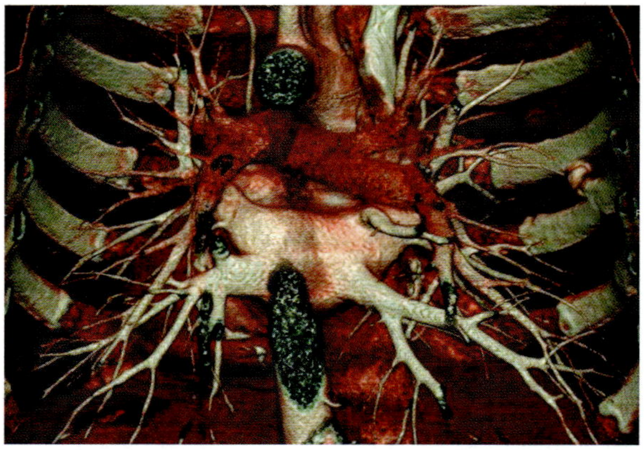

Fig. 22.14. Volume-rendered multidetector-row CT study of a patient scheduled to undergo radio-frequency ablation of an arrhythmogenic focus in the left atrium. Posterior view on the left atrium demonstrating topographic anatomy prior to the procedure

is currently unknown and therefore requires further prospective studies.

Further indication for MDCT includes non-invasive assessment of coronary artery bypass grafts (Fig. 22.13), of anomalous coronary arteries, assessment of left atrial geometry, and post-therapeutic monitoring in the course of radio-frequency ablation of arrhythmogenic foci (Fig. 22.14), and if in selective angiography, it was impossible to enter the ostium of the RCA.

References

Achenbach S, Giesler T, Ropers D et al. (2001) Detection of coronary artery stenoses by contrast-enhanced, retrospectively electrocardiographically gated, multislice spiral computed tomography. Circulation 103:2535–2538

Austen WG, Edwards JE, Frye RL et al. (1975) A reporting system on patients evaluated for coronary artery disease. Report of the Ad Hoc Committee for Grading of Coronary Artery Disease, Council on Cardiovascular Surgery, American Heart Association. Circulation 51 (Suppl 4):5–40

Becker CR, Knez A, Ohnesorge B, Schoepf UJ, Reiser MF (2000) Imaging of noncalcified coronary plaques using helical CT with retrospective ECG gating. Am J Roentgenol 175: 423–424

Boyd D (1983) Computerized transmission tomography of the heart using scanning electron beams. In: Higgins C (ed) CT of the heart and the great vessels: experimental evaluation and clinical application. Futura, Mount Kisco N.Y.

Gibbons R, Chatterjee K, Daley J et al. (1999) ACC/AHA/ACP-ASIM guidelines for the management of patients with chronic stable angina: a report of the American College of Cardiology/American Heart Association Task Force on Practice Guidelines (Committee on Management of Patients With Chronic Stable Angina). J Am Coll Cardiol 33:2092–2197

Glagov S, Weisenberg E, Zarins C, Stankunavicius R, Kolettis G (1987) Compensatory enlargement of human atherosclerotic coronary arteries. N Engl J Med 316:1371–1375

Haage P, Schmitz-Rode T, Hubner D, Piroth W, Gunther RW (2000) Reduction of contrast material dose and artifacts by a saline flush using a double power injector in helical CT of the thorax. Am J Roentgenol 174:1049–1053

Herzog C, Abolmaali N, Balzer JO et al. (2002) Heart-rate-adapted image reconstruction in multidetector-row cardiac CT: influence of physiological and technical prerequisite on image quality. Eur Radiol 12:2670–2678

Hittmair K, Fleischmann D (2001) Accuracy of predicting and controlling time-dependent aortic enhancement from a test bolus injection. J Comput Assist Tomogr 25:287–294

Hong C, Becker CR, Huber A et al. (2001) ECG-gated reconstructed multi-detector row CT coronary angiography: effect of varying trigger delay on image quality. Radiology 220:712–717

Hong C, Becker C, Schoepf UJ, Ohnesorge B, Bruening R, Reiser M (2002) Absolute quantification of coronary artery calcium in non-enhanced and contrast enhanced multidetector-row CT studies. Radiology 223:474–480

Hopper KD, Mosher TJ, Kasales CJ, Ten Have TR, Tully DA, Weaver JS (1997) Thoracic spiral CT: delivery of contrast material pushed with injectable saline solution in a power injector. Radiology 205:269–271

Horton KM, Post WS, Blumenthal RS, Fishman EK (2002) Prevalence of significant noncardiac findings on electron-beam computed tomography coronary artery calcium screening examinations. Circulation 106:532–534

Huber D, Lapray J, Hessel S (1981) In vivo evaluation of experimental myocardial infarcts by ungated computed tomography. AJR 136:469–473

Jakobs TF, Becker CR, Ohnesorge B et al. (2002) Multislice helical CT of the heart with retrospective ECG gating: reduction of radiation exposure by ECG-controlled tube current modulation. Eur Radiol 12:1081–1086

Johnson M (1996) Principles and practice of coronary angiography. In: Skorton D, Schelbert H, Wolf G, Brundage B (eds) Marcus cardiac imaginng: a companion to Braunwald's heart disease, vol 1. Saunders, Philadelphia, pp 220–250

Kajinami K, Seki H, Takekoshi N, Mabuchi H (1997) Coronary calcification and coronary atherosclerosis: site by site comparative morphologic study of electron beam computed tomography and coronary angiography. J Am Coll Cardiol 29:1549–1556

Knez A, Becker C, Leber A et al. (2001) Usefulness of multislice spiral computed tomography angiography for determination of coronary artery stenoses. Am J Cardiol 88:1191–1194

Knez A, Becker C, Ohnesorge B, Haberl R, Reiser M, Steinbeck G (2000) Noninvasive detection of coronary artery stenosis by multislice helical computed tomography. Circulation 101:E221–E222

Masuda Y, Yoshida H, Morooka N, Watanabe S, Inagaki Y (1984) The usefulness of X-ray computed tomography for the diagnosis of myocardial infarction. Circulation 70: 217–225

Moshage WE, Achenbach S, Seese B, Bachmann K, Kirchgeorg M (1995) Coronary artery stenoses: three-dimensional imaging with electrocardiographically triggered, contrast agent-enhanced, electron-beam CT. Radiology 196:707–714

Nakanishi T, Ito K, Imazu M, Yamakido M (1997) Evaluation of coronary artery stenoses using electron-beam CT and multiplanar reformation. J Comput Assist Tomogr 21:121–127

Nieman K, Oudkerk M, Rensing B et al. (2001) Coronary angiography with multi-slice computed computed tomography. Lancet 357:599–603

Nieman K, Cademartiri F, Lemos PA, Raaijmakers R, Pattynama PM, de Feyter PJ (2002) Reliable noninvasive coronary angiography with fast submillimeter multislice spiral computed tomography. Circulation 106:2051–2054

Ryan T, Anderson J, Antman E et al. (1996) ACC/AHA guidelines for the management of patients with acute myocardial infarction. A report of the American College of Cardiology/American Heart Association Task Force on Practice Guidelines (Committee on Management of Acute Myocardial Infarction). J Am Coll Cardiol 28:1328–1428

Schmermund A, Rensing BJ, Sheedy PF, Bell MR, Rumberger JA (1998) Intravenous electron-beam computed tomographic coronary angiography for segmental analysis of coronary artery stenosis. Am J Cardiol 31:1547–1554

Schroeder S, Kopp A, Baumbach A et al. (2001) Noninvasive detection and evalutation of atherosclerotic coronary plaque with multislice computed tomography. J Am Coll Cardiol 37:1430–1435

Virmani R, Kolodgie FD, Burke AP, Frab A, Schwartz SM (2000) Lessons from sudden coronary death. A comprehensive morphological classification scheme for atherosclerotic lesions. Arterioscler Thromb Vasc Biol 20:1262–1275

Vogl TJ, Abolmaali ND, Diebold T et al. (2002) Techniques for the detection of coronary atherosclerosis: multi-detector row CT coronary angiography. Radiology 223:212–220

Wexler L, Brundage B, Crouse J et al. (1996) Coronary artery calcification: pathophysiology, epidemiology, imaging methods, and clinical implications. A statement for health professionals from the American Heart Association. Circulation 94:1175–1192

Ziada K, Kapadia S, Tuzcu E, Nissen S (1999) The current status of intravascular ultrasound imaging. Curr Prob Cardiol 24:541–566

Data Management

23 Workflow Design for MDCT of the Thorax

R. Loose, S. Schaller, M. Oldendorf

CONTENTS

23.1 Introduction

Since the introduction of the powerful tool of CT into clinical radiology approximately 30 years ago (Hounsfield 1973), technical improvements have been made with steps of 20–50% with regard to the speed of scanning or image reconstruction (Nagel 2000; Kalender et al. 1990). Two major leaps were the introduction of the slip-ring technique with continuous rotation of X-ray tube and detector and the spiral technique (Kalender et al. 1990). The first two-detector spiral scanner was introduced by Elscint (Haifa, Israel) in 1994. The introduction of the first 4-row multi-detector CT systems (MDCT) in 1998 with 0.5-s rotation time increased both, scanning speed and scan volume, up to 800% in comparison with standard single-detector scanners with 1-s rotation time and by 600% in comparison with the fastest 0.75-s scanners. Within 2 years several manufacturers developed 16-row scanners with rotation times down to 0.4 s. Presently, MDCT scanners with 2, 4, 6, 8, 10, and 16 rows are available with rotation times of approximately 0.4 s. Whereas the advantages of increased scanning speed, fewer motion artifacts, and more thinner slices are obvious, it is less clear how to deal with the massive amounts of data generated by MDCT. Major unresolved issues relate to data storage, access and transfer across networks, remote access, viewing of images, and workflow. Besides general considerations, personal results are based on 3 years of experience with a 4-row MDCT system (Somatom VolumeZoom, Siemens, Erlangen, Germany) and some weeks of experience with a new 6-row MDCT system (Emotion 6, Siemens) at the Hospital Nuremberg-North with an annual frequency of 11,000 examinations at both CT scanners. The following considerations focus on scan protocols, postprocessing, network communication, storage, and workflow.

R. Loose, MD, PhD
Institut für diagnostische und interventionelle Radiologie, Klinikum Nürnberg-Nord, Prof.-Ernst-Nathan-Strasse 1, 90419 Nürnberg, Germany
S. Schaller, PhD
Siemens Medical Systems, Siemensstrasse 1, 91301 Forchheim, Germany
M. Oldendorf, MD
Institut für diagnostische und interventionelle Radiologie, Klinikum Nürnberg-Nord, Prof.-Ernst-Nathan-Strasse 1, 90419 Nürnberg, Germany

23.2 Scan Protocols and Data Volumes

If MDCT is used in clinical routine and not only in scientific research projects, most of the thorax examinations can be performed with only two different collimations. Table 23.1 shows as an example different combinations of beam collimation and readout of adaptive detector arrays for 16-row scanners which are provided by General Electric (Milwaukee, Wis.), Philips (Eindhoven, The Netherlands), Siemens (Erlangen, Germany), and Toshiba (Tokyo, Japan). Spiral data sets can be acquired in a range from 16×0.5 to 16×2 mm with these systems. In over 90% of all examinations we use the wider of both available collimations if only axial slices have to be generated. If any 3D postprocessing, such as multiplanar reconstruction (MPR), maximum intensity projection (MIP), or Volume Rendering Technique (VRT), is planned, the thinner collimation is recommended

Table 23.1. Specification of 16-row MDCT scanners

Manufacturer	Scanner	Minimum rotation time (s)	Rows	Detection length (mm)	Collimations (mm)
GE	LightSpeed-16	0.5	16	20	16 0.63, 16 1.25
Philips	Mx8000 Infinite	0.4	16	24	16 0.75, 16 1.5
Siemens	Sensation-16	0.4	16	24	16 0.75, 16 1.5
Toshiba	Aquilion-16	0.4	16	32	16 0 .5, 16 1, 16 2

as long as the scan time does not exceed the patient's maximal breath-hold time. Furthermore, aspects of data volume, X-ray tube load, and patient dose have to be considered when scan protocols with thin slices are used. The smaller detectors in the center of an adaptive array have a slightly lower geometric efficiency than the detectors at the margin of the array which results in higher patient dose for constant signal-to-noise ratio. Data volume and X-ray tube load both increase with decreasing slice width.

As an example, the raw and slice data volume of a 16-row MDCT thorax examination is estimated (scan length 300 mm, collimation 16×0.75 mm, pitch 1.5, reconstruction increment 0.5 mm). The number of reconstructed slices will be 300/0.5=600 if no additional postprocessing is done. In case of reconstructions with different kernels or generation of MPR or MIP images, the volume of image data may easily exceed 1000 slices or 500 Megabytes. The MDCT scanner Sensation 16 (Siemens) uses 672 channels with 1160 samples per rotation at 0.5-s rotation speed and 2320 samples at 0.75 s (flying focal spot). After 17 tube rotations, the whole scan volume is covered with a raw data volume of 1160 samples 672 channels 16 rows 2 bytes/pixel 17 rotations = 424 Megabytes at 0.5 s or 848 Megabytes at 0.75 s. With an assumed frequency of 40 patients, the daily data volume of one MDCT scanner is in the range of 40 Gigabyte.

23.3 Postprocessing

After an incremental or spiral scan with a single- or multidetector CT, the raw data set holds the highest degree of information and is used for reconstruction of slices with individual parameters such as slice thickness, reconstruction increment, and filter (kernel). After the raw data have been deleted, any further postprocessing has to be done with the reconstructed images with fewer capabilities. The need for images with good spatial resolution (bone, HR lung) and good contrast detectability (soft tissue) is the reason why raw data sets have to be processed several times with different filters. In addition, MDCT scanners allow the reconstruction of images with a wide range of the slice thickness. As MDCT scanners are not only used to improve the scanning speed, but also to acquire more and thinner slices, the data volume of the same examination is two to four times higher with MDCTs. Table 23.2 gives a survey of the typical number of slices for different examinations and postprocessings. Normally, CT images are reconstructed with reconstruction increments, which are in the range of the slice thickness with gaps, contiguous or overlapping slices. If one tries to achieve coronal, sagittal, or oblique slices – like MRI – with highest image quality, the reconstruction increments have to be small (50–70%) in comparison with the slice thickness. These widely overlapping slices are used as temporary data for further reconstructions in any orientation and, in fact, such a complex examination can easily exceed a total number of 1000 images (Deichen et al. 2000; Oldendorf et al. 2000; Loose et al. 2000).

The CT examinations of skull base, temporal bone, or facial sinuses often require two scans, one axial and one coronal, if single-slice scanners are used. As CT examinations of the thorax can be performed only with axial scans, all MPR or MIP postprocessings with coronal, sagittal, or oblique orientations need a large data set of thin axial slices.

Another postprocessing technique, which is well known from MR angiography, is the MIP. Without application of a threshold, the contiguous images of a volume data set are superimposed. This technique is used, for example, for a better detectability of pulmo-

Table 23.2. Typical number of slices for different MDCT scan protocols of the thorax and optional postprocessing. *MIP* maximum intensity projection, *VRT* Volume Rendering Technique

Reconstruction increment 1 mm, scan length 300 mm	300 slices
Reconstruction increment 0.5 mm, scan length 300 mm	600 slices
Additional coronal and sagittal reconstructions	200–600 slices
Oblique reformations, MIPs, or VRT	200–400 slices

nary nodules in lung cancer screening. In an animal osteosarcoma model, the detection rate of pulmonary nodules with MIP technique was twice as high as with MPR technique (Coakley et al. 1998). To avoid a misregistration of nodules at borderlines of MIP slabs, the slabs should be reconstructed with a 10–20% overlap.

Volume Rendering Technique (VRT) enables a very good pseudorealistic visualization of anatomical structures, but the creation of these images was time-consuming. Certain colors or gray levels are mapped to certain ranges of Hounsfield units with the additional option of cutting off unnecessary anatomical details. In clinical routine the number of patients where we use VRT is below 1% of all examinations.

23.4 Network Communication and Storage

In clinical networks MDCT scanners produce a very high network load. The large number of slices requires networks with a high bandwidth and archives with high storage capacity, as one MDCT scanner can easily produce several Terabyte of data per year. As mentioned previously, data volumes of 500 Megabyte per examination or more have to be managed. The transmission of such data packages in a 10-Megabit Ethernet would produce an unacceptable long continuous burst of data over 8 min with 100% network load. Furthermore, such high network loads over several minutes may cause timeouts or a crash of other software applications in the same segment of the network. Hence, it is highly recommended to operate MDCT scanners in "intelligent" networks with appropriate segmentation (min. switched Ethernet with 100 Mbit/s) and fast backbones (min. 1 Gigabit/s). The network load of imaging modalities should be kept out of all segments where images are not needed. Even under real conditions in a switched 100-Mbit/s network, we observed transfer rates of approximately 10 CT slices per second which is 50% of the maximum speed. The transmission time of a 500-image data set to a workstation is in the range of 1 min. As the transmission speed over external networks (wireless LAN, DSL, ISDN) for teleradiology is approximately two magnitudes slower, only selected and reduced data sets should be transferred.

When CT data sets are acquired with non-isotropic voxels (wide collimation and large slice thickness), only the raw data sets of these CT examinations provide all capabilities of slice reconstructions. As additional clinical questions may arise 1 or 2 days after the examination, the temporary storage of the raw data is extremely important. The CT raw data are not DICOM-compatible, and hence, storage in PACS archives is not possible. With normal configuration and patient throughput the internal hard disk of an MDCT holds the raw data for less than 1 day. In fact, we have doubled the raw data storage space in our MDCT.

A solution to reduce the storage volume is image compression. "Lossless" algorithms allow a reduction of storage volumes by a factor of 2–3, whereas "lossy" algorithms, such as JPEG, JPEG2000, or Wavelet, enable a reduction factor of 10 or more without visible reduction of image quality. Whereas there are many studies about image compression, no clear guidelines about compression algorithm and compression level exist for the daily routine.

In a clinical network with a PACS archive, laser imagers, reporting workstations, postprocessing workstations, workstations for clinical conferences, and the ward image viewers, different data sets have to be sent to these destinations. All the very thin slices with small reconstruction increments could be used as temporary data only for further reconstructions and hence need not be archived. Nevertheless, PACS archives are overloaded with all these images as there is no definition or recommendation as to which images are for temporary and which are for permanent use. All steps of image reconstruction, postprocessing, storage, and network communication have been done manually in the past and were very time-consuming. Current developments are combined protocols for data acquisition, postprocessing, and network distribution, which can be configured individually with regard to the workflow, the anatomical structures, and the questions of the referring physicians (Loose et al. 2000).

23.5 Workflow

23.5.1 General Developments in Routine Workflow

Historically, in CT we distinguish between inplane (or x–y) resolution and longitudinal (or z-) resolution. In the days of single-slice CT, the z-resolution was determined before the data acquisition by selecting an appropriate collimation. The x–y resolution could still be changed retrospectively during the image reconstruction by selecting the desired kernel (Kalender 1995).

Starting with the introduction of multi-slice CT systems in 1998, the workflow changed towards routine thin-slice acquisition. This led to a change in paradigm, because the desired slice width could now be selected after the data had been acquired by choosing it appropriately in the spiral image reconstruction (Klingenbeck-Regn et al. 1999; Hu et al. 2000; Ohnesorge et al. 1999; Flohr et al. 2000a, 2000b; Schaller et al., in press). As an example, the SureView image reconstruction concept allowed reconstruction of a variety of slice thicknesses even after a data set had been acquired at a given collimation. Yet, the x–y resolution and the z-resolution were still treated differently: one was selected via slice-thickness, the other via the kernel. This is also reflected in specifications, where in-plane resolution is characterized by a resolution measured in terms of line pairs per centimeter visible (lp/cm) and longitudinal resolution is given by specifying the full width at half maximum (FWHM) of the slice profile in the z-direction.

Presently, many users routinely perform multiple reconstructions with several different kernels and slice widths on a single data set. As an example, consider a thorax CT scan. The choice of reconstruction settings always is a tradeoff between image noise and resolution in x–y and z. For high-resolution lung images, it is desirable to reconstruct narrow slices using a fairly sharp kernel. These images are commonly viewed using wide window settings. Therefore, noise is not a major concern. However, when looking at the mediastinum, narrower window settings are used; hence, lower noise levels are desired. This is typically achieved by using larger slice thicknesses and smoother kernels. Furthermore, sometimes one set of thin-slice images is reconstructed for use on a postprocessing workstation, whereas a few thicker images are used for filming or archiving.

It has been shown that all of these different results can also be generated from one suitably reconstructed high-resolution set of volume data. If one stack of thin-slice images is reconstructed as an isotropic set of quasi-raw data, then thicker images can be generated by calculating thick MPRs, i.e., by averaging multiple images. Similarly, images corresponding to smoother kernels can be generated by using image filters on the high-resolution images; therefore, in the future, we anticipate a workflow where one standard reconstruction is performed, resulting in a high-resolution isotropic data set. All other manipulations will be performed on this volume data. All three spatial dimensions will be treated the same way.

23.5.2 Workflow Automation

Modern multi-slice CT scanners allow reconstruction of high-resolution reformatted images in the coronal or sagittal or oblique orientation. To this end, users must reconstruct several hundred thin-slice images, load these images into a 3D card, and produce the MPRs there. New software platforms have efficiently simplified these operations for routine use: images of a certain study type can be autoloaded into the 3D task after image reconstruction. There, predefined protocols are automatically called upon for further processing of the data; thus, for example, a thorax study can trigger reconstruction of many hundreds of images, these are autoloaded into 3D, and there automatic generation of few thick sagittal slices is performed. These sagittal slices are then archived. Figure 23.1 shows the automation task cards supplied by the Syngo software platform. To further simplify this routine procedure, a recent software version released on the Siemens Somatom Sensation 16 completely changes the paradigm and incorporates selection of the slice orientation into the acquisition platform. With this new software interface, the user directly selects an arbitrarily oriented slice as the primary output of the scan. Intermediate axial reconstruction results are hidden from the user for the sake of simplified usage and to avoid data congestion related to the need to reconstruct many hundreds of slices as an intermediate result.

One of the applications where this is of particular interest is cardiac CT imaging, where frequently short-axis images of the heart are desired. If reconstructions are to be performed in several different heart phases, the old paradigm meant reconstructing several sets of thin-slice images for all desired heart phases, loading each of those sets into a 3D application and performing the reformation, ideally all at the same orientation. The new paradigm makes the workflow a lot more efficient. One can now select the reconstruction range with arbitrary orientation of the primary images and then start reconstruction of all desired heart phases. Figure 23.2 shows the user interface.

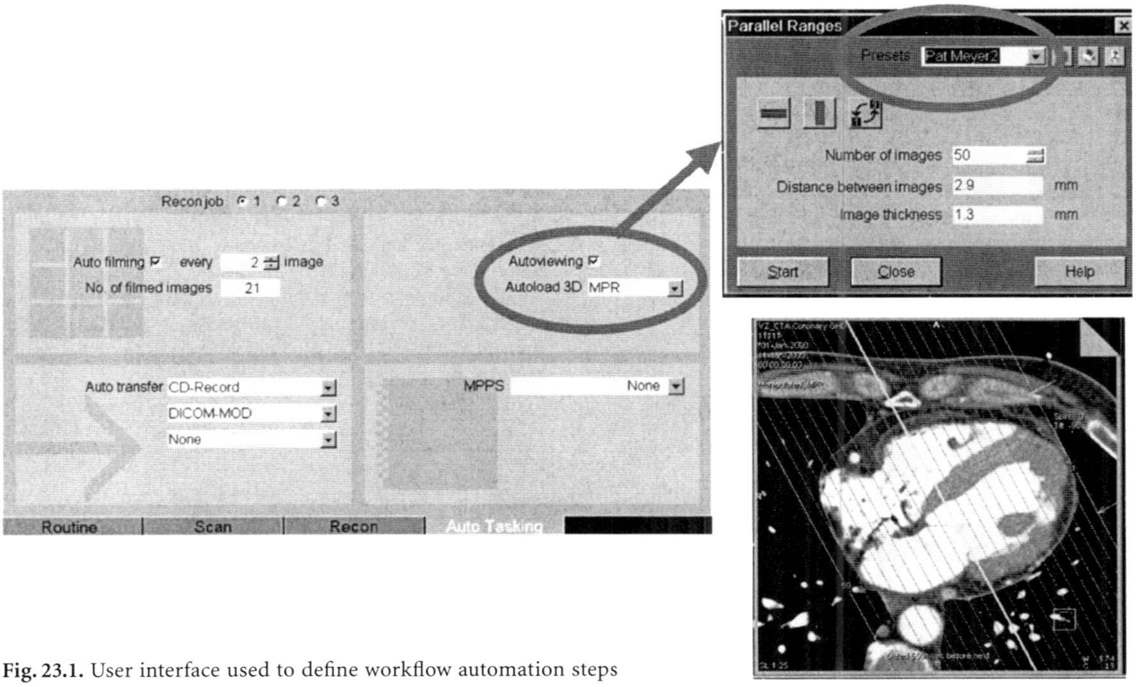

Fig. 23.1. User interface used to define workflow automation steps

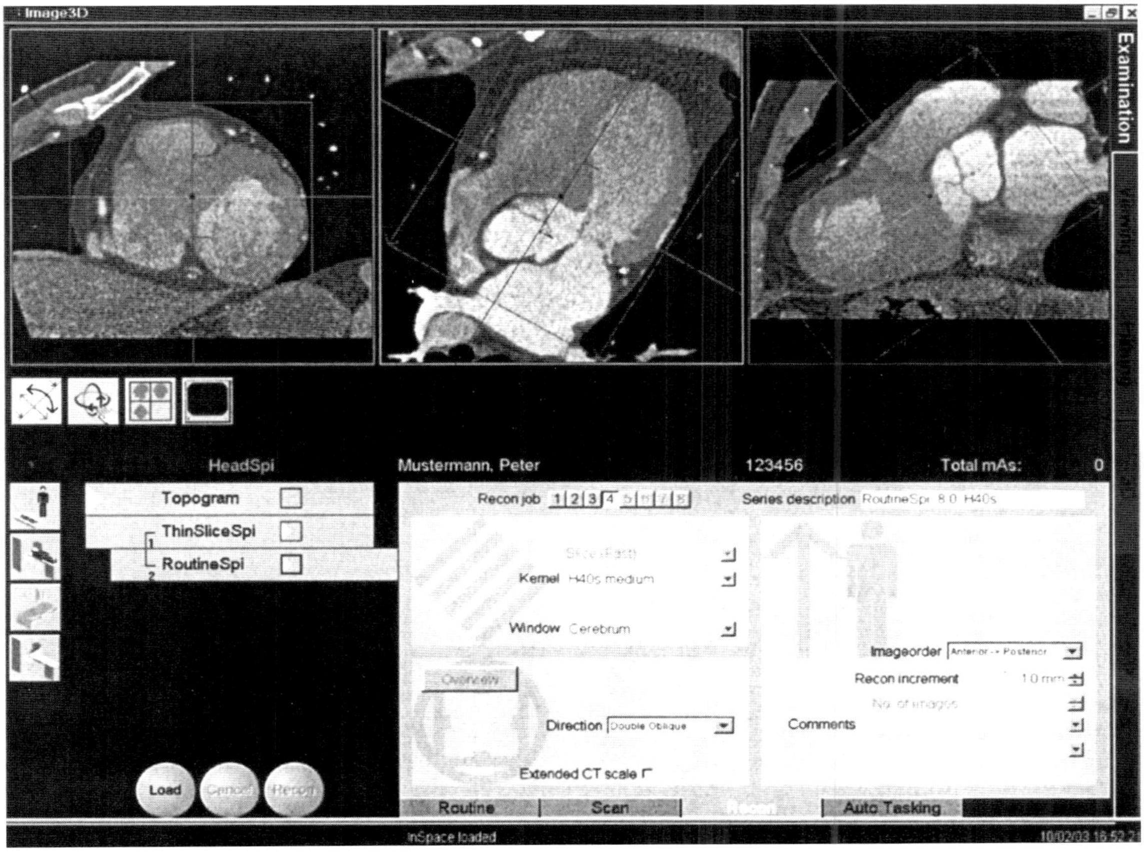

Fig. 23.2. Scan user interface for selection of arbitrarily oriented primary slices

References

Coakley FV, Cohen MD, Johnson MS, Gonin R, Hanna MP (1998) Maximum intensity projection images in the detection of simulated pulmonary nodules by spiral CT. Br J Radiol 71:135–140

Deichen JT, Detmar K, Oldendorf M, Loose RWR (2000) Multislice CT: image quality of primary coronal acquired images compared with secondary reformatted coronal images of primary axial acquired data. Eur Radiol 10 (Suppl 1):189

Flohr T, Stierstorfer K, Bruder H, Simon J, Schaller S (2002a) New technical developments in multislice CT. Part 1: Approaching isotropic resolution with sub-millimeter 16-slice scanning. Fortschr Röntgenstr 174:839–845

Flohr T, Bruder H, Stierstorfer K, Simon J, Schaller S, Ohnesorge B (2002b) New technical developments in multislice CT. Part 2: Sub-millimeter 16-slice scanning and increased gantry rotation speed for cardiac imaging. Fortschr Röntgenstr 174:1022–1027

Hounsfield GN (1973) Computerized transverse axial scanning (tomography). 1. Description of system. Br J Radiol 46:1016–1022

Hu H, He HD, Foley WD, Fox SH (2000) Four multidetector-row helical CT: image quality and volume coverage speed. Radiology 215:55–62

Kalender W (1995) Thin-section three-dimensional spiral CT: Is isotropic imaging possible? Radiology 197:578–580

Kalender WA, Vock P, Polacin A, Soucek M (1990) Spiral-CT: a new technique for volumetric scans. I. Basic principles and methodology. Rontgenpraxis 43:323–330

Klingenbeck-Regn K, Schaller S, Flohr T, Ohnesorge B, Kopp AF, Baum U (1999) Subsecond multi-slice computed tomography: basics and applications. Eur J Radiol 31:110–124

Loose R, Oldendorf M, Deichen JT, Wucherer M (2000) Management des Datenvolumens von Multizeilen-CT-Scannern. Fortschr Röntgenstr 172:133

Nagel HD (2000) Factors influencing patient dose in CT. In: Nagel HD (ed) Radiation exposure in computed tomography. COCIR c/o ZVEI Fachverband Elektromedizinische Technik, pp 25–43

Ohnesorge B, Flohr T, Schaller S, Klingenbeck-Regn K, Becker C, Schöpf UJ, Brüning R, Reiser MF (1999) Technische Grundlagen und Anwendungen der Mehrschicht-CT. Radiologe 39:923–931

Oldendorf M, Loose R, Wucherer M (2000) Mehrzeilen Spiral-CT des Thorax. Neue Scanprotokolle und sekundäre Nachverarbeitungstechniken. Fortschr Röntgenstr 172:18

Schaller S, Wildberger JE, Raupach R, Niethammer M, Klingenbeck-Regn K, Flohr T (in press) Spatial domain filtering for fast modification of the tradeoff between image sharpness and pixel noise in computed tomography. IEEE Trans Med Imaging

24 2D and 3D Visualization of Thoracic MDCT Data

L. P. LAWLER and E. K. FISHMAN

CONTENTS

24.1 Introduction

Multidetector-row CT (MDCT) data sets improve on the already established prowess of single-detector helical CT (SDCT) for thoracic imaging (HU et al. 2000; KLINGENBECK-REGN et al. 1999; KALENDER et al. 1990a,b; KALENDER and POLACIN 1991). Many anatomical features of the chest do not conform to a single two-dimensional (2D) axial plane and full exploitation of the isotropic and near isotropic MDCT data requires 2D and three-dimensional (3D) post-processing techniques to harness the added advantage of improved z-axis resolution and coverage (RAVENEL et al. 2001; REMY et al. 1998; LAWLER and FISHMAN 2001a; FISHMAN et al. 1991; KIRCHGEORG and PROKOP 1998). Data acquisition and processing as it relates to constructing the appropriate substrate for post-processing as well as the various 2D and 3D techniques are discussed. The clinical application of 2D and 3D visualization to bronchovascular structures, lung parenchyma, chest wall and diaphragm are addressed.

L. P. LAWLER, MD, FRCR
The Russell H. Morgan Department of Radiology and Radiological Science, Johns Hopkins Medical Institutions, 601 N. Caroline Street, Baltimore, MD 21287, USA
E. K. FISHMAN, MD, FACR
The Russell H. Morgan Department of Radiology and Radiological Science, Johns Hopkins Medical Institutions, 601 N. Caroline Street, Baltimore, MD 21287, USA

24.2 Two- and Three-Dimensional Post-Processing

Both optimal 2D and 3D studies require careful selection of the protocol for data acquisition (NEUMANN et al. 2000; RODENWALDT et al. 1997). Most current 2D and 3D studies are obtained from an 8-detector adaptive array system using 4-channel data acquisition though the principles of 2D and 3D visualization are the same for 16-detector arrays. For the majority of patients we employ the 1- or 2.5-mm detectors producing 1.25- or 3-mm slice widths, respectively. The larger detectors can be used with faster table translation for poor breathholders or where greater scan coverage is required. The 2D reconstructions can be made at any slice position or reconstruction interval. Unlike single detector systems, the slice width is not inextricably linked to the beam collimation and data acquired may be assimilated into larger slice widths, which are of higher quality than similarly sized single-detector slices. The smallest slice width available is equal to the smallest detector applied. Cardiac images with decreased motion may be obtained using the fast temporal resolution of MDCT together with prospective or retrospective cardiac gating.

The 2D slices with a 512 matrix are fashioned from the helical data by a number of techniques of interpolation, which aim to approximate a true planar slice from the helical data set. Although there is some widening of the slice-sensitivity profile, increased pitch has less deleterious effects on effective slice width compared with single-detector systems (KLINGENBECK-REGN et al. 1999; BRINK et al. 1992). Both 180 or 360° linear interpolation deduces the slice data from adjacent helices 180 and 360° apart. The 2D data from 180° linear interpolation has a higher temporal resolution and smaller effective slice width (LOUBEYRE et al. 1997). Filter width interpolation is an MDCT technique that derives the slice data from a series of detector information not just the helices immediately adjacent to the designated slice. For high-resolution imaging (e.g. interstitial lung disease or chest wall bone imaging) a high spatial frequency reconstruction kernel is used, whereas a soft tissue kernel is best for most other protocols including routine chest, mediastinal and angiographic imaging. Multiplanar and curved multiplanar (MPR and CMPR) are 2D techniques that provide alternate viewing perspectives usually with conventional window settings (Richenberg and Hansell 1998). These images are a re-ordering of the voxels into 1-voxel-thick tomographic sections excluding those voxels outside the imaging plane, and they require minimal computer power. A curved line may be drawn to include an entire structure that does not lie in a single plane (CMPR).

The 3D visualization provides both a means to manage the large data sets of MDCT and to obtain novel perspectives on diseases of the chest with near-isotropic and isotropic data sets. The main 3D techniques currently available include shaded-surface display (SSD), maximum intensity projection (MIP), minimum intensity projection (MinIP) and volume rendering (VR; Remy et al. 1998; Richenberg and Hansell 1998; Calhoun et al. 1999; Johnson et al. 1996, 1998; Schreiner et al. 1996; Pavone et al. 2001). Shaded-surface display reformats the data around a threshold that defines the interface of tissues. The 3D surface is then simulated using polygon building-block reconstructions and lighting models (Ravenel et al. 2001; Remy et al. 1998). The SSD does not reveal internal detail and is used mainly for imaging the musculoskeletal components of the chest and can be used to show the mucosa surface of the airways (Hopper et al. 2000). The MIP casts a ray through the data and then only displays the data above a certain assigned value, reducing all the data in the ray to a single plane. It is most akin to a projectional technique and has been applied mainly to vascular imaging, although it has been mentioned to be of use for nodule detection. The MIP does not have any depth cues and the 3D relationships of structures are only appreciated by moving the image (Richenberg and Hansell 1998; Calhoun et al. 1999). The MinIP is the opposite of MIP and by displaying only data *below* a designated threshold is best suited for showing areas of lower density such as cystic change, emphysema or air trapping. The SSD, MIP and MinIP only display 10–20% of the data actually present and thus do not require large computer power (Napel et al. 1993).

Volume rendering is a quite unique form of 3D visualization of high fidelity to the originally acquired data with preservation of depth cues and spatial relationships (Fishman et al. 1991; Calhoun et al. 1999; Johnson et al. 1996, 1998; Kuszyk et al. 1996). In this process a ray is cast through the data and a weighted representation of all the Hounsfield units encountered is displayed depending on their representation within the tissues including voxels only partially filled with a density of interest. A histogram representation of the data may be generated (trapezoid) and then manipulated through various tools that display the data to best effect such as internal or external perspectives (Ferretti et al. 2001). There is depth information present and various levels of opacity can be assigned to tissues of interest. Volume rendering has been applied to all areas of chest CT.

Regardless of the 3D processing technique employed the editing steps must be quick and efficient. Laborious segmentation of data using slice-by-slice regions of interest is not acceptable in clinical practice. With volume rendering a region of interest may be drawn on a large volume of data at once. Clip plane editing is used to remove slabs of data in an infinite number of planes and can be performed in a real-time manner to remove overlying chest wall and can be customized to isolate individual bronchi. Sliding thin-slab (STS) MIP and MinIP can be used to provide a scrolling projection of extreme attenuation values contained within multiple sections of lung tissue of 5- to 10-mm thickness (Napel et al. 1993). Infinite manipulation of viewing perspective with frame rates over 20 frames per second are also a requisite for a viable 3D tool.

The choice of image display is hard or soft copy. Hard-copy imaging is satisfactory for routine axial planar imaging, but picture archiving and communications systems with cine scrolling are preferred with smaller slice widths and intervals where larger image numbers are generated. All 3D studies are interpreted on soft-copy workstations, which allow real-time clinical consultation, although select hard-copy images can be generated to go with the report or into the patient file.

24.3 High-Resolution Chest Imaging

When high-resolution chest CT is requested the clinical question usually relates to interstitial lung disease. Our interest centers on the secondary pulmonary lobule, the functional unit of the lung made up of terminal bronchovascular structures and alveoli gathered within connective tissue septations that carry lymphatic drainage (Bergin et al. 1988). The 2D MDCT can visualize these units with a detail that approximates gross pathological inspection (Engeler et al. 1994). Unlike single-detector imaging, MDCT using 1-mm detectors can generate both the low-noise larger slice widths necessary for general chest evaluation as well as the high-resolution 1.25-mm slice widths required for interstitial study. It is not necessary to perform a second acquisition at preselected levels and dedicated reconstruction of areas of interest is possible before the raw data is deleted. This has practical implication with regard to many of the interstitial disease processes, which have static and dynamic patterns of distribution that may favor various disparate parts of the lung. Inspiratory and expiratory scans are performed to assess for air trapping and mosaic pattern, whereas alternate prone and supine imaging can differentiate true disease from basal atelectasis (Kinsella et al. 1990). Some authors advocate printing or displaying high-resolution images with a smaller field of view dedicated to one lung with side-by-side display of alternate phase or posture images to aid direct comparison.

The 2D reconstructions have high sensitivity for the detection of many of the signs of interstitial and airspace disease including septal lines, fibrosis, bronchiectasis, and alveolar filling. By their nature, many interstitial lung diseases are multifocal with asymmetry both superior to inferior and right to left. These complex distributions of disease can be reduced to single succinct images with MPR and VR which can better depict the relative severity of certain areas of disease and may provide better reproducibility for longitudinal follow-up of response to therapy or progression (Figs. 24.1–24.4). The MinIP reconstructions have been shown to be sensitive for the detection of areas of low attenuation such as cystic change or air trapping (e.g. emphysema; Fig. 24.5; Park et al. 1999; Kauczor et al. 1996; Mergo et al. 1998) and it has been suggested that MIP and STS–MIP images better depict centrilobular nodules (Remy-Jardin et al. 1996a; Bhalla et al. 1996). For focal severe bron-

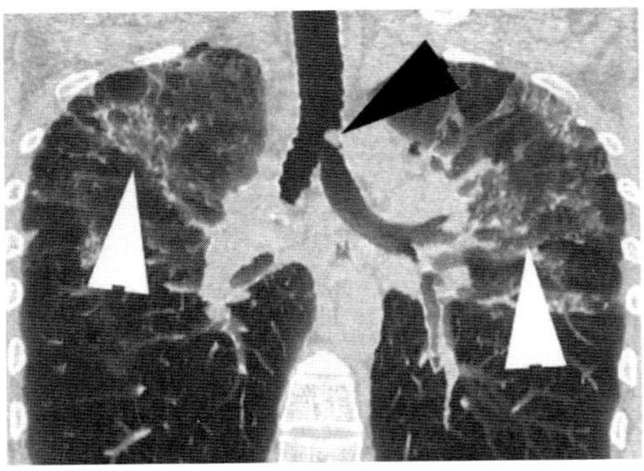

Fig. 24.1. Volume-rendered (VR) anteroposterior (AP) view of upper lobe predominant interstitial fibrosis (*white arrowheads*). Filling defect in trachea (*black arrowhead*)

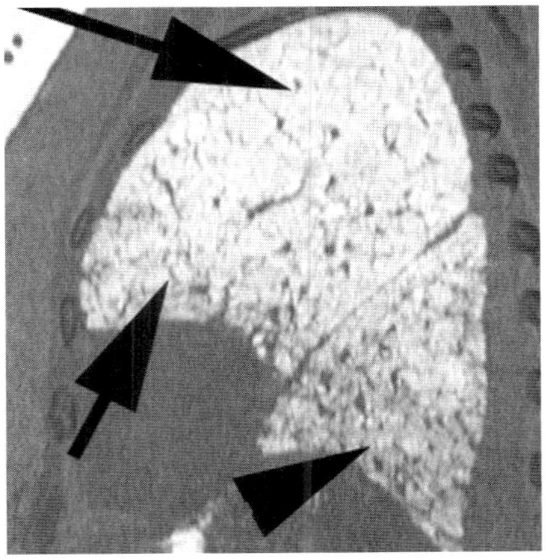

Fig. 24.2. A VR lateral view of lower lobe (*arrowhead*) and lingular (*short arrow*) fibrosis with relative sparing of the upper lung (*long arrow*)

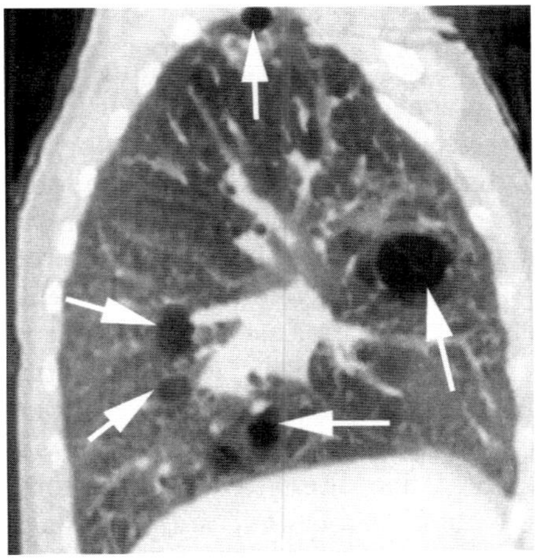

Fig. 24.3. Right lateral VR image of cystic change related to tuberous sclerosis (*arrows*)

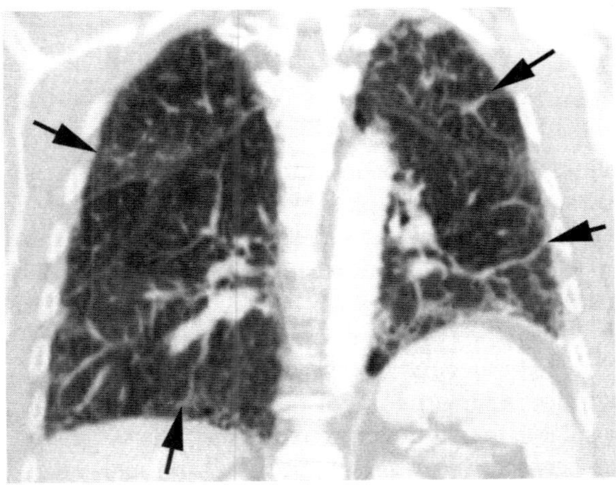

Fig. 24.4. An AP VR view of interstitial lung disease demonstrating greater loss of volume on the left and septal lines throughout (*arrows*)

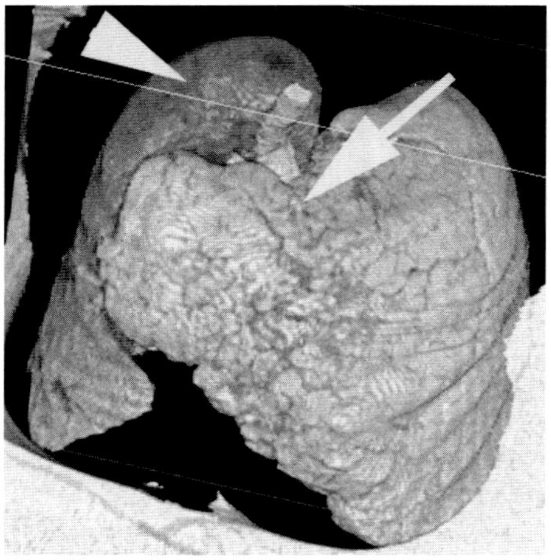

Fig. 24.5. A left lateral oblique view of a hyperinflated emphysematous left lung (*arrow*) using solid trapezoids. Right lung normal volume noted (*arrowhead*)

chiectatic or emphysematous change limited lung resection can be planned and followed up (Holbert et al. 1996) using VR data to establish the anatomical distribution of disease and normal lung and tailored images can be correlated with selected nuclear medicine ventilation/perfusion images (Thurnheer et al. 1999). The CT density and volume measurements (Brown et al. 1999) do correlate with pulmonary function tests (Mergo et al. 1998; Hoffmann et al. 1995), and it is hoped that through volume and perfusion measurements of the lung in various phases of respiration MDCT may ultimately provide a comprehensive evaluation of anatomic and functional derangements in a single examination (Park et al. 1999; Hoffman et al. 1995; Arakawa et al. 2001).

24.4 Airway Imaging

Both CT and endoscopic bronchoscopy contributed to the demise of conventional bronchography (Newmark et al. 1994). Whereas 2D CT can provide much of the information on lumen, wall and extramural structures of the tracheobronchial tree, bronchoscopy can better discern mucosal detail, sample tissues and intervene when necessary. Airway studies require the use of the narrowest collimation available for the coverage required with overlapping reconstruction. Although most fields of view extend from above the thoracic inlet to diaphragm, any clinical questions regarding the glottic or subglottic area require extension to the hypopharynx. In an effort to limit dose exposure, dynamic inspiratory and expiratory imaging is reserved for those patients with a clear clinical suspicion of bronchomalacia where a management benefit can be demonstrated (Goldin and Aberle 1997). The 2D interpretation of caliber change, irregularity and the anatomic distribution of abnormality are best achieved on lung windows, whereas mediastinal windows better depict mural thickening or calcification or the extramural relationship of pathology (Curtin et al. 1998).

The CT of the airways can best serve the pulmonologist and bronchoscopist when interpreted together with 3D reconstructions, which improve accuracy and confidence in the readings (Quint et al. 1995; LoCicero et al. 1996; Lacrosse et al. 1995; Ney et al. 1990). These images provide sophisticated maps of tracheobronchial abnormalities and their exact relation to recognized anatomic landmarks that can be seen on endoscopy. In select cases 3D CT can obviate the need for bronchoscopy, in particular for follow-up of caliber change. Although MPR can be helpful (Quint et al. 1995; Remy-Jardin et al. 1996b), the preferred technique is either SSD or VR using a wide range of trapezoids, projections and clip planes tailored to individual oblique branching airways to increase the conspicuity of disease (Figs. 24.6, 24.7; Remy-Jardin et al. 1998). Solid- or luminal-view trapezoids with increased opacity are best to depict airway filling defects, whereas these and bronchography-like images can be used for mapping caliber change such as stenoses or bronchiectasis. Surface rendering and VR have been used to produce endoscopic simulations of the airway, and technologies that aid in finding the centerline for fly-through evaluation have been explored (Ferretti et al. 1996, 2000, 2001; Naidich and Harkin 1996; Naidich et

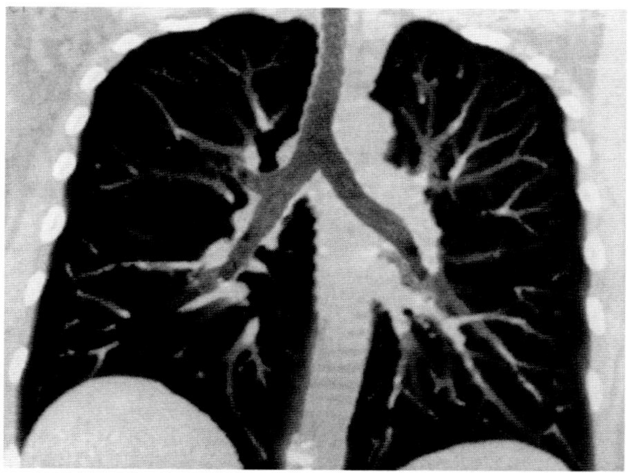

Fig. 24.6. A VR AP view of the airways using a luminal trapezoid

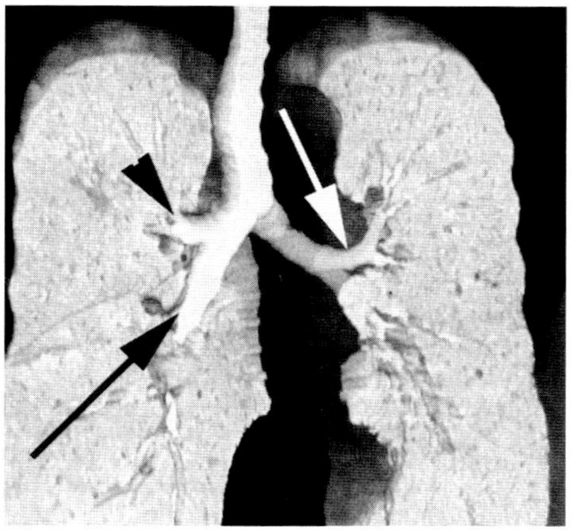

Fig. 24.7. Airway anatomy with solid trapezoids, AP view. Right upper lobe (*arrowhead*), lingual/left upper lobe (*white arrow*), right lower lobe (*black arrow*)

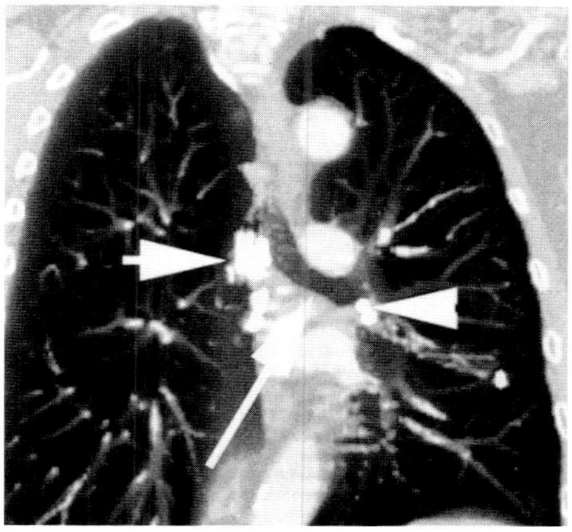

Fig. 24.8. A broncholith (*arrowhead*) is seen eroding into the left lower lobe bronchus (*long arrow*) on this AP VR image of a patient with extensive calcified mediastinal lymph nodes (*short arrow*)

al. 1997; Fleiter et al. 1997; Gluecker et al. 2001; Becker 1999; Colt et al. 2001; Haponik et al. 1999). Such virtual endoscopic or perspective VR images (Liewald et al. 1998) are not widely applied as they seldom give added information in a patient who has already had bronchoscopy, and they cannot reproduce the hue and texture accurately (Aquino and Vining 1999); however, virtual CT bronchoscopy incorporated into 3D information of extraluminal information can provide unique additional information such as safe routes for tracheobronchial biopsy (McAdams et al. 1998a; Bricault et al. 1998). There is an increasing use of expandable endoprostheses for benign and malignant disease and trapezoids to depict the stent and the airway can be designed (Lehman et al. 1998).

Congenital abnormalities of the airway can be difficult to discern on 2D images alone and endoscopic evaluation can be limited by small airway caliber (Manson et al. 1994); however, accessory and atretic bronchi or bronchi with abnormal angulation (e.g. bridging bronchus) are conspicuous on 3D studies and together with 3D CT angiography bronchovascular evaluation of rings and slings (Katz et al. 1995; Hopkins et al. 1996) can be achieved (Dunham and Wolf 1996). Airway filling defects are usually detected on close inspection of 2D studies with lung windows. Volume-rendered studies better define such abnormalities as filling defects within otherwise normal airway images (Figs. 24.8, 24.9). Secondary invasion of the airway can be evaluated using 2D axial and MPR mediastinal windows or VR reconstructions that display both airway and extrinsic tissues to best effect. Defects in the wall due to tracheoesophageal fistula

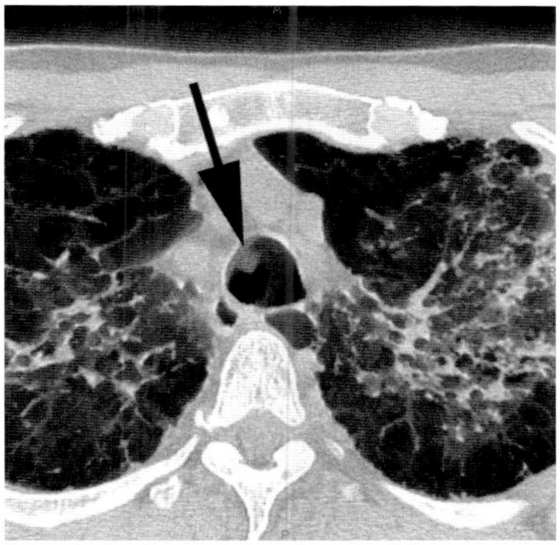

Fig. 24.9. A fibrovascular polyp (*arrow*) is seen on a VR image with a perspective down the airway

can be mapped for possible resection and reconstruction (Fig. 24.10). Coronal or sagittal MPR and 3D studies are of particular value to demonstrate thin in-plane webs of the upper airway (Quint et al. 1995; LoCicero et al. 1996). Tracheobronchial stenoses are optimally seen with 3D reconstructions (Figs. 24.11, 24.12; McAdams et al. 1998b). Although discrete caliber change of tracheobronchial tree can be appreciated on serial axial 2D images, more subtle tapering and bronchiectasis is best demonstrated with 3D coronal or sagittal reconstructions using bronchography or solid airway trapezoids (Kauczor et al. 1996). Dedicated clip planes and projections are superior to measure the exact length of oblique running airways and are useful to provide consistent images for follow-up inflamma-

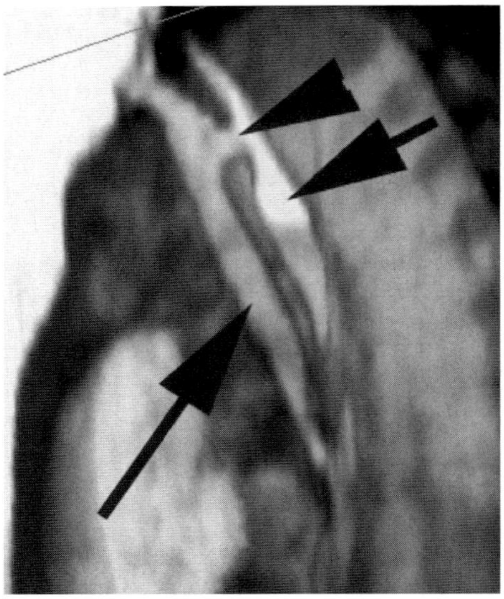

Fig. 24.10. A tracheo-esophageal fistula in the upper trachea due to carcinoma is seen (*arrowhead*) extending between the trachea (*long arrow*) and esophagus (*short arrow*) on this lateral VR image

tory stenoses (e.g. Wegener's). With the increasing use of self-expandable endoprostheses to restore or maintain airway patency for benign and malignant conditions 2D and 3D CT is of value (Fig. 24.13; Wilson et al. 1996; Doi et al. 1999; Nicholson 1998) . The 2D visualization can provide at thorough assessment of the etiology and complications of stenoses and assess the parenchyma for likelihood of benefit from attempts to relieve the obstruction. The 3D reconstructions are used to determine the ability of the bronchoscopist to traverse the narrowing and to customize the stent graft (Zwischenberger et al. 1997). Non-invasive follow-up can be provided by CT using internal and external VR and bronchoscopic exams can be reserved for stent salvage or replacement. Airway dilatation (bronchiectasis) can be mapped in relation to remaining normal lung parenchyma to assess response to therapy and aid possible surgical resection (Fig. 24.14)

24.5 Nodules and Masses

Lung nodules and masses can be well evaluated using 2D interpretation. Three-millimeter slice widths from 2.5-mm detectors with a soft tissue reconstruction kernel usually provide all the information on shape, size, borders, multiplicity and attenuation profile. Some authors have suggested that the 2D contrast dynamics of lung nodules can aid the differentiation

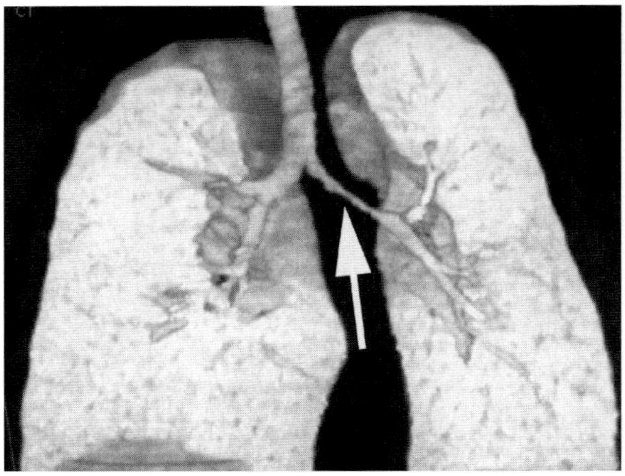

Fig. 24.11. A long left lower lobe stenosis (*arrow*) due to Wegener's granulomatosis is seen on this solid trapezoid, AP VR view

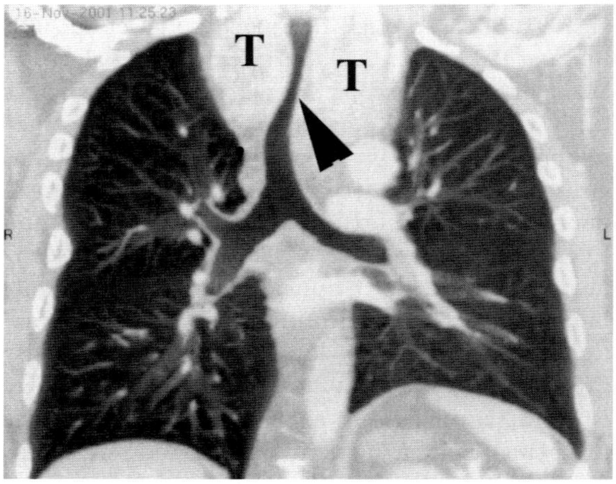

Fig. 24.12. Tracheal stenosis (*arrowhead*) due to a substernal goiter (*T*) is depicted on this AP VR view

of benign and malignant disease. The MIP has been shown to improve depiction and diagnosis of small nodules compared with axial 2D and MPR image interpretation (Eibel et al. 2001). Superior sulcus tumors (Pancoast tumors) are best seen with coronal reformations of the chest apex (Fig. 24.15). Likewise, diaphragmatic surface lesions that can be hard to differentiate from liver lesions can be discriminated on sagittal plane interpretation (Fig. 24.16). For both benign and malignant small nodules surgical consultation for the resection approach is facilitated by a multidimensional map which can facilitate segment-sparing surgery (Fig. 24.17). The MPR images are used to map PET studies to CT either by computer fusion of data from different machines or with synchronous

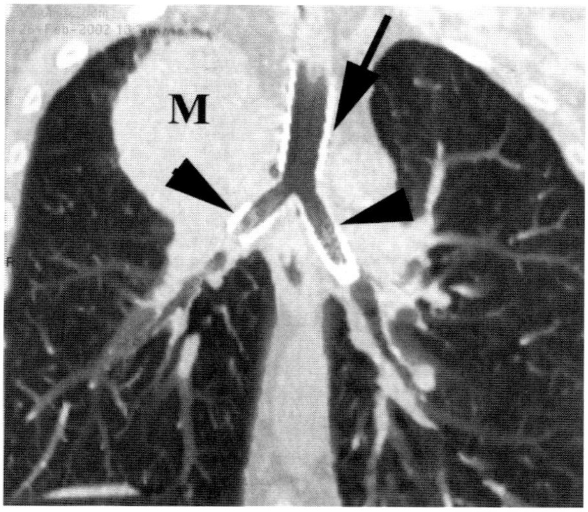

Fig. 24.13. Tracheal (*arrow*) and bronchial (*arrowheads*) stents were placed in this patient to prevent compromise by an encroaching right upper lung mass (*M*)

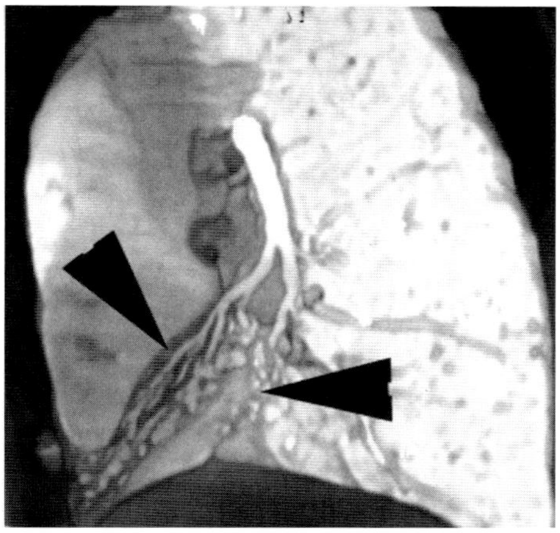

Fig. 24.14. Focal bronchiectatic change (*arrowheads*) in the right lung is seen on this left lateral VR view

PET and CT scanning on a single machine. The images are usually visualized with planar axial, coronal, and sagittal reformations, although there is great potential for 3D volume studies to be used in the future.

For TNM staging of lung cancer off-coronal VR that shows the central extent of a medial lung mass and accurately names the lymph node chain involved can better serve the surgeon and oncologist in deciding on possible sleeve resection or alternate therapy (Fig. 24.18). All lung mass locations can be described indirectly with reference to landmarks on the patient body surface or on the chest X-ray to aid definition of the field for 3D radiation therapy that aims to treat the tumor with minimal ill effects to the normal tis-

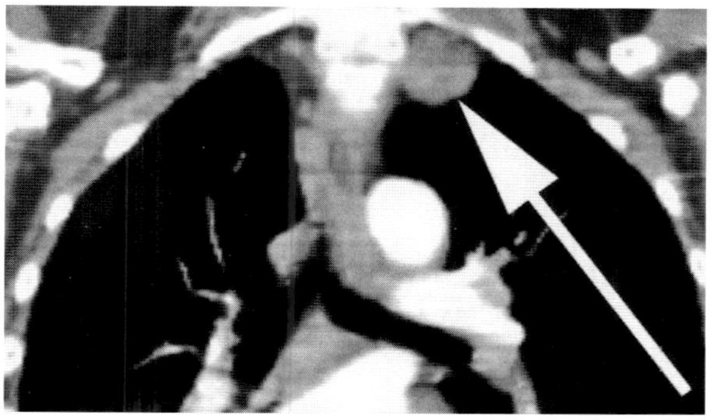

Fig. 24.15. In this patient a left apical lesion (*arrow*) consistent with a nerve sheath tumor is seen on coronal MPR

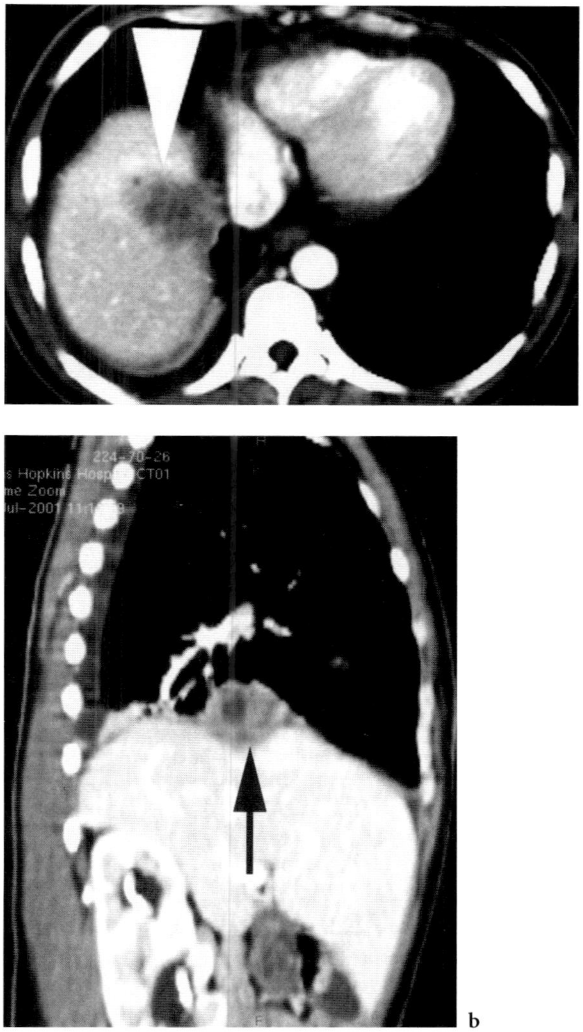

a

b

Fig. 24.16. **a** It is unclear whether this lesion is in the lower lung or in the dome of diaphragm (*arrowhead*). **b** A right sagittal MPR clearly shows this lesion (*arrow*) to be in the lower lung making an impression on the liver, not vice versa

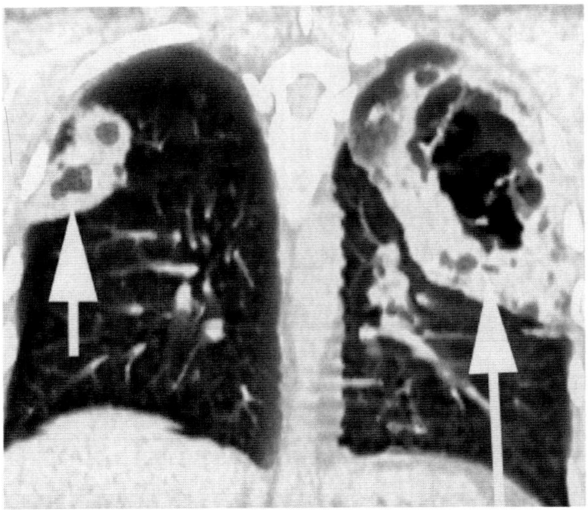
a

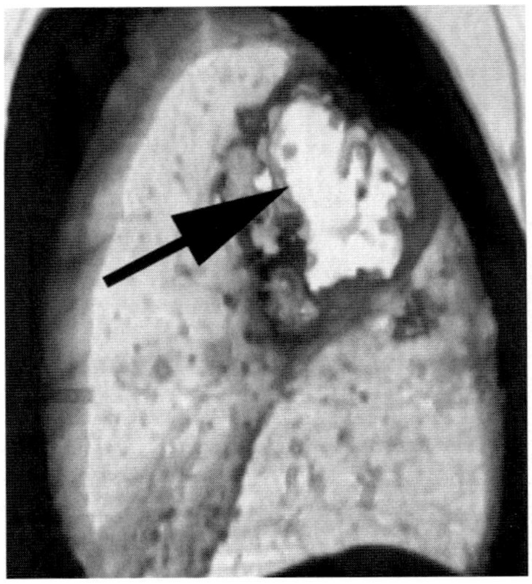
b

Fig. 24.17. **a** Cavitary masses in the right and left upper lungs (*arrows*) seen on this AP VR view. **b** A left lateral VR image better demonstrates the site of the cavitary lesion in the left upper lung (*arrow*)

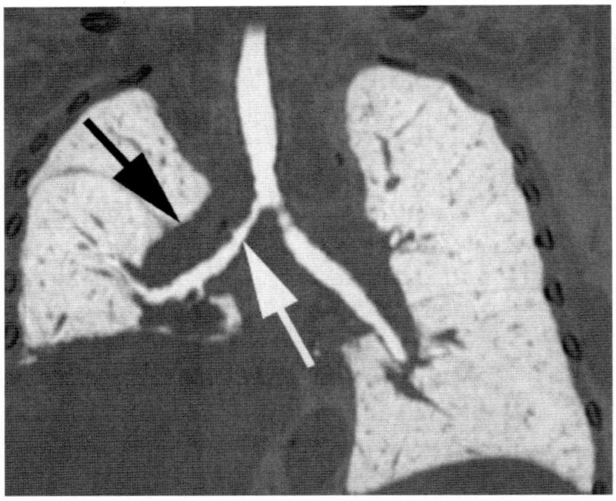
a

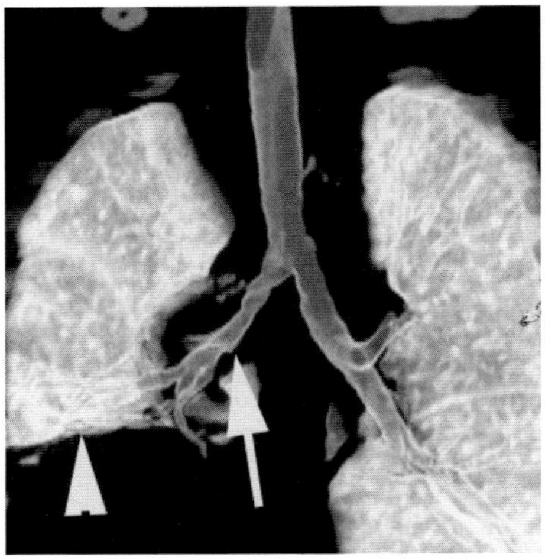
b

Fig. 24.18. **a** A right hilar mass (*black arrow*) extends medially causing significant stenosis of the right lower bronchus (*white arrow*) causing partial lung collapse and precluding surgical resection (solid trapezoid). **b** A right hilar mass (*black arrow*) extends medially causing significant stenosis of the right lower bronchus (*white arrow*) causing partial lung collapse and precluding surgical resection (bronchography trapezoid)

sues (Vuong et al. 2000; Armstrong 1998; Leibel et al. 1992). Most CT-guided biopsies use limited 2D with static or CT fluoroscopic acquisition. Individual bronchi can be followed on 2D CT and 3D visualization to provide maps for bronchoscopic, mediastinoscopy or limited surgical approaches for lymph node and lung biopsy (McAdams et al. 1998a; Asano et al. 2002; Midthun 2001).

Lung nodules and masses are rarely spherical leading to inter-scan and inter-observer measurement inaccuracy (van de Steene et al. 2002). It is thought that volume measurements which are independent of shape may be more accurate and can sensitively demonstrate temporal change that may predict doubling time and biological behavior (Yankelevitz et al. 2000).

24.6 Chest Wall and Diaphragm

Computed tomography is used to evaluate chest wall and diaphragm pathology (Leitman et al. 1983), and in general 3D visualization is superior for the bone, muscle, pleura and diaphragm. The SSD and VR are used primarily for bony chest wall evaluation (Kuszyk et al. 1996). Primary tumors (e.g., Askin or osteosarcoma) and secondary invasion of the chest wall can be better seen in relation to the normal chest on 3D reformations. Similarly, congenital abnormalities, such as pectus excavatum, can be better measured for surgical planning with inferior and sagittal perspectives (Fig. 24.19; Remy-Jardin et al. 1995; Pretorius and Fishman 1999a,b; Pretorius et al. 1998). Sternal trauma can be very difficult to see on axial images and sagittal MPR or VR is more sensitive (Fig. 24.20; Pretorius and Fishman 1999a). Similarly, the step-off of sternoclavicular dislocation or clavicle fracture is shown on coronal VR images rather than 2D studies. The extent of pleural disease (e.g. mesothelioma) and any change over time is best achieved with serial coronal comparisons using MPR or VR (Kuriyama et al. 1994). Diaphragmatic rupture can be difficult to differentiate from eventration with 2D axial visualization, but discontinuity of the muscle and any mesentery or bowel herniation can be clearly seen with coronal or sagittal MPR (Brink et al. 1994; Killeen et al. 1999; Israel et al. 1996).

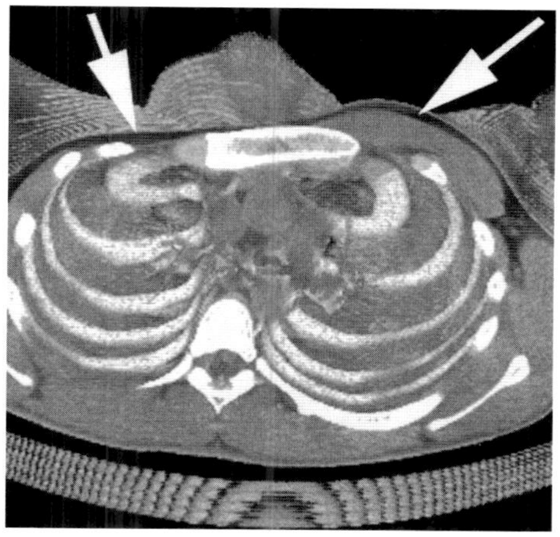

Fig. 24.19. Right chest wall deformity due to Poland's syndrome with absent right pectoral muscles (*short arrow*) and normal left pectoral muscles (*long arrow*). VR inferior image

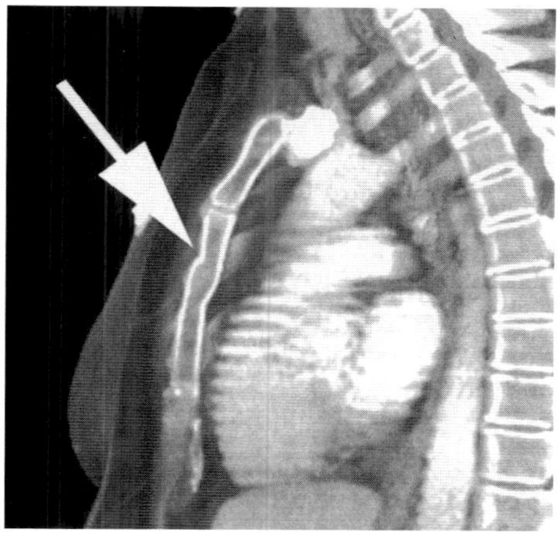

Fig. 24.20. Sagittal VR image demonstrates a subtle sternal fracture (*arrow*)

24.7 Vascular Imaging

Chest CT for vascular imaging includes studies of the systemic and pulmonary venous and arterial systems. The standard evaluation of all these vessels includes CT angiography (CTA) using contrast-enhanced studies with cine and multidimensional interpretation (Kalender and Prokop 2001; Prokop et al. 1993; Prokop 2000; Kawamoto et al. 1998; Remy-Jardin and Remy 1999; Rubin et al. 1995; Rubin 2000). MPR and CMPR can provide limited additional information to the axial 2D visualization. MIP and SSD suffer many of the shortcomings of digital subtraction angiography whereas volume rendering is preferred to discriminate the endoluminal contrast from vessel wall and bony thorax and may be more accurate (Johnson et al. 1998; Costello et al. 1992; Addis et al. 2001). Endoscopic modes can show the relation of pathology to branch vessel origins such as subclavian relationship to thoracic aneurysms but have not found widely application or utility (Smith et al. 1998; Kimura et al. 1996).

The systemic veins of the thorax form a complex inter-connection of vessels between the chest wall and mediastinal structures, which have highly variable branching patterns. CT angiography can obtain better contrast opacification from a single bolus than conventional venographic studies. Contrast injection will preferentially opacify ipsilateral veins and contralateral opacification may require delayed imaging or alternate vein injection. Most commonly patients are referred for evaluation of complete or partial lumen compromise. 3D techniques are useful to measure the length of thrombosis or occlusion, to depict the relation of an impinging mass and to map collateral formation, which may aid recanalization procedures (LAWLER and FISHMAN 2001b; QANADLI et al. 1999a,b). Coronal and right anterior oblique views are best for the superior vena cava and the azygos and accessory hemiazygos systems are better seen with sagittal perspective. Since the veins tend to be close to the thoracic vertebrae volume rendering will show them better than SSD or MIP techniques. The pulmonary veins have become increasingly important of late with the use of ablative techniques to treat arrhythmogenic foci in their myocardial sleeves (WELLENS 2000). This requires an accurate map of the number and branch pattern of the veins to guide catheter based therapy and follow-up for stenoses. Though large anomalies can be seen on 2D axial images these vessels are best seen with volume rendering using posterior perspectives (VANHERREWEGHE et al. 2000; HEYNEMAN et al. 2001; INOUE et al. 2002).

Pulmonary thrombo-embolic disease is the primary reason for pulmonary artery CT. Most emboli are well seen with 2D as low attenuation filling defects with possibly some asymmetric vessel enlargement (QANADLI et al. 2000). The ability of MDCT to capture the bolus is such that on may need to alter window width and level settings compared with SDCT so as not to obscure a small clot. Cine 2D scrolling can increase sensitivity to detection and MPR or 3D can on occasion help discriminate false positives due to obliquely coursing vessels (PARK et al. 1999; KAUCZOR et al. 1996; MERGO et al. 1998; REMY-JARDIN et al. 1995). If the pulmonary embolism study is done together with an examination for DVT axial images from the iliac bifurcation to the deep femoral vessels are obtained. 5 mm slice widths are adequate to survey the area and the attenuation difference of clot within the veins is best appreciated on 2D review. Chronic thrombo-embolic disease represents and build-up of thrombus along the walls of the pulmonary arteries gradually narrowing their lumen and distorting their walls. This condition is often treated surgically with an attempt made to remove the entire thrombus, as a cast and 3D mapping of the extent of disease can be useful in pre-operative planning.

CT examinations of the thoracic systemic arterial system center largely on aortic aneurysm and dissection including intramural hematoma, penetrating atherosclerotic ulcer and acute traumatic aortic injury (PRETRE and VON SEGESSER 1997; RYDBERG et al. 2000a,b) (Figs. 24.21–24.24). CT has a key role in the prompt evaluation and diagnosis of these conditions. For the most part in the emergency room setting 2D with cine scrolling of soft copy images can accurately depict an aneurysm or pseudoaneurysm, show dissection flaps with entry or re-entry tears and vascular

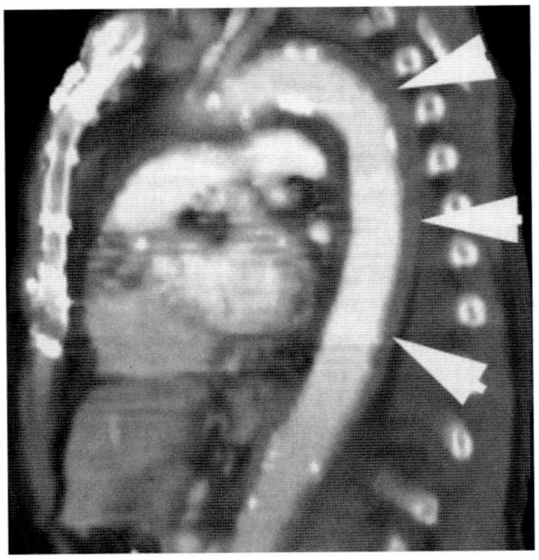

Fig. 24.21. A VR lateral view of an intramural hematoma (*arrowheads*)

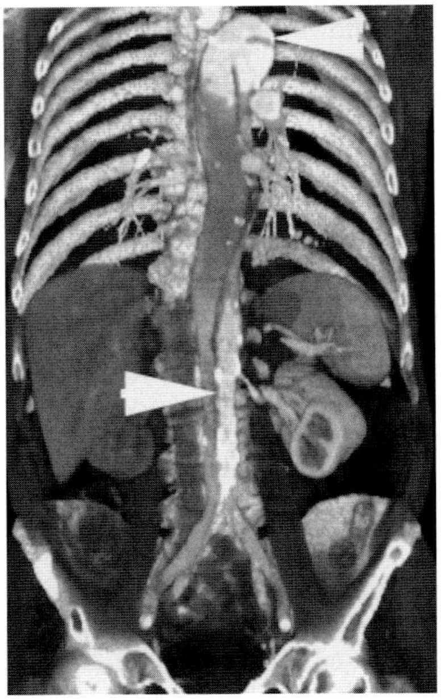

Fig. 24.22. A VR AP view of a type-B dissection (*arrowheads*) extending to the iliac vessels

complications such as organ ischemia (ERRINGTON et al. 1997). The subtle kink of traumatic injury may require multiplanar, MIP or volume rendered images. For therapeutic decisions both aneurysms and dissections benefit from 3D reformations (ADACHI et al. 1994) and volume rendering is preferred to display all the density values of intimal calcification, contrast, thrombus and slow flow (WU et al. 1999). MIP and SSD will only contain a portion of the data and may not depict an intimal flap or mural thrombus. 3D

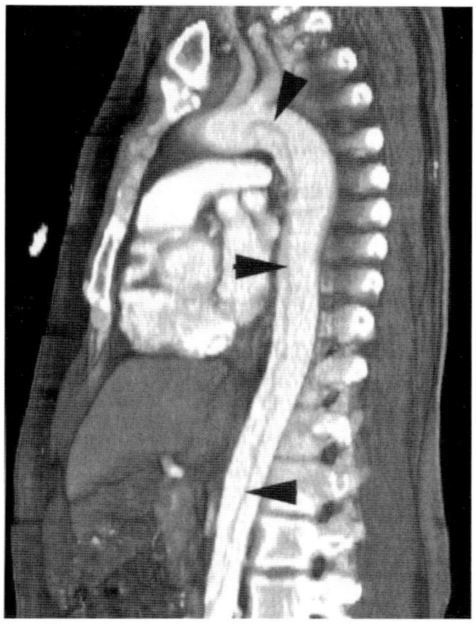

Fig. 24.23. A VR lateral view of a type-B dissection (*arrowheads*)

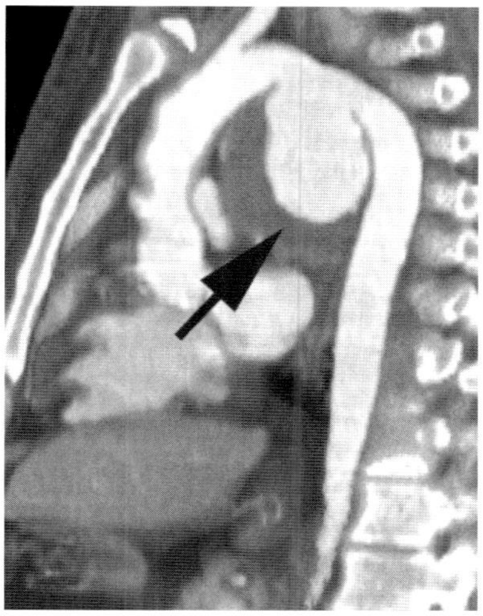

Fig. 24.24. A VR lateral view of a post-traumatic pseudoaneurysm (*arrow*)

visualization can better depict aortic tortuosity and provide true orthogonal measurements of true and false lumina and may provide better localization of entry and re-entry tears (Zeman et al. 1995; Quint et al. 1996; Sommer et al. 1996). 180 degree linear interpolated 2D and 3D reconstructions may be helpful to assess possible false positive dissections such as pulsation artifact (Posniak et al. 1993a,b), which will appear as a regular irregularity on sagittal MPR or 3D studies (Loubeyre et al. 1997a,b). One can better appreciate the optimal location for clamp placement and graft or stent design (Bortone et al. 2001; Dake et al. 1999) and the burden of mural thrombus is clearly shown. The size of the neck of a pseudoaneurysm and its thrombus cap can be accurately measured and its often-complex shape can be appreciated. Increasingly both aneurysms and dissection CT studies must have coverage that includes the femoral vessels for an endovascular approach and 3D techniques provide a sense of their tortuosity and any subtle caliber change. Routinely antero-posterior and left anterior oblique images of the aorta are produced and oblique views of the femoral vessels just as in conventional angiography. Then additional perspectives tailored to the individual patient are generated.

Arteriovenous malformations can be easily diagnosed on 2D CT (Gupta et al. 2002). However they can have complex tortuous blood supply and drainage, which cannot be fully discerned on 2D imaging alone. Failure to fully map the abnormal blood vessels can lead to recanalization and recurrence in

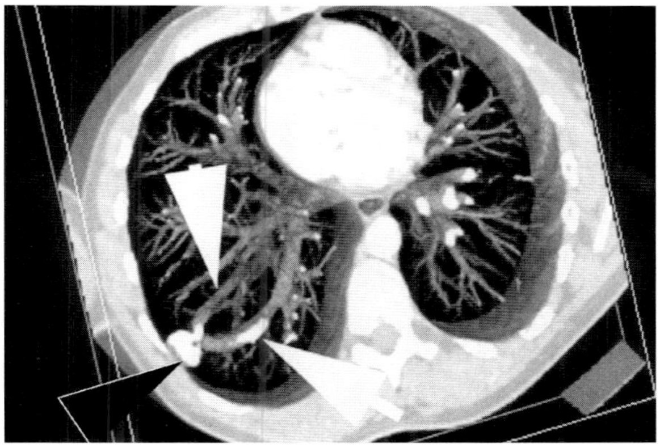

Fig. 24.25. A VR inferior view of an arteriovenous malformation (*arrowheads*)

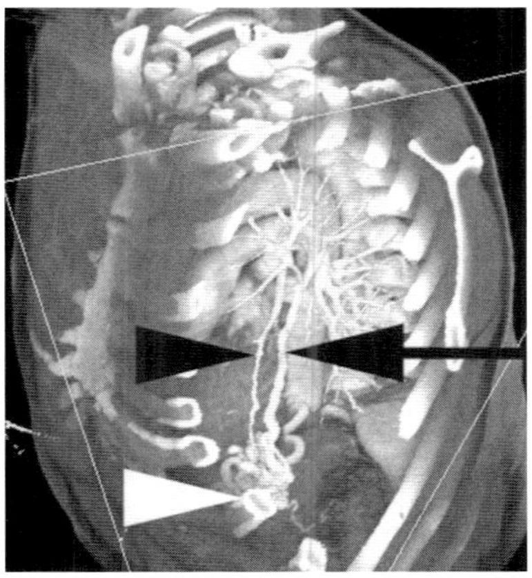

Fig. 24.26. VR left lateral oblique view of a complex left arteriovenous malformation (*white arrowhead*) with feeders from the left pulmonary artery (*arrow*) and drainage to the left superior pulmonary vein (*black arrowhead*)

those patients treated by intravascular embolic therapy (WHITE et al. 1983). 3D visualization has been shown to better assess their angioarchitecture in a way that positively affects outcome with decreased contrast requirements compared with conventional angiography (HOFMANN et al. 2000; REMY et al. 1994; LAWLER and FISHMAN 2002) (Figs. 24.25, 24.26).

There is much current interest in the role of MDCT for cardiac imaging. Axial 2D interpretation is used for coronary artery calcium scoring and estimating pericardial effusions. Multidimensional techniques are used for cardiac masses to better localize their site with the chambers. It is unclear which will be the most efficacious way to evaluate coronary artery (KNEZ et al. 2001; RUMBERGER 2001) and perfusion abnormalities but algorithms are likely to include multidimensional visualization including cine studies and techniques to segment the coronary arteries to measure caliber change (HA et al. 1999; FALLENBERG et al. 2002; BECKER et al. 2000; SCHROEDER et al. 2002).

24.8 Conclusion

As data acquisition continues to improve with MDCT there is a greater need to manage the large data sets and exploit their potential through the use of post-processing tools for two and three-dimensional visualization (RAVENEL et al. 2001; REMY et al. 1998; LAWLER and FISHMAN 2001a; KIRCHGEORG and PROKOP 1998). The immediate future will be contінal change and refinements in data aquisition and post-processing tool. Though two-dimensional axial interpretation will remain fundamental in practice for some time the concept of both volume acquisition and interpretation as a means to tailor chest CT studies to individual patients and pathology plays an increasing role.

References

Adachi H, Ino T, Mizuhara A, Yamaguchi A, Kobayashi Y, Nagai J (1994) Assessment of aortic disease using three-dimensional CT angiography. J Card Surg 9:673–678

Addis KA, Hopper KD, Iyriboz TA et al. (2001) CT angiography: in vitro comparison of five reconstruction methods. Am J Roentgenol 177:1171–1176

Aquino SL, Vining DJ (1999) Virtual bronchoscopy. Clin Chest Med 20:725–730, vii–viii

Arakawa A, Yamashita Y, Nakayama Y et al. (2001) Assessment of lung volumes in pulmonary emphysema using multidetector helical CT: comparison with pulmonary function tests. Comput Med Imaging Graph 25:399–404

Armstrong JG (1998) Target volume definition for three-dimensional conformal radiation therapy of lung cancer. Br J Radiol 71:587–594

Asano F, Matsuno Y, Matsushita T, Kondo H, Saito Y, Seko A, Ishihara Y (2002) Transbronchial diagnosis of a pulmonary peripheral small lesion using an ultrathin bronchoscope with virtual bronchoscopic navigation. J Bronchol 9:108–111

Becker CR, Ohnesorge BM, Schoepf UJ, Reiser MF (2000) Current development of cardiac imaging with multidetector-row CT. Eur J Radiol 36:97–103

Becker HD (1999) Heading into a virtual world-bronchoscopy at the turn of the century. J Bronchol 6:151–152

Bergin C, Roggli V, Coblentz C, Chiles C (1988) The secondary pulmonary lobule: normal and abnormal CT appearances. Am J Roentgenol 151:21–25

Bhalla M, Naidich DP, McGuinness G, Gruden JF, Leitman BS, McCauley DI (1996) Diffuse lung disease: assessment with helical CT – preliminary observations of the role of maximum and minimum intensity projection images. Radiology 200:341–347

Bortone AS, Schena S, Mannatrizio G et al. (2001) Endovascular stent-graft treatment for diseases of the descending thoracic aorta. Eur J Cardiothorac Surg 20:514–519

Bricault I, Ferretti G, Cinquin P (1998) Registration of real and CT-derived virtual bronchoscopic images to assist transbronchial biopsy. IEEE Trans Med Imaging 17:703–714

Brink JA, Heiken JP, Balfe DM, Sagel SS, DiCroce J, Vannier MW (1992) Spiral CT decreased spatial resolution in vivo due to broadening of section-sensitivity profile. Radiology 185:469–474

Brink JA, Heiken JP, Semenkovich J, Teefey SA, McClennan BL, Sagel SS (1994) Abnormalities of the diaphragm and adjacent structures: findings on multiplanar spiral CT scans. Am J Roentgenol 163:307–310

Brown MS, McNitt-Gray MF, Goldin JG et al. (1999) Automated measurement of single and total lung volume from CT. J Comput Assist Tomogr 23:632–640

Calhoun PS, Kuszyk BS, Heath DG, Carley JC, Fishman EK (1999) Three-dimensional volume rendering of spiral CT data: theory and method. Radiographics 19:745–764

Colt HG, Crawford SW, Galbraith O III (2001) Virtual reality bronchoscopy simulation: a revolution in procedural training. Chest 120:1333–1339

Costello P, Dupuy DE, Ecker CP, Tello R (1992) Spiral CT of the thorax with reduced volume of contrast material: a comparative study. Radiology 183:663–666

Curtin JJ, Innes NJ, Harrison BD (1998) Thin-section spiral volumetric CT for the assessment of lobar and segmental bronchial stenoses. Clin Radiol 53:110–115

Dake MD, Kato N, Mitchell RS et al. (1999) Endovascular stent-graft placement for the treatment of acute aortic dissection. N Engl J Med 340:1546–1552

Doi M, Miyazawa T, Mineshita M, Suei S, Kurata T, Fukuhara N, Ochiai M (1999) Three-dimensional bronchial imaging by spiral computed tomography as applied to tracheobronchial stent placement. J Bronchol 6:155–158

Dunham ME, Wolf RN (1996) Visualizing the pediatric airway: three-dimensional modeling of endoscopic images. Ann Otol Rhinol Laryngol 105:12–17

Eibel R, Turk TR, Kulinna C, Herrmann K, Reiser MF (2001)

Multidetector-row CT of the lungs: multiplanar reconstructions and maximum intensity projections for the detection of pulmonary nodules. Rofo Fortschr Geb Rontgenstr Neuen Bildgeb Verfahr 173:815–821

Engeler CE, Tashjian JH, Engeler CM, Geise RA, Holm JC, Ritenour ER (1994) Volumetric high-resolution CT in the diagnosis of interstitial lung disease and bronchiectasis: diagnostic accuracy and radiation dose. Am J Roentgenol 163:31–35

Errington ML, Ferguson JM, Gillespie IN, Connell HM, Ruckley CV, Wright AR (1997) Complete pre-operative imaging assessment of abdominal aortic aneurysm with spiral CT angiography. Clin Radiol 52:369–377

Fallenberg M, Juergens KU, Wichter T, Scheld HH, Fischbach R (2002) Coronary artery aneurysm and type-A aortic dissection demonstrated by retrospectively ECG-gated multislice spiral CT. Eur Radiol 12:201–204

Ferretti GR, Bricault I, Coulomb M (2001) Virtual tools for imaging of the thorax. Eur Respir J 18:381–392

Ferretti GR, Vining DJ, Knoplioch J, Coulomb M (1996) Tracheobronchial tree: three-dimensional spiral CT with bronchoscopic perspective. J Comput Assist Tomogr 20:777–781

Ferretti GR, Knoplioch J, Bricault I, Brambilla C, Coulomb M (1997) Central airway stenoses: preliminary results of spiral-CT-generated virtual bronchoscopy simulations in 29 patients. Eur Radiol 7:854–859

Ferretti GR, Thony F, Bosson JL, Pison C, Arbib F, Coulomb M (2000) Benign abnormalities and carcinoid tumors of the central airways: diagnostic impact of CT bronchography. Am J Roentgenol 174:1307–1313

Fishman EK, Magid D, Ney DR et al. (1991) Three-dimensional imaging. Radiology 181:321–337

Fleiter T, Merkle EM, Aschoff AJ et al. (1997) Comparison of real-time virtual and fiberoptic bronchoscopy in patients with bronchial carcinoma: opportunities and limitations. Am J Roentgenol 169:1591–1595

Gilkeson RC, Ciancibello LM, Hejal RB, Montenegro HD, Lange P (2001) Tracheobronchomalacia: dynamic airway evaluation with multidetector CT. Am J Roentgenol 176: 205–210

Gluecker T, Lang F, Bessler S et al. (2001) 2D and 3D CT imaging correlated to rigid endoscopy in complex laryngo-tracheal stenoses. Eur Radiol 11:50–54

Goldin JG, Aberle DR (1997) Functional imaging of the airways. J Thorac Imaging 12:29–37

Gupta H, Mayo-Smith WW, Mainiero MB, Dupuy DE, Abbott GF (2002) Helical CT of pulmonary vascular abnormalities. Am J Roentgenol 178:487–492

Ha JW, Cho SY, Shim WH et al. (1999) Noninvasive evaluation of coronary artery bypass graft patency using three-dimensional angiography obtained with contrast-enhanced electron beam CT. Am J Roentgenol 172:1055–1059

Haponik EF, Aquino SL, Vining DJ (1999) Virtual bronchoscopy. Clin Chest Med 20:201–217

Heyneman LE, Nolan RL, Harrison JK, McAdams HP (2001) Congenital unilateral pulmonary vein atresia: radiologic findings in three adult patients. Am J Roentgenol 177: 681–685

Hoffman EA, Tajik JK, Kugelmass SD (1995) Matching pulmonary structure and perfusion via combined dynamic multislice CT and thin-slice high-resolution CT. Comput Med Imaging Graph 19:101–112

Hofmann LV, Kuszyk BS, Mitchell SE, Horton KM, Fishman EK (2000) Angioarchitecture of pulmonary arteriovenous malformations: characterization using volume-rendered 3-D CT angiography. Cardiovasc Intervent Radiol 23:165–170

Holbert JM, Brown ML, Sciurba FC, Keenan RJ, Landreneau RJ, Holzer AD (1996) Changes in lung volume and volume of emphysema after unilateral lung reduction surgery: analysis with CT lung densitometry. Radiology 201:793–797

Hopkins KL, Patrick LE, Simoneaux SF, Bank ER, Parks WJ, Smith SS (1996) Pediatric great vessel anomalies: initial clinical experience with spiral CT angiography. Radiology 200:811–815

Hopper KD, Iyriboz AT, Wise SW, Neuman JD, Mauger DT, Kasales CJ (2000) Mucosal detail at CT virtual reality: surface versus volume rendering. Radiology 214:517–522

Hu H, He HD, Foley WD, Fox SH (2000) Four multidetector-row helical CT: image quality and volume coverage speed. Radiology 215:55–62

Inoue T, Ichihara M, Uchida T, Sakai Y, Hayashi T, Morooka S (2002) Three-dimensional computed tomography showing partial anomalous pulmonary venous connection complicated by the scimitar syndrome. Circulation 105:663

Israel RS, McDaniel PA, Primack SL, Salmon CJ, Fountain RL, Koslin DB (1996) Diagnosis of diaphragmatic trauma with helical CT in a swine model. Am J Roentgenol 167:637–641

Johnson PT, Fishman EK, Duckwall JR, Calhoun PS, Heath DG (1998) Interactive three-dimensional volume rendering of spiral CT data: current applications in the thorax. Radiographics 18:165–187

Johnson PT, Heath DG, Bliss DF, Cabral B, Fishman EK (1996) Three-dimensional CT: real-time interactive volume rendering. Am J Roentgenol 167:581–583

Kalender WA, Polacin A (1991) Physical performance characteristics of spiral CT scanning. Med Phys 18:910–915

Kalender WA, Prokop M (2001) 3D CT angiography. Crit Rev Diagn Imaging 42:1–28

Kalender WA, Vock P, Polacin A, Soucek M (1990a) Spiral-CT: a new technique for volumetric scans. I. Basic principles and methodology. Rontgenpraxis 43:323–330

Kalender WA, Seissler W, Klotz E, Vock P (1990b) Spiral volumetric CT with single-breath-hold technique, continuous transport, and continuous scanner rotation. Radiology 176:181–183

Katz M, Konen E, Rozenman J, Szeinberg A, Itzchak Y (1995) Spiral CT and 3D image reconstruction of vascular rings and associated tracheobronchial anomalies. J Comput Assist Tomogr 19:564–568

Kauczor HU, Wolcke B, Fischer B, Mildenberger P, Lorenz J, Thelen M (1996) Three-dimensional helical CT of the tracheobronchial tree: evaluation of imaging protocols and assessment of suspected stenoses with bronchoscopic correlation. Am J Roentgenol 167:419–424

Kawamoto S, Johnson PT, Fishman EK (1998) Three-dimensional CT angiography of the thorax: clinical applications. Semin Ultrasound CT MR 19:425–438

Killeen KL, Mirvis SE, Shanmuganathan K (1999) Helical CT of diaphragmatic rupture caused by blunt trauma. Am J Roentgenol 173:1611–1616

Kimura F, Shen Y, Date S, Azemoto S, Mochizuki T (1996) Thoracic aortic aneurysm and aortic dissection: new endoscopic mode for three-dimensional CT display of aorta. Radiology 198:573–578

Kinsella M, Muller NL, Abboud RT, Morrison NJ, DyBuncio A (1990) Quantitation of emphysema by computed tomography using a "density mask" program and correlation with pulmonary function tests. Chest 97:315–321

Kirchgeorg MA, Prokop M (1998) Increasing spiral CT benefits with postprocessing applications. Eur J Radiol 28:39–54

Klingenbeck-Regn K, Schaller S, Flohr T, Ohnesorge B, Kopp AF, Baum U (1999) Subsecond multi-slice computed tomography: basics and applications. Eur J Radiol 31:110–124

Knez A, Becker CR, Leber A et al. (2001) Usefulness of multislice spiral computed tomography angiography for determination of coronary artery stenoses. Am J Cardiol 88:1191–1194

Kuriyama K, Tateishi R, Kumatani T et al. (1994) Pleural invasion by peripheral bronchogenic carcinoma: assessment with three-dimensional helical CT. Radiology 191:365–369

Kuszyk BS, Heath DG, Bliss DF, Fishman EK (1996) Skeletal 3-D CT: advantages of volume rendering over surface rendering. Skeletal Radiol 25:207–214

Lacrosse M, Trigaux JP, van Beers BE, Weynants P (1995) 3D spiral CT of the tracheobronchial tree. J Comput Assist Tomogr 19:341–347

Lawler LP, Fishman EK (2001a) Multi-detector row CT of thoracic disease with emphasis on 3D volume rendering and CT angiography. Radiographics 21:1257–1273

Lawler LP, Fishman EK (2001b) Pericardial varices: depiction on three-dimensional CT angiography. Am J Roentgenol 177:202–204

Lawler LP, Fishman EK (2002) Arteriovenous malformations and systemic lung supply: evaluation by multidetector CT and three-dimensional volume rendering. Am J Roentgenol 178:493–495

Lehman JD, Gordon RL, Kerlan RK Jr et al. (1998) Expandable metallic stents in benign tracheobronchial obstruction. J Thorac Imaging 13:105–115

Leibel SA, Kutcher GJ, Mohan R et al. (1992) Three-dimensional conformal radiation therapy at the Memorial Sloan-Kettering Cancer Center. Semin Radiat Oncol 2:274–289

Leitman BS, Firooznia H, McCauley DI et al. (1983) The use of computed tomography in evaluating chest wall pathology. J Comput Tomogr 7:399–405

Liewald F, Lang G, Fleiter T, Sokiranski R, Halter G, Orend KH (1998) Comparison of virtual and fiberoptic bronchoscopy. Thorac Cardiovasc Surg 46:361–364

LoCicero J III, Costello P, Campos CT et al. (1996) Spiral CT with multiplanar and three-dimensional reconstructions accurately predicts tracheobronchial pathology. Ann Thorac Surg 62:818–823

Loubeyre P, Grozel F, Carrillon Y et al. (1997a) Prevalence of motion artifact simulating aortic dissection on spiral CT using a 180 degree linear interpolation algorithm for reconstruction of the images. Eur Radiol 7:320–322

Loubeyre P, Angelie E, Grozel F, Abidi H, Minh VA (1997b) Spiral CT artifact that simulates aortic dissection: image reconstruction with use of 180 degrees and 360 degrees linear-interpolation algorithms. Radiology 205:153–157

Manson D, Babyn P, Filler R, Holowka S (1994) Three-dimensional imaging of the pediatric trachea in congenital tracheal stenosis. Pediatr Radiol 24:175–179

McAdams HP, Goodman PC, Kussin P (1998a) Virtual bronchoscopy for directing transbronchial needle aspiration of hilar and mediastinal lymph nodes: a pilot study. Am J Roentgenol 170:1361–1364

McAdams HP, Palmer SM, Erasmus JJ et al. (1998b) Bronchial anastomotic complications in lung transplant recipients: virtual bronchoscopy for noninvasive assessment. Radiology 209:689–695

Mergo PJ, Williams WF, Gonzalez-Rothi R et al. (1998) Three-dimensional volumetric assessment of abnormally low attenuation of the lung from routine helical CT: inspiratory and expiratory quantification. Am J Roentgenol 170:1355–1360

Midthun DE (2001) Pulmonary nodules: reach for the imaging – not the scope. J Bronchol 8:159–160

Naidich DP, Harkin TJ (1996) Airways and lung: CT versus bronchography through the fiberoptic bronchoscope. Radiology 200:613–614

Naidich DP, Gruden JF, McGuinness G, McCauley DI, Bhalla M (1997) Volumetric (helical/spiral) CT (VCT) of the airways. J Thorac Imaging 12:11–28

Napel S, Rubin GD, Jeffrey RB Jr (1993) STS-MIP: a new reconstruction technique for CT of the chest. J Comput Assist Tomogr 17:832–838

Neumann K, Winterer J, Kimmig M et al. (2000) Real-time interactive virtual endoscopy of the tracheo-bronchial system: influence of CT imaging protocols and observer ability. Eur J Radiol 33:50–54

Newmark GM, Conces DJ Jr, Kopecky KK (1994) Spiral CT evaluation of the trachea and bronchi. J Comput Assist Tomogr 18:552–554

Ney DR, Kuhlman JE, Hruban RH, Ren H, Hutchins GM, Fishman EK (1990) Three-dimensional CT-volumetric reconstruction and display of the bronchial tree. Invest Radiol 25:736–742

Nicholson DA (1998) Tracheal and oesophageal stenting for carcinoma of the upper oesophagus invading the tracheobronchial tree. Clin Radiol 53:760–763

Park KJ, Bergin CJ, Clausen JL (1999) Quantitation of emphysema with three-dimensional CT densitometry: comparison with two-dimensional analysis, visual emphysema scores, and pulmonary function test results. Radiology 211:541–547

Pavone P, Luccichenti G, Cademartiri F (2001) From maximum intensity projection to volume rendering. Semin Ultrasound CT MR 22:413–419

Posniak H, Olson M, Demos T (1993a) Motion artifact simulating aortic dissection. Am J Roentgenol 160:420

Posniak H, Olson MC, Demos TC (1993b) Aortic motion artifact simulating dissection on CT scans: elimination with reconstructive segmented images. Am J Roentgenol 161: 557–558

Pretorius ES, Fishman EK (1999a) Spiral CT and three-dimensional CT of musculoskeletal pathology. Emergency room applications. Radiol Clin North Am 37:953–974, vi

Pretorius ES, Fishman EK (1999b) Volume-rendered three-dimensional spiral CT: musculoskeletal applications. Radiographics 19:1143–1160

Pretorius ES, Haller JA, Fishman EK (1998) Spiral CT with 3D reconstruction in children requiring reoperation for failure of chest wall growth after pectus excavatum surgery. Preliminary observations. Clin Imaging 22:108–116

Pretre R, von Segesser LK (1997) Aortic dissection. Lancet 349: 1461–1464

Prokop M (2000) Multislice CT angiography. Eur J Radiol 36: 86–96

Prokop M, Schaefer C, Kalender WA, Polacin A, Galanski M (1993) Vascular imaging with spiral-CT. The path to CT-angiography. Radiologe 33:694–704

Qanadli SD, El Hajjam M, Bruckert F et al. (1999a) Helical CT phlebography of the superior vena cava: diagnosis and evaluation of venous obstruction. Am J Roentgenol 172:1327–1333

Qanadli SD, El Hajjam M, Mignon F et al. (1999b) Subacute and chronic benign superior vena cava obstructions: endovascular treatment with self-expanding metallic stents. Am J Roentgenol 173:159–164

Qanadli SD, Hajjam ME, Mesurolle B et al. (2000) Pulmonary embolism detection: prospective evaluation of dual-section helical CT versus selective pulmonary arteriography in 157 patients. Radiology 217:447–455

Quint LE, Whyte RI, Kazerooni EA et al. (1995) Stenosis of the central airways: evaluation by using helical CT with multiplanar reconstructions. Radiology 194:871–877

Quint LE, Francis IR, Williams DM et al. (1996) Evaluation of thoracic aortic disease with the use of helical CT and multiplanar reconstructions: comparison with surgical findings. Radiology 201:37–41

Ravenel JG, McAdams HP, Remy-Jardin M, Remy J (2001) Multidimensional imaging of the thorax: practical applications. J Thorac Imaging 16:269–281

Remy J, Remy-Jardin M, Giraud F, Wattinne L (1994) Angioarchitecture of pulmonary arteriovenous malformations: clinical utility of three-dimensional helical CT. Radiology 191:657–664

Remy J, Remy-Jardin M, Artaud D, Fribourg M (1998) Multiplanar and three-dimensional reconstruction techniques in CT: impact on chest diseases. Eur Radiol 8:335–351

Remy-Jardin M, Remy J (1999) Spiral CT angiography of the pulmonary circulation. Radiology 212:615–636

Remy-Jardin M, Remy J, Cauvain O, Petyt L, Wannebroucq J, Beregi JP (1995) Diagnosis of central pulmonary embolism with helical CT: role of two-dimensional multiplanar reformations. Am J Roentgenol 165:1131–1138

Remy-Jardin M, Remy J, Gosselin B, Copin MC, Wurtz A, Duhamel A (1996a) Sliding thin slab, minimum intensity projection technique in the diagnosis of emphysema: histopathologic-CT correlation. Radiology 200:665–671

Remy-Jardin M, Remy J, Deschildre F, Artaud D, Ramon P, Edme JL (1996b) Obstructive lesions of the central airways: evaluation by using spiral CT with multiplanar and three-dimensional reformations. Eur Radiol 6:807–816

Remy-Jardin M, Remy J, Artaud D, Fribourg M, Naili A (1998) Tracheobronchial tree: assessment with volume rendering – technical aspects. Radiology 208:393–398

Richenberg JL, Hansell DM (1998) Image processing and spiral CT of the thorax. Br J Radiol 71:708–716

Rodenwaldt J, Kopka L, Roedel R, Margas A, Grabbe E (1997) 3D virtual endoscopy of the upper airway: optimization of the scan parameters in a cadaver phantom and clinical assessment. J Comput Assist Tomogr 21:405–411

Rubin GD (2000) Data explosion: the challenge of multidetector-row CT. Eur J Radiol 36:74–80

Rubin GD, Dake MD, Semba CP (1995) Current status of three-dimensional spiral CT scanning for imaging the vasculature. Radiol Clin North Am 33:51–70

Rumberger JA (2001) Tomographic (plaque) imaging: state of the art. Am J Cardiol 88:66E–69E

Rydberg J, Kopecky KK, Fleiter TR (2000a) Multislice CT improves diagnosis, management of aortic disease. Diagn Imaging (San Franc) 22:159–163, 165

Rydberg J, Buckwalter KA, Caldemeyer KS et al. (2000b) Multisection CT: scanning techniques and clinical applications. Radiographics 20:1787–1806

Schreiner S, Paschal CB, Galloway RL (1996) Comparison of projection algorithms used for the construction of maximum intensity projection images. J Comput Assist Tomogr 20:56–67

Schroeder S, Kopp AF, Ohnesorge B et al. (2002) Virtual coronary angioscopy using multislice computed tomography. Heart 87:205–209

Smith PA, Heath DG, Fishman EK (1998) Virtual angioscopy using spiral CT and real-time interactive volume- rendering techniques. J Comput Assist Tomogr 22:212–214

Sommer T, Fehske W, Holzknecht N et al. (1996) Aortic dissection: a comparative study of diagnosis with spiral CT, multiplanar transesophageal echocardiography, and MR imaging. Radiology 199:347–352

Thurnheer R, Engel H, Weder W et al. (1999) Role of lung perfusion scintigraphy in relation to chest computed tomography and pulmonary function in the evaluation of candidates for lung volume reduction surgery. Am J Respir Crit Care Med 159:301–310

Van de Steene J, Linthout N, de Mey J et al. (2002) Definition of gross tumor volume in lung cancer: inter-observer variability. Radiother Oncol 62:37–49

Vanherreweghe E, Rigauts H, Bogaerts Y, Meeus L (2000) Pulmonary vein varix: diagnosis with multi-slice helical CT. Eur Radiol 10:1315–1317

Vuong T, Parker W, Patrocinio HJ et al. (2000) An alternative mantle irradiation technique using 3D CT- based treatment planning for female patients with Hodgkin's disease. Int J Radiat Oncol Biol Phys 47:739–748

Wellens HJ (2000) Pulmonary vein ablation in atrial fibrillation: hype or hope? Circulation 102:2562–2564

White RI Jr, Mitchell SE, Barth KH et al. (1983) Angioarchitecture of pulmonary arteriovenous malformations: an important consideration before embolotherapy. Am J Roentgenol 140:681–686

Wilson GE, Walshaw MJ, Hind CR (1996) Treatment of large airway obstruction in lung cancer using expandable metal stents inserted under direct vision via the fibreoptic bronchoscope. Thorax 51:248–252

Wu CM, Urban BA, Fishman EK (1999) Spiral CT of the thoracic aorta with 3-D volume rendering: a pictorial review of current applications. Cardiovasc Intervent Radiol 22: 159–167

Yankelevitz DF, Reeves AP, Kostis WJ, Zhao B, Henschke CI (2000) Small pulmonary nodules: volumetrically determined growth rates based on CT evaluation. Radiology 217:251–256

Zeman RK, Berman PM, Silverman PM et al. (1995) Diagnosis of aortic dissection: value of helical CT with multiplanar reformation and three-dimensional rendering. Am J Roentgenol 164:1375–1380

Zwischenberger JB, Wittich GR, van Sonnenberg E et al. (1997) Airway simulation to guide stent placement for tracheobronchial obstruction in lung cancer. Ann Thorac Surg 64: 1619–1625

25 Computer-Aided Diagnosis

S. A. Wood

CONTENTS

25.1 Introduction

There has been no technological advance for imaging of the thorax with as profound impact on the way data is visualized, diagnosed and managed than multidetector-row CT (MDCT). The fast acquisition times and higher resolution have forever changed imaging of the lung, an organ whose dynamic nature demands rapid acquisition and whose complex anatomy demands isotropic resolution for fine anatomic detail and true three-dimensional analysis. Multidetector-row (MDCT) allows shorter breathholds, fewer breathing and motion artifacts, and reduced contrast delivery for CT angiography studies. It is with this anatomic detail that we can better clarify pulmonary anatomy and detect change in pulmonary anatomy as an indicator of disease.

The rapid uptake of MDCT scanners in the clinical marketplace is indication of their significant technological advance. The number and complexity of procedures now possible with MDCT is increasing and will continue to increase as new protocols emerge that take advantage of the unique properties of the scanner. The uptake of MDCT scanners in the United States between 1998 and 2001 had a compound annual growth rate of 160% (Fig. 25.1) in an otherwise dormant CT market in the mid to late 1990s. This dramatic increase is likely because of the increased clinical value provided with faster, higher resolution scanners (IMV, Medical Information Division, Des Plaines, IL).

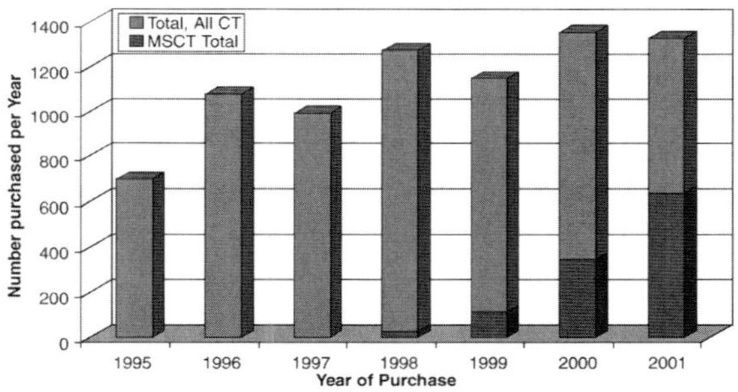

Fig. 25.1. American College of Radiology data indicating the rapid decrease in job seekers in diagnostic radiology combined with the increase in available jobs.

The finer resolution data produced by MDCT, however, comes with the consequence of a massive explosion of data. While the increase in resolution of data and acquisition speed brings greater interpretive potential and variety of applications capable of being performed with CT, the enormity of the acquired image volume has resulted in significant workflow challenges to the radiologist accustomed to diagnosing from axial slices.

The increase in generated data also comes at a time when radiology departments are increasingly resource constrained. Availability of radiologists increased just 3% in 2000, while CT procedures increased 19.4% in the same year, second only to positron emission tomography (PET, at 48%) in procedural increase (Margulis 2001). Figure 25.2 illustrates the decline of radiology related job seekers

S. A. Wood, PhD
Vice President, CT Products, R2 Technology, Inc., 1195 West Fremont Avenue, Sunnyvale, CA 94087, USA

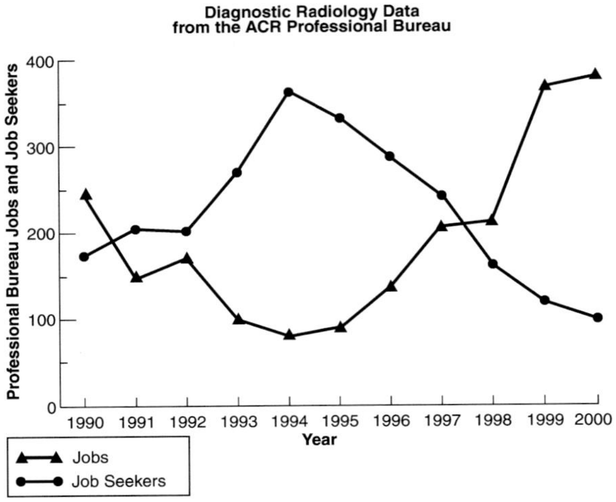

Fig. 25.2. Graph showing the influx of MDCT scanners intot he US market. Since their debut in 1998, MDCT scanners have experienced a 160% compound annual growth rate (CAGR) from 1998 through 2001. Their influx into the marketplace is an indication of their profound incremental clinical value.

since the mid 1990s and a steady increase in available jobs. Because of increased case demand and decreased resources, radiologists are literally flooded with data and desperately require better interpretive tools to analyze it quickly and accurately.

Softcopy review, while more prevalent in CT than in any other modality, has already been shown to increase radiologists productivity when compared to film reading (Reiner et al. 2001). Softcopy review is a minimal requirement with MDCT. The number of axial slices now generated with MDCT precludes their efficient review using two-dimensional viewing techniques alone, and because of sheer numbers of images, are often read at a lower resolution. Volumetric postprocessing tools have been available for over a decade (Napel et al. 1992, 1993; Croisille et al. 1995; Johnson et al. 1998; Fan et al. 2002; Gruden et al. 2002) and while currently readily available in a softcopy environment, are rarely used for primary diagnosis (Fishman 2001). This phenomenon is in part because current volumetric analysis tools are not currently as efficient and accurate as axial review (Rubin 2003). While acquired volumetric image resolution is accessible at the expense of many transverse images, true volumetric reconstruction with better postprocessing tools are required to help the radiologist. The long-awaited paradigm shift from two-dimensional to three-dimensional review (Rubin et al. 1996), may indeed be coming, spearheaded by the rapid market uptake of MDCT scanners and the subsequent demand for computer assistance to interpret these multidimensional exams.

25.2 Computer-Aided Detection (CAD) in Medical Imaging

One measure of effective computer assistance in radiological exams is their ability to focus valuable radiologists' time on interpretation of images. With increasing volume of single and multimodality data generated, the radiologist will have little time to spend on each examination, and will need to focus their attention on interpretation. CAD has the potential to take the time-consuming tasks of the radiologist and minimize their involvement in those areas where their expertise is not required (i.e., image registration, automatic measurement). CAD can accomplish this feat by directing the radiologist's review and to automatically generate quantitative information about the finding for faster interpretation.

Another measure of the effectiveness of CAD systems is the consistency and repeatability of a CAD system to identify patterns that indicate abnormalities. When this consistency is synergized with the variability of human observation, the accuracy of the radiologist can increase, and may increase at different rates for the same observer depending on environmental conditions. It also has the ability to effect readers of different experience levels differently (Das et al. 2002, 2003c).

Volumetric imaging will be essential with MDCT acquisitions of the thorax, and CAD will bring the added clinical utility to volumetric imaging to warrant its more routine use in a diagnostic setting. Instead of volumetric imaging alone, CAD directed volumetric imaging brings added clinical utility and purpose to 3D imaging.

25.3 Current State of CAD Technology

In their current form, Computer-Aided Detection (CAD) systems are used for automatic detection in medical images and are currently positioned as a second review for radiologists. They target the problem of improved accuracy of clinical detection and provide other analysis tools to aid clinical interpretation. Given a consistent set of patterns, CAD systems can identify potential abnormalities, but the diagnosis of the finding remains the responsibility of the radiologist. A radiologist reads the case, queries the CAD system and the CAD system highlights areas that may require a second review. The radiologist can react to the CAD mark if it was overlooked in the original interpretation, or dismiss it altogether. As a second review, CAD systems can complement the inherent variability of human observation by finding oversights that were missed in the original review. The CAD system does not tire, get phone calls, change moods, or need to rush out of the door to get to dinner. Therefore the consistency of a CAD system combined with the variability of the human observer can have a positive impact on detection accuracy. It is likely that the CAD system does not need the sensitivity of the radiologist to be valuable (GIGER and MACMAHON 1996), but the consistency of detection can help the radiologist (WARREN BURHENNE et al. 2000).

25.3.1 Evolution of a CAD System: Mammography as a Case Study

Computer-aided detection (CAD) techniques have been researched for over a decade with initial work mostly concentrating on CAD for two-dimensional modalities of mammography and projection chest radiography (CHAN, DOI et al. 1987; Chan, Doi et al. 1990; MACMAHON, DOI et al. 1990; DOI, GIGER et al. 1992; ABE, DOI et al. 1993; GIGER, DOI et al.; GIGER, BAE and MACMAHON, 1994). The first commercially available CAD product was approved in the United States in 1998 by the Food and Drug Administration for screening mammography (WARREN BURHENNE et al. 2000). Presently, the number of mammography CAD systems in routine clinical use for both film-based and digital mammography approaches 1000. It is, therefore, only mammographic CAD systems that have transitioned from concept, to product to common clinical use. The mammography model has the longevity that can best be used as a measure of the impact of CAD on clinical efficacy.

Figure 25.3a illustrates a model for the evolution of a CAD system for mammography from automatic detection of abnormalities to its impact on clinical decision making. At its base, a CAD system *detects regions that are consistent with suspicion of disease* with detection often measured as stand-alone sensitivity. Evaluating the stand-alone sensitivity of mammographic CAD algorithms is measured against a gold standard database of biopsy-proven cancers. The sensitivity is defined as the number of CAD detected cancers compared to all cancers in the gold standard database. CAD is displayed to the radiologist as a subsampled mammographic image with overlays on the image where CAD found features suspicious of disease. An asterisk (*) is an indication of a potential mass finding in a mammogram and a triangle (▵) is an indication of a potential calcification finding (Fig. 25.3b). The CAD stand-alone performance for one screening mammographic system

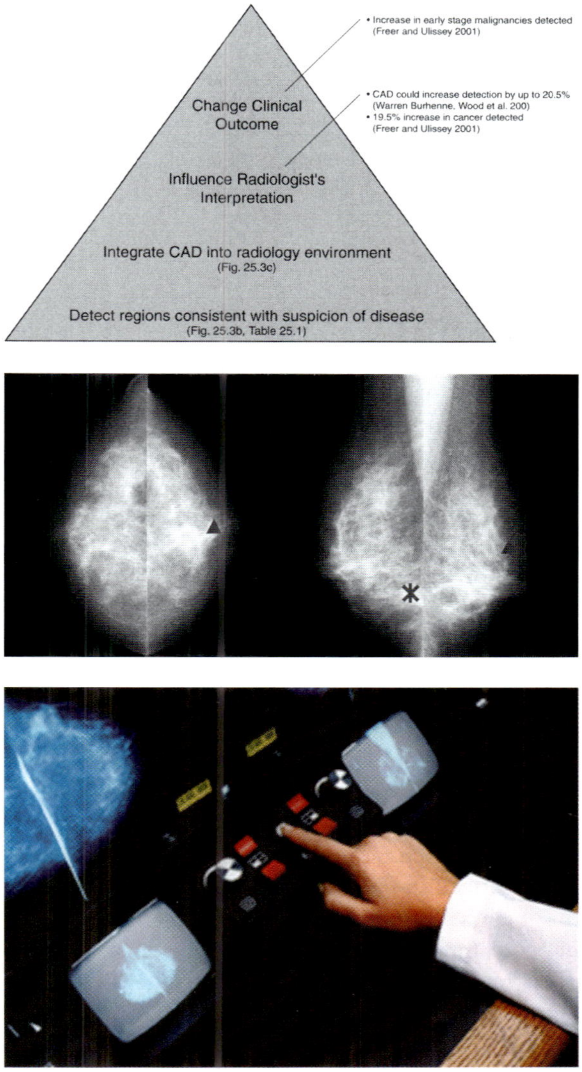

a

b

c

Fig. 25.3a–c. a Evolution of a CAD system. Detection algorithms lead to a change in clinical outcome, ut detection algorithms alone are not enough. **b** Two view (Cranial-Caudal (CC) and Medial-lateral oblique (MLO) screening mammograms. The overlays are areas where the CAD tool found lesions suspicious of disease. The asterix (*) indicates a mass finding and the triangle (▲) indicates a calcification. At the base of the pyramid or the platform of what we do is algorithmic development. **c** The ImageChecker™ was designed with a one-button workflow. The radiologist reads normally, presses the white button (shown above) and maps any CAD findings to the original image. For CAD to be adopted routinely, it must not inhibit the workflow of the radiologist. CAD also has the potential to help the radiologist's workflow.

on the market is shown in Table 25.1. The CAD algorithmic base has evolved over its nearly 10-year commercial development cycle to have overall high sensitivity for detecting breast cancer with a low false positive rate. This high performance is a baseline for a clinically acceptable CAD system.

Table 25.1. Performance results on 1083 screening mammograms (Warren Burhenne et al. 2000)

Type	Sensitivity
Microcalcifications	97.8% (397/406)
Masses	87.7% (594/677)
Combined*	91.5% (991/1083)

*1.6 false positive markings per case

The utility of CAD is limited; however, even at high detection performance levels if CAD is not properly *integrated into the environment of the radiologist*. A CAD system must present its information in a way that is intuitive to the radiologist and not hinder normal workflow. Figure 25.3c illustrates one component of a mammographic CAD system easing its utility in the workflow of screening mammography. The one-button approach is intuitive to the radiologist and quickly integrates into their reading workflow. After the radiologist reads his or her cases normally, he or she presses a button and compares the CAD findings to the already read images. The simplicity of the one-button approach eases the utility of CAD.

At its next level of maturity, CAD has the potential to *influence the decision of the radiologist*. That is, if CAD alerts the radiologist to a potential area of abnormality, the radiologist will react to the finding if overlooked in the initial read, or determine that it is not clinically relevant. CAD has shown potential to increase the radiologists accuracy in breast cancer detection by over 20%, retrospectively without an increase in radiologists' workup rate (Warren Burhenne et al. 2000) and more recently prospectively, in a study of over 12,000 screening cases (Freer and Ulissey 2001). In the prospective study, Freer showed an increase in detection rate of 19.5% with the aid of a CAD system as a second review.

Finally, at its highest level of maturity, a CAD system has the potential to detect disease earlier and at an earlier stage, and therefore could *change clinical outcome*. Freer showed an increase in early stage cancers found with CAD (Freer and Ulissey 2001) and by detecting these cancers earlier, would likely have a positive impact on patient outcome. As mammography CAD systems continue to be used in clinical practice, more data will become available to assess the CAD system's influence on clinical practice and the model would be strengthened with more clinical data. The maturity of new CAD applications like those presently being evaluated for MDCT of the chest can be evaluated using a similar model as that for mammography.

25.4 CAD for MDCT of the Thorax

MDCT has such a transformational impact on clinical workflow that the clinical community is clamoring for a solution to the data management problem. Potential CAD solutions are quickly moving from research to marketplace. With the size and complexity of current MDCT exams, automatic detection has the potential to provide a key component to the workflow difficulties facing current MDCT users. CAD systems are currently being prototypically evaluated for the automatic detection of lung nodules using MDCT (Lawler et al. 2003, submitted), but unlike mammography and projection chest, no CAD systems are currently available to the market and therefore are not used in routine clinical practice. CAD can target patterns indicative of lung nodules after an initial clinical evaluation, automatically measure lesion size and density, and make comparisons over time. This combination of tools makes a more efficient review for the radiologist.

Most CAD systems being evaluated now concentrate on lung nodule detection (Das et al. 2002; Wood et al. 2002; Das et al. 2003a,b; Wood et al. 2003a,b) and more recent work has concentrated on CAD for pulmonary embolism (PE) detection (Schoepf et al. 2002; Das et al. 2003). Both disease states lend themselves nicely to the help of CAD because they have proven difficulty in detection and potentially increased reading time with MDCT examinations read with transverse sections, because of the volume of images and anatomical complexities. The evolution of CAD in both disease states of the thorax will be detailed in the sections below.

25.4.1 CAD for Lung Nodule Detection with MDCT

Traditional computed tomography (CT) and single-detector helical CT were previously shown to be significantly better at detecting and diagnosing focal lung disease than chest radiographs (Muhm et al. 1977, 1983). However, even with the increased anatomical clarity of the lung using CT, cancers are still missed (GURNEY 1996; HAZELRIGG et al. 1997; RUSINEK et al. 1998; KAKINUMA et al. 1999).

Earlier methods developed to automatically detect lung nodules using single-detector-row CT (SDCT) were composed largely of two-dimensional analyses with some compensation for the three dimensionality of CT datasets. (GIGER et al. 1994; KANAZAWA et al. 1998; ARMATO et al. 1999, 2001, 2002). With the transition to isotropic resolution with MDCT of the chest, these techniques may not scale to true three-dimensional analysis.

25.4.1.1
The Evolution of CAD for Lung Nodule Detection

The use of CAD in MDCT for analysis of lung nodules and other disease states is less mature than mammography because of the limited time that MDCT has been available to the market and because there is no CAD system for MDCT currently available for commercial use. The same model illustrated in Fig. 25.2a can be applied to the automatic detection of lung nodules with MDCT, but the individual components of the model are less advanced.

At the base of the CAD system are the automatic detection algorithms, algorithms that *detect regions consistent with suspicion of disease*. Most reported techniques have shown high sensitivity for lung nodule detection (ARMATO et al. 2001; Ko and BETKE 2001; SCHOEPF et al. 2002; WOOD et al. 2002; BROWN et al. 2003; DAS et al. 2003; WOOD et al. 2003a,b). Table 25.2 shows the stand-alone CAD performance for one CAD system developed for the MDCT environment (WOOD et al. 2002, 2003a,b). Preliminary results indicate that the CAD performance with high sensitivity and low false positive rates, could be acceptable performance for routine clinical practice.

Table 25.2. CAD performance for lung nodule detection (WOOD et al. 2003a,b)

Database type	CAD sensitivity
Training	90.3% (287/318)
Test	81.4% (114/140)
Combined*	87.6% (401/458)

*Median of 2.0 false positive markings per case

25.4.1.2
The Gold Standard for Lung Nodule Detection

Measuring stand-alone CAD performance for lung nodule detection; however, varies from mammography. A comparable standard of biopsy proof is not only difficult, but may not apply for the detection of lung nodules. Firstly, the biopsy of nodules as small as three and four millimeters in diameter is not common and therefore a database of small cancers is difficult, but it is likely that smaller abnormalities pose the larger detection problem. Secondly, detection algorithms designed to detect lung nodules as an abnormality are not designed to detect malignancies since not all lung nodules are malignant, but may none-the-less be important clinical findings. Biopsy proof, while objective, may not be a scalable reference criteria for lung nodule detection.

Generally, gold standard algorithms for the detection of lung nodules are defined by consensus panels (DAS et al. 2002; WOOD et al. 2002; DAS et al. 2003a,b), but by their very nature, are a more subjective standard than biopsy. Getting a repeatable reference dataset with consensus panels relies on a very tight definition of the reference measurement. However, radiologists in test environments, removed from their normal clinical environment, may overcall lesions because of the lack of clinical consequence or patient impact of their decision making (E.K. Fishman 2003, personal communication). All factors contribute to the difficulty in defining the reference dataset.

One method of producing a repeatable reference dataset is through the insertion of artificial nodules with properties similar to the true nodules into the original imaging database (CROISILLE, SOUTO et al. 1995; RUSINEK, NAIDICH et al. 1998; DAS, SCHNEIDER et al. 2003) (Fig. 25.4a, b). This tighter standard may prove to be valuable in the evaluation of standalone performance in CAD systems, but has yet to be tested on a wider scale.

25.4.1.3
The Integration of CAD for Lung Nodule Detection into the Clinical Workflow Using MDCT

The *integration of CAD in the current radiological environment* of MDCT is challenging, partly because MDCT has so significantly impacted the clinical workflow that it requires fundamental change (RUBIN 2003). CAD is in a position to facilitate that change. Figure 25.5 shows the review component of an investigational CAD system. The inset image shows the detected nodule, its automatically detected contour, and the automatically generated two-dimensional and volumetric measurement of the nodule. These measurements can be saved and tracked over time to automatically evaluate nodule progression or regression. Once the nodule is automatically detected, these workflow enhancements,

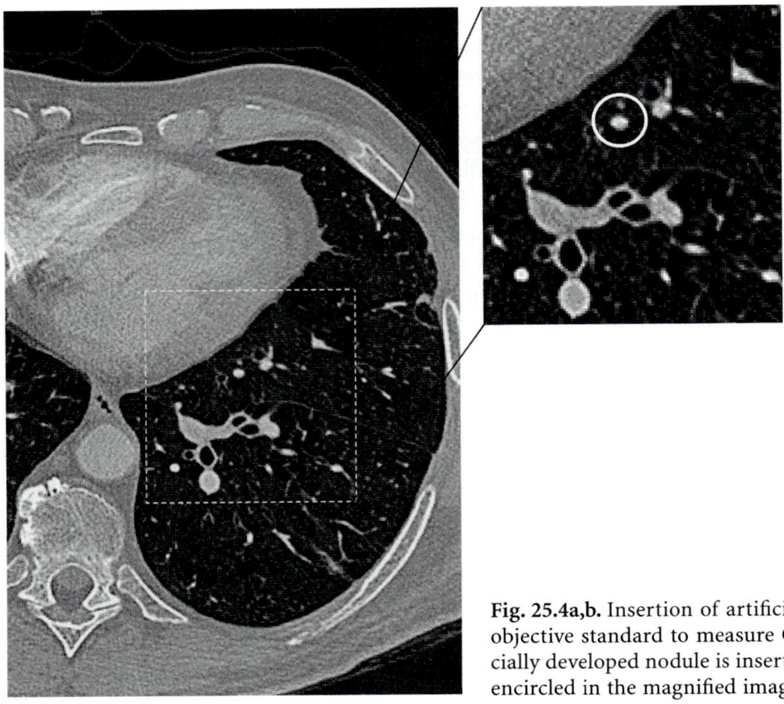

a b

Fig. 25.4a,b. Insertion of artificial nodules is a possible way to develop an objective standard to measure CAD stand-alone performance. The artificially developed nodule is inserted into the original CT image (**a**) in shown encircled in the magnified image (**b**).

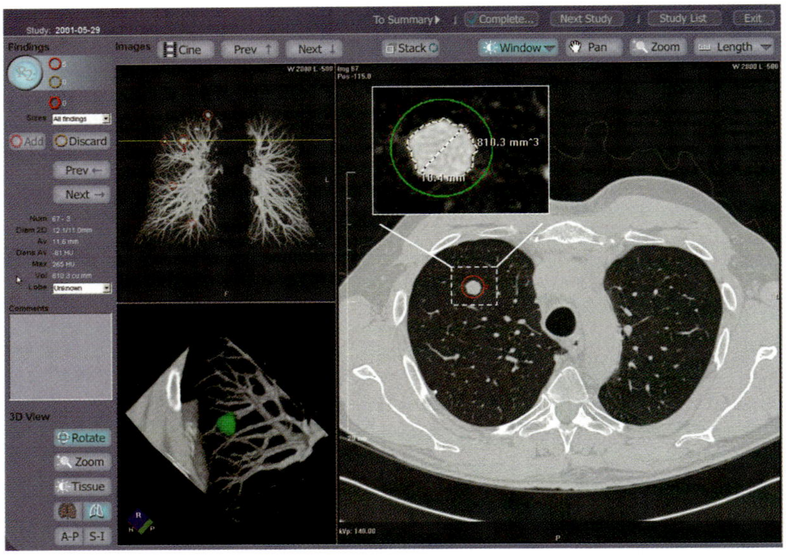

Fig. 25.5. A CAD application for the automatic detection and analysis of lung nodules. The application displays the automatically detected nodules with synchronized 2D and 3D views. The automatically detected region encircled in the axial view is shown with automatic contouring of the border of the detected region and associated measurement of the detected region.

often done manually otherwise, are available to the user. These automatically generated measurements could save time and produce more repeatable results than human interaction. CAD therefore has immediate potential to focus the radiologist's energy on interpretation of images and increasing the efficiency of a radiologist in a MDCT environment (Armato et al. 2002; Das et al. 2002, 2003; Wood et al. 2003b; Fan et al. 2002).

Other workflow enhancements driven by MDCT and by CAD are the ability to retrospectively reconstruct axial slices at varying slice thicknesses (Wood et al. 2003a). CAD will always read the highest resolution image available, but because it remains routine to read MDCT data using transverse reconstructions, the user may choose to read fewer slices at a lower resolution. Figure 25.6a shows a CAD system in which the axial image is retrospectively reconstructed at 5 mm

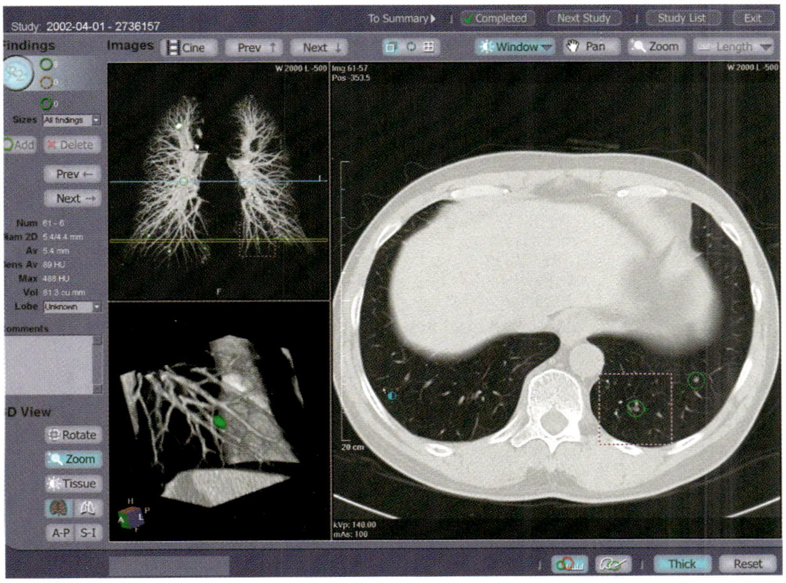

a

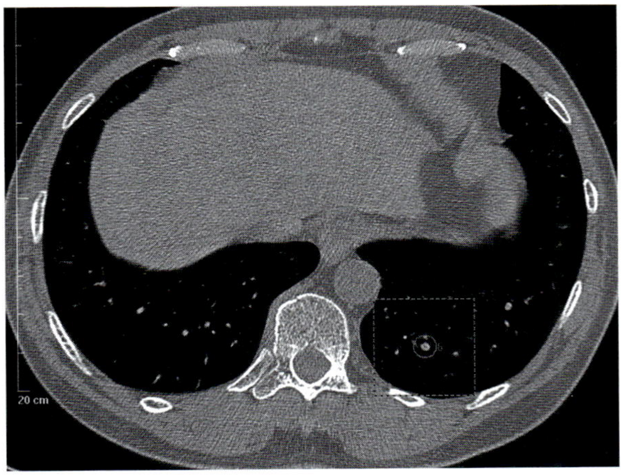

b

Fig. 25.6a,b. With the ability of CAD algorithms to retrospectively reconstruct at multiple collimations enable the user to view the image data at a lower resolution than its reconstruction acquired. CAD reads and displays in 3D the highest acquired resolution and prompts the reader on the lower resolution axial image (**a**). The user can then toggle the axial data to the higher resolution (**b**). This reading paradigm enables the user to read fewer axial images on initial review.

slice thickness. CAD, however, analyzed the data at the higher resolution (1.25 mm) collimation. The volumetric rendering using the higher resolution data in the lower left viewport of Fig. 25.6a clearly indicates an isolated finding, but the location of that finding encircled in the axial image at lower resolution is less clearly identified. Toggling the axial data from lower (5 mm) resolution to higher (1.25 mm) resolution (Fig. 25.6b) a feature allowed by MDCT, the isolated finding is more clearly identified and the radiologist is able to make a more informed decision.

Ideally, CAD could have the potential to *influence the radiologist's interpretation* if lung nodules are overlooked in a normal clinical setting. Wood et al. (2002) reported a 7.3% increase in the detection of actionable lung nodules after the double reading of MDCT datasets, indicating the potential for a higher increase in detection from CAD after just a single read. The value of CAD for increased accuracy of detection is found in the clinically significant findings not originally found with the double read.

Das et al. reported the effectiveness of CAD for readers of different experience levels. Table 25.3 indicates two readers performance, one with six years experience reading chest CT images and the other with one year of experience reading chest CT images, before and after the use of the CAD system. With CAD, the performance of the inexperienced reader approached that of the experienced reader, clearly more positively influencing the inexperienced reader. CAD therefore has the potential to level the playing field among users of different experience levels producing a more consistent performance.

The observer performance of CAD for the detection of lung nodules is not well enough developed to determine its *effect on clinical outcome*. When these systems become available for routine clinical use, these data will become more readily available.

25.4.2 CAD for Pulmonary Embolism (PE) Detection

One area where MDCT has made the greatest impact is for its use in vascular applications (Schoepf et al. 2001; Rubin 2003a,b). MDCT used for PE diagnosis can potentially reestablish the gold standard from more expensive and invasive methods like traditional angiography. CAD is ideally suited for the detection of pulmonary embolus because the tortuous nature of the pulmonary arterial tree. The tracking of its branching structure to identify emboli is time consuming and tedious, especially when using the more common mode of reviewing CT angiography examinations with transverse slices. Once an abnormality is found; however, its diagnosis is reasonably straightforward. Identifying PE in CT angiography examinations is a problem of detection, making it an ideal use of CAD. CAD can potentially reduce tracking time, increase accuracy of detection, and is a valuable safety net for physicians making an emergent and critical diagnosis. CAD with MDCT makes this application clinically feasible in a resource-constrained environment. Table 25.4 shows the performance of a prototype pulmonary embolism detection system for segmental and subsegmental emboli. CAD has shown a high level of performance in initial studies (Schoepf et al. 2002, 2003) that approach clinical acceptability. CAD combined with CT angiography studies using MDCT, could produce a more accurate and less invasive clinical evaluation for pulmonary embolus than traditional angiography.

Figure 25.7 shows the CAD system for pulmonary embolism detection. The detected emboli are shown encircled in the axial image, and those detected emboli map to the demarcations in the volumetric viewports. The PE detection program was designed to run concurrently with the lung nodule detection system. A lung nodule found in a PE study, for example, would demarcate the regions suspicious for a lung nodule even though those nodules may not be visible in the PE review window. To again optimize the clinical workflow in a MDCT environment, the automatic detection of both PE and lung nodules are available on the same application.

Table 25.3. Differences in observer performance for lung nodule detection with and without CAD (Das et al. 2002, 2003)

Sensitivity	No CAD	With CAD
Novice reader	78.1%	86.5%
Expert reader	93.3%	95.5%

Table 25.4. CAD used for the automatic detection of pulmonary embolism (Schoepf et al. 2002; Das et al. 2003)

Vessel type	CAD sensitivity
Segmental artery	91% (118/130)
Subsegmental artery	66% (99/150)

25.5 Other Applications for MDCT of the Thorax

CAD applications focus on the detection of abnormalities of the thorax rather than the diagnosis of these abnormalities. In their current state, CAD algorithms are a great benefit as a safety net to radiologists for increased accuracy of detection and for driving workflow-enhancing automations to aid in the diagnosis. However, as CAD systems become more advanced, their output will likely be of more diagnostic quality. The transition of these devices from detection devices to diagnostic devices will likely be led by mammography systems (Giger et al. 2002) because of the longevity of mammographic systems in clinical practice and the familiarity of mammographic systems to regulatory agencies. A computer-aided diagnosis product will likely be commercially acceptable after its proven commercial use as a detection product.

Similarly, CAD has the potential to be a first reader in some clinical applications and the sensitivity of computerized detection may surpass human observation for some disease states (i.e., calcifications). Computerized detection is currently being used as a first reader for PAP smears and may in time be used as a first reader in some screening environments where the radiologist reads predominately normal cases. These first reader applications would again be led by CAD devices with more common clinical acceptance as a second reader before approaching the workflow of a first reader. Because the workflow in the current MDCT environment is changing, CAD could have value as a concurrent reader, where the CAD marks are available to the radiologist as he or she makes the initial review of the case. CAD's acceptance as a second review, however, would need to be well established before approaching the standard of a concurrent reader.

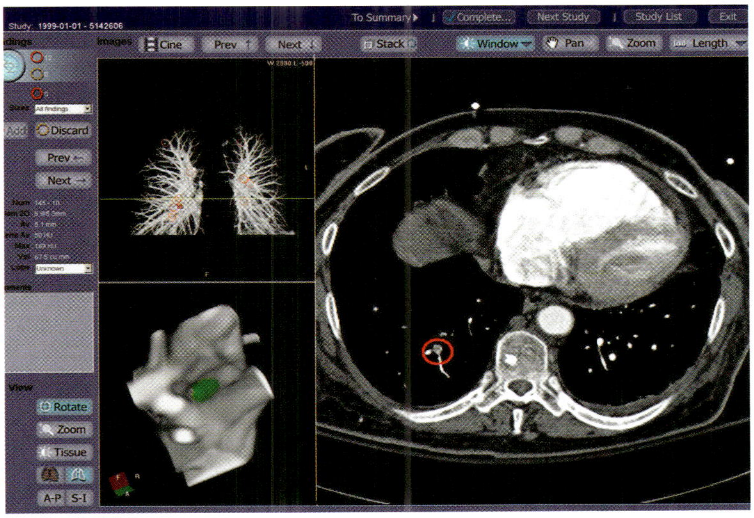

Fig. 25.7. CAD detection algorithm for PE using same user interface as CAD for lung nodule detection. The PE is encircled in the axial image. The user can toggle between lung and PE detection windows.

The combination of automatic detection for abnormalities of the thorax could in future be combined with surgical navigation since both of these technologies are independently well established. Similarly, the integration of CAD information with information from multiple modalities of anatomic (MDCT) and functional (i.e., positron emission tomography (PET)) will play a key role in facilitating the unification and workflow from these two technologies.

25.6 Conclusion

Present day CAD systems complement human observation by consistency and repeatability without fatigue and therefore complement the natural variability of human observation. However, in their present form, they lack the judgment of the human observer. It therefore remains the assessment of the radiologist, once detected, to determine the clinical course of the patient.

With the dynamic nature and anatomical complexity of the organs in the thorax, faster and higher resolution acquisitions significantly impact the quality of the examination. MDCT, therefore, has the potential to fundamentally change the way CT is performed in the thorax if the workflow problems associated with larger and larger datasets are solved. With the known miss rates associated with human observations added to the complexity of image overload using MDCT, observational oversights could become more prevalent with higher-resolution data. Workflow issues associated with MDCT therefore may be forcing the requirement for CAD in a clinical setting to increase accuracy of detection, assuredness and consistency of review, and productivity. These improvements may enable volumetric imaging to reach its true clinical potential.

References

Abe K, Doi K, MacMahon H, Giger M. L, Jia H, Chen X et al (1993) Computer-aided diagnosis in chest radiography. Preliminary experience. Invest Radiol 28:987–993

Armato SG III, Giger ML, Moran CJ, Blackburn JT, Doi K, MacMahon H (1999) Computerized detection of pulmonary nodules on CT scans. Radiographics 19:1303–1311

Armato SG III, Giger ML, MacMahon H (2001) Automated detection of lung nodules in CT scans: preliminary results. Med Phys 28:1552–1561

Armato SG III, Li F, Giger ML, MacMahon H, Sone S, Doi K (2002) Lung cancer: performance of automated lung nodule detection applied to cancers missed in a CT screening program. Radiology 225:685–692

Brown MS, Goldin JG, Suh RD, McNitt-Gray MF, Sayre JW, Aberle DR (2003) Lung micronodules: automated method for detection at thin-section CT–initial experience. Radiology 226:256–262

Chan HP, Doi K, Galhotra S, Vyborny CJ, MacMahon H, Jokich PM (1987) Image feature analysis and computer-aided diagnosis in digital radiography. I. Automated detection of microcalcifications in mammography. Med Phys 14:538–548

Chan HP, Doi K, Vyborny CJ, Schmidt RA, Metz CE, Lam KL et al (1990) Improvement in radiologists' detection of clustered microcalcifications on mammograms. The potential of computer-aided diagnosis. Invest Radiol 25:1102–1110

Croisille P, Souto M, Cova M, Wood S, Afework Y, Kuhlman JE et al (1995) Pulmonary nodules: improved detection with vascular segmentation and extraction with spiral CT. Work in progress. Radiology 197:397–401

Das M, Jacobson F, Schneider A, Wood S, Schoepf U (2002) CAD of lung nodules on multidetector-row CT: impact on readers with variable levels of experience. Radiology 225:476

Das M, Schneider A, Anderson M, Herzog P, Judy P, Jacobson F et al (2003a) Computer-aided detection (CAD) of lung nodules in high resolution multidetector-row CT (MDCT) chest scans. Eur Radiol 13:169

Das M, Schneider A, Bonneau V, Mamisch C, Herzog P, Wood S et al (2003b) CAD of segmental and subsegmental pulmonary emboli on 1-mm multidetector-row CT studies. Eur Radiol 13:138

Das M, Schneider A, Jacobson F, Wood S, Schoepf U (2003c) CAD of lung nodules on multidetector-row CT: impact on readers with variable levels of experience. Eur Radiol 13:315

Doi K, Giger ML, MacMahon H, Hoffmann KR, Nishikawa RM, Schmidt RA et al (1992) Computer-aided diagnosis: development of automated schemes for quantitative analysis of radiographic images. Semin Ultrasound CT MR 13:140–152

Fan L, Qian J, Wei G-Q, Naidich DP (2002) Pulmonary nodule detection using cartwheel projection analysis. CARS, Springer, Berlin Heidelberg New York

Fishman EK (2001) International Society for Strategic Studies in Radiology (ISSSR), San Francisco, CA

Freer TW, Ulissey MJ (2001) Screening mammography with computer-aided detection: prospective study of 12,860 patients in a community breast center. Radiology 220:781–786

Giger M, MacMahon H (1996) Image processing and computer-aided diagnosis. Radiol Clin North Am 34:565–596

Giger ML, Doi K, MacMahon H, Nishikawa RM, Hoffmann KR, Vyborny CJ et al (1993) An "intelligent" workstation for computer-aided diagnosis. Radiographics 13:647–656

Giger ML, Bae KT, MacMahon H (1994) Computerized detection of pulmonary nodules in computed tomography images. Invest Radiol 29:459–465

Giger M, Huo Z, Vyborney C, Lan L, Nishikawa RM, Rosenborough I (2002) Results of an observer study with an intelligent mammographic workstation for CAD. In: Peitgen H-O (ed) Digital mammography IWDM 2002. Springer, Berlin Heidelberg New York, pp 297–303

Gruden JF, Ouanounou S, Tigges S, Norris SD, Klausner TS (2002) Incremental benefit of maximum-intensity-projection images on observer detection of small pulmonary nodules revealed by multidetector CT. AJR Am J Roentgenol 179:149–157

Gurney JW (1996) Missed lung cancer at CT: imaging findings in nine patients. Radiology 199:117–122

Hazelrigg SR, Boley TM, Weber D, Magee MJ, Naunheim KS (1997) Incidence of lung nodules found in patients undergoing lung volume reduction. Ann Thorac Surg 64:303–306

Henschke CI, Yankelevitz DF, Mateescu I, Brettle DW, Rainey TG, Weingard FS (1997) Neural networks for the analysis of small pulmonary nodules. Clin Imaging 21:390–399

Johnson PT, Fishman EK, Duckwall JR, Calhoun PS, Heath DG (1998) Interactive three-dimensional volume rendering of spiral CT data: current applications in the thorax. Radiographics 18:165–187

Kakinuma R, Ohmatsu H, Kaneko M, Eguchi K, Naruke T, Nagai K et al (1999) Detection failures in spiral CT screening for lung cancer: analysis of CT findings. Radiology 212:61–66

Kanazawa K, Kawata Y, Niki N, Satoh H, Ohmatsu H, Kakinuma R et al (1998) Computer-aided diagnosis for pulmonary nodules based on helical CT images. Comput Med Imaging Graph 22:157–167

Ko JP, Betke M (2001) Chest CT: automated nodule detection and assessment of change over time – preliminary experience. Radiology 218:267–273

Lawler L, Wood S, Fishman E (2003) Computer-assisted detection of pulmonary nodules: preliminary observations using a prototype system with multidetector row CT datasets. J Dig Imaging (submitted)

MacMahon H, Doi K, Chan HP, Giger ML, Katsuragawa S, Nakamori N (1990) Computer-aided diagnosis in chest radiology. J Thorac Imaging 5:67–76

Margulis A (2001) International Society of Strategic Studies in Radiology (ISSSR), San Francisco, CA

Muhm JR, Brown LR, Crowe JK (1977a) Detection of pulmonary nodules by computed tomography. AJR Am J Roentgenol 128: 267–270

Muhm JR, Brown LR, Crowe JK (1977b) Use of computed tomography in the detection of pulmonary nodules. Mayo Clin Proc 52:345–348

Muhm JR, Miller WE, Fontana RS, Sanderson DR, Uhlenhopp MA (1983) Lung cancer detected during a screening program using four-month chest radiographs. Radiology 148: 609–615

Napel S, Marks MP, Rubin GD, Dake MD, McDonnell CH, Song SM et al (1992) CT angiography with spiral CT and maximum intensity projection. Radiology 185:607–610

Napel S, Rubin GD, Jeffrey RB Jr (1993) STS-MIP: a new reconstruction technique for CT of the chest. J Comput Assist Tomogr 17:832–838

Reiner BI, Siegel EL, Hooper FJ, Pomerantz S, Dahlke A, Rallis D (2001) Radiologists' productivity in the interpretation of CT scans: a comparison of PACS with conventional film. AJR Am J Roentgenol 176:861–864

Rubin GD (2003a) 3-D imaging with MDCT. Eur J Radiol 45 [Suppl 1]:S37–S41

Rubin GD (2003b) MDCT imaging of the aorta and peripheral vessels. Eur J Radiol 45 [Suppl 1]:S42–S49

Rubin GD, Napel S, Leung AN (1996) Volumetric analysis of volumetric data: achieving a paradigm shift. Radiology 200: 312–317

Rusinek H, Naidich DP, McGuinness G, Leitman BS, McCauley DI, Krinsky GA et al (1998) Pulmonary nodule detection: low-dose versus conventional CT. Radiology 209:243–249

Schoepf UJ, Kessler MA, Rieger CT, Herzog P, Klotz E, Wiesgigl S et al (2001) Multislice CT imaging of pulmonary embolism. Eur Radiol 11:2278–2286

Schoepf U, Das M, Schneider A, Anderson M, Wood S, Costello P (2002) CAD of segmental and subsegmental pulmonary emboli on 1-mm multidetector-Row CT studies. Radiology 225:384

Schwartz, LH, Ginsberg MS, DeCarato D, Rothenberg LN, Einstein S, Kijewski P, et al. (2000) Evaluation of tumor measurements in oncology: use of filmbased and electronic techniques. J Clin Oncol 18(10):2179–2184

Warren Burhenne LJ, Wood SA, D'Orsi CJ, Feig SA, Kopans DB, O'Shaughnessy KF et al (2000) Potential contribution of computer-aided detection to the sensitivity of screening mammography. Radiology 215:554–562

Wood S, Stapleton S, Schneider A, Herold C, Castellino R (2002) CAD of actionable lung nodules using MSCT scans of the lung: sensitivity and false marker rates. Radiology 225:477

Wood S, Schneider A, Gamboa-Aldeco A, Castellino R (2003a) The ImageChecker-CT: computer-aided detection (CAD) for chest MSCT. Eur Radiol 13:574

Wood S, Stapleton S, Schneider A, Herold C, Castellino R (2003b) CAD of actionable lung nodules using MSCT scans of the lung: sensitivity and false marker rates. J Eur Radiol 13:169

Miscellaneous

26 Pediatric Multislice Computed Tomography of the Chest

M. J. Siegel

CONTENTS

M. J. Siegel, MD
Mallinckrodt Institute of Radiology, Washington University School of Medicine, 510 South Kingshighway Blvd., St. Louis, MO 63110, USA

26.1 Introduction

In the early 1980 s the introduction of single-slice helical CT into clinical radiology dramatically improved the diagnosis of thoracic diseases in children. The introduction of multislice CT has again advanced diagnostic imaging of the pediatric chest. The benefits of multislice CT– improved temporal and spatial resolution, greater anatomic coverage, optimal contrast enhancement, and higher quality three-dimensional renderings– have practical applications for virtually the entire spectrum of thoracic disease. This chapter addresses the areas in which multislice CT has already proved of value in the pediatric chest. The technical factors for optimizing the CT examination also are reviewed.

26.2 Patient Preparation

Pediatric patients have several inherent problems that are not present in adults, in particular patient motion, small body size, and lack of perivisceral fat. These problems can be minimized or eliminated by appropriate use of sedation and oral and intravenous contrast medium.

26.2.1 Sedation

As the speed of CT increases, the need for sedation in the pediatric age group decreases (Kaste et al. 1997; White 1995; Pappas et al. 2000). Although the frequency has diminished, sedation has not been eliminated. Sedation will likely still be required for some infants and children 5 years of age and younger to prevent motion artifacts during scanning. Children older than 5 years of age generally will cooperate after verbal reassurance and explanation of the procedure and will not need immobilization or sedation.

Standards of care for sedation are based on recommendations from the Committee on Drugs, American Academy of Pediatrics (AAP) (1992) and the American Society of Anesthesiologists (ASA) Task Force (1996). Sedation for imaging examinations is nearly always conscious sedation. Conscious sedation is defined as a minimally depressed level of consciousness that retains the patient's abilities to maintain a patent airway, independently and continuously, and respond appropriately to physical stimulation and/or verbal command.

26.2.1.1 Pre-sedation Preparation

All patients need to be screened for past and current illness prior to receiving sedation. This evaluation includes (a) a review of past health history and previous hospitalizations; (b) review of systems; (c) physical examination; and (d) assessment of baseline vital signs (temperature, pulse, respiratory rate, and blood pressure), weight, level of consciousness and motor function.

As part of the preparation process, intravenous access should be obtained, and preparatory guidelines appropriate to sedation, particularly oral and solid intake status, reviewed. Aspiration is a major clinical concern in sedated children and NPO (non per os or "nothing by mouth") guidelines should be as stringent as those used for general anesthesia.

26.2.1.2 Parenteral Sedation Drugs and Techniques

The sedatives used most widely for CT are oral chloral hydrate and intravenous pentobarbital sodium. Oral chloral hydrate (Pharmaceutical Associates, Inc., Greenville, S.C.) is the drug of choice for children younger than 18 months. It is given in a dose of 50 to 100 mg/kg, with a maximum dosage of 2,000 mg. Onset of action is usually within 20 to 30 min. Intravenous pentobarbital (Nembutal, Abbot Laboratories, North Chicago, IL) is preferred in children 18 months of age and older. Intravenous pentobarbital, up to 6 mg/kg, with a maximum dose of 200 mg, is injected slowly in aliquots, starting at 2–3 mg/kg, and is titrated against the patient's response. Onset of action is usually within 5 to 10 minutes.

Regardless of the choice of drug, the use of parenteral sedation requires personnel experienced in maintaining adequate cardiorespiratory support during and after the examination. Intravenous access must be continuously maintained and continuous monitoring of vital signs must be performed and recorded.

26.2.2 Intravenous Contrast Medium

Nearly all CT examinations of the chest are performed with administration of intravenous contrast material. An intravenous line should be in place before the child arrives in the CT suite. This reduces patient agitation that otherwise would be associated with a venipuncture performed immediately prior to administration of contrast material and thus increases patient cooperation. The largest gauge cannula that can be placed is recommended.

26.3 Imaging Techniques

Prior to initiation of scanning, decisions must be made about the anatomic coverage required to answer the clinical question, the protocol for contrast administration, and the CT acquisition parameters.

In general, the anatomic coverage should extend from just above the thoracic inlet to 1 to 2 cm below the diaphragm. A greater degree of coverage to include the upper abdomen may be warranted occasionally, particularly in the setting of assessment of sequestration or aneurysm.

Contrast medium may be administered by hand injection or a mechanical injector (Kaste and Young 1995; Siegel 1999). Hand injections are used when the intravenous access is via a peripheral vein placed in the dorsum of the hand or foot. Power injectors are used when a 22-gauge or larger cannula can be placed in an antecubital vein. The contrast injection rate is determined by the caliber of the intravenous catheter. For a 22 gauge catheter, the flow rate is 1.5 to 2.0 mL/sec; for a 20 gauge catheter, flow rates are 2.0 to 3.0 mL sec. The site of injection is closely monitored during the initial injection of contrast in order to minimize the risk of contrast extravasation Power injection through a central venous catheter or a 24 gauge catheter has been shown to be safe, provided that there is proper intravascular positioning of the access line, verified by the unimpeded return of blood and the unimpeded delivery of a saline flush (Kaste and Young 1995; Herts et al. 2001) and the rate of injection is slow (1 ml/sec). The benefit of power injection is the uniformity of contrast delivery which allows for maximal enhancement. The complication rates for manual and power injections are similar (<0.4%), provided that the catheter is positioned properly and functions well (Herts et al. 2001). The iodinated contrast material should be nonionic (Cohan et al. 1996; Stockberger et al. 1998) and administered in a volume of 2mL/kg (not to exceed 125 mL).

The final and crucial step for optimizing delivery of the contrast medium is the determination of the scan delay time after the initiation of the contrast medium bolus. In general, a 20 to 30 second delay is sufficient for routine chest CT examinations (i.e., tumor staging, evaluation of a mediastinal or pulmonary mass, trauma). The shorter delays (20 s) are used in neonates and infants (under 2 years of age), who have higher cardiac output, with longer delay times used in older children and adolescents. For CT angiography (i.e., evaluation of cardiovascular anomalies, sequestration, arteriovenous malformation, and hypogenetic lung), a 12 to 15 second scan delay after the start of the contrast administration produces excellent vascular enhancement in patients under 2 years of age. A 20 to 25 second delay is used in older children.

Because of the additional radiation exposure, unenhanced scans are not obtained routinely prior to contrast administration. They are indicated when assessing stent grafts and dissections. In the assessment of the former, they help to identify perigraft calcifications which can mimic a leak on contrast-enhanced scans. In the setting of dissection, unenhanced sections are useful for localizing high attenuation hematoma in the false lumen.

Alternatively, a semi-automated bolus-tracking method can be used to optimize contrast enhancement. This method allows continuous monitoring of the attenuation within a large target vessel (e.g., aorta or pulmonary artery) by use of a series of low-dose axial images. Once a predetermined threshold is reached, the low-dose scanning is terminated and the diagnostic examination is automatically initiated. A default delay can be programmed in case the desired threshold is not achieved. This technology has proven particularly useful in CT angiography.

26.3.1 CT Protocol

For CT examinations performed with a four detector row scanner with an adaptive array design, a nominal section (collimator) thickness of 2.5 mm coupled with a table speed of 15 to 20 mm per rotation (pitch of 1.5 to 2.0) is adequate. A 1.0 mm collimation thickness may be of value when a detailed evaluation of small vessels is indicated. For examinations performed with a 16 detector row scanner, the collimation is 1.5 with a table speed of 24 to 36 mm per rotation. A 2.0 to 5.0 mm effective slice thickness is used for viewing thoracic structures.

The CT study should be performed with a single breath hold whenever possible. This can usually be done in children older than 5 or 6 years of age. If breath-holding is not possible, scanning should be performed during quiet respiration.

For the vast majority of thoracic CT studies in children, a single phase study in the arterial phase is sufficient. However, for evaluation of stent-graft repair of coarctation, a second set of images, 60 to 70 seconds after the initiation of the contrast injection, can be important to assess for endoleak.

Finally adjustments in tube current must be made in pediatric patients to save radiation exposure (Donnelly et al. 2001; Haaga 2001; Lucaya et al. 2000; Patterson et al. 2001; Rogalla et al. 1999; Slovis 2002) (Table 26.1). Because children are more radiosensitive than adults to the same organ dose and because they have a longer life span, a potential for development of radiation-included malignancies exists. CT should be performed with parameters which provide acceptable image quality and the lowest possible radiation exposure. We typically use the lowest possible milliamperage (mA) and kilovoltage (kV). In patients with smaller body habitus, studies can be performed with 80KV, which lowers the radiation dose to the patient (compared to the standard 120 kV protocols) by a factor of approximately 30%. A higher kV (100 to 120) will be needed in children with large body habitus.

Table 26.1. Chest CT Acquisitions Factors

Weight (Kg)	mA	kV
<15	25	80
16–24	30	80
25–34	45	80
35–44	75	80
45–54	90–100	100–120
>54	120 or >	100–120

26.4 Reconstruction Techniques

When multiplanar or 3D imaging is contemplated, the 2.5 mm and 1.5 mm thick volumetric data are reconstructed with a section thickness of 3 and 2 mm respectively and an interval of 1 to 2 mm. A standard reconstruction algorithm usually suffices for routine CT examinations and CT angiograms, while a high resolution (bone) algorithm is best for examinations of the airway and diffuse lung disease.

A detailed description of the two- and three-dimensional reconstruction techniques is beyond the scope of this chapter. In general, multiplanar reformations and 3D volume renderings are most useful in the assessment of the mediastinal great vessels and central airways. Thick-slab maximum and minimum intensity projections may be useful in evaluation of small airway or vessel disease. A more detailed discussion of multiplanar reformation and three-dimensional reconstruction techniques can be found elsewhere in this textbook and in the literature (Boiselle et al. 2002; Cody 2002; Lawler and Fishman 2001; Ravenel et al. 2001; Ruben 2000).

26.5 Clinical Applications: Chest

The cross-sectional and 3D CT images are helpful in detecting or clarifying abnormalities in the lungs, mediastinum, chest wall and peridiaphragmatic regions. The information provided by these techniques can directly affect treatment or aid in determining the prognosis of a patient.

The common clinical applications for CT of the pediatric chest are: a) oncologic screening (evaluation of lung metastases); b) congenital lung anomalies, c) mediastinal masses; d) cardiovascular anomalies; e) airway disease; f) diffuse lung disease, and g) complex chest wall abnormalities.

26.6 Evaluation Of Pulmonary Metastases (Protocol 1)

26.6.1 Metastases

CT is a valuable technique for detection of pulmonary metastases in patients with known malignancies with a high propensity for lung dissemination, such as Wilms' tumor, osteogenic sarcoma, and rhabdomyosarcoma. Demonstration of one or more pulmonary nodules in such patients, or documentation of additional nodules in a patient with an apparent solitary metastasis for whom surgery is planned, may be critical to treatment planning. In the first instance, such detection may lead to additional treatment (surgery, chemotherapy, or radiation), whereas in the latter setting, demonstration of several metastatic nodules may negate surgical plans.

The temporal and spatial resolution afforded by CT improves the detection and characterization of pulmonary nodules. The use of thin collimation allows retrospective reconstructions to be obtained through suspected nodules without the need for rescanning, which decreases radiation dose and optimizes the characterization of focal lesions (Remy-Jardin et al. 1993; Wright et al. 1996).

26.6.2 Other Focal Lung Nodules

Other causes of nodular lung lesions, besides metastases, include granuloma, opportunistic infections, lymphoproliferative disorders, intrapulmonary lymph node, and some of the congenital anomalies (Fig. 26.1). Congenital lesions, such as bronchial atresia or those with abnormal vessels (arteriovenous malformation or pulmonary varix), can be diagnosed confidently with CT. In other instances, clinical history or a repeat CT after waiting 6 to 8 weeks may needed before a specific diagnosis can be made. In a patient with a primary neoplasm, an increase in number or size of nodules can be assumed to represent evidence of metastatic disease.

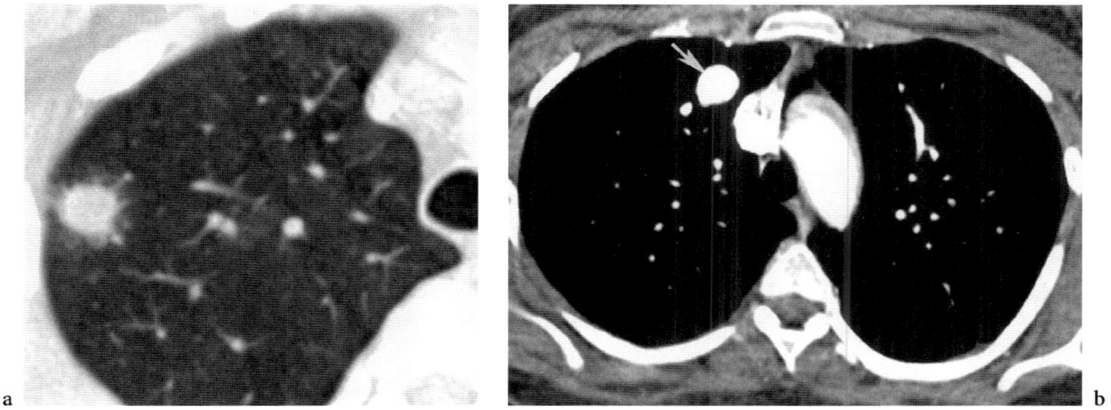

Fig. 26.1. Pulmonary nodules. **a:** Invasive aspergillosis. CT scan at lung window setting shows a well-circumscribed nodule surrounded by hazy opaque infiltrate (halo sign) in the right upper lobe. **b:** Arteriovenous malformation. CT scan shown at soft-tissue setting shows a well-circumscribed enhancing nodule (arrow) in the right upper lobe

26.7 Congenital Lung Anomalies (Protocols 1 and 2)

Congenital lung anomalies include a variety of conditions involving the pulmonary parenchyma, the pulmonary vasculature, or a combination of both. Because these conditions are associated with either a parenchymal lesion or anomalous vessels, they are well suited for evaluation by CT scanning (Siegel and Siegel 1999a; Gupta et al. 2002).

26.7.1 Anomalies with Normal Vasculature

Congenital lobar emphysema, cystic adenomatoid malformation, and bronchial atresia are anomalies resulting from abnormal bronchial development. The role of CT is to confirm the diagnosis and to determine the extent of abnormality in patients in whom surgery is contemplated.

26.7.1.1 Congenital Lobar Emphysema

Congenital lobar emphysema is characterized by hyperinflation of a lobe. The CT findings are an overinflated lobe with attenuated vascularity, compression of ipsilateral adjacent lobes, and mediastinal shift to the opposite side. The left upper lobe is involved in about 45% of cases, the right middle lobe in 30%, the right upper lobe in 20%, and two lobes in 5% of cases.

26.7.1.2 Cystic Adenomatoid Malformation

Cystic adenomatoid malformation is characterized by an overgrowth of distal bronchial tissue that results in the formation of a cystic mass rather than normal alveoli. Three types of cystic adenomatoid malformation have been described on pathologic examination: Type I (50% of cases) contains a single or multiple large cysts (>2 cm in diameter); type II (40%) contains multiple small cysts (1 to 20 mm in diameter) ; type III (10%) is a solid lesion to visual inspection, but it contains tiny cysts microscopically. The anomaly occurs with equal frequency in both lungs, although there is a slight upper lobe predominance. On CT, cystic adenomatoid malformation appears as a parenchymal mass that may be predominantly cystic or solid or contain an admixture of cystic and solid components (Siegel and Siegel 1999a; Kim et al. 1997) (Fig. 26.2). Cystic adenomatoid malformation can occur in association with sequestration.

26.7.1.3 Bronchial Atresia

Bronchial atresia results from abnormal development of a segmental or subsegmental bronchus. CT features of bronchial atresia include overaerated lung distal to the atresia and a round, ovoid or branching density near the hilum, representing mucoid impaction just beyond the atretic bronchus.

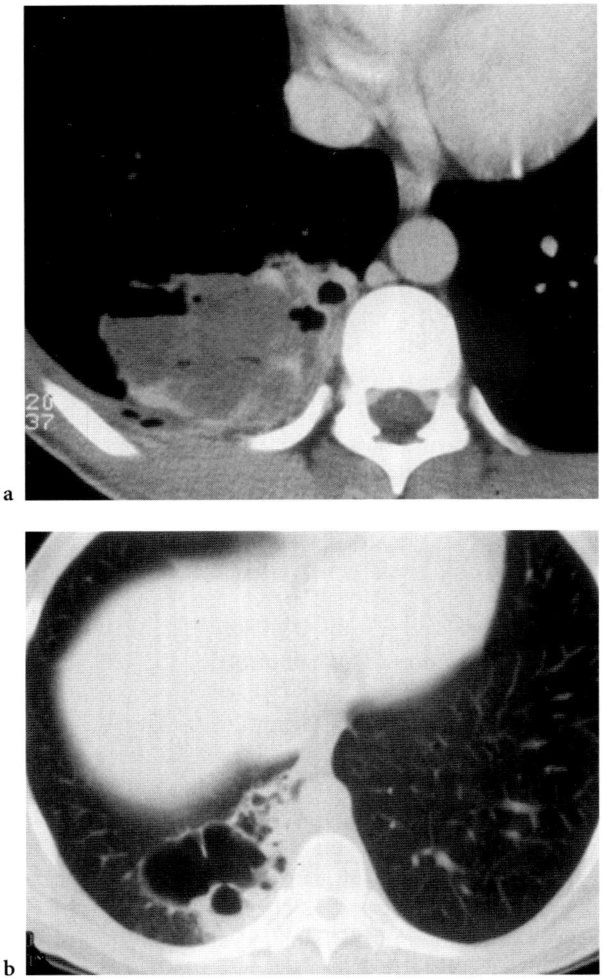

Fig. 26.2. Cystic adenomatoid malformation. **a:** Axial image at mediastinal windows shows a predominantly fluid-filled mass in the right lower lobe. Some-air-filled areas are also present. **b:** A scan at a more caudal level with lung windows shows a complex mass with several air-filled cysts

26.7.2 Anomalies with Abnormal Vasculature

Sequestration, hypogenetic lung syndrome, and arteriovenous malformation (AVM) are congenital anomalies with abnormal vasculature.

26.7.2.1 *Bronchopulmonary Sequestration*

Bronchopulmonary sequestration is a congenital mass of pulmonary tissue that has no normal connection with the tracheobronchial tree and is supplied by an anomalous artery, usually arising from the aorta. When the sequestered lung is confined within the normal visceral pleura and has venous drainage to the pulmonary veins, it is termed congenital or intralobar (Frazier et al. 1997). The sequestered lung is termed acquired or extralobar when it has its own pleura and venous drainage to systemic veins.

CT scanning after an injection of contrast material demonstrates opacification of the anomalous vessel immediately following peak aortic enhancement (Frazier et al. 1997; Ko et al. 2000) (Fig. 26.3). The anomalous vessel usually arises from the aorta, but upper abdominal vessels can be a source of the arterial supply. The CT appearance of the pulmonary parenchyma depends on whether or not the sequestered lung is aerated. When the sequestration communicates with the remainder of the lung, usually after being infected, it appears cystic; a sequestration that does not communicate appears as a homogeneous density, usually in the posterior portion of the lower lobe.

26.7.2.2 *Hypogenetic Lung Syndrome*

Hypogenetic lung, also known as venolobar or scimitar syndrome, refers to the combination of a small lung, which is nearly always on the right, and anomalous pulmonary venous. Other findings include a corresponding small pulmonary artery and ipsilateral mediastinal displacement (Woodring et al. 1994; Zwetsch et al. 1995). The anomalous return is usually into the inferior vena cava, although it may enter the suprahepatic portion of the inferior vena cava, the hepatic veins, portal veins, azygous vein or right atrium. Associated anomalies include systemic arterial supply to the hypogenetic lung and horseshoe lung. Horseshoe lung is a rare anomaly in which the posterobasal segments of both lungs are fused behind the pericardial sac.

26.7.2.3 *Pulmonary Arteriovenous Malformation (AVM)*

Pulmonary AVM is characterized by a direct communication between a pulmonary artery and vein without an intervening capillary bed. At CT, AVMs appear as rounded or lobular masses with rapid enhancement and washout after intravenous contrast medium administration (Lawler and Fishman 2002; Hoffman et al. 2000; Remy et al. 1994) (Fig. 26.4).

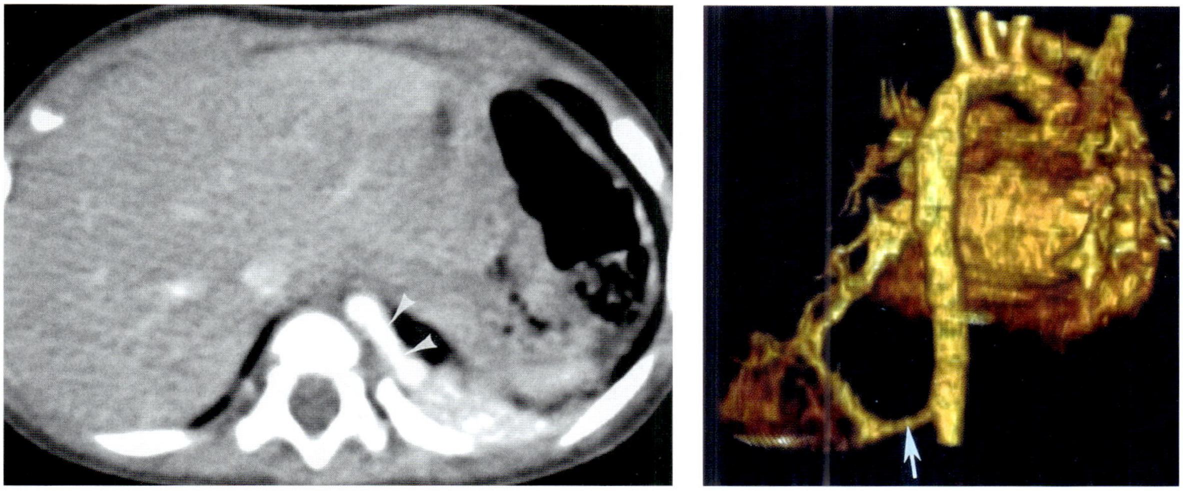

a b

Fig. 26.3. Intralobar pulmonary sequestration. A: Axial contrast-enhanced CT section demonstrates a vessel (arrowheads) arising laterally from the descending thoracic aorta and extending to an area of left lower lobe opacity. B: Three-dimensional volume rendering shows the feeding artery (arrow) arising from the aorta and extending to the lower lobe sequestration. Drainage was via a pulmonary, which entered the left atrium

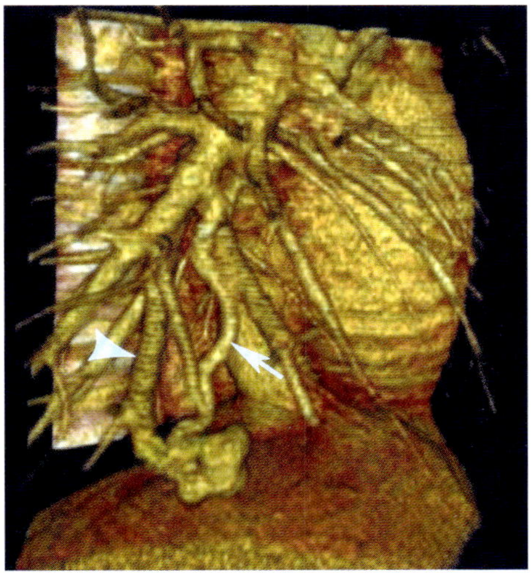

Fig. 26.4. Pulmonary arteriovenous malformation. 3D volume rendering. The feeding artery (arrow) originates from the right lower lobe artery. The draining vein (arrowhead) drains into the right inferior pulmonary vein

Enhancement typically occurs immediately after enhancement of the right ventricle. Axial images can establish the diagnosis of a vascular ring, but 3D reconstructions are of value in demonstrating the precise anatomy of the malformation, including the number of feeding arteries and draining veins, which is critical information for treatment planning. This anomaly can occur in isolation or with Rendu-Osler-Weber disease.

26.8 Mediastinal Mass Evaluation (Protocol 1)

A widened mediastinum in infants and children often is due to a mass lesion (Bower and Kiesewetter 1996; Merten 1992; Meza et al. 1993). The role of CT in the evaluation of mediastinal and lung masses is lesion characterization and definition of extent. In general, axial images alone can provide this information. The use of multiplanar reformations in coronal, sagittal, and oblique planes can provide information about the longitudinal extent of disease, which can be valuable in patient management, particularly in planning surgical and radiation therapy.

CT appearances of the most common mediastinal masses in children are discussed below.

26.8.1 Anterior Mediastinal Masses

Lymphoma, thymic hyperplasia, teratoma, and cystic hygroma are the most common anterior mediastinal masses in children. Rarer causes of anterior mediastinal masses include thymoma, an enlarged thyroid, thymolipoma, lipoblastoma, and thymic cysts.

Protocol 1

INDICATION:	Standard Lung/Mediastinum (Oncologic staging, detection of metastases, characterization of mediastinal or pulmonary mass, evaluation of trauma)
Extent	Lung apices to caudal bases
Scanner settings:	kVp: 80; mA: lowest possible based on patient weight
Detector collimation	2.5 mm for 4-row scanner 1.5 mm for 15-row scanner
Table speed (Pitch)	15–20 mm/rotation (1.5–2) for 4-row scanner 24–36 mm/rotation for 16-row scanner
Slice thickness	3–5 mm for 4-row scanner 2–5 mm for 16-row scanner
IV Contrast	Nonionic 280–320 mg iodine/mL
Contrast volume	2 mL/kg (maximum of 4 mL/kg or125 mL, whichever is lower)
Contrast injection rate **	Hand injection: rapid push bolus Power injector: 22 gauge: 1.5 -2.0 mL/sec 20 gauge: 2.0 -3.0 mL/sec
Scan delay	20 to 30 s
Miscellaneous	1. If the child is sedated or uncooperative, CT scans are obtained at quite breathing. 2. Contrast medium used at discretion of radiologist in the evaluation of metastases. Routinely given for evaluation of mediastinal and pulmonary masses and trauma 3. Higher kVp (100 to 120) may be needed in larger patients (>50 kg). 4. Use a standard reconstruction algorithm.

26.8.1.1
Lymphoma

Lymphoma, including Hodgkin's disease and non-Hodgkin's lymphoma, is the most common cause of an anterior mediastinal mass. Approximately 65% of pediatric patients with Hodgkin disease have intrathoracic involvement at clinical presentation, and the superior mediastinal nodes and/or thymus are involved in almost all cases (>95%) (Hudson and Donaldson 1997). Additional sites of involvement are the lung parenchyma (10%) and pleura (10%). About 40% of pediatric patients with non-Hodgkin lymphoma have chest disease at diagnosis, and only 50% of this disease involves the superior mediastinum. Other common sites of involvement in non-Hodgkin's lymphoma are the hilar and subcarinal node. The frequency of parenchymal and pleural involvement in non-Hodgkin's lymphoma is about the same as in Hodgkin's disease (Hammrick-Turner et al. 1994).

Lymphomatous masses in Hodgkin disease are most common in the anterior mediastinum and reflect either infiltration and enlargement of the thymus or lymphadenopathy. The enlarged thymus has a quadrilateral shape with convex, lobular lateral borders (Siegel and Siegel 1999b; Siegel 1993) (Fig. 26.5). The attenuation of the lymphomatous organ is equal to that of soft tissue. Additional findings include mediastinal or hilar lymph node enlargement, airway narrowing and compression of vascular structures.

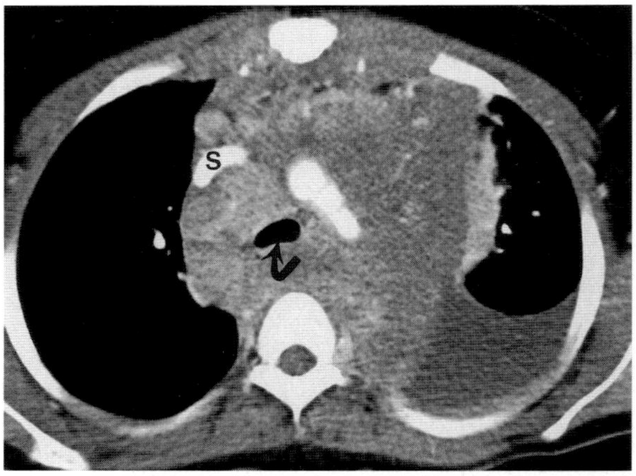

Fig. 26.5. Thymic Hodgkin's disease. A large anterior mediastinal mass, representing massive infiltration of the thymus by lymphoma, displaces the carina (arrow) posteriorly. The superior vena cava (S) is also compressed. Concomitant enlargement of right paratracheal lymph nodes is present. The tumor extends posteriorly to the left paraspinal area and there is a left pleural effusion. Because most mediastinal masses are large, axial images suffice for diagnosis. Multiplanar images can be useful to show longitudinal tumor extent.

Lymphadenopathy is the other common intrathoracic manifestation of lymphoma. The appearance varies from mildly enlarged nodes in a single area to large conglomerate soft tissue masses in multiple regions. Typically, the enlarged nodes have well-defined margins and show little enhancement after intravenous administration of contrast medium. Hodgkin disease usually causes enlargement of the thymus or anterior mediastinal nodes, whereas non-Hodgkin lymphoma predominantly affects middle mediastinal lymph nodes.

26.8.1.2
Thymic Hyperplasia

Thymic hyperplasia is another cause of diffuse thymic enlargement. In childhood, it has been associated with myasthenia gravis, red cell aplasia, hyperthyroidism, but the most frequent cause is rebound hyperplasia. Rebound hyperplasia may be observed during the course of chemotherapy or after the completion of therapy. On CT, hyperplasia appears as diffuse enlargement of the thymus with preservation of the normal triangular shape. The attenuation value of the hyperplastic thymus is similar to that of the normal organ. It is the absence of other active disease and a gradual decrease in size of the thymus on serial CT scans that supports the diagnosis of rebound hyperplasia as the cause of thymic enlargement.

26.8.1.3
Germ Cell Tumors

Germ cell tumors are the most common cause of a fat-containing mediastinal mass in children. They are derived from one or more of the three embryonic germ cell layers and usually arise in the thymus. Approximately 90% are benign and histologically are either dermoid cysts (containing only ectodermal elements) or teratomas (containing tissue from all three germinal layers). On CT, both lesions are well-defined, thick-walled, predominantly cystic (fluid-filled) masses containing a variable admixture of tissues: calcium, fat, and soft tissue. A fat-fluid level occasionally can be seen within these tumors.

A malignant teratoma generally appears as a poorly defined, predominantly soft tissue mass, sometimes containing calcification and fat. Local infiltration into the adjacent mediastinum with encasement or invasion of mediastinal vessels or airways also is frequent.

26.8.1.4
Cystic Hygroma

Cystic hygromas are lymphogenous cysts that occur in the antero-superior mediastinum and are almost always inferior extensions of cervical hygromas. The CT appearance is that of a thin-walled, multiloculated mass of near-water attenuation value. The surrounding fascial planes are obliterated if the tumor infiltrates the adjacent soft tissues. Hemorrhage can increase the CT attenuation value.

26.8.2
Middle Mediastinal Masses

The frequent causes of middle mediastinal masses are congenital foregut cysts and lymph node enlargement.

26.8.2.1
Bronchopulmonary Foregut Cysts

Bronchopulmonary foregut malformations include bronchogenic, enteric and neurenteric cysts (Siegel and Siegel 1999b; Haddon and Bowen 1991). Bronchogenic cysts are lined by respiratory epithelium, and most are located in the subcarinal or right paratracheal regions. Enteric cysts, also known as esophageal duplications are lined by gastrointestinal mucosa and usually are located close to or within the esophageal wall. Neurenteric cysts are posterior mediastinal lesions that are connected to the meninges through a midline defect in one or more vertebral bodies and are lined by gastrointestinal epithelium.

CT findings of foregut cysts include a non-enhancing round or tubular mass with well-defined margins and thin or imperceptible walls (Fig. 26.6). The cyst contents usually are homogeneous and of

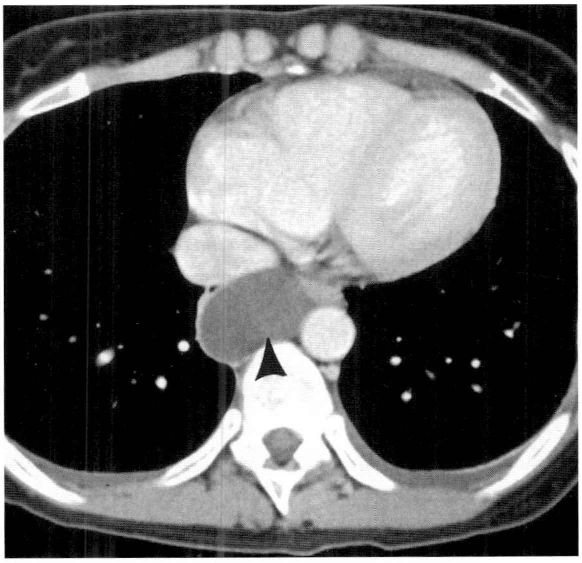

Fig. 26.6. Enteric cyst. Axial contrast-enhanced CT shows a well-defined, homogeneous water-attenuation mass (arrowhead) filling the azygoesophageal recess

near-water attenuation, reflecting their serous nature. Some foregut cysts will have higher attenuation values because the contents contain proteinaceous fluid, hemorrhage, mucus, or calcium.

26.8.2.2
Lymphadenopathy

Lymph node enlargement, as a cause of a middle mediastinal mass, is usually caused by lymphoma or granulomatous disease. On CT, adenopathy can appear as discrete soft tissue masses, or as a single soft tissue mass with ill defined margins. Calcification within lymph nodes suggests old granulomatous disease, such as histoplasmosis or tuberculosis. Low attenuation areas suggest tuberculosis.

26.8.3
Posterior Mediastinal Masses

26.8.3.1
Neurogenic Tumors

Neurogenic tumors are the most common cause of a posterior mediastinal mass. Neuroblastoma and ganglioneuroblastoma are more common in infants and children, while ganglioneuroma, neurofibroma and schwannoma increase in frequency in adolescents and adults. Rarer causes of posterior mediastinal masses in children include paraspinal abscess, lymphoma, neurenteric cyst, lateral meningocele, and extramedullary hematopoiesis.

On CT, ganglion cell tumors appear as fusiform or elongated paraspinal masses, extending over the length of several vertebral bodies (Siegel and Siegel 1999b). They are of soft tissue attenuation and contain calcifications in up to 50% of cases (Fig. 26.7). Nerve root tumors tend to be smaller, spherical, and occur near the junction of a vertebral body with an adjacent rib. Both types of tumors may cause pressure erosion of a rib. Because of their origin from neural tissue, neurogenic tumors have a tendency to invade the spinal canal. Intraspinal extension is extradural in location, displacing and occasionally compressing the cord. Identification of intraspinal invasion is important because affected patients require radiation therapy or a laminectomy prior to tumor debulking.

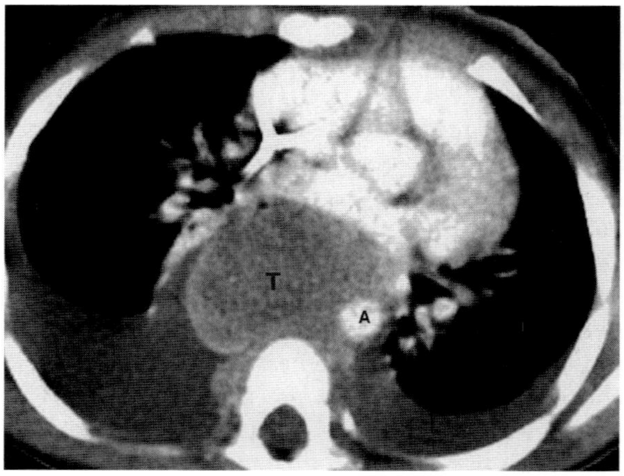

Fig. 26.7. Posterior mediastinal mass, neuroblastoma. Axial CT scan through the lower thorax shows a large soft tissue tumor (T) in a paravertebral location. The tumor extends around the descending aorta (A). Also seen are bilateral pleural effusions

26.9
Vascular Assessment (CT Angiography) (Protocol 2)

The evolution of multislice CT has led to a changing role for CT angiography in the evaluation of cardiovascular anomalies in children. CT angiography can clearly demonstrate the morphology of the pulmonary vessels and aorta and thus, it has gained increasing acceptance as an alternative method to MR imaging and conventional catheter angiography in the diagnosis of vascular anomalies (Hopkins et al. 1996; Katz et al. 1995). An important advantage of CT angiography over MR angiography relates to the shorter scan time which means reduction in the need for sedation and the ability to scan extremely ill patients who cannot tolerate the long imaging times for MR examinations. There is the risk of radiation exposure in CT angiography, but in the critically ill patient the risk of prolonged sedation may be greater than that of radiation. Compared with the radiation dose for angiography, the radiation dose for CT angiography is at least two to three times less.

While routine axial images are usually sufficient for diagnosis, the reconstructed images can provide better anatomic detail about anatomic relationships between the great vessels and tracheobronchial tree and provide a more reliable assessment of airway compromise. With regard to the assessment of vascular narrowing, multiplanar volume reformation and 3D reconstructions can aid in the detection of mild coarctations and improve the accuracy of determining the length of coarctation. In addition, these images can aid in the planning of surgery or stent placement.

Protocol 2

INDICATION:	CT Angiography (Mediastinal vascular anomalies, dissection, aneurysm, post-operative shunts)
Extent	Lung apices to caudal bases
Scanner settings:	kVp: 80; mA: lowest possible based on patient weight
Detector collimation	2.5 mm for 4-row scanner 1.5 mm for 15-row scanner
Table speed (Pitch)	15–20 mm/rotation (1.5–2) for 4-row scanner 24–36 mm/rotation for 16-row scanner
Slice thickness	3–5 mm for 4-row scanner 2–5 mm for 16-row scanner
IV Contrast	Nonionic 280–320 mg iodine/mL
Contrast volume	2 mL/kg (maximum of 4 mL/kg or150 mL, whichever is lower)
Contrast injection rate	Hand injection: rapid push bolus Power injector: 22 gauge: 1.5–2.0mL/sec 20 gauge: 2.0–3.0 mL/sec
Scan delay	Patient weight <15 kg: 12 to 15 s Patient weight >15 kg: 20 to 25 s
Miscellaneous	1. If the child is sedated or uncooperative, CT scans are obtained at quite breathing. 2. Higher kVp (100 to 120) may be needed in larger patients (>50 kg). 3. If sequestration is suspected, scanning should extend through the upper abdominal aorta. 4. Precontrast images are not needed for most examinations, but they are used in the evaluation of endovascular stents. 5. Use standard reconstruction algorithm.

26.9.1 Congenital Heart Disease

Most congenital and acquired cardiac lesions are evaluable by echocardiography, but CT can be of use when echocardiography provides inadequate information. The major indications for CT in congenital cardiac anomalies include: (a) evaluation of the size and patency of the pulmonary arteries in patients with cyanotic heart disease, such as pulmonary atresia and tetrology of Fallot, (b) detection of anomalous origin of the coronary artery (Fig. 26.8), (c) determination of the extracardiac anatomy in patients with complex congenital heart disease (e.g. great vessel relationships, bronchial collateral vessels, abdominal situs), and (d) evaluation of surgically created systemic-to-pulmonary artery shunts in patients with complex anatomic heart diseases, such as truncus arteriosus, tetrology of Fallot, hemitruncus, and pulmonary atresia. Vessel anatomy, shunt patency, and the presence of collateral vessel formation are clearly depicted with 3D volume rendering techniques.

Because multislice CT can be performed rapidly, artifacts from cardiac pulsation are eliminated or minimized. In addition, the use of 3D volume rendering allows for more confident depiction of vessels that course obliquely through the imaging planes.

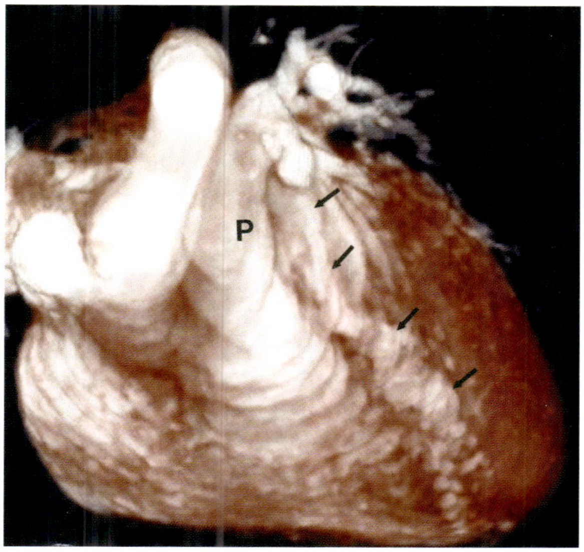

Fig. 26.8. Anomalous origin of the left coronary artery. Three dimensional volume-rendered images. The left coronary artery (arrows) originates from the main pulmonary artery (P)

26.9.2 Pulmonary Arteries and Vein

26.9.2.1 Pulmonary Arteries

The two common abnormalities of the pulmonary arteries are the obstructive lesions (i.e., pulmonary artery atresia, stenosis and hypoplasia) and the pulmonary sling.

The role of CT angiography in patients with obstructive lesions of the pulmonary artery is to determine the presence, caliber and confluence of the main pulmonary arteries and the presence and distribution of collateral vessels (Fig. 26.9). Collateral vessels can originate from brachiocephalic arteries, the descending thoracic aorta, or the subdiaphragmatic aorta. These collateral arteries can anastomose with intrapulmonary vessels.

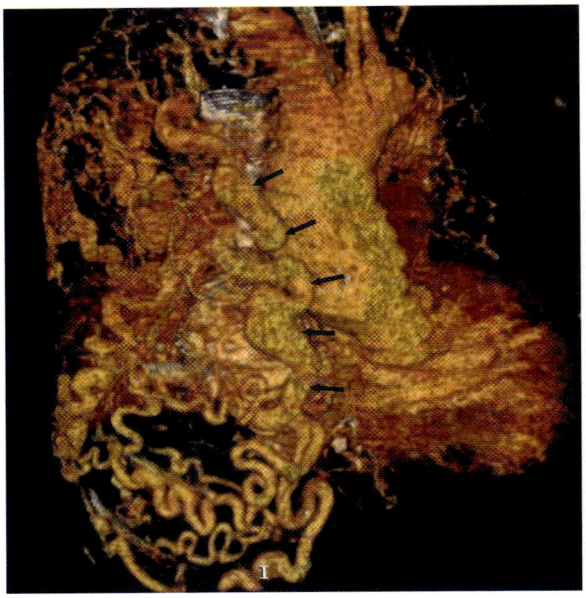

Fig. 26.9. Pulmonary stenosis with a failed right Blalock-Taussig shunt. Coronal volume rendered image demonstrates multiple transpleural collateral vessels arising from a dilated, tortuous right mammary (internal thoracic) artery (arrows)

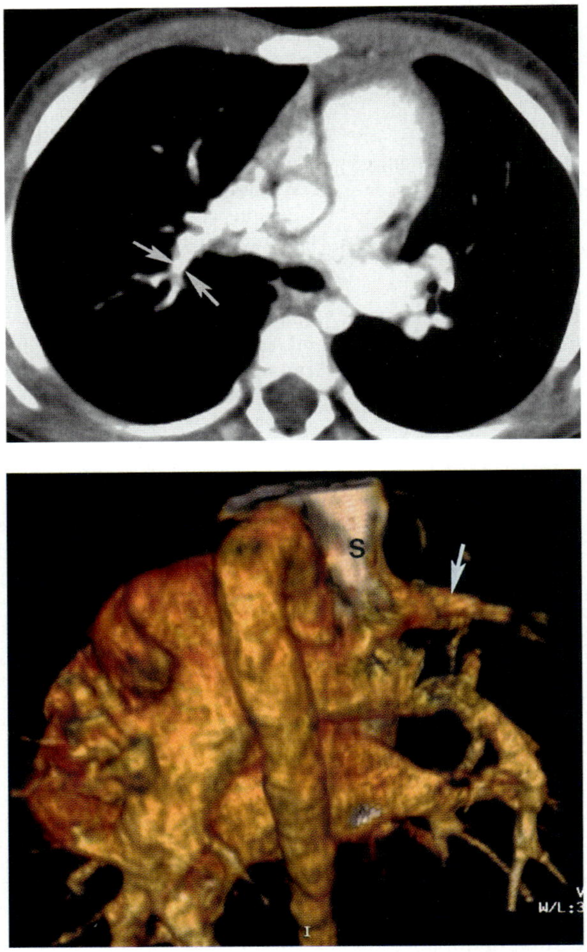

Fig. 26.10. Partial anomalous venous return. A: Axial CT scan at the level of the superior mediastinum shows part of the anomalous pulmonary vein draining the right upper lobe. B: 3D volume rendered image, viewed from behind, shows the anomalous vessel entering the superior vena cava (S). Arrow=anomalous vein

In patients with pulmonary sling, the left pulmonary artery originates from the right pulmonary artery and crosses the mediastinum, extending between the trachea and esophagus to reach the left hilum. Patients typically present with respiratory symptoms due to compression of the airway by the left pulmonary artery or associated stenosis of the trachea or main bronchi.

26.9.2.2
Pulmonary Veins

Partial anomalous return is the most common abnormality of the pulmonary veins. Anomalous drainage of the pulmonary veins can occur in isolation or with hypogenetic lung syndrome (Fig. 26.10). The anomalous drainage commonly involves the left superior and right inferior pulmonary veins. The anomalous left superior pulmonary vein drains into the left brachiocephalic vein, producing a vertical vein that courses lateral to the aortic arch and aortopulmonary window. The anomalous right inferior pulmonary vein drains cephalad into the azygous vein or caudal into the subdiaphragmatic inferior vena cava or portal vein, producing a scimitar vein.

26.9.3
Aortic Anomalies

The common anomalies of the aorta are the vascular rings and non-valvar stenotic lesions (coarctation, interrupted arch, supravalvular stenosis). Aneurysm formation and dissection are rare in children.

26.9.3.1
Vascular Rings

Vascular rings result from an abnormal development of the aortic arch system, which results in derivatives of the arch encircling the trachea and esophagus. The diagnosis of a vascular ring is usually suggested on conventional chest radiography. CT is used to define the anatomy for surgical planning. Axial images can establish the diagnosis of a vascular ring, but coronal images are of value in demonstrating the precise anatomy of the rings and their relationship to adjacent structures.

The common symptomatic vascular rings are the double aortic arch and the right aortic arch with an aberrant left subclavian artery. In double aortic arch, there are two aortic arches, both of which arise from a single ascending aorta. Each arch gives rise to a subclavian and carotid artery, before uniting to form a single descending aorta. The right arch tends to be higher and larger than the left (Fig. 26.11). The two components of the arch encircle the trachea and esophagus, resulting in airway compromise or dysphagia.

Right aortic arches are classified into two major subtypes: the right arch with an aberrant left subclavian artery and the right arch with mirror-imaging branching. The former type is rarely associated with congenital heart disease. In a right aortic arch anomaly with an aberrant left subclavian artery, the aberrant subclavian artery originates from an aortic diverticulum (Kommerell diverticulum), and the vascular ring is completed by the ligamentum arteriosum. Patients are symptomatic because the trachea and esophagus are encircled by mediastinal vessel or because the descending aorta compresses the trachea (Donnelly et al. 2002). On CT, the aberrant subclavian artery is seen as the last branch vessel to arise from the right aortic arch; it is often dilated at its origin (Fig. 26.12). A right aortic arch with mirror image branching has a high incidence of heart disease, but stridor and dysphagia are usually absent because there is not structure posterior to the trachea of the esophagus.

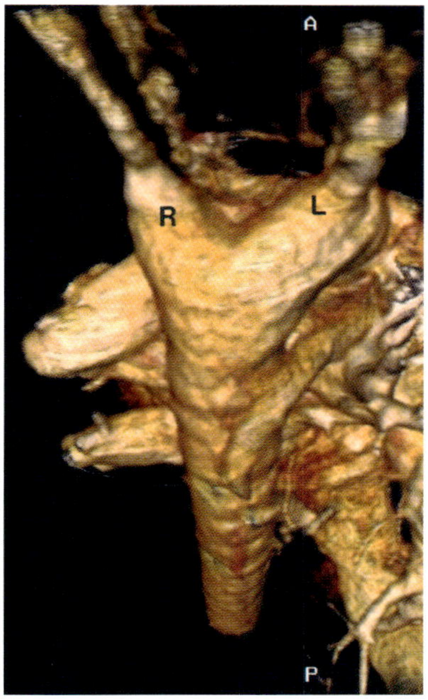

Fig. 26.11. Double aortic arch. Coronal volume rendered image shows a double arch. R = right arch; L = left arch

26.9.3.2
Non-valvar Stenosis of the Aorta

Aortic Coarctation

Coarctation of the aorta refers to a constriction or obliteration of a segment of that vessel. The segment of aorta just distal to the left subclavian artery is the most common site of coarctation. If the coarctation occurs between the left subclavian artery and the ductus arteriosus, it is termed preductal or infantile coarctation. This type may be associated with aortic arch hypoplasia. The second type of coarctation occurs distal to the ductus arteriosus and is referred to as adult coarctation (Fig. 26.13). In this anomaly, the aortic arch is usually of normal diameter, and collateral vessel formation is common.

Following surgical repair or balloon angioplasty, CT is useful to demonstrate aneurysm or restenosis.

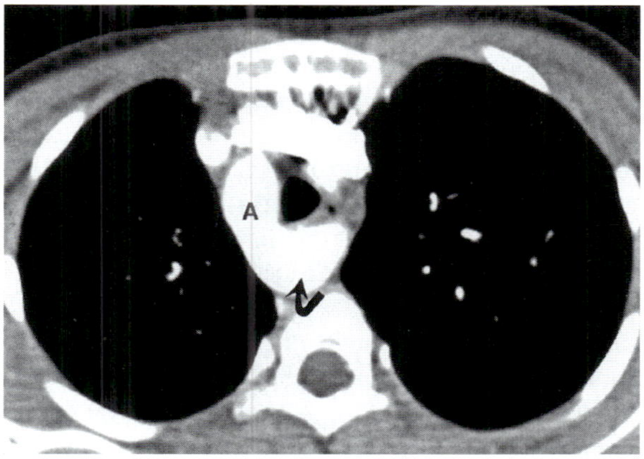

Fig. 26.12. Right aortic arch. Axial contrast-enhanced image shows the right arch (A) and aberrant left subclavian artery (arrow) crossing behind the trachea. Mild compression of the right wall of the trachea is seen

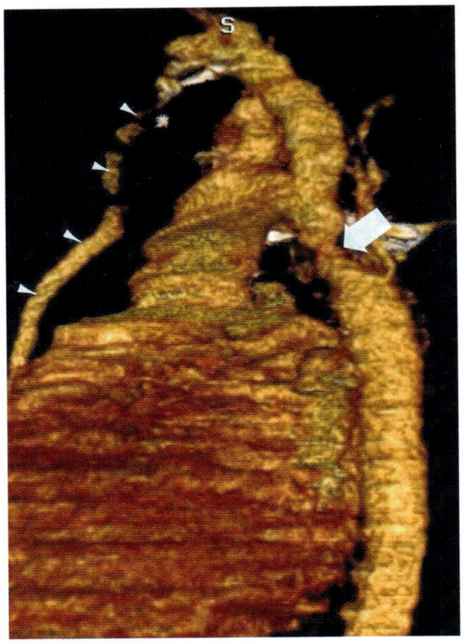

Fig. 26.13. Aortic coarctation. Volume rendered 3D reconstruction demonstrates focal narrowing (arrow) of the proximal descending aorta. Also note the large mammary artery collateral vessel (arrowheads)

Patients who have had repair of coarctation using prosthetic patches have an approximately 25% risk of developing aneurysms at the coarctation repair site (Bromberg et al. 1989).

Interruption of the Aortic Arch

Interruption of the aortic arch is characterized by complete discontinuity between the ascending and the descending aorta. There are three basic types of interrupted arch, which in descending order of frequency are: Type A: interruption of the aortic arch distal to the left subclavian artery, Type B: interruption of the arch between the left common carotid artery and the left subclavian artery, and Type C: interruption of the arch proximal to the left carotid artery. CT angiography can demonstrate the interrupted transverse arch and the patent ductus arteriosus supplying the descending aorta (Fig. 26.14). It is important not to mistake the dilated patent ductus arteriosus for the transverse arch.

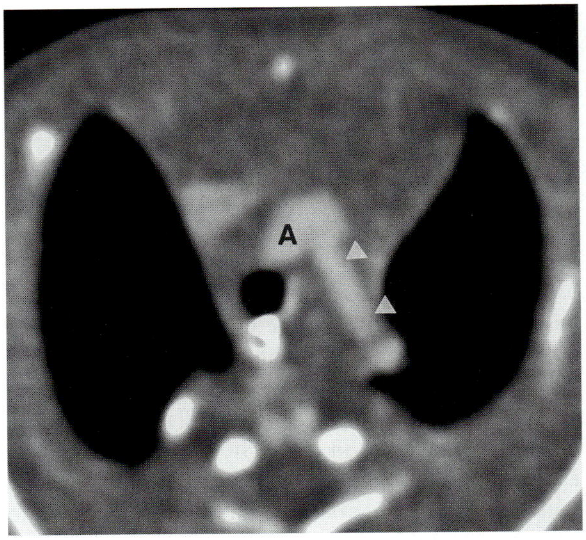

a

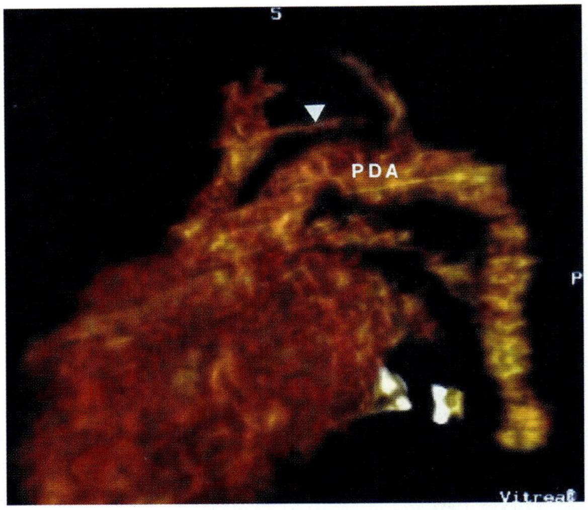

b

Fig. 26.14. Interrupted aortic arch. A Axial CT section in a 2 kg neonate demonstrates a normal caliber proximal aorta (A). The vessel latter and inferior to the aorta is a dilated patent ductus arteriosus (arrowheads). B: Volume-rendered reconstruction shows a markedly hypoplastic transverse arch (arrowhead) and a large patent ductus arteriosus (PDA) which supplies the distal aorta

Aortic Stenosis

Aortic narrowing can be seen in patients with arteritis, such as Takayasu arteritis, and William's syndrome. Takayasu arteritis is a primary arteritis of unknown origin that commonly affects the aorta and its major branches as well as the pulmonary artery. William's syndrome is characterized by the combination of supravalvar aortic stenosis, peripheral pulmonary arterial stenosis, mental retardation, and an "elfin facies". CT angiography can delineate the site and length of the aortic narrowing and a thickened arterial wall (Yamada et al. 1998).

26.9.3.3
Aortic Aneurysms and Dissections

Aortic aneurysms and associated dissections are rare in children. When they occur, they are usually associated with predisposing conditions, such as Turner syndrome, aortic coarctation, Marfan's syndrome (Fig. 26.15), Ehlers-Danlos syndrome, Kawasaki's disease, prior surgery, or trauma.

The diagnosis of aneurysm can be made when the diameter of the aorta is greater than 50% of the normal diameter of the aorta or when the diameter of the proximal descending aorta is 1.5 times the diameter of the descending thoracic aorta at the level of the diaphragm (Fig. 26.15). The CT diagnosis of dissection is based on demonstration of an intimal flap (Fig. 26.15). In general, the true aortic lumen is smaller than the false lumen, has an oval shape, follows the inner curve of the aorta, and contains faster flowing blood. The false lumen is usually larger than the true lumen, is crescent shaped, follows the outer curve of the aorta, and contains slower flowing blood.

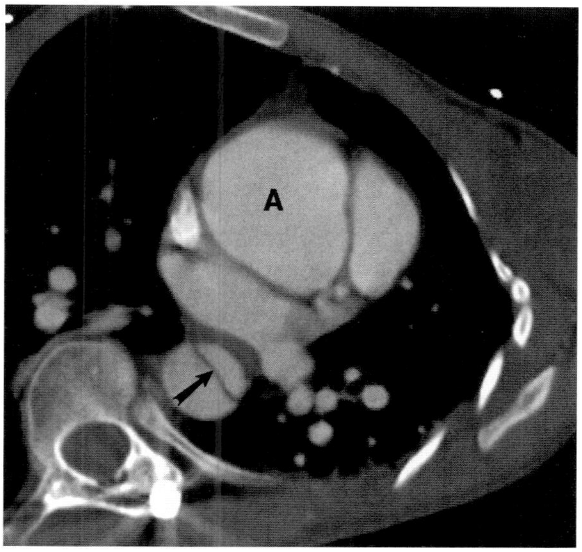

Fig. 26.15. Annuloaortic ectasia and dissection secondary to Marfan's disease. Axial CT scan shows a dilated proximal descending aorta (A) and an intimal flap (arrow) in the distal descending aorta, due to an acute dissection

26.9.4
Systemic Veins

The common venous anomalies include: duplicated superior vena cava and interruption of the inferior vena cava with azygous/hemiazygous continuation. A persistent left superior vena cava can occur in the general population, but it is more likely to occur in patients with congenital heart disease. The left superior vena cava lies lateral to the aortic arch as it descends along the left side of the mediastinum. As it courses inferiorly, it passes lateral to the main pulmonary artery and anterior to the left hilum to enter the coronary sinus that wraps around the bottom of the left atrium.

Inferior vena caval interruption results when the suprarenal, infrahepatic segment of the inferior vena cava fails to develop. Blood from the lower half of the body then returns to the heart via persistent subcardinal veins, termed the azygos and hemiazygous veins. Azygous and hemiazygous continuation of the inferior vena cava can be an isolated abnormality or it can coexist with congenital heart disease. CT findings are dilatation of the azygos arch, the azygos vein, and the superior vena cava caudal to the azygos junction; enlargement of the azygos and hemiazygous veins in the paraspinal and retrocrural areas; and absence of the suprarenal and intrahepatic portions of the inferior vena cava.

26.10
Evaluation of the Airway (Protocol 3)

26.10.1
Central Airway Disease

Axial CT images remain the standard for evaluating the central airways. However, multiplanar and 3D reconstructions can provide additional useful information and more precise depiction of tracheobronchial abnormalities (Hoppe et al. 2002; Lee et al. 1997; Remy-Jardin et al. 1998a,b; Sorantin et al. 2002).

Axial images are indispensable for assessing extraluminal disease, including the lung parenchyma and mediastinal structures. Multiplanar reformations aid in the detection of mild stenoses and tracheomalacia, provide a more reliable assessment of the extent of narrowing in the craniocaudal direction, and aid in the planning of stent placement or surgery (Boiselle et al. 2002). For the evaluation of tracheomalacia, scans are acquired at both end-inspiration and end-expiration and then reformatted in coronal and sagittal planes. This technique is limited to cooperative patients or to patients who are on assisted ventilation. In most uncomplicated cases, 3D reconstructions are of minimal value and only supplement multiplanar reformations. However, they can help to depict complex congenital airway abnormalities,

Protocol 3

INDICATION:	Tracheobronchial tree (Congenital anomalies; stricture, tumor, tracheomalacia)
Extent	Vocal cords to mainstem bronchi, just below carina
Scanner settings:	kVp:80; mA: lowest possible
Detector collimation	2.5 mm for 4-row scanner 1.5 mm for 15-row scanner
Table speed (Pitch)	15–20 mm/rotation (1.5–2) for 4-row scanner 24–36 mm/rotation for 16-row scanner
Slice thickness	3–5 mm for 4-row scanner 2–5 mm for 16-row scanner
Patient Instructions	Suspended inspiration
Contrast type	None
Comments	1. Aim for a single breath hold. Select pitch so that the area of interest can be scanned in a single breath hold in cooperative patients. 2. Use high spatial resolution reconstruction (bone) algorithm 3. Multiplanar and 3D reconstructions are useful to provide an overview of anatomy for surgical planning. 4. If small airway obstruction or tracheomalacia is suspected, obtain scans in inspiration and expiration 5. If child sedated or uncooperative, CT scans obtained at quiet breathing. 6. Higher kVp (100 to 120) may be needed in larger patients (>50 kg).

such as abnormal origins of the bronchi or broncho-esophageal fistulas, and they can help to improve the detection of subtle airway stenosis (Remy-Jardin et al. 1998a,b). In addition, they can provide information about the shape, length and extent of airway stenosis (Boiselle et al. 2002). Virtual bronchoscopy has a rather limited application, but it is indicated when there is a high-grade stenosis or large intraluminal tumor. This technique allows evaluation of the airways beyond the site of stenosis or neoplasm, which otherwise can be difficult to visualize by conventional bronchoscopy.

The indications for CT of the pediatric trachea and large bronchi include: evaluation of congenital bronchial anomalies (e.g., accessory bronchi, bronchial hypoplasia and atresia (McGuiness et al. 1993; Al-Nakshabandi et al. 2000), assessment of the extent of tracheal stricture (Quint et al. 1995) (Fig. 26.16) or tumor (Fig. 26.17), and detection and confirmation of tracheomalacia (Fig. 26.18) (Gilkeson et al. 2001).

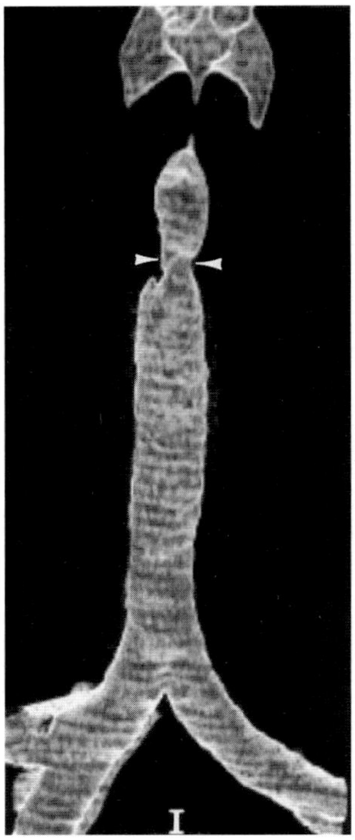

Fig. 26.16. Tracheal stricture secondary to prior intubation. Coronal multiplanar reformation shows focal narrowing of the proximal airway (arrowheads)

26.10.2 Peripheral Airway Disease

Bronchiolitis obliterans is the most common peripheral airway disease in children. It primarily affects the terminal and respiratory bronchioles and is the result of submucosal and peribronchiolar inflammation and fibrosis; parenchymal inflammation is absent. Bronchiolectasia with inspissated secretions is another common finding at histologic examination.

There are three predominant CT patterns of disease: (a) a tree-in-bud pattern; (b) poorly defined centrilobular nodules; and (c) decreased lung attenuation (Aquina et al. 1996; Collins et al. 1998; Lau et al. 1998; Muller and Miller 1995).

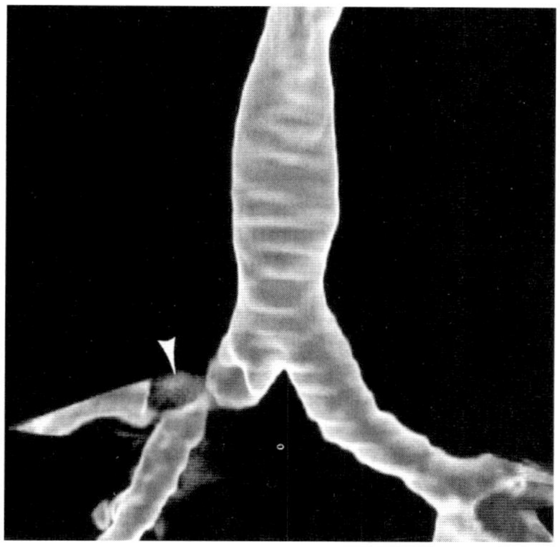

Fig. 26.17. Central airway tumor in a young adult following lung transplantation. Coronal 3D volume rendered reconstruction shows a soft-tissue mass (arrowhead) in the right mainstem bronchus. Final diagnosis was post-transplant lymphoproliferative disease

The decreased lung attenuation represents a combination of oligemia and air-trapping (SIEGEL et al. (2001); STERN and FRANK 1994). This appearance has been termed mosaic perfusion or mosaic attenuation. The presence of air trapping can be confirmed by acquisition of images in both inspiration and expiration, either at a single level or through select lung volumes (Fig. 26.19).

26.11 Diffuse Lung Disease (Protocol 4)

Chest radiography remains the imaging study of choice for evaluating most diffuse parenchymal lung disease. CT, however, can be useful to better define and characterize an abnormality suspected on conventional chest radiography, especially when the CT examination is performed with high resolution technique using 1 mm collimation every 10 to 20 mm. In most instances, axial images suffice for diagnosis. Multiplanar and 3D maximum intensity projection (MIP) and minimum intensity projection (minIP) images can help to characterize some diffuse lung diseases. MIP images can increase small nodule detection and help in characterizing the location of centrilobular and peribronchovascular nodules, whereas minIP images can improve depiction of the lumen of small airways and centrilobular emphysema. Recent reports have suggested that automated segmentation techniques may further improve the identification of diffuse lung disease and perhaps aid in the ability to quantify lung volumes and pulmonary function (BANKIER 1999; GENEVOIS 1996).

The indications for high-resolution CT of the lung parenchyma in children include: (a) detection of disease in children who are at increased risk for lung disease (e.g., immunocompromised patients) and who have respiratory symptoms but a normal

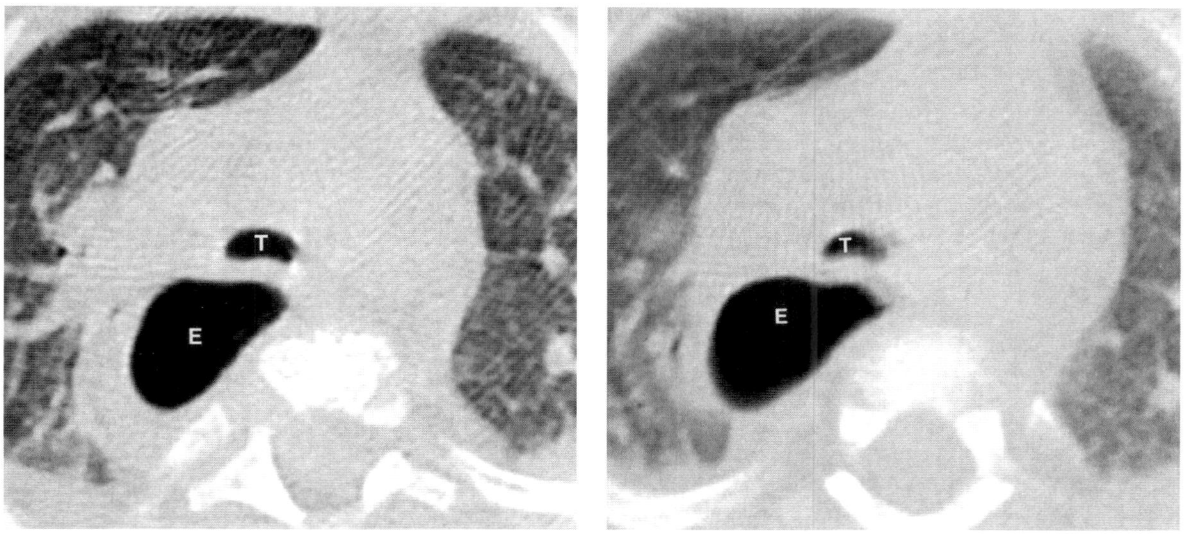

Fig. 26.18. Tracheomalacia in a 1-month-old girl who had undergone an esophageal pull-through for repair of esophageal atresia and who had marked dyspnea on attempts to extubate. The patient was intubated during the CT scan, allowing images to be obtained in inspiration and expiration. A: CT scan during end inspiration and B: during end expiration demonstrates a dilated esophagus (E) and marked collapse of the intrathoracic trachea (T), consistent with tracheomalacia, which was confirmed at fiberoptic bronchoscopy

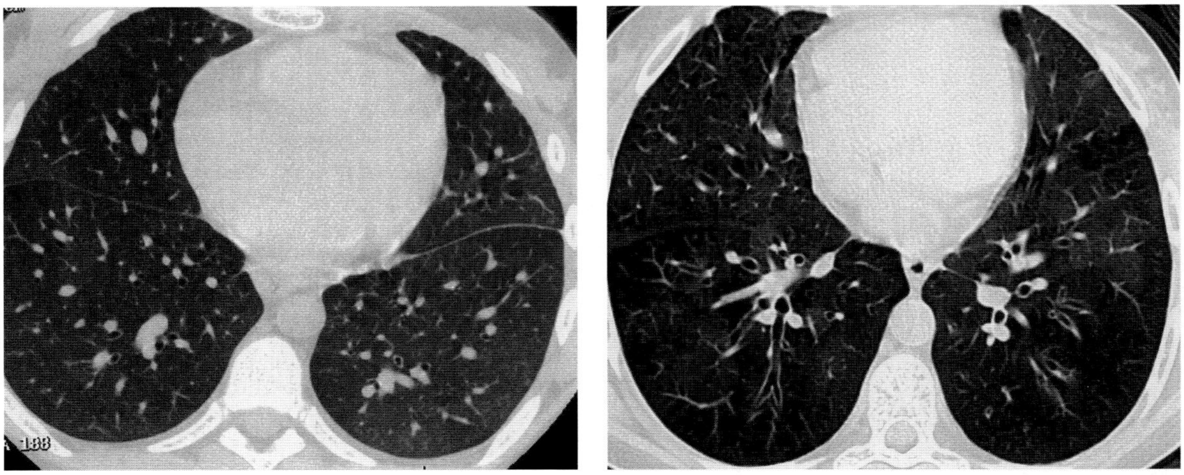

a b

Fig. 26.19. Bronchiolitis obliterans in a 14-year-old girl after bilateral lung transplantation. **a:** Axial section through the lower lungs at inspiration shows several areas of mild bronchial dilatation. **b:** Scan during expiration shows mosaic attenuation. The lower attenuation areas indicate air trapping and small airway obstruction. Bronchial dilatation is again noted

Protocol 4

INDICATION:	Combined Chest/High Resolution CT) (Suspected interstitial disease)
Extent	Lung apices to caudal bases
Scanner settings:	kVp: 80; mA: lowest possible
Detector collimation	1 mm
Table Speed	10–20 mm
Slice thickness	5 mm for initial survey, 1.25 mm for HRCT
Patient Instructions	Suspended inspiration
IV Contrast	None
Miscellaneous	1. Expiration imaging can be useful to evaluate suspected areas of air trapping. 2. If child sedated or uncooperative, CT scans obtained at quiet breathing. 3. Higher kVp (100 to 120) may be needed in larger patients (>50 kg).

chest radiograph; (b) determination of the extent, distribution, and character of diffuse lung diseases; (c) localization of abnormal lung for biopsy; and (d) assessment of the response to treatment.

26.12 Chest Wall

Multislice CT can also be applied to imaging of the thoracic cage (Pretorius and Fishman 1999). The complex anatomy of the thoracic cage is particularly well suited to multiplanar and 3 D volume-rendering imaging. These techniques can be of value in the imaging of a variety of chest wall abnormalities. In particular, they can help in evaluating congenital and postsurgical changes (Fig. 26.20), assessing the relationship of peripheral masses to the chest wall and in surgical planning of repair of pectus excavatum deformities

26.13 Summary

In summary, multislice CT is an important noninvasive tool for imaging the pediatric thorax. The clear delineation of anatomy, the high levels of contrast enhancement, and the continued refinement of 3D techniques have increased the applications of CT in chest imaging. Despite the obvious impact that multislice CT has already has on thoracic imaging, it cannot be overstated that attention must be paid to patient preparation and radiation doses.

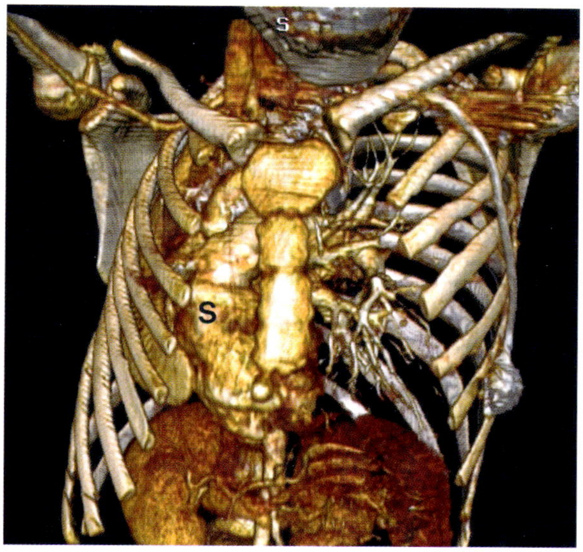

Fig. 26.20. Chest wall deformity secondary to prior pneumonectomy. A pre-operative CT scan was done to assess the volume of the right hemithorax prior to insertion of a chest prosthesis. Coronal volume rendered image shows a small right hemithorax and dextroscoliosis of the thoracic spine (S)

References

Al-Nakshabandi N, Lingawi S, Muller NL (2000) Congenital bronchial atresia. Can Assoc Radiol 51:47–48

American Society of Anesthesiologists Task Force (1996) Practice guidelines for sedation and analgesia by non-anesthesiologist: a report by the American Society of Anesthesiologists Task Force on sedation and analgesia by non-anesthesiologists. Anesthesiology 84:459–471

Aquina SL, Gamsu G, Webb R, Kee ST (1996) Tree-in-bud pattern: frequency and significance on thin section CT. J Comput Assist Tomogr 20:594–599

Bankier (1999) Pulmonary emphysema: subjective visual grading vs. objective quantification with macroscopic morphometry and thin-section CT densitometry. Radiology 211:851–858

Boiselle PM, Reynolds KF, Ernst A (2002) Multiplanar and three-dimensional imaging of the central airways with multidetector CT. AJR 179:301–308

Bower RJ, Kiesewetter WB (1996) Mediastinal masses in infants and children. Arch Surg 112:1003–1009

Bromberg BI, Beekman RH, Rocchini AP et al (1989) Aortic aneurysm after patch aortoplasty repair of coarctation: a prospective analysis of prevalence, screening tests and risks. J Am Coll Cardiol 14:734–741

Cody DD (2002) Image processing in CT. RadioGraphics 2: 1255–1268

Cohan RH, Ellis JH, Garner WL (1996) Extravasation of radiographic contrast material: recognition, prevention and treatment. Radiology 200:593–604

Collins J, Blankenbaker, Stern EJ (1998) CT patterns of bronchiolar disease: what is "tree-in-bud"? AJR 171:365–370

Committee on Drugs, American Academy of Pediatrics (1992) Guidelines for monitoring and management of pediatric patients during and after sedation for diagnostic and therapeutic procedures. Pediatrics 89:1110–1115

Donnelly LF, Emery KH, Brody AS et al (2001) Minimizing radiation dose for pediatric body applications for single-detector helical CT: strategies at a large children's hospital. AJR 176:303–306

Donnelly LF, Fleck RJ, Pacharn P, Ziegler MA, Fricke BL, Cotton RT (2002) Aberrant subclavian arteries: cross-sectional imaging findings in infants and children referred for evaluation of extrinsic airway compression. AJR 178: 1269–1274

Frazier AA, Rosado de Christenson ML, Stocker JT et al (1997) Intralobar sequestration: radiologic-pathologic correlation. RadioGraphics 17:725–745

Genevois (1996) Pulmonary emphysema: quantitative CT during expiration. Radiology 199:825–829

Gilkeson RC, Ciancibello LM, Hejal RB, Montenegro HD, Lange P (2001) Tracheobronchomalacia dynamic airway evaluation with multidetector CT. AJR 176:205–210

Gupta H, Mayo-Smith WW, Mainiero MB, Dupuy DE, Abbott GF (2002) Helical CT of pulmonary vascular abnormalities. AJR 178:487–492

Haaga JR (2001) Commentary. Radiation dose management weighing risk versus benefit. AJR 177:289–291

Haddon MJ, Bowen A (1991) Bronchopulmonary and neurenteric forms of foregut anomalies. Imaging for diagnosis and management. Radiol Clin North Am 29:241–254

Hammrick-Turner JE, Saif MF, Powers CI, Blumenthal BI, Royal SA, Iyer RV (1994) Imaging of childhood non-Hodgkin lymphoma: assessment by histologic subtype. RadioGraphics 14:11–28

Herts BR, O'Malley CM, Wirth SL et al (2001) Power injection of contrast media using central venous catheter feasibility, safety, and efficacy. AJR 176:447–453

Hoffman LV, Kuszyk BS, Mitchell SE et al (2000) Angioarchitecture of pulmonary AVM malformation characterization using volume-rendered 3D CT angiography. Cardiovasc Intervent Radiol 23:165 AVM

Hopkins KL, Patrick LE, Simoneaux SF et al (1996) Pediatric great vessel anomalies: initial clinical experience with spiral CT angiography. Radiology 200:811–815

Hoppe H, Walder B, Sonnenschein M, Vock P, Dinkel H-P (2002) Multidetector CT virtual bronchoscopy to grade tracheobronchial stenosis. AJR 178:1195–2000

Hudson MM, Donaldson SS (1997) Hodgkin's disease. In: Pizzo PA, Poplack DG (eds) Principles and practice of pediatric oncology, 3rd edn. Lippincott/Raven, Philadelphia, pp 523–543

Kaste SC, Young CW (1995) Safe use of power injectors with central and peripheral venous access devices for pediatric CT. Pediatr Radiol 26:499–501

Kaste SC, Young CW, Holmes TP, Baker DK (1997) Effect of helical CT on the frequency of sedation in pediatric patients. AJR 168:1001–1003

Katz M, Konen E, Rozenman et al (1995) Spiral CT and 3D image reconstruction of vascular rings and associated tracheobronchial anomalies. J Comput Assist Tomogr 19: 564–568

Kim WS, Lee KS, Kim IO et al (1997) Congenital cystic adenomatoid malformation of the lung: CT-pathologic correlation. AJR 168:47–53

Ko SF, Ng SH, Lee TY et al (2000) Noninvasive imaging of bronchopulmonary sequestration. AJR 175:1005–1012

Lau DM, Siegel MJ, Hildebolt CF, Cohen AH (1998) Bronchiolitis obliterans syndrome: thin-section CT diagnosis of obstructive changes in infants and young children after lung transplantation. Radiology 208:783–788

Lawler LP, Fishman EK (2001) Multi-detector row CT of thoracic disease with emphasis on 3D volume rendering and CT angiography. RadioGraphics 21:1257–1273

Lawler LP, Fishman EK (2002) Arteriovenous malformations and systemic lung supply: evaluation by multidetector CT and three-dimensional volume rendering. AJR 178: 493–494

Lee KS, Yoon JH, Kim TK, Kim JS, Chung MP, Kwon OJ (1997) Evaluation of tracheobronchial disease with helical CT with multiplanar and three-dimensional reconstruction: correlation with bronchoscopy. RadioGraphics 17:555–567

Lucaya J, Piqeunas J, Garcia-Pena P et al (2000) Low-dose high resolution CT of the chest in children and young adults: dose, cooperation artifact, incidence and image quality. AJR 175:985–992

McGuiness G, Naidich D, Garay S, Davis AL, Boyd AD, Mizrachi HH (1993) Accessory cardiac bronchus: CT features and clinical significance. Radiology 189:563–566

Merten DF (1992) Diagnostic imaging of mediastinal masses in children. AJR 158:825–832

Meza MP, Benson M, Slovis TL (1993) Imaging of mediastinal masses in children. Radiol Clin North Am 31:583–604

Muller NL, Miller RR (1995) Diseases of the bronchioles: CT and histopathologic findings. Radiology 196:3–12

Pappas JN, Donnelly LF, Frush DP (2000) Reduced frequency of sedation of young children using new multi-slice helical CT. Radiology 215:897–899

Patterson A, Frush DP, Donnelly L (2001) Helical CT of the body: are settings adjusted for pediatric patients. AJR 176: 297–301

Pretorius ES, Fishman EK (1999) Volume-rendered three-dimensional spiral CT: musculoskeletal applications. Radiographics 19:1143–1160

Quint LE, Whyte RI, Kazerooni EA et al (1995) Stenosis of the central airways: evaluation by using helical CT with multiplanar reconstructions. Radiology 194:871–877

Ravenel JG, McAdams HP, Remy-Jardin M, Remy J (2001) Multidimensional imaging of the thorax. Practical applications. J Thor Imaging 16:279–281

Remy J, Remy-Jardin M, Giraud F et al (1994) Angiotecture of pulmonary arteriovenous malformation: clinical utility of three-dimensional helical CT. Radiology 191:657–664

Remy-Jardin M, Remy J, Artaud D, Fribourg M, Naili A (1998a) Tracheobronchial tree: assessment with volume rendering – technical aspects. Radiology 208:393–398

Remy-Jardin M, Remy J, Artaud D, Fribourg M, Duhamel A (1998b) Volume rendering of the tracheobronchial tree: clinical evaluation of bronchographic images. Radiology 208:761–770

Remy-Jardin M, Remy J, Giraud F, Marquette CH (1993) Pulmonary nodules: detection with thick-section spiral CT versus conventional CT. Radiology 187:513–520

Rogalla P, Stover B, Scheer I, Juran R, Gaedicke G, Hamm B (1999) Low-dose spiral CT: applicability to paediatric chest imaging. Pediatr Radiol 29:565–569

Ruben GD (2000) Data explosion: the challenge of multidetector CT. Eur J Radiol 36:74–81

Siegel MJ, Bhalla S, Gutierrez FR, Hildebolt C (2001) Post-lung transplantation bronchiolitis obliterans syndrome: usefulness of expiratory thin-section CT for diagnosis. Radiology 220:455–462

Siegel MJ (1993) Diseases of the thymus in children and adolescents. Postgrad Radiol 13:106–132

Siegel MJ (1999) Techniques. In: Siegel MJ (ed) Pediatric body CT. Lippincott Williams and Wilkins, Philadelphia, pp 1–41

Siegel MJ (1999a) Lungs, pleura and chest wall. In: Siegel MJ (ed) Pediatric body CT. Lippincott Williams and Wilkins, Philadelphia, pp 201–225

Siegel MJ (1999b) Mediastinum. In: Siegel MJ (ed) Pediatric body CT. Lippincott Williams and Wilkins, Philadelphia, pp 65–100

Slovis TL (2002) The ALARA concept in pediatric CT: myth or reality. Radiology 223:5–6

Sorantin E, Geiger B, Lindbichler F, Eber E, Schimph G (2002) CT based virtual tracheobronchoscopy in children – comparison with axial CT and multiplanar reconstructions: preliminary results. Pediatr Radiol 32:8–15

Stern EJ, Frank MS (1994) Small airway disease of the lungs: findings at expiratory CT. AJR 163:37–41

Stockberger SM, Hickling JA, Liang Y, Ambrosius WT (1998) Spiral CT with ionic and nonionic contrast material: evaluation of patient motion and scan quality. Radiology 206:631–636

White KS (1995) Reduced need for sedation in pediatric patients undergoing helical CT of the chest and abdomen. Pediatr Radiol 25:344–346

Woodring JH, Howard TA, Kanga JF (1994) Congenital pulmonary venolobar syndrome revisited. RadioGraphics 14: 349–369

Wright AR, Collie DA, Williams JR, Hasemi-Malayeri, Stevenson AJM, Turnbull CM (1996) Pulmonary nodules: effect on detection of spiral CT pitch. Radiology 199:837–841

Yamada I, Nakagawa T, Himeno Y, Numano F, Shibuya H (1998) Takayasu arteritis: evaluation of the thoracic aorta with CT angiography. Radiology 209:103–109

Zwetsch B, Wicky S, Meuli R et al (1995) Three-dimensional image reconstruction of partial anomalous pulmonary venous return to the superior vena cava. Chest 108:1743–1745

27 Diaphragm, Chest Wall, Pleura

J. Verschakelen

CONTENTS

27.1 Diaphragm

27.1.1 Introduction

The diaphragm is a thin, flat musculotendinous structure that separates the thoracic cavity from the abdominal cavity and that, being a respiratory muscle, has an important role in respiration.

Although diseases of the diaphragm itself are relatively infrequent, knowledge of radiographic appearance of the diaphragm and the peridiaphragmatic region is mandatory. It is important to differentiate between pathology originating from the diaphragm itself and pathological processes located immediately above or below the diaphragm. Since diaphragmatic disease is also often benign, it is important to be able to differentiate between abnormalities that have no clinical relevance and abnormalities that need further exploration.

Unfortunately, radiology of the diaphragm is difficult (Panicek et al. 1988; Tarver et al. 1989), in part because many diaphragmatic and also peridiaphragmatic abnormalities are obscure clinically, but also and mainly because there is no imaging technique that can clearly and entirely visualize the diaphragm. Moreover, the radiological appearance of the diaphragm is variable since it depends on the function and integrity of the diaphragmatic muscle and is related to the thoracic and abdominal volumes and contents and to the motion of rib cage and abdomen.

Although we usually speak of the top of the opaque abdominal mass (usually composed of liver, spleen, stomach, or colon) as being the diaphragm on a conventional chest film, the diaphragmatic muscle as such is only visible when air is present above and below it.

Ultrasound (Lewandowski and Winsberg 1983; Oyen et al. 1984; Pery et al. 1984; Verschakelen et al. 1989b), CT (Gale 1986; Kleinman and Raptopoulos 1985; Shin and Berland 1985), and magnetic resonance imaging (MRI; Yamashita et al. 1993) are the only imaging modalities that can visualize the diaphragm itself. Although visualization is mostly partial and depends on the presence of pleural disease in ultrasound (Verschakelen et al. 1989b) and subdiaphragmatic fat in CT (Fig. 1) and MRI (Gale 1986; Kleinman and Raptopoulos 1985). Both MR and CT have the ability to image the diaphragm in imaging planes other than the axial plane. Visualization of the diaphragm in the sagittal and frontal plane is indeed often helpful in the study of diaphragmatic and especially of peridiaphragmatic disease (Fig. 2; Brink et al. 1994). Since the introduction of spiral CT and multidetector CT, it has become possible to obtain high-quality multiplanar and even 3D reconstructions of the diaphragmatic area (Fig. 2; Cassart et al. 1999; Pettiaux et al. 1997). Moreover, the ability to perform

J. Verschakelen, MD
Department of Radiology, University Hospitals, Herestraat 49, 3000 Leuven, Belgium

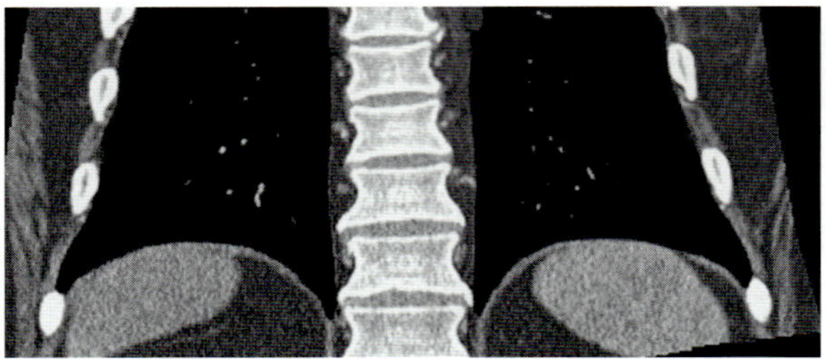

a

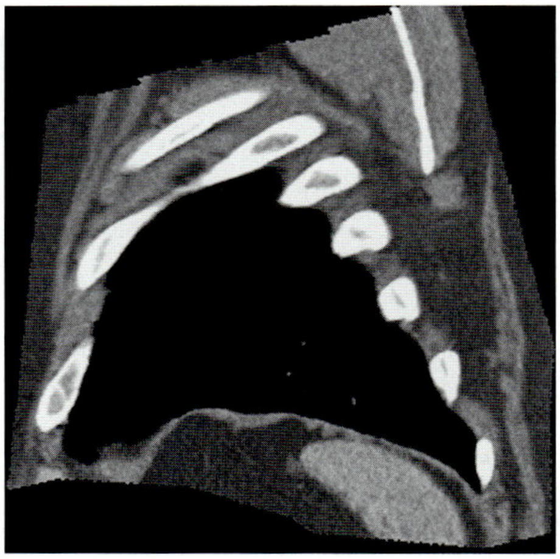

b

Fig. 27.1. A MDCT of the diaphragm **a** frontal and **b** sagittal reconstructions. The costal part of the diaphragm is visible as a thin line between the fat below and the lung above; however, when there is no fat separating the diaphragm from the liver, the spleen, the stomach, or the heart, the diaphragm is not visible. The CT protocol: acquisition 4×1mm; pitch 1.75; slice thickness for frontal and sagittal reformations 1 m

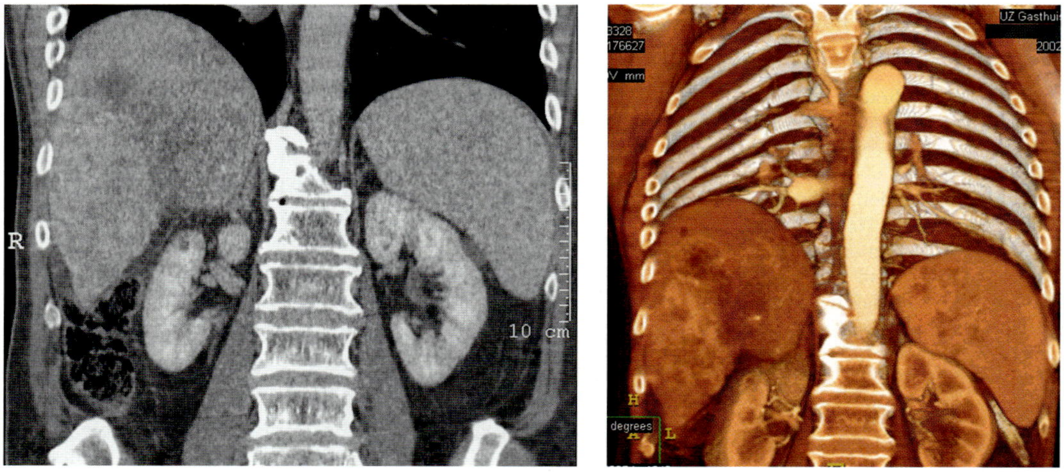

a b

Fig. 27.2. A MDCT of the diaphragm **a** frontal and **b** 3D reconstructions. Patient with a large malignant tumor in the right lobe of the liver causing elevation of the right hemidiaphragm. Note that the diaphragmatic crura are visible as smooth linear opacities originating from the central tendon and oriented downward, parallel to the vertebral column. The CT protocol: acquisition 16×0.75 mm; pitch 1.75; slice thickness for frontal reformation 1 mm

image acquisition during one breath hold allows elimination of respiratory motion artifacts which improves image quality and also makes it possible to visualize the diaphragm at different levels of respiration. Study of the diaphragmatic function, initially only possible with fluoroscopy and ultrasound, can now also be performed using dynamic MRI and spiral- and multidetector CT (Cassart et al. 1997, 1999, 2001).

27.1.2 Acquisition and Injection Techniques

Since high detail is necessary to identify the diaphragm correctly, a scanning protocol should be chosen that offers the highest image quality (Brink et al. 1994). A thin detector set should be chosen to allow reconstruction of high-detail contiguous or overlapping thin sections and, when necessary, to make targeted reconstructions through the region of interest. A specific advantage of MDCT is that, choosing a thin detector set, detailed characterization of the diaphragm remains possible, even though it was initially planned to view the images with thicker slices. In this way a second high-resolution acquisition through the region with thin collimation, which is usual with spiral CT, is obviated. In the setting of a trauma, when rapid and accurate diagnosis is critical and examination technique is limited due to patient positioning and clinical situation, MDCT allows a rapid and comprehensive screening of the diaphragm and peridiaphragmatic regions.

In general, the administration of contrast is not necessary in every patient. Contrast is given in order to better locate or identify peridiaphragmatic masses and abnormalities. The diaphragm itself does not show marked enhancement and its visualization depends more on the presence or absence of subdiaphragmatic fat.

In order to have good opacification of atelectatic lung tissue or lung tumor adjacent to the diaphragm, and in order to have good enhancement of the liver, a long scan delay (45–60 s) is preferred.

The administration of oral contrast can be necessary when there is suspicion of herniated bowel or stomach.

27.1.3 Normal CT Appearance

On CT scans the costal part of the diaphragm can be visible as a soft tissue stripe between the fat below and the aerated lung above. The diaphragm is not visible when it is tangential to the scanning plane or where there is no fat separating it from soft tissue structures such as the liver, spleen, stomach, or colon (Fig. 1; Gale 1986; Kleinman and Raptopoulos 1985). The MDCT-generated multiplanar reconstructions can resolve to a certain degree the first problem, but a good visualization of the diaphragm is only achieved when enough fat separates it from adjacent tissue even when high-detail reformations are available. In some cases it is possible with CT to differentiate between the muscular part of the diaphragm and the central tendon. The muscular part presents as a double line representing the muscle layers, whereas the central tendon presents as a single line. Unlike in ultrasound, pleural disease needs not to be present in order to differentiate these two parts of the diaphragm (Verschakelen et al. 1989b). The diaphragm can appear nodular because of the visualization of hypertrophic muscular bundles. Using high-detail acquisition techniques small anatomic structures, such as the inferior phrenic arteries, can become visible (Smith 2002; Ujita et al. 1993).

In most patients the diaphragmatic crura can easily be recognized both on axial and on reformatted images (Fig. 2a). They appear mostly as smooth linear opacities originating from the central tendon oriented downward parallel and lateral to the aorta. They usually appear smooth but can also have a nodular appearance (Caskey et al. 1989). These pseudotumors increase in number and severity with age. Defects in the crura can also be present and are seen more in older patients and patients with emphysema (Caskey et al. 1989).

27.1.4 Pathology of the Diaphragm

27.1.4.1 Diaphragmatic Hernia

Bochdalek hernia, Morgagni hernia and hiatus hernia are the most frequently occurring herniations of the diaphragm.

Large Bochdalek hernias usually become evident in the neonatal period because they cause respiratory symptoms (Snyder and Greany 1965). Small Bochdalek hernias, however, only rarely have symptoms and are often an incidental finding in adults (Gale 1985; Wilbur et al. 1994). They are usually without any clinical importance, but they should be differentiated from diaphragmatic and peridiaphragmatic masses. These hernias often first present in the same way as tumors do: a single focal bulge on the diaphragmatic contour. However, this finding is very suggestive for Bochdalek hernia when the patient has no symptoms and when the bulge is centered approximately 4–5 cm anterior to either posterior diaphragmatic insertion. The CT can make the diagnosis in case of doubt (Gale 1985). The hernia presents as a soft tissue or fatty mass abutting the surface of the posteromedial aspect of either hemidiaphragm (Fig. 3). This mass is in continuity with subdiaphragmatic structures through a diaphragmatic defect presenting as a discontinuity of the soft tissue line of the diaphragm. The fact that the defect is located in the posteromedial aspect of the diaphragm makes it usually visible on axial scans. In some cases, sagittal reformations give additional information because the diaphragmatic stripe is better identified (Yamana and Ohba 1994). Also 3D imaging can be useful for stereographic perception of the hernia (Yamana and Ohba 1994).

The incidence of Morgagni hernia detected in the neonatal period because of symptoms is low. In older children and adults, Morgagni hernia is often an incidental finding. Although the weak area at the fibrotendinous elements between the costal and the crural part of the diaphragm is congenital, Morgagni hernia can be acquired. Increase in abdominal pressure due to severe effort, trauma or obesity is probably responsible (Paris et al. 1973; Thomas and Clitherow 1977;

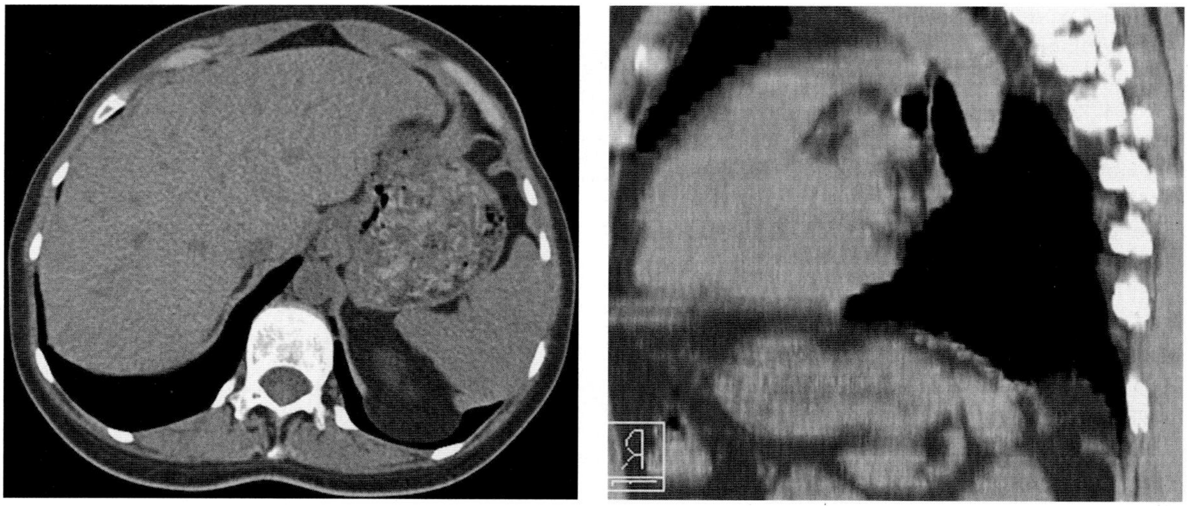

a b

Fig. 27.3. A MDCT of the diaphragm **a** axial and **b** sagittal reconstructions. Small Bochdalek hernia presenting as a fatty mass in continuity with subdiaphragmatic structures through a diaphragmatic defect presenting as a discontinuity of the soft tissue line of the diaphragm. The CT protocol: acquisition 4×2.5 mm; pitch 1.38; slice thickness for axial slice and sagittal reformation 5 mm

Wilbur et al. 1994). When bowel is herniated to the chest, the diagnosis can usually be made with conventional chest-film and barium studies. Herniated liver or fat can be identified with CT. Because there is very often fat above and below the diaphragm in that area, the diaphragmatic defect is frequently visible on axial scans or on sagittal and frontal reformations.

The diagnosis of hiatus hernia can be made on conventional posteroanterior chest film, but its presence is usually confirmed by a barium study. Hiatus hernias are often an incidental finding on CT. Multiplanar reconstructions can be helpful in some selected cases in order to better demonstrate the exact position of the diaphragm (Bogaert et al. 1995).

Multiplanar reconstructions can also be helpful in determining the nature, relationship of the herniated organs, the precise side and size of the diaphragmatic defect in patients with non-traumatic acquired defects (Coulier et al. 1999).

27.1.4.2 *Traumatic Diaphragmatic Rupture*

Blunt trauma and penetrating wounds of the chest are the most frequent causes of traumatic diaphragmatic rupture. In blunt trauma the tear is left sided in 70–90% of all cases (Dee 1992). This is probably due to the protective function of the liver (Fataar et al. 1979; van Daele et al. 1987). Injuries from penetrating wounds may be found in any area of the diaphragm (Cotter and Tyndal 1986).

Although in the majority of patients with diaphragmatic rupture, abnormalities are demonstrated on the chest radiograph at the time of the injury, diagnosis is often delayed. Aspecific clinical symptoms and radiographic findings are responsible for the fact that some patients are first seen within 3 years of the time the injury occurred with symptoms of bowel herniation (Carter et al. 1951; Heiberg et al. 1980).

Most hemodynamically stable patients with blunt diaphragmatic injury as a result of severe polytrauma require an admission CT examination to evaluate the extent and anatomical sites of coexisting thoracoabdominal injuries (Linsenmaier et al. 2002; Shanmuganathan et al. 2000); however, there is disagreement in the literature about the use of CT in the diagnosis of traumatic diaphragmatic rupture. Several case reports have demonstrated that traumatic diaphragmatic rupture can be identified at CT (Demos et al. 1989; Gurney et al. 1985; Heiberg et al. 1980; Holland and Quint 1991); however, in a series of seven patients reported by Gelman et al. (1991), CT made the correct diagnosis in only one patient. On the other hand, Worthy et al. (1995) found diagnostic features with CT in 9 of 11 patients. This contradiction is not surprising since, as discussed previously, it is often difficult to identify the diaphragm on CT scan, especially when it is immediately adjacent to abdominal organs. The CT is generally more diagnostic when herniated abdominal organs or bowel can be demonstrated but is less diagnostic when there is a small tear without herniation of abdominal content. In a retrospective study of 35 patients with surgically confirmed diaphragmatic rupture, CT was able to demonstrate diaphragmatic rupture in all cases where thoracic herniation of the abdominal organs was present; however, CT findings were questionable in 25% of the cases when no herniation was seen (Scaglione et al. 2000). Similar findings were reported by Killeen et al. (1999). In their study CT had a sensitivity of 78% and a specificity of 100% for the detection of left-sided diaphragmatic rupture, whereas these figures were respectively 50 and 100% for right-sided diaphragmatic rupture. The CT signs of diaphragmatic rupture include: discontinuity of the diaphragm with direct visualization of the diaphragmatic injury, herniation of abdominal organs with liver, bowel, or stomach in contact with the posterior ribs ("dependent viscera sign"; Bergin et al. 2001) thickening of the crus ("thick crus sign"; Leung et al. 1999) constriction of the stomach or bowel ("collar sign"; Gurney et al. 1985; Naidich et al. 1991), active arterial extravasation of contrast material near the diaphragm and in case of a penetrating diaphragmatic injury depiction of a missile or puncturing instrument trajectory. In a recent study Larici et al. (2002) found that the dependent viscera sign had the highest sensitivity, whereas the collar sign, extravasation of contrast material and a trajectory were the most specific manifestations of diaphragmatic injury. In this study coronal and sagittal reconstructions were of limited use in establishing or refuting the diagnosis of acute diaphragmatic injury. This is in contradiction with the findings of others who have shown that multiplanar reformations can increase diagnostic accuracy (Killeen et al. 1999). The detection of small diaphragmatic defects requires high detail and it can be expected that MDCT giving these detailed images can provide additional information. This is especially true for small tears in the dome and at the musculotendinous junction where spiral CT was not successful in one study (Scaglione et al. 2000).

When the rupture is missed at the time of the trauma and patient has recovered from the associated lesions a "latent "phase of diaphragmatic rupture can occur. Symptoms and signs are then caused by recurrent herniation of abdominal structures through the diaphragmatic defect and are again often aspecific. The MDCT might again be helpful in detecting these missed tears.

27.1.4.3 Tumors of the Diaphragm

Tumors of the diaphragm are rare lesions that are often difficult to assess and classify both clinically and roentgenographically (Anderson and Forrest 1973). Malignant tumors are more frequent than benign tumors and can be primary or secondary (Anderson and Forrest 1973; Tarver et al. 1989). Benign tumors (lipomas, fibromas, angiofibromas, neurofibromas, and neurolemmomas) are mostly asymptomatic and often found at post-mortem examination (Anderson and Forrest 1973; Schwartz and Wechsler 1989). The majority of the primary malignant tumors are of fibrous origin (fibrosarcoma, fibromyosarcoma, fibroangioendothelioma) or are undifferentiated sarcomas (Anderson and Forrest 1973; Schwartz and Wechsler 1989). In contrast to benign tumors, malignant tumors mostly induce symptoms (pleuritic chest pain, pain referred to the epigastrium) and are often associated with pleural effusion. Secondary malignant tumors are mostly due to direct invasion from adjacent lesions originating from the lung, the stomach, the pancreas, the adrenals, the colon, and the liver (Fig. 4; Anderson and Forrest 1973; Schwartz and Wechsler 1989). Metastatic implants are rare and only found in cases of widely disseminated disease. Thin sections MDCT performed during one breath hold and multiplanar reformations generated from MDCT data allow a better delineation of the diaphragm and of the relationship between the mass and the diaphragmatic muscle. Even when the diaphragmatic muscle as such is not visible (because of the absence of fat between the diaphragm and the subdiaphragmatic organ), contact between a mass and the diaphragm or diaphragmatic invasion by a tumor can often be diagnosed by looking at the expected contour of the diaphragm.

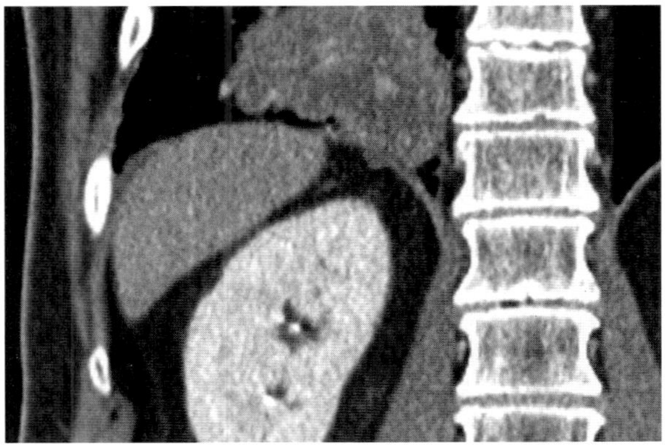

Fig. 27.4. Malignant lung tumor invading in the diaphragm. Coronal reconstruction shows close contact between the tumor and the diaphragm and the extension of the tumor into the subdiaphragmatic fat. The CT protocol: acquisition 16×0.75 mm; pitch 0.950; slice thickness 3 mm

27.1.4.4
Eventration

Eventration of the diaphragm is defined as an abnormally high or elevated position of one leaf of the intact diaphragm as a result of paralysis, aplasia, or atrophy of varying degrees of muscle fibers (Bisgard 1947). In the area of eventration the normal diaphragmatic muscle fibers are replaced by a thin layer of connective tissue and a few scattered muscle fibers. Eventration can be congenital resulting from congenital failure of proper muscularization of a part or of the entire diaphragmatic leaf (Lindstrom and Allen 1966; Tarver et al. 1989). Eventration can also be acquired and is then the result of long-lasting paralysis causing atrophy and scarring of the diaphragmatic muscle (Bovornkitti et al. 1960; McNamara et al. 1968; Michelson 1961). Total eventration of one hemidiaphragm is more often seen on the left side. Partial eventrations are usually right sided with a predilection for the anteromedial portion; however, diaphragmatic eventration may occur almost anywhere along the diaphragmatic surface and is commonly multifocal.

Since eventration usually is asymptomatic, the role of CT is mostly limited to the differentiation of this entity from a tumoral mass in a patient presenting with a focal bulge on the diaphragmatic contour. In contrast to a herniation, where there is a defect in the diaphragm and where abdominal fat or an abdominal organ is protruding into the chest, in eventration the diaphragm, although thin and only consisting of a thin layer of connective tissue, is not interrupted. Differential diagnosis is often easy because of typical localization of both congenital hernias and eventrations, but can be more difficult when herniation is the result of a posttraumatic diaphragmatic tear. Differential diagnosis with focal eventually reversible paralysis is, however, mostly impossible.

27.1.4.5
Paralysis of the Diaphragm

The role of CT in the diagnosis of diaphragmatic paralysis is limited. The radiological evaluation of paralysis requires chest radiographs, adequate fluoroscopic tests or when not possible ultrasound together with a good knowledge of the clinical history of the patient. The CT can be helpful in the diagnosis of intrathoracic causes of phrenic nerve injury (Ujita et al. 1993). The CT and especially MDCT can also be valuable in the differential diagnosis of a paralyzed (hemi)diaphragm and peridiaphragmatic pathology (subpulmonary pleural effusion, ascites, lung atelectasis, lung or liver mass adjacent to the diaphragm). As mentioned previously, the differential diagnosis with eventration can be difficult and is often impossible.

27.1.5
Conclusions

Because of its capability to scan the diaphragm and the peridiaphragmatic region during one breath hold, and especially because of its ability to perform high-detail multiplanar reformations, MDCT can become very important in the study of the diaphragm and of its adjacent structures. Especially sagittal and coronal reformations can be very important to localize abnormalities to the diaphragm itself, to the intraabdominal viscera, the cardiophrenic space, the pleura, the lung, or the pericardium.

27.2
Chest Wall and Pleura

27.2.1
Introduction

The use of CT in the study of diseases of the chest wall is usually limited to the evaluation of tumor extension: detection of pleural and chest wall invasion of peripheral bronchogenic carcinoma or determination of tumor extension in patients with tumor of breast or mesothelioma. However, it is well known that 2D CT scans generally have a low sensitivity and specificity when invasion of the parietal pleura and chest wall by a lung or pleura tumor is examined (Epstein et al. 1986; Grenier et al. 1989; Pearlberg et al. 1987; Pennes et al. 1985; Webb et al. 1991). Studies have shown that 2D or 3D reformations obtained with spiral CT can add some valuable information (Kuriyama et al. 1994a). Moreover, the ability offered by spiral CT to observe a tumor during its different phases of contrast enhancement has been used to study tumors of the breast (Teifke et al. 1994). It can be expected that MDCT, because of its ability to produce high-detail images in different imaging planes, will further increase the role of CT in the study of pleura and chest wall abnormalities.

27.2.2 Acquisition and Injection Techniques

Since the added value of MDCT is related to its ability to perform reformations, and since high detail is necessary, scans should be performed with a thin detector set and reconstructed with overlap. Of course these parameters have to be adapted to the scan volume and to the possibility of the patient to stop breathing.

When intravenous contrast is given, an appropriate delay between the start of the injection and the scan should be chosen in order to allow enhancement of the tumor, but also, when present, of the thickened pleura and atelectatic lung tissue.

27.2.3 Pathology of the Chest Wall

27.2.3.1 Congenital Deformation of the Chest Wall

In evaluating congenital disease of the chest wall, one needs to use CT only occasionally (Gouliamos et al. 1980; Toombs et al. 1981); however, conditions such as congenital absence of a pectoral muscle, deformities of the sternum, the ribs, and the vertebrae can sometimes be assessed to advantage in transaxial images (Laufer et al. 1999). In addition, when surgical correction is considered, 3D reconstruction of the bony chest can probably help the surgeon to better understand the deformation of the chest and to chose the best surgical procedure to correct it (Haller et al. 1989; Hurwitz et al. 1994).

27.2.3.2 Trauma to the Chest Wall

Most osseous injuries are easily evaluated on plain films, but sometimes CT imaging adds significant information (Dee 1992; Mirvis and Templeton 1992; Stark and Jaramillo 1986). Although the presence of life-support devices and orthopedic devices can make it difficult to position a traumatized patient, and although cooperation of the patient is often limited, MDCT has the advantage over conventional and spiral CT that scanning time can be further reduced. In this way it can eventually help to detect and locate multiple fragments of bones, hematomas in soft tissues, foreign bodies, subluxations, damage to the spinal canal, and extrapleural air collections (Fig. 5; Kurihara et al. 1997).

27.2.3.3 Invasion of the Chest Wall by Tumor

Assessment of pleural and chest wall invasion is an important component of lung cancer staging; however, the accuracy of 2D CT in those cases where the tumor is adjacent to the chest wall without any bone destruction is low (Epstein et al. 1986; Grenier et al. 1989; Pearlberg et al. 1987; Pennes et al. 1985; Webb et al. 1991). A first reason for this is the axial format not allowing to evaluate lesions in contact with the apex of the chest and the diaphragm. A second reason is the fact that features such as a large contact (>3 cm) between the mass and the pleura, an obtuse angle between the tumor and the chest wall, an associated pleural thickening, and the presence of pleural tags, mostly considered as signs of chest wall invasion, also occur with benign lesions. Three-dimensional techniques have been used successfully to study lung tumors, peripheral pulmonary vessels, and pleural surface (Kuriyama et al. 1994a,b). In a study where they reviewed 2D and 3D images obtained with spiral CT in 42 patients with peripheral bronchogenic carcinoma, Kuriyama and co-workers (1994b) found that 3D-reconstruction imaging was superior to 2D CT in the assessment of pleural invasion. Three-dimensional reconstructions allowed them to correctly predict pleural involvement and to differentiate between visceral pleura and parietal pleural involvement or chest wall invasion. According to their results, it was possible to differentiate between simple pleural

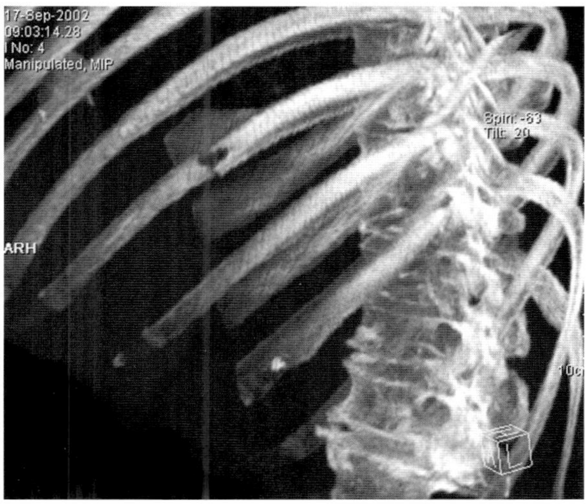

Fig. 27.5. A MDCT of the chest. Three-dimensional reformatted image very clearly shows the osteolytic lesion with a pathological fracture of the rib

tags (i.e., fibrotic bands extending from the lesion to the visceral pleura) from visceral pleural invasion (i.e., pleural puckering associated with an indrawn locally thickened pleura). Another way of evaluating parietal pleural invasion of lung masses was proposed by SHIRAKAWA and co-workers (1994). These investigators performed spiral CT scans of the chest during deep inspiration and expiration in patients with peripheral lung tumors in contact with the chest wall. They found the presence of respiratory phase shift to be a reliable indicator of the lack of parietal pleural invasion for tumors in middle and lower lung lobes.

In cases where tumor invasion in the chest wall or the diaphragm is obvious, 2D sagittal or frontal reformatted images can be helpful in studying the extent of the mass (Fig. 6; DESCHILDERE et al. 1994). It is not determined yet whether these reformatted images give more information than sagittal or frontal magnetic resonance images. The MRI is at this moment still considered as the image modality of choice in studying superior sulcus tumors and their extension to the chest wall (TAKASUGI et al. 1989). It can be expected that MDCT, due to the lack of motion artifacts and the better evaluation of invasion in the bony cortex of the ribs, will play a more important role than either CT and spiral CT. Three-dimensional image reconstruction methods can also be used in selected cases to clarify a complex relationship between a tumor invading the chest wall and vascular structures of the thoracic inlet (Fig. 7; TELLO et al. 1993).

27.2.4 Pleural Abnormalities

The combination of axial scans and 2D and 3D reformations can be helpful in selected cases to study the extent of pleural disease and to estimate the total surface that is involved (Fig. 8; MEIER et al. 1993). The MDCT can also be helpful in cases where it is difficult to differentiate pleural disease from lung or diaphragmatic abnormalities (Fig. 9). Sagittal and coronal reformations can better show the curvation of bronchovascular structures toward a pleural-based area of lung atelectasis (comet tail sign): an additional diagnostic feature of rounded atelectasis that previously could only be shown by sagittal conventional tomograms or MRI (Fig. 10; VERSCHAKELEN et al. 1989a).

27.2.5 Tumors of the Breast

Computed tomography is often performed in patients with a tumor of the breast when tumor infiltration in the chest wall is suspected or to look for axillary, parasternal, and mediastinal adenopathy.

The development of spiral CT in the early 1990s induced a renewed interest to use this technique not only for staging but also for detection of breast carcinoma (TEIFKE et al. 1994; SARDANELLI et al. 1995). Spiral CT has the advantage that it can examine the breasts and axillary areas in a short time with high

a 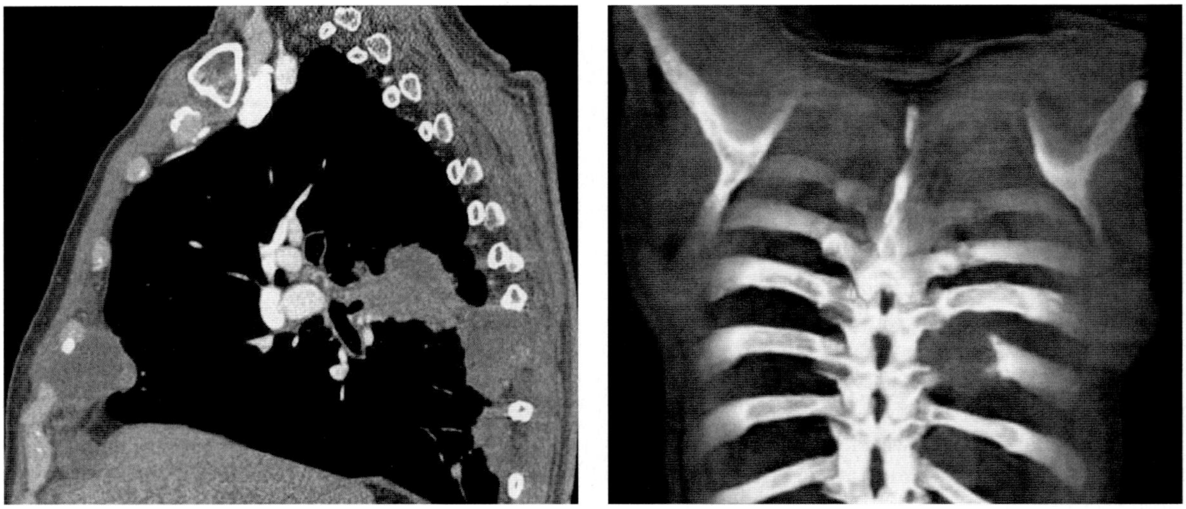 b

Fig. 27.6. A MDCT of the chest and chest wall **a** sagittal and **b** 3D reformations. Reformatted image shows tumor extension in the anterior and posterior chest wall. Bony destruction is best demonstrated on the 3D reconstruction

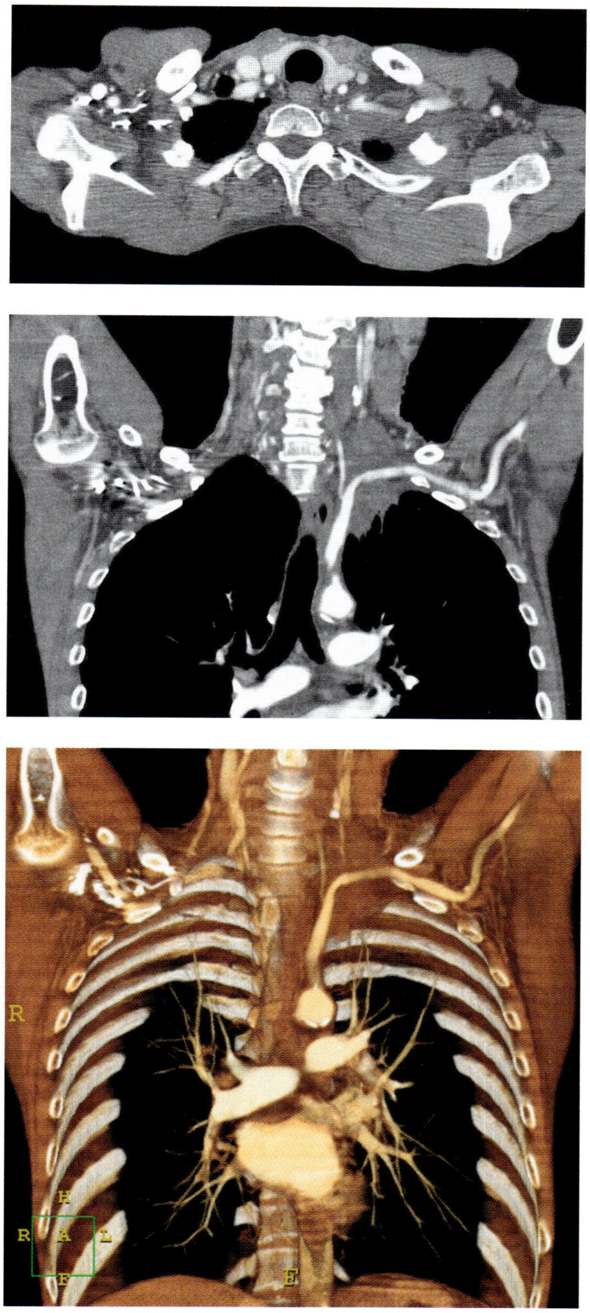

a

b

c

Fig. 27.7a–c. Superior sulcus tumor invading the chest wall. **a** Axial slice, **b** coronal, and **c** 3D reconstructions show the tumor extending into the apical soft tissues and surrounding the left subclavian artery which is narrowed. The CT protocol: acquisition 16×0.75 mm; pitch 0.950; slice thickness, axial slice 5 mm; coronal reformation 3 mm

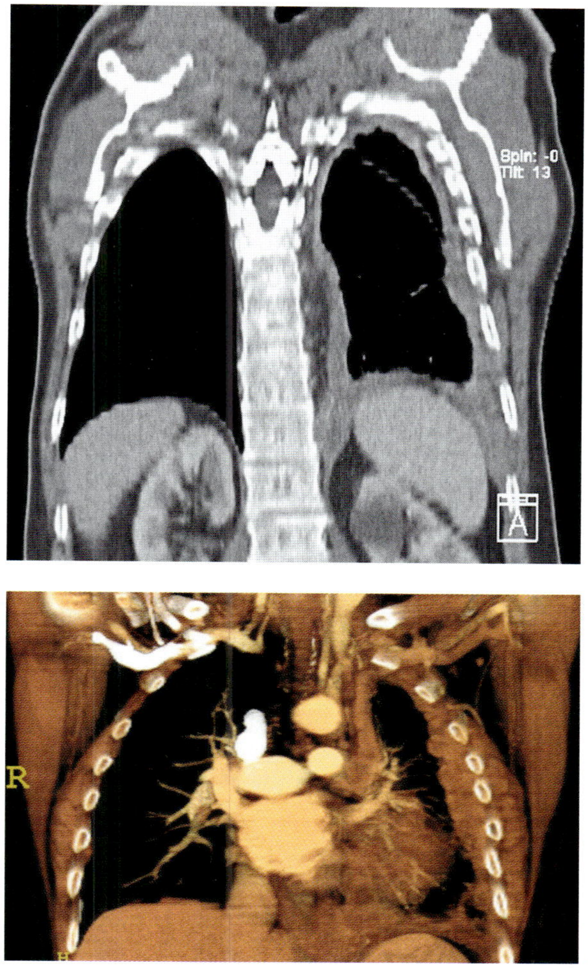

a

b

Fig. 27.8a, b. Malignant mesothelioma. **a** Coronal and **b** 3D reconstruction. The MDCT is very helpful in studying the extent of pleural involvement and in estimating the total pleural surface that is involved. The CT protocol: coronal slice acquisition 4×2.5 mm; pitch 5 mm; 3D view acquisition 16×0.75 mm; pitch 0.950

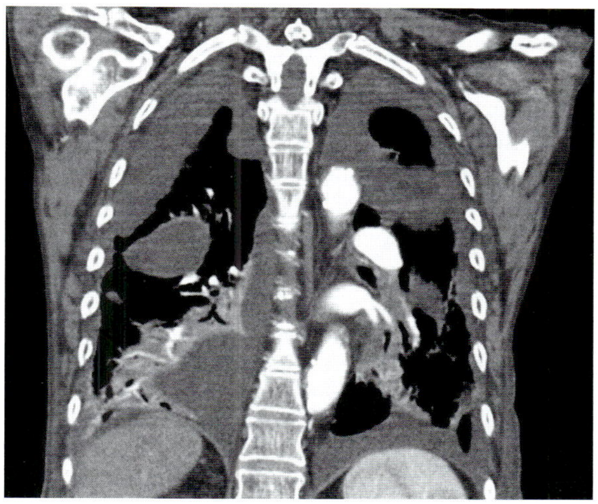

Fig. 27.9. Bilateral pleural effusion with extension into the fissure. Coronal reformation shows the extent of the pleural effusion and helps in differentiating this pleural effusion from the atelectatic lung tissue in both lower lobes. The CT protocol: acquisition 16×0.75 mm; pitch 0.950; slice thickness 3 mm

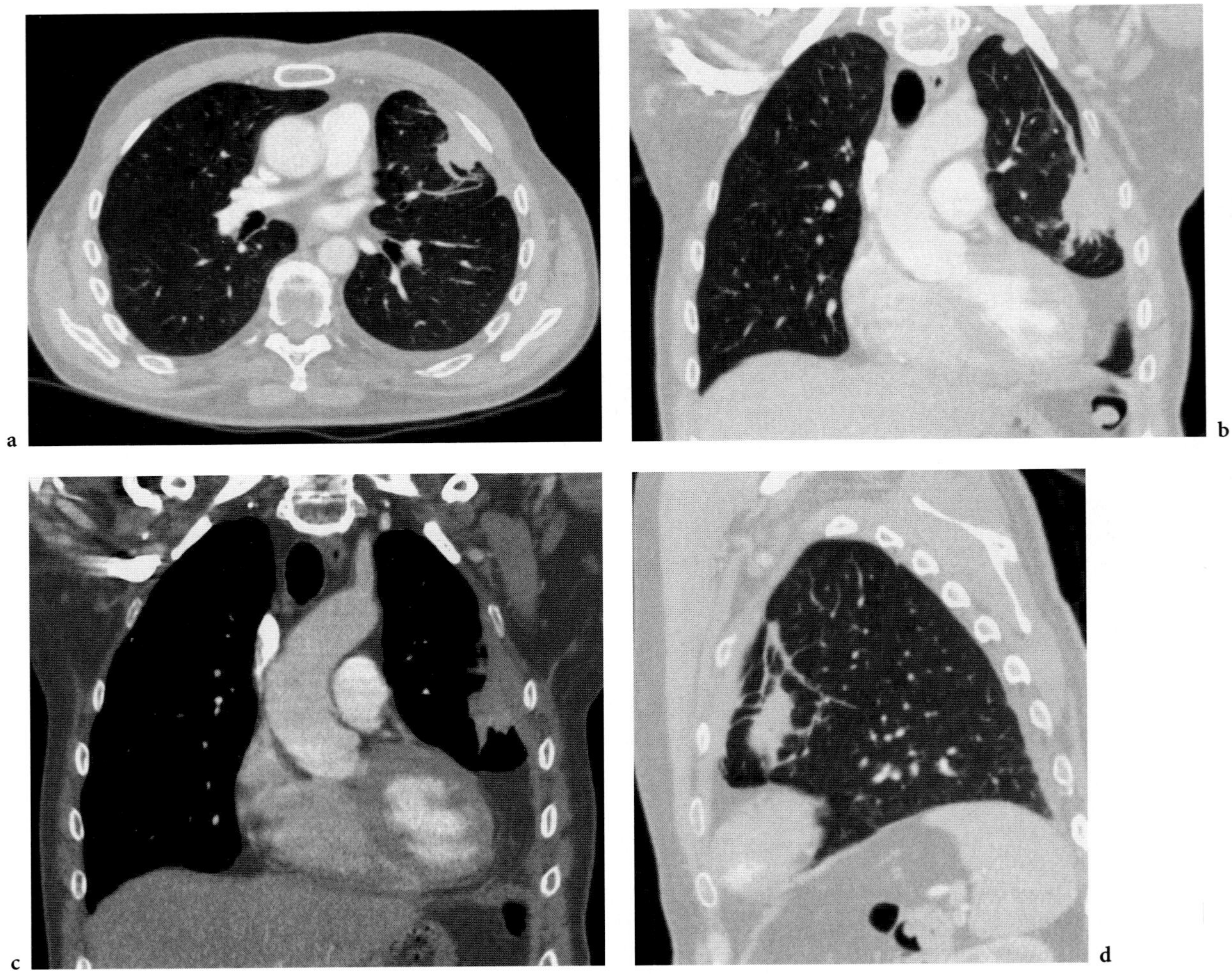

Fig. 27.10a–d. Rounded atelectasis of the lung. **b, c** Coronal and **d** sagittal reformations add information to **a** the axial slice by showing additional curvilinear opacities extending towards the pleural based mass. The CT protocol: acquisition 16×0.75 mm; pitch 0.950; slice thickness, coronal and sagittal reformations 3 mm

detail during optimal enhancement of the tumor. Teifke and co-workers (1994) found spiral CT very helpful for elucidating problems in the diagnosis of breast lesions. They appreciated especially the speed of the method, the comfort for the patient, the absence of movement artifacts, the easy standardization, and the wide applicability of the method making it a good alternative for MRI when this technique is not available. These authors compared spiral scans performed before and 50 s after injection of contrast. A mass showing increase in density of less than 30 Hounsfield units (HU) is very likely to be a benign lesion (fibroadenoma), whereas lesions with an increase in density of more than 60 HU are very suggestive for malignant tumors. For lesions with an enhancement between 30 and 60 HU the differential diagnosis between benign and malignant disease was difficult and should be based on other criteria such as delineation of the tumor. Presently, however, spiral CT is only occasionally used and most institutions use MRI to explore breast tumors after a mammogram and an ultrasound have been performed. It is not sure whether MDCT will change this, but this technique has some advantages over MRI. Examination time is shorter, reducing motion artifacts, invasion in the bony chest wall is better seen, and the examination can be performed in the same body position as the surgical procedure (Fig. 11).

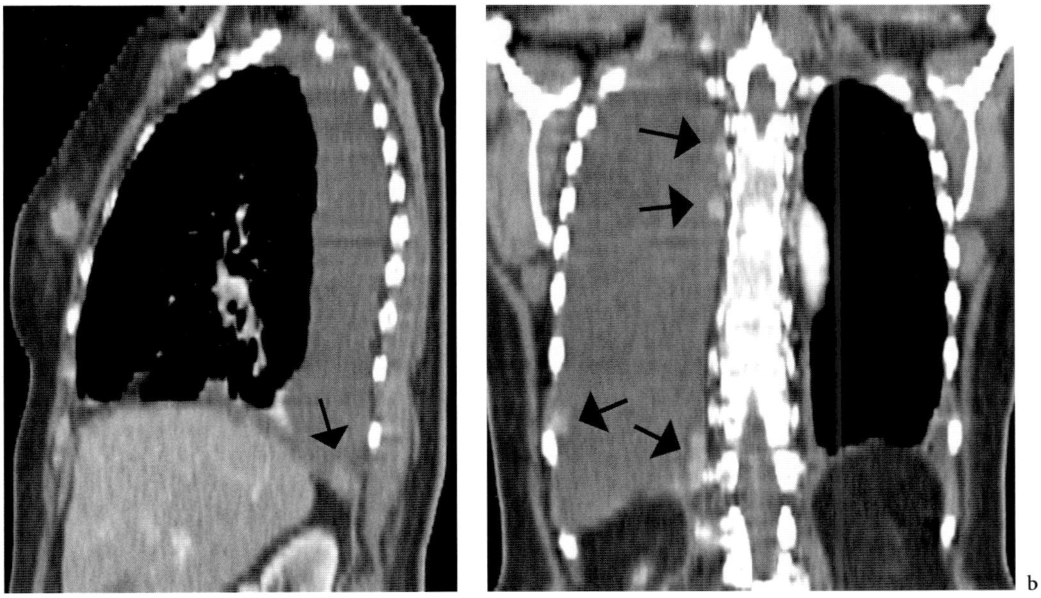

Fig. 27.11a, b. Malignant tumor of the breast. **a** Sagittal reformation shows the mass which is separated from the pectoralis muscle by a small amount of fat. On this sagittal image and also on the **b** coronal view an important pleural effusion and several pleural metastases are seen (*arrows*). The CT protocol: acquisition 4×2.5 mm; pitch 1.38; slice thickness for coronal and sagittal reformations 3 mm

27.2.6 Conclusions

The advantage of MDCT in the study of chest wall and pleura is related to its ability to perform high-detail images in a very short time. In this way motion artifacts and respiratory motion artifacts, often occurring with conventional CT of these areas, can be avoided. The value of 2D and 3D reformations is not yet fully determined.

References

Anderson LS, Forrest JV (1973) Tumors of the diaphragm. Am J Roentgenol 119:259–265

Bergin D, Ennis R, Keogh C et al. (2001) The"dependent viscera" sign in CT diagnosis of blunt traumatic diaphragmatic rupture. Am J Roentgenol 177:1137–1140

Bisgard JD (1947) Congenital eventration of the diaphragm. J Thorac Surg 16:484–488

Bogaert J, Weemaes K, Verschakelen JA et al. (1995) Spiral CT findings in a postoperative intrathoracic gastric herniation: a case report. Eur Radiol 5:192–195

Bovornkitti S, Kangsadal P, Sandvichien S et al. (1960) Neurogenic muscular aplasia (eventration) of the diaphragm. Am Rev Respir Dis 82:876–880

Brink JA, Heiken JP, Semenkovich J et al. (1994) Abnormalities of the diaphragm and adjacent structures: findings on multiplanar spiral CT scans. Am J Roentgenol 163:307–310

Carter B, Giuseffi J, Felson B (1951) Traumatic diaphragmatic hernia. Am J Roentgenol 65:56–71

Caskey CI, Zerhouni EA, Fishman EK et al. (1989) Aging of the diaphragm: a CT study. Radiology 171:385–389

Cassart M, Pettiaux N, Gevenois PA et al. (1997) Effect of chronic hyperinflation on diaphragm length and surface area. Am J Respir Crit Care Med 156:504–508

Cassart M, Verbandt Y, de Francquen P et al. (1999) Diaphragm dimensions after single-lung transplantation for emphysema. Am J Respir Crit Care Med 159:1992–1997

Cassart M, Hamacher J, Verbandt Y et al. (2001) Effects of lung volume reduction surgery for emphysema on diaphragm dimensions and configuration. Am J Respir Crit Care Med 163:1042–1043

Coulier B, Ramboux A, Mailleux P et al. (1999) Diagnosis of non-hiatal diaphragmatic hernia using helical computed tomography. JBR BTR 82:1–5

Cotter CP, Tyndal EC (1986) Traumatic diaphragmatic injuries. Arch Fr Pediatr 33:197–203

Dee PM (1992) The radiology of chest trauma. Radiol Clin North Am 30:291–306

Demos TC, Solomon C, Posniak HV et al. (1989) Computed tomography in traumatic defects of the diaphragm. Clin Imaging 13:62–67

Deschildre F, Petyt L, Rémy-Jardin M et al. (1994) Evaluation de la TDM par balayage spirale volumique (BSV) vs IRM dans le bilan d'extension pariétal des masses thoraciques. Rev Im Med 6:188

Epstein DM, Stephenson LW, Gefter WB et al. (1986) Value of CT in the preoperative assessment of lung cancer: a survey of thoracic surgeons. Radiology 161:423–427

Fataar S, Rad FF, Schulman A (1979) Diagnosis of diaphragmatic tears. Br J Radiol 52:375–381

Gale ME (1985) Bochdalek hernia: prevalence and CT characteristics. Radiology 156:449–452
Gale ME (1986) Anterior diaphragm: variations in the CT appearance. Radiology 161:635–639
Gelman R, Mirvis SE, Gens D (1991) Diaphragmatic rupture due to blunt trauma: sensitivity of plain chest radiographs. Am J Roentgenol 156:51–57
Gouliamos AD, Carter BL, Enami B (1980) Computed tomography of the chest wall. Radiology 134:433–436
Grenier P, Dubray B, Carette MF et al. (1989) Preoperative thoracic staging of lung cancer: CT and MR evaluation. Diagn Intervent Radiol 1:23–28
Gurney J, Harrison NL, Anderson JC (1985) Omental fat simulating pleural fluid in traumatic diaphragmatic hernia: CT characteristics. J Comput Assist Tomogr 9:1112–1114
Haller JA, Scherer LR, Turner CS et al. (1989) Evolving management of pectus excavatum based on a single institutional experience of 664 patients. Ann Surg 209:578–582
Heiberg E, Wolverson MK, Hurd RN et al. (1980) CT recognition of traumatic rupture of the diaphragm. Am J Roentgenol 135:369–372
Holland DG, Quint LE (1991) Traumatic rupture of the diaphragm without visceral herniation: CT diagnosis. Am J Roentgenol 157:17–18
Hurwitz DJ, Stofman G, Curtin H (1994) Three-dimensional imaging of Poland's syndrome. Plast Reconstr Surg 94: 719–723
Killeen KL, Mirvis SE, Shanmuganathan K (1999) Helical CT of diaphragmatic rupture caused by blunt trauma. Am J Roentgenol 173:1611–1616
Kleinman PK, Raptopoulos V (1985) The anterior diaphragmatic attachments: an anatomic and radiologic study with clinical correlates. Radiology 155:289–293
Kuriyama K, Hosomi N, Sawai Y et al. (1994a) Three-dimensional imaging of focal lung disease using spiral volumetric CT. Jpn J Clin Radiol 39:9–13
Kuriyama K, Tateishi R, Kumatani T et al. (1994b) Pleural invasion by peripheral bronchogenic carcinoma: assessment with three-dimensional helical CT. Radiology 191:365–369
Kurihara Y, Nakajima Y, Niimi H et al. (1997) Extrapleural air collections mimicking pneumothorax: helical CT finding. J Comput Assist Tomogr 21:771–772
Larici AR, Gotway MB, Litt HI et al. (2002) Helical CT with sagittal and coronal reconstructions: accuracy for detection of diaphragmatic injury. Am J Roentgenol 179:451–457
Laufer L, Schulman H, Hertzanu Y (1999) Intrathoracic rib demonstrated by helical CT with three-dimensional reconstruction. Eur Radiol 9:60–61
Leung JC, Nance ML, Schwab CW et al. (1999) Thickening of the diaphragm: a new computed tomography sign of diaphragm injury. J Thorac Imaging 14:126–129
Lewandowski B, Winsberg F (1983) Echographic appearance of the right hemidiaphragm. J Ultrasound Med 2:243–249
Lindstrom CH, Allen RP (1966) Bilateral congenital eventration of the diaphragm. Am J Roentgenol 97:216–221
Linsenmaier U, Krotz M, Hauser H et al. (2002) Whole-body computed tomography in polytrauma: techniques and management. Eur Radiol 12:1728–1740
McNamara JJ, Paulson DL, Urschel HC et al. (1968) Eventration of the diaphragm. Surgery 64:1013–1021
Meier RA, Marianacci EB, Costello P et al. (1993) 3D image reconstruction of right subclavian artery aneurysms. J Comput Assist Tomogr 17:887–890
Michelson E (1961) Eventration of the diaphragm. Surgery 49:410–422
Mirvis SE, Templeton P (1992) Imaging in acute thoracic trauma. Semin Roentgenol 27:184–210
Naidich DP, Zerhouni EA, Siegelman SS (1991) Computed tomography and magnetic resonance of the thorax. Raven Press, New York
Oyen R, Marchal G, Verschakelen J et al. (1984) Sonographic aspect of hypertrophic diaphragmatic muscular bundles. J Clin Ultrasound 12:121–123
Panicek DM, Benson CB, Gottlieb RH et al. (1988) The diaphragm: anatomic, pathologic and radiologic considerations. Radiographics 8:385–425
Paris F, Tarazona V, Casillas M et al. (1973) Hernia of Morgagni. Thorax 28:631
Pearlberg JL, Sandler MA, Beute GH et al. (1987) Limitations of CT in evaluation of neoplasms involving chest wall. J Comput Assist Tomogr 11:290–293
Pennes DR, Glazer GM, Wimbish KJ et al. (1985) Chest wall invasion by lung cancer: limitations of CT evaluation. Am J Roentgenol 144:507–511
Pery M, Kaftori J, Rosenberger A (1984) Causes of abnormal right diaphragmatic position diagnosed by ultrasound. J Clin Ultrasound 12:121–123
Pettiaux N, Cassart M, Paiva M et al. (1997) Three-dimensional reconstruction of human diaphragm with the use of spiral computed tomography. Appl Physiol 82:998–1002
Sardanelli F, Melani E, Calabrese M et al. (1995) Dynamic spiral CT of suspected breast tumors. Eur Radiol 5 (Suppl):280
Scaglione M, Pinto F, Grassi R et al. (2000) Diagnostic sensitivity of computerized tomography in closed trauma of the diaphragm. Retrospective study of 35 consecutive cases. Radiol Med (Torino) 99:46–50
Schwartz EE, Wechsler RJ (1989) Diaphragmatic and paradiaphragmatic tumors and pseudotumors. J Thorac Imaging 4:19–28
Shanmuganathan K, Killeen K, Mirvis SE et al. (2000) Imaging of diaphragmatic injuries. J Thorac Imaging 15:104–111
Shin MS, Berland LL (1985) Computed tomography of retrocrural spaces: normal, anatomic variants and pathologic conditions. Am J Roentgenol 145:81–86
Shirakawa T, Fukuda K, Miyamoto Y et al. (1994) Parietal pleural invasion of lung masses: evaluation with CT performed during deep inspiration and expiration. Radiology 192:809–811
Smith TR (2002) Demonstration of inferior phrenic arteries on spiral CT. Clin Imaging 26:27–29
Snyder WH, Greany EM (1965) Congenital diaphragmatic hernia; 77 consecutive cases. Surgery 57:576–588
Stark P, Jaramillo D (1986) CT of the sternum. Am J Roentgenol 147:72–77
Takasugi JE, Rapoport S, Shaw C (1989) Superior sulcus tumors: the role of imaging. J Thorac Imaging 4:41–48
Tarver RD, Cones DJ, Cory DA et al. (1989) Imaging the diaphragm and its disorders. J Thorac Imaging 4:1–18
Teifke A, Schweden F, Cagil H et al. (1994) Spiral-Computertomographie der Mamma. Fortschr Roentgenstr 161: 495–500
Tello R, Scholz E, Finn JP et al. (1993) Subclavian vein thrombosis detected with spiral CT and three-dimensional reconstruction. Am J Roentgenol 160:33–34
Thomas GG, Clitherow NR (1977) Herniation through the foramen of Morgagni in children. Br J Surg 64:215–217

Toombs BD, Sandler CM, Lester RG (1981) Computed tomography of chest trauma. Radiology 140:733–738
Ujita M, Ojiri H, Ariizumi M et al. (1993) Appearance of the inferior phrenic artery and vein on CT scans of the chest: a CT and cadaveric study. Am J Roentgenol 160:745–747
Van Daele G, Joris L, Eyskens E (1987) Traumatische diafragmaruptuur. Tijdschr Geneeskd 43:1649–1653
Verschakelen JA, Demaerel P, Coolen J et al. (1989a) Rounded atelactasis of the lung: MR appearance. Am J Roentgenol 152:965–966
Verschakelen JA, Marchal G, Verbeken E et al. (1989b) Sonographic appearance of the diaphragm in the presence of pleural disease: a cadaver study. J Clin Ultrasound 17: 222–227
Webb WR, Gatsonis C, Zerhouni EA et al. (1991) CT and MR imaging in staging non-small cell bronchogenic carcinoma: report of the radiologic diagnostic oncology group. Radiology 178:705–713
Wilbur AC, Gorodetsky A, Hibbeln JF (1994) Imaging findings of adult Bochdalek hernias. Clin Imaging 18:224–229
Worthy SA, Kang EY, Hartman TE et al. (1995) Diaphragmatic rupture: CT findings in 11 patients. Radiology 194:885–888
Yamana D, Ohba S (1994) Three-dimensional image of Bochdalek diaphragmatic hernia; a case report. Radiat Med 12: 39–41
Yamashita K, Minemori K, Matsuda H et al. (1993) MR imaging in the diagnosis of partial eventration of the diaphragm. Chest 104:328

28 MDCT of Chest Trauma

M. Wintermark and P. Schnyder

CONTENTS

28.1 Demographics of Chest Trauma

In industrialized countries, trauma is the third leading cause of death, immediately behind cardiovascular diseases and cancers (Nourjah 1999). Trauma thus represents a major concern, since it mainly affects young patients. Indeed, trauma is the main cause of death in the age bracket of 25–44 years (Schnyder and Wintermark 2000; Peng et al. 1998).

Chest injuries are encountered in approximately 20% of trauma patients. They are associated with head trauma in 69%, abdominal and pelvic lesions in 43%, and limb fractures in 52% of cases (Nourjah 1999; Schnyder and Wintermark 2000). Chest trauma mortality amounts to 20% (Zinck and Primack 2000). Fifty percent of the casualties die from head injuries and 20% from hemodynamic or respiratory complications, both at an early stage after trauma. The remaining 30% die later, from infection and sepsis, with subsequent adult respiratory distress syndrome and multiple-organ failure (Leidner et al. 1998; van Hise et al. 1998; Collins 2000). Furthermore, trauma is responsible for considerable morbidity and has a major socio-economic impact. Globally, it induces 30,000 disability days per 100,000 persons annually in the United States (Schnyder and Wintermark 2000; Peng et al. 1998). Two billion U.S. dollars are the estimated total short-, mid-, and long-term costs of trauma in Switzerland, where 30,000 severe injuries and 600 deaths are recorded annually for a population of 7,600,000 inhabitants and 4,600,000 motor vehicles (Siegel et al. 1993).

Since trauma affects mainly young patients and thus has a considerable socio-economic impact, chest trauma, as well as its management, constitute a major challenge. The purpose of this chapter is to focus on the radiological management of chest trauma patients, and to show how the advent of MDCT has induced dramatic modifications.

28.2 Biomechanics of Blunt Chest Trauma

In the western European countries and United States, trauma most often results from traffic accidents, whereas falls, mainly at the work site, recreational accidents, and violence account for the other causes (Zinck and Primack 2000; Siegel et al. 1993; Shanmuganathan and Mirvis 1999). In traffic accidents, chest injuries result from changes in pressure and shear forces produced by three mechanisms: direct blow to the chest, crushing, and deceleration, which most often combine into windscreen syndrome, dashboard syndrome, side-door syndrome, and seat-belt syndrome. The observed syndrome depends on the circumstances and characteristics of the accident, the position of the victim, driver or passenger, the design of the car, with or without lateral reinforcement, the presence of active protective devices such as frontal or lateral inflatable airbags, the use of frontal or rear seat belts, etc. (Schnyder and Wintermark 2000; Siegel et al. 1993).

Trauma consecutive to motor vehicle accidents or to violence is clearly related to alcohol consumption:

M. Wintermark, MD
Department of Diagnostic and Interventional Radiology, University Hospital (CHUV), 1011 Lausanne, Switzerland
P. Schnyder, MD
Professor, Department of Diagnostic and Interventional Radiology, University Hospital (CHUV), 1011 Lausanne, Switzerland

up to 65% of the victims of traffic accidents are found with positive alcoholemia, 26–50% exceeding the legal limit of 0.5–0.8‰ (Guerrero-Lopez et al. 2000; Voggenreiter et al. 2000).

28.3 Modern Design of Emergency Radiology Units

Trauma patients' admission in the emergency room is characterized by the intervention of a multidisciplinary teamwork involving anesthetists, neurosurgeons, thoracic and abdominal surgeons, as well as orthopedists. Among all these specialists, radiology plays an increasingly preponderant role, both in the selection of trauma patients according to the severity of their injuries and in the taking of clinical decisions at each management step. This growing role of imaging does not only have to be coped with in the emergency room, but also in the resuscitation room, in the operating room, and in the intensive care unit; thus, when admitted in the resuscitation room, trauma patients undergo a cervical spine radiograph before possible endotracheal intubation, as well as screening chest X-ray and abdominal sonography. Once hemodynamic stabilization is obtained, a CT survey is performed to assess possible head, thoracic, and abdominal visceral injuries. The admission survey ends up with analog or digitized radiographs for limb fractures. Some surgical procedures in the operating room are performed under fluoroscopic or sonographic guidance. Furthermore, conventional radiological or CT follow-up examinations are mandatory after surgery or during the intensive care unit stay, in order to afford early detection of complications and check-up of tube and line position. Fluoroscopic, sonographic, and CT guidance is increasingly more often required in interventional procedures such as tube positioning. Finally, information provided by CT regarding, for instance, the site and importance of an active hemorrhage, constitute a useful guide for diagnostic and therapeutic interventional maneuvers.

Availability and proximity of emergency radiology units are evidenced by this increasingly preponderant role of imaging in the management of trauma patients.

Availability of fully equipped radiology units located within the emergency room, where emergency patients can immediately be evaluated, without interfering with scheduled outpatients, goes along with the mandatory around-the-clock presence of an experienced radiologist in the emergency radiology unit. The latter's role is to direct technologists in the selection and performance of imaging protocols. They are also in charge of rapidly providing clinicians with a diagnosis regarding the trauma patients' condition. Moreover, the radiologist is responsible for the coordination of trauma patient management in the emergency radiology unit, where non-urgent diagnostic and nursing procedures often interfere with imaging examinations and slow down trauma patients' imaging survey as well as subsequent mandatory, sometimes life-saving, therapeutic procedures.

Proximity must govern the architectural design of emergency rooms and of its four components: resuscitation room, emergency radiology unit, operating room, and intensive care unit, which should ideally be next to each other. Every effort should be made to reduce transportation times, since the fitting-out of trauma patients and their monitoring for transportation are challenging and time-consuming. At our institution, transportation of trauma patients used to represent 30–50% of the total time spent in the emergency radiology unit.

Monitoring of trauma patients during transportation is often more complicated and supervening complications more difficult to manage, with possible life-threatening consequences. Moreover, in order to prevent displacement of fractures, mainly of unstable spine fractures, trauma patient transportation, for instance, form his bed onto the CT or angiography table, requires a minimum of four persons. These people have to be recruited among the technologist and nursing pools. Yet, their number is presently limited for economic reasons, which is a further argument in favor of the proximity of the emergency room components. Our 13-year experience demonstrates that preparation and transportation times, for instance, in a CT unit, can be reduced by 50% with an adequate organization and training of the technologist team.

28.4 Computed Tomography: the Cornerstone of Trauma Radiology

Management of trauma patients relies on a simple but obvious concept: time is life! The challenge for the emergency radiologist in his evaluation of the radiological admission survey of severe chest trauma patients is to reach the correct diagnosis, and this as soon as possible upon admission. The ideal imaging survey in an efficient emergency radiology unit must neither interfere with the monitoring of hemodynamically unstable trauma patients nor delay other diagnostic and therapeutic procedures. It must afford simultaneous and accurate evaluation of head, chest, abdomen and pelvis.

Spiral computed tomography (SCT), and, even better, multidetector-row SCT (MDCT), show all these advantages and has asserted itself as the gold standard imaging technique in the emergency radiology unit. Clinical relevance of CT compared with plain films is high. It represents an adequate screening test to depict hemomediastinum, aortic injuries, pericardial effusions, occult pneumothoraces or pleural effusions, free peritoneal fluid, hepatic, splenic and renal trauma, as well as spine fractures. When compared with plain chest films, it displays up to 83% of additional lesions requiring undelayed treatment, chest tube insertion for occult pneumothorax being the most common procedure (Schnyder and Wintermark 2000; Leidner et al. 1998; Guerrero-Lopez et al. 2000; Voggenreiter et al. 2000; Trupka et al. 1997).

Other imaging techniques are progressively replaced by MDCT.

Conventional radiographs are required for the assessment of the cervical spine on admission. It is usually limited to a lateral view, with consideration for a possible urgent endotracheal intubation; however, if plain lateral views of the cervical spine are reliable in depicting severe unstable fractures or dislocations, they are not accurate enough to rule out more subtle ones, which makes CT mandatory. Similarly, CT shows more accuracy than plain films in the screening for thoraco-lumbar spine fractures, as discussed below (Crim et al. 2001; Mirvis and Shanmuganathan 1995).

Supine chest X-ray remains the most important imaging examination for the initial assessment of thoracic lesions and their management. Its sensitivity is indeed very high with respect to mediastinal hemorrhage, tension pneumothoraces, large hemothoraces, and flail chests. On the other hand, plain films fail in the detection of occult pneumothoraces, pulmonary contusions, and lacerations. Furthermore, the specificity of supine chest X-rays is low. This is illustrated by the multiple possible origins for mediastinal widening, including mediastinal lipomatosis, aortic tortuosity in the elderly, and hemomediastinum originating from small arterial branches and veins, commonly associated with sternal and/or vertebral fractures. Aortic traumatic lesions account for only 15% of traumatic enlarged mediastinal shadows (Schnyder and Wintermark 2000; Lacqua and Sahdev 1994; Dalldorf et al. 1990).

Finally, conventional radiographs are used in the assessment and characterization of limb fractures.

Sonography can be easily, quickly, and safely performed in trauma patients at their bedside with a small mobile ultrasound unit. It has precise but rather limited indications in the emergency setting. It can detect free peritoneal fluid, but its sensitivity in depicting hepatic, splenic, and renal trauma in the acute phase is limited (Rose et al. 2001; Stengel et al. 2001). Echocardiography, with transthoracic and transesophageal probes, finds particular applications in the identification of cardiac and aortic injuries (Garcia-Fernandez et al. 1998; Vignon et al. 1998); however, sonography in the evaluation of severe trauma patients is usually suboptimal, due to possible chest and/or abdominal wall pain, subcutaneous emphysema, wounds, and dressings.

Angiography represents the gold standard in the detection of traumatic aortic and vascular injuries. Development of new interventional procedures affords alternatives to invasive surgery. Percutaneous positioning of endovascular balloon-expandable stents under angiographic guidance thus constitutes a recent and promising therapeutic tool in the management of blunt traumatic aortic lesions. Bleeding from small- and mid-size arterial lesions may be embolized, constituting a substitute for or a preparation to surgery.

For the time being, magnetic resonance imaging has few applications in the emergency management of blunt chest trauma. Development of rapid acquisition sequences and spreading of open magnets will perhaps allow MR to play a growing role in the emergency radiology unit.

28.5 Imaging Algorithms Dedicated for Trauma Patients

Trauma patients admitted in the emergency room are often confused, unconscious, or even intubated. The examiner's suspicion must rely on the trauma mechanism rather than on the patients' complaints. The fundamental concept underlying trauma biomechanics is that a severe trauma usually overlaps anatomically defined areas, thus explaining, for instance, that each trauma patient shows an average of 1.5 lesions. Similarly, severe head trauma is associated with an occult pneumothorax in 20% and with pulmonary contusions in 23%, whereas chest trauma is associated with extrathoracic injuries in up to 80% of cases

(Schnyder and Wintermark 2000; Karaaslan et al. 1995).

In agreement with others (Leidner et al. 1998; Haydel et al. 2000; Linsenmaier et al. 2002), we propose a standardized screening MDCT survey dedicated for trauma patients, based on the trauma mechanism and its severity. Of course, this MDCT survey can only be performed once the trauma patient has been hemodynamically stabilized, whereas supine chest X-ray and abdominal echography are obtained in unstable trauma patients.

In case of significant but non-severe trauma, including traffic accidents at a speed below 50 km/h and falls from a height exceeding 1 m, we recommend to perform a head MDCT, a cervical spine MDCT including the petrous pyramids, as well as ten incremental 5-mm CT slices on the chest. In cases of severe trauma, such as traffic accidents at a speed higher than 50 km/h, substantial car deformity, falls from a height exceeding 3 m, and/or any crush accident, head MDCT should be performed, followed by cervical spine MDCT including the petrous pyramids as well as by thoraco-abdomino-pelvic MDCT. Head MDCT affords brain evaluation, which is mandatory in unconscious or intubated patients who cannot be evaluated neurologically. Cervical MDCT allows for a survey of the whole cervical spine and superior aero-digestive structures, of the petrous pyramids, and even of the skeletal face in case of clinical facial trauma. The few chest CT sections obtained in the "minimal" chest survey protocol are dedicated to the identification of occult pneumothoraces, whereas the complete thoraco-abdomino-pelvic MDCT in the "extensive" survey is intended to detect aortic injuries, which are usually clinically silent until the sudden onset of a hemodynamic decompensation. As detailed below, thoraco-abdomino-pelvic MDCT has also shown its superiority to plain films in the detection of thoraco-lumbar spine fractures.

The fundamental motivation for the use of these MDCT screening protocols is to obtain a complete and comprehensive assessment of the trauma patients' condition upon their admission. They will afford categorization of trauma patients according to the severity of their injuries, and to set up the chronology of the required therapeutic procedures. Furthermore, such screening MDCT surveys spare the time wasted in moving the patients from the CT unit to the conventional radiology room or to the operating room, and vice versa, when the latter present new symptoms or sudden hemodynamic instability. As in every screening test, the excessive character of this MDCT survey for a single trauma patient is largely compensated for by the benefit for a population of trauma patients. At our institution, we have definitely convinced our surgeons of the validity of such MDCT survey protocols, which are used on a daily basis in our emergency radiology unit. They are available on our web site: http://www.hospvd.ch/public/chuv/rad/home.htm.

The CT examination in a trauma patient is performed with his arms placed along his sides, since the patient's arms cannot be positioned above his head due to the frequently associated upper limb fractures. The subsequent streak artifacts are minimized by spiral data acquisition, especially with multidetector-row technology, and do not interfere with the interpretation of the so-acquired MDCT survey. Minor streak artifacts may be induced by metallic components such as skin EKG electrodes, naso-gastric or naso-tracheal tubes, or life-support equipment, but never justify their removal (Schnyder and Wintermark 2000; Leidner et al. 1998; Guerrero-Lopez et al. 2000; Voggenreiter et al. 2000; Trupka et al. 1997).

At our institution, complete performance of a cerebral, cervical, thoracic, and abdominal MDCT survey used to average 40 min, with the following distribution: 45% for transportation; 35% for CT data acquisition itself; and 20% for data management by the technologist, including two-dimensional (2D) sagittal and coronal reconstructions. The 14 min required for CT data acquisition is much longer than the performance of the cerebral, cervical, thoracic, and abdominal MDCT series themselves, which account for less than 3 min when added to each other. The 11-min mismatch result from the frequent interruptions of data acquisition required by the monitoring of trauma patients, their frequent motion and/or agitation, and resuscitation procedures required by hemodynamic instability. The 14 min required for CT data acquisition can hardly be shortened. On the other hand, our experience has revealed a possible saving of up to 20–25 min in the duration of the MDCT survey in trauma patients by improving technologist work ergonomics and especially by a systematic overlapping of patient transportation to his bed and data management; thus, in daytime at least, one technologist should be in charge of the MDCT data processing and printing, whereas another one should collaborate with the emergency room nursing team to transport the patient.

The MDCT affords multiple advantages relating to the voluminous character of data acquisition; however, it involves a substantially higher radiation dose to the patient than conventional radiology (Verdun et al., in press). Our MDCT protocols have been designed for adults of average body build. Acquisition parameters, notably kVp, must be constantly optimized, which is automatically realized by some MDCT units. Most often, they have to be lowered, especially in children, in order to reduce the effective dose. For instance, low kVp (80 kVp) can be used in children for bone evaluation such as in cervical spine surveys, affording significant dose reduction to the thyroid gland.

Besides the radiation dose, MDCT raises several questions relating to the MDCT data volume. The first question relates to the method of interpretation for MDCT examinations. The cerebral, cervical, and thoraco-abdomino-pelvic MDCT survey represents several hundred images, and up to 1000 images when including reformats with pulmonary and bone window settings. The emergency radiologist has to interpret them in less than 15 min, and this under the constant pressure of consulting neurosurgeons, thoracic, abdominal, and orthopedic surgeons, each of them arguing about the priority of their field of interest over the others. Such a setting may be difficult to manage by training junior radiologists who have to face experienced senior consultants; therefore, an experienced radiologist's support is mandatory, at least during the junior radiologist's first months in the emergency radiology unit. The latter radiologist has no choice indeed but to learn how to manage these uncomfortable situations very quickly.

With respect to the MDCT data volume, hard-copy interpretation becomes a nonsense, and soft-copy interpretation on dedicated workstations becomes mandatory. Soft-copy interpretation has proved as reliable as hard-copy interpretation (Kundel et al. 2001). The contrast loss due to the maximal brightness of video monitors is largely compensated for by the multiple adjustment possibilities of window and level settings. Soft-copy interpretation also simplifies 2D and 3D reformat processing and reading. Interpretation methods also evolve significantly: from a slice-to-slice hard-copy interpretation, emergency radiologists, mainly junior ones, frequently adopt an organ-to-organ soft-copy interpretation. In the future, ergonomic planning of the emergency radiology unit working station should start with the architectural design of the reading room, including positioning of the windows and lights, noise shielding, and air conditioning.

The MDCT technology also questions the strategy for result transmission. Film printing becomes debatable, all the more when considering the production and reproduction of films to maintain availability of images to multiple consulting teams. The 2D and 3D reconstructions become preponderant to summarize the imaging findings and to give a synthetic representation of the diagnosis to the surgical consultants (Fig. 28.1).

The third question raised by MDCT technology relates to data storage. The MDCT examination printing generates a huge volume of hard copies

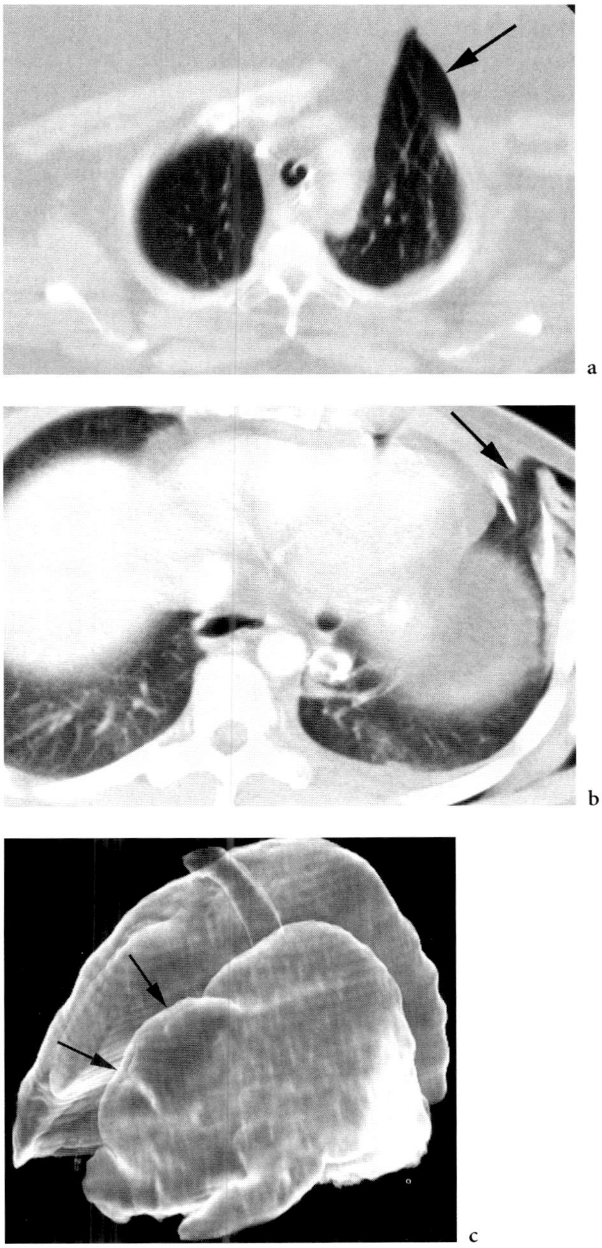

Fig. 28.1. Traumatic left pulmonary hernia *(arrows)* through a chest wall defect, diagnosed on **a**, **b** axial images but better demonstrated to the surgical consultants on a **c** tridimensional (3D) surface-shaded-display (SSD) reconstruction

and thus represents a high financial cost that cannot be considered in the long run, also considering the limited size of archiving rooms. Hard-copy archiving is compelled to be replaced by picture archiving and communication systems (PACS), which constitute the companion piece for soft-copy interpretation of MDCT examinations on workstations. A typical PACS uses a hierarchical architecture with different storage media, depending on the amount and duration of storage and the expected retrieval frequency. It may easily be integrated to radiological and hospital information systems (RIS and HIS, respectively; Foord 1999; Junck et al. 1998; Redfern et al. 2000). At our institution, when we moved from single-slice CT (SSCT) to MDCT, we observed a 400% increase in acquired data volume. As a result, our PACS central storage capacity, which had been initially chosen at 3.7 Terabytes on a 4-year time basis, had to be changed and increased to 21 Terabytes, which we expect to be sufficient for the next 5–6 years.

28.6 Radiological Semiology of Blunt Chest Trauma

The radiological semiology of blunt chest trauma has not been modified by the advent of MDCT. It relates to the different anatomical compartments of the chest: chest wall (Fig. 28.2), diaphragm, pleura (Fig. 28.3), lung parenchyma (Fig. 28.4) and mediastinum (Schnyder and Wintermark 2000; Wintermark and Schnyder 2001).

However, since MDCT affords increased ability to perform 2D and 3D reformats, major progress has been achieved in the result representation for the surgical consultants. Sagittal and coronal 2D reformats are moreover likely to be associated with increased diagnostic value, notably for flail chest (Fig. 28.5), sternal fractures (Fig. 28.6), diaphragmatic rupture (Fig. 28.7), and tracheo-bronchial injuries (Fig. 28.8), although this has not been

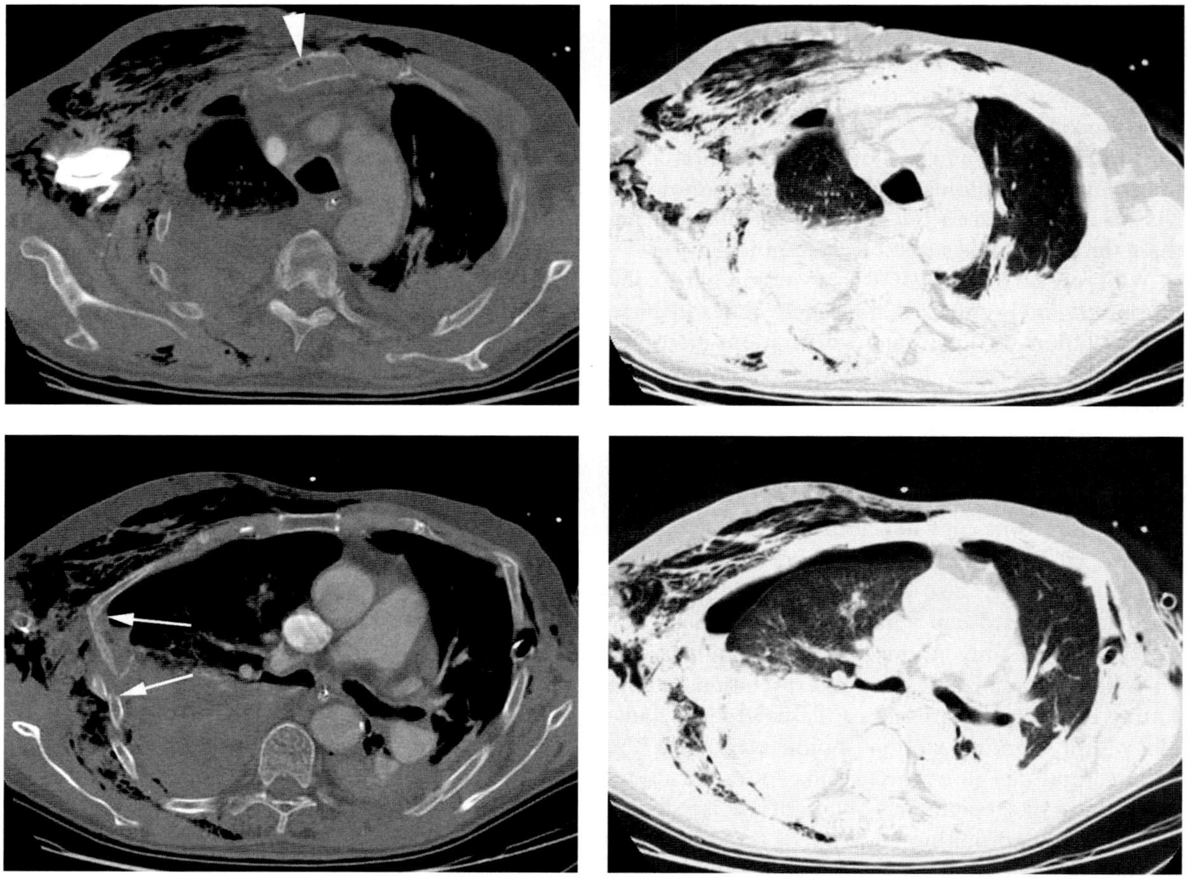

a b c d

Fig. 28.2a–d. Several rib fractures (*arrows*) responsible for extensive subcutaneous emphysema and right hemopneumothorax, portraying an air-fluid level. A right lower lobe bronchoaspiration is also present. A left pneumothorax consecutive to rib fractures has already been drained. Finally, a sternal fracture is featured by the presence of intrasternal air (*arrowhead*)

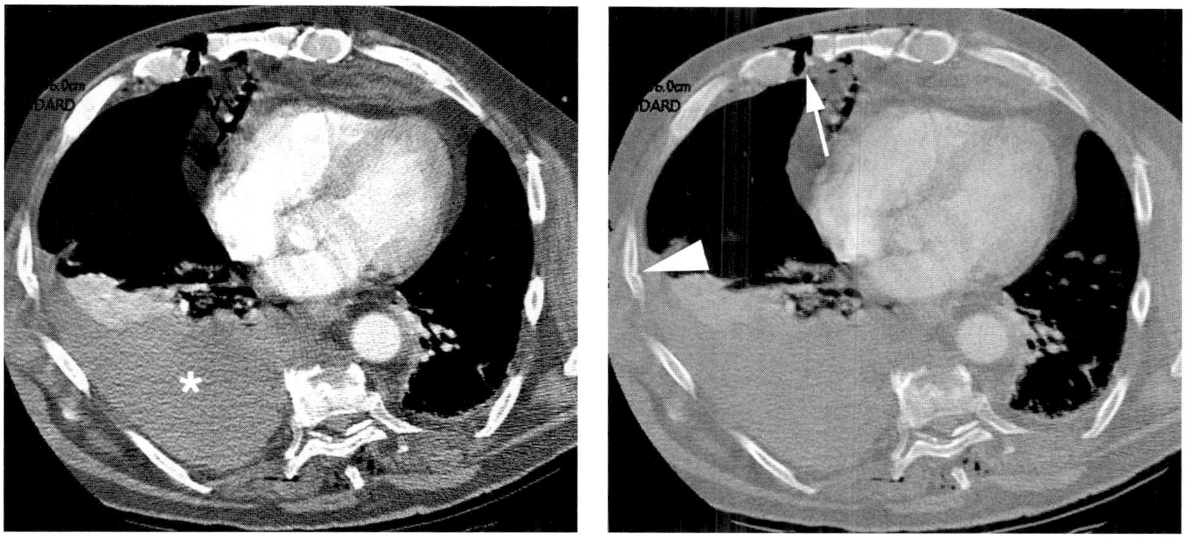

a b

Fig. 28.3a, b. Right hemothorax (*star*) resulting from rib fracture (*arrowhead*) and right chondrosternal dislocation (*arrow*), the latter also being responsible for retrosternal hematoma. Vertebral fracture was suspected upon the presence of perivertebral free-air collections

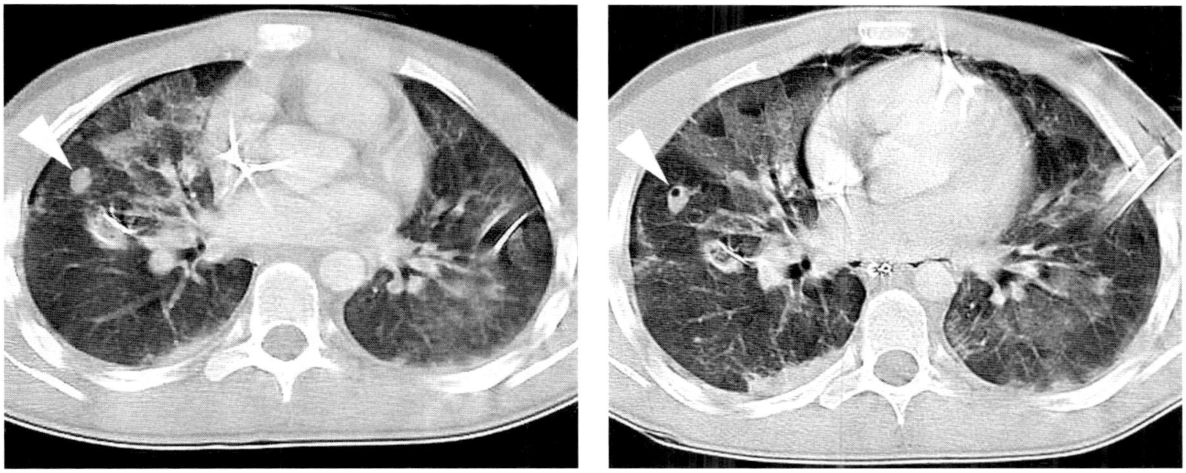

a b

Fig. 28.4a, b. Bilateral pulmonary contusions, characterized by their rapid migration, their radiological pattern evolving hourly and being worsened by medical treatment, notably by exaggerated perfusions, oxygenation and mechanical ventilation, as featured by these two MDCT examinations obtained 24 h apart. A small pulmonary hematoma (*arrowhead*) on **a** the first MDCT has evolved into **b** a pneumatocele on the second MDCT

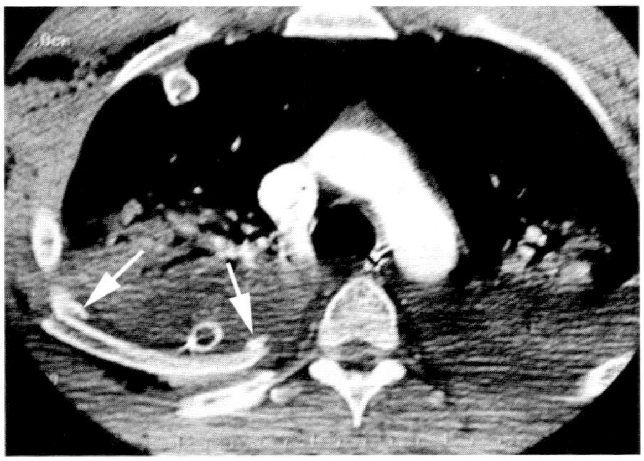

Fig. 28.5. Right flail chest (*arrows*), relating to three or more adjacent fractured ribs, each being broken at least on two separate sites. This flail chest has induced subcutaneous emphysema, as well as right hemopneumothorax, which has already been treated by chest tube insertion. Bilateral atelectases are also present

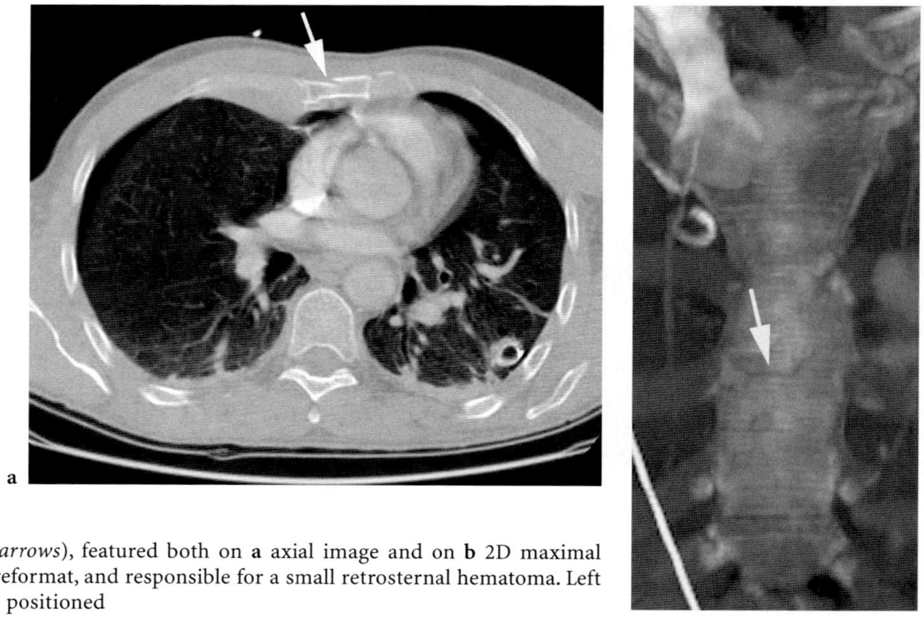

Fig. 28.6. Sternal fracture (*arrows*), featured both on **a** axial image and on **b** 2D maximal intensity projection (MIP) reformat, and responsible for a small retrosternal hematoma. Left chest tube has already been positioned

confirmed by dedicated randomized studies for the moment.

The MDCT has also led to considerable progress in the field of CT angiography (CTA), notably for coronary arteries (Nieman et al. 2002). Multidetector-row CTA (MDCTA) offers reduced acquisition times and enables increased arterial opacification, through improved coincidence between MDCTA data acquisition and iodinated contrast material passage within the volume of interest (Reiser et al. 2001). The impact of MDCTA on the management of patients with suspected blunt aortic lesion is illustrated below.

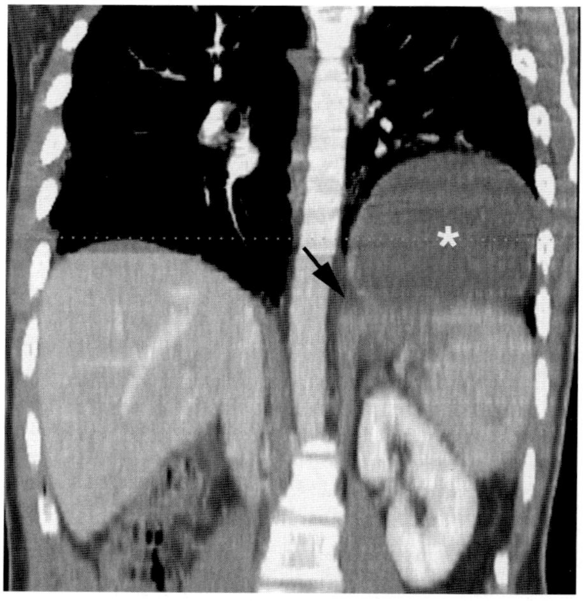

Fig. 28.7. Left traumatic diaphragmatic rupture, with interruption of the left hemidiaphragmatic outline (*arrow*) and gastric herniation through this gap (*asterisk*) as a result of the negative intrathoracic pressure

28.7 MDCT Assessment of Blunt Aortic Lesions

Blunt traumatic aortic lesions are a major concern in the setting of high-speed deceleration accidents, since they are associated with a very high mortality rate. Approximately 80% of patients with blunt traumatic aortic lesion die from exsanguination at the scene of the accident. In the remaining 20%, the mortality rate of acute traumatic aortic lesion in the absence of surgical correction is also high: 30% die within 6 h, 50% within 24 h, and 90% within 4 months (Frick et al. 1997; Williams et al. 1994); however, with prompt diagnosis and surgery, 70% of the patients with a blunt aortic lesion who reach the hospital alive will survive (Frick et al. 1997; Symbas et al. 1998; Mirvis 1997; Hunink and Bos 1995). This statement challenges the emergency radiologist in his evaluation of the radiological admission survey in a severe chest trauma patient.

Aortic lesions represent the most lethal condition among chest injuries and are responsible for up to 40% of fatalities occurring in traffic accidents (Mirvis

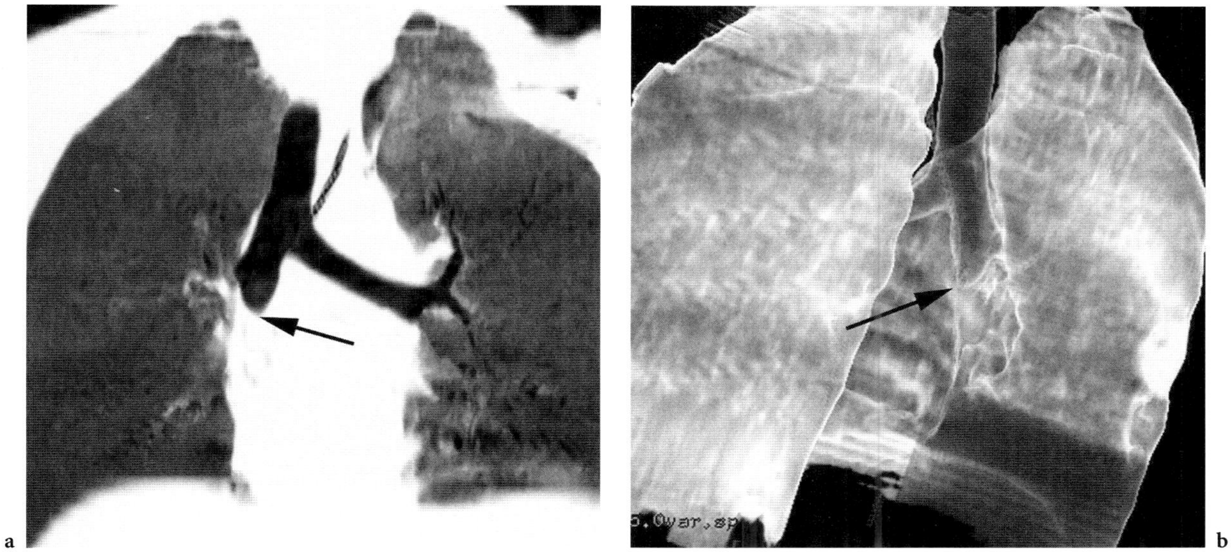

Fig. 28.8. Traumatic injury of the right inferior bronchus (*arrow*), well demonstrated on the **a** 2D minimal intensity projection and on the **b** 3D surface-shaded-display (SSD) reconstruction. This bronchial lesion was responsible for a downward atelectasis of the right lower lobe. It was confirmed by bronchoscopy

1997; FECZKO et al. 1992). Head-on and lateral motor vehicle accidents at speeds greater than 50 km/h, or associated with substantial car deformity, are the main cause (76%) of blunt traumatic aortic injuries, followed by falls from heights - usually exceeding 3 m - and crush injuries (WICKY et al. 2000; WILLIAMS et al. 1994; KATYAL et al. 1997; LOO et al. 1996).

Three mechanisms are hypothesized to explain blunt lesions to the thoracic aorta (SCHNYDER and WINTERMARK 2000; ECKERT 1977). Sudden antero-posterior or lateral deceleration superior to 80 g induces anterior cardiac displacement, leading to shearing forces, and sometimes rupture, at the aortic isthmic level (SCHNYDER and WINTERMARK 2000; FECZKO et al. 1992). The "water-hammer effect" relates to a low thoracic or abdominal compression. The resultant sudden raise of the intra-aortic pressure may be responsible for ascending aortic injuries immediately above the aortic valve. A pressure peak of 80–350 kPa (600–2500 mmHg) is required to rupture a normal aorta (WILLIAMS et al. 1994). Finally, the "osseous pinch" hypothesis assumes a compression of the heart and the aorta between the sternum and vertebral column, for instance, under a violent front impact against the steering wheel. The resultant left posterior displacement of the heart generates an aortic torsion, which may result in a traumatic aortic lesion, sometimes associated with thoracic vertebral fractures (COHEN et al. 1992).

Most blunt traumatic aortic injuries consist of transverse aortic lesions. They are rarely longitudinal, spiral, or ragged. They are segmental in 55% and circumferential in 45% of cases. Aortic lesions may either be partial (65%) or transmural (35%; FECZKO et al. 1992; BEN-MENACHEM 1993; CREASY et al. 1997). Partial blunt aortic lesions may rarely be limited to intimal (Fig. 28.9) and/or medial hemorrhage with intact overlying adventitia or consist of traumatic aortic dissection or intramural hematoma, especially in young patients. More often, intima and media are completely disrupted and sometimes drawn apart over several centimeters, whereas the adventitia remains intact. Bleeding from the aorta or from intramural vasa vasorum generates a pseudoaneurysm, which features a saccular pulsating outpouching, separated from the aortic lumen by a collar and limited by a thin layer of adventitia and by neighboring tissues, usually surrounded by a hemomediastinum. It may rupture at any moment (FECZKO et al. 1992; BEN-MENACHEM 1993; CREASY et al. 1997; CLEVERLEY et al. 2002; HEYSTRATEN et al. 1986).

Ninety percent of blunt traumatic aortic injuries occur on the antero-medial aspect of the aortic isthmus. Seven to eight percent of blunt traumatic aortic lesions are located on the ascending aorta, above the aortic valve. Such injuries are usually associated with aortic valve tears, cardiac contusions or ruptures, coronary artery tears or hemopericardium with cardiac tamponade. They are almost always fatal (SYMBAS et al. 1998; FECZKO et al. 1992; BEN-MENACHEM 1993; CREASY et al. 1997). Blunt traumatic lesions of the descending aorta at the level of the diaphragm are

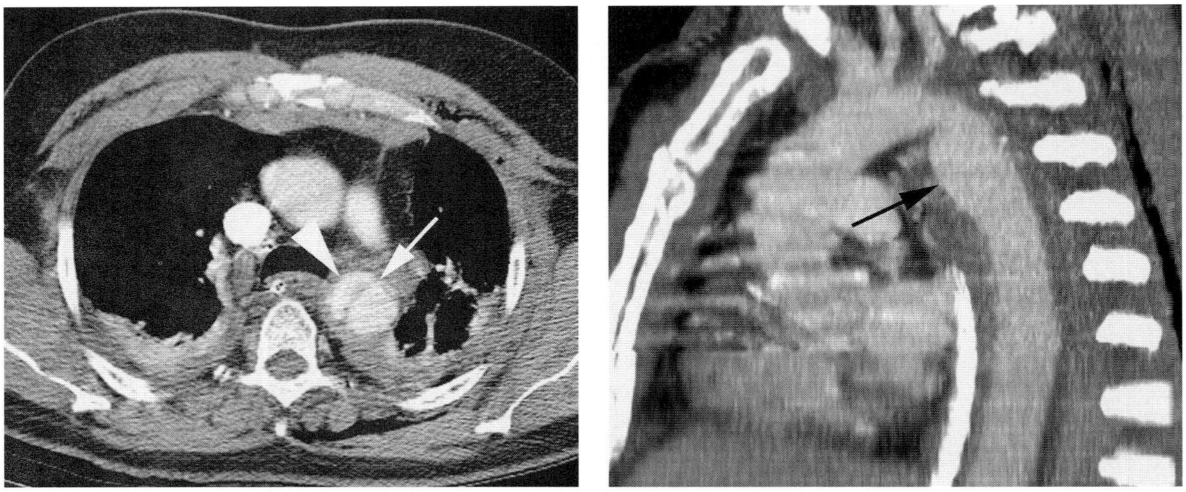

Fig. 28.9. **a** Blunt traumatic aortic lesion at the isthmic level, featuring an intimal flap (*arrow*) associated with an anteromedial pseudoaneurysm (*arrowhead*), surrounded by hemomediastinum. Bilateral small hemothoraces can also be depicted. **b** The 2D maximal intensity projection reformat shows the pseudoaneurysm as a focal bulge (*arrow*) of the contrast-enhanced aortic lumen

observed in 2–3% of cases. In 10% of cases they occur simultaneously with diaphragmatic ruptures, both sharing similar biomechanics (Feczko et al. 1992; Ben-Menachem 1993; Creasy et al. 1997; Rizoli et al. 1994).

With a 90% sensitivity, a 25% specificity, and a 95% negative predictive value for the identification of blunt traumatic aortic injuries, the supine chest X-ray is a worthy screening tool for mediastinal hemorrhage, but affords little as far as a definite diagnosis is concerned (Schnyder and Wintermark 2000; Hunink and Bos 1995; Wintermark et al. 2002; Patel et al. 1998; Fishman 2000). If aortography has classically been considered as the gold standard, it has a low positive response ranging to less than 15% when performed on the basis of trauma mechanism, clinical data, and chest X-ray findings (Hunink and Bos 1995). The MDCTA is presently not only considered as a screening method to select patients for thoracic aortography, but also as an alternative diagnostic procedure in the identification of blunt traumatic aortic lesions, at least in hemodynamically stable trauma patients (Schnyder and Wintermark 2000; Hunink and Bos 1995; Wintermark et al. 2002; Patel et al. 1998; Fishman 2000). In our series of 1150 MDCTA examinations and 28 traumatic aortic injuries, MDCTA has demonstrated a 96.4% sensitivity, a 99.8% specificity, and a 99.8% accuracy. Hemomediastinum is an indirect sign of blunt traumatic aortic lesion, whereas direct SCTAo signs of blunt traumatic aortic injuries include curvilinear intimal flap, intramural hematoma or dissection, and pseudoaneurysm. An unequivocally normal mediastinum on MDCTA, with a regular aorta surrounded by normal fat and no mediastinal hematoma, has a 99.9% negative predictive value for aortic injury (Wicky et al. 2000; Wintermark et al. 2002).

28.8 MDCT Assessment of Thoracic Spine Fractures

Another example of the superiority of MDCT in the management of trauma patients, and of the significant modifications resulting from its advent in the emergency radiology unit, relates to the assessment of possible thoraco-dorsal spine fractures.

Spinal cord injuries annually affect 10,000 patients in the U.S. Motor vehicle accidents and falls account for most of these injuries. Approximately one-third of the patients with spinal cord damage resulting from trauma develop complete paraplegia or quadriplegia (Pathria and Petersilge 1991). The cost of treatment for such acute spinal cord injury patients in the U.S. has been estimated at 2 billion dollars annually (Sarant and Chipman 1982). Given these potentially devastating consequences, especially for an individual in whom a spine injury has been missed, and the potential medical legal consequences for the involved physicians, all trauma patients have to be assessed for possible spine fractures. Ideally, the spine should be cleared within minutes after the trauma patient's admission into the emergency room. In many cases, however, severe trauma patients are frequently uncooperative, obtunded, or unstable, and thus difficult to examine clinically; thus, a rapid yet accurate and thorough imaging assessment of the spine must be performed.

We have demonstrated that MDCT is better than conventional radiography for the identification of thoraco-lumbar spine fractures. It can replace conventional radiographs and be performed alone in severe trauma patients. The MDCT sensitivity is 2.5 times that of conventional radiology in the findings of thoraco-lumbar spine fractures. More precisely, MDCT detects 50% additional thoraco-lumbar spine fractures that are overlooked on plain films. Its sensitivity for unstable fractures is almost 100% (Fig. 28.10; Wintermark et al. 2003). At our institution, severe trauma patients undergo cerebral, cervical, and thoraco-abdomino-pelvic MDCT survey for visceral injury. Dedicated axial, sagittal and coronal reconstructions are obtained on the thoraco-lumbar spine, with adequate windowing, and is evaluated for possible spine fractures. If such a fracture is diagnosed, a localized lateral plain film is obtained on the fractured vertebra, in order to facilitate follow-up. If MDCT shows no thoraco-lumbar spinal fracture, its diagnosis is considered as fully ruled out. No conventional radiographs are obtained in such cases, affording a substantial reduction in the duration of the admission imaging evaluation, trauma patients' manipulation, as well as in the radiation dose of the patients.

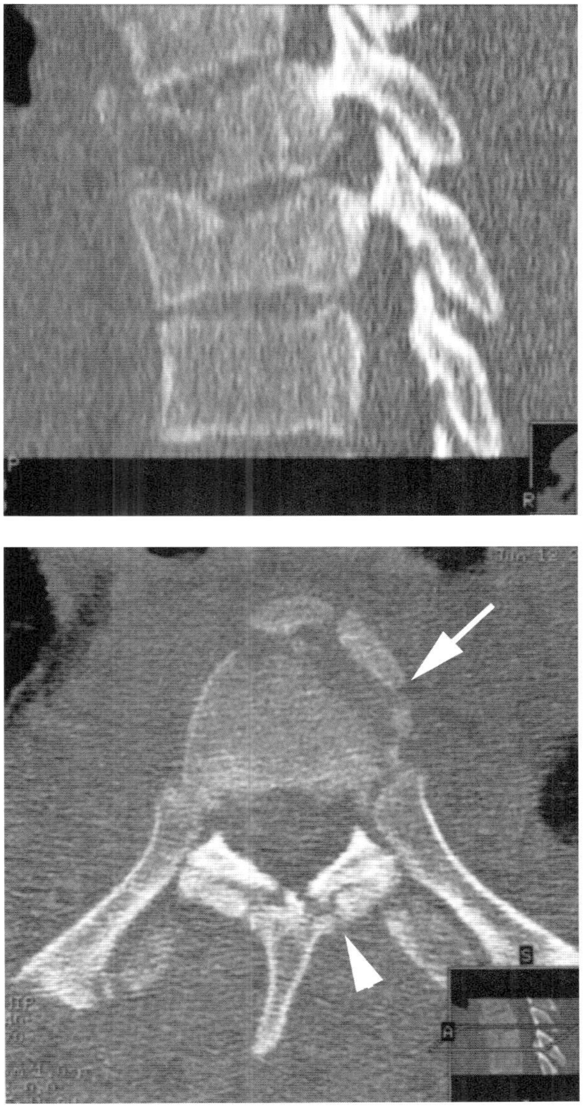

a

b

Fig. 28.10. T3- and T4-vertebral fractures, featured both by **a** sagittal reformat and **b** axial raw image, and demonstrated as unstable since involving both the anterior vertebral wall (*arrow*) and the left lamina of the vertebral arch (*arrowhead*). Those fractures could not be identified on the plain films, notably on the lateral views, due to the superimposition of the shoulders

28.9 Conclusion

The MDCT is meant to play a growing role in the management of trauma patients. It indeed represents the major diagnostic tool in the emergency room; its use for a comprehensive assessment of trauma patients and for their categorization according to the severity of traumatic injuries will inexorably grow. This challenges the emergency radiologist, who will go foreground in the management of trauma patients, all the more so since development of interventional radiology will afford alternative therapeutic procedures to surgery. Trauma radiology, and emergency radiology on the whole, will assert themselves as a consistent and thorough area of specialization.

References

Ben-Menachem Y (1993) Rupture of the thoracic aorta by broadside impacts in road traffic and other collisions: further angiographic observations and preliminary autopsy findings. J Trauma 35:363–367

Cleverley JR, Barrie JR, Ramond GS, Primack SL, Mayo JR (2002) Direct findings of aortic injury on contrast-enhanced CT in surgically proven traumatic aortic injury: a multi-centre review. Clin Radiol 57:281–286

Cohen AM, Crass JR, Thomas HA et al. (1992) CT evidence for the "osseous pinch" mechanism of traumatic aortic injury. AJR 159:271–274

Collins J (2000) Chest wall trauma. J Thorac Imaging 15: 112–119

Creasy JD, Chiles C, Routh WD, Dyer RB (1997) Overview of traumatic injury of the thoracic aorta. Radiographics 17: 27–45

Crim JR, Moore K, Brodke D (2001) Clearance of the cervical spine in multitrauma patients: the role of advanced imaging. Semin Ultrasound CT MRI 22:283–305

Dalldorf PG, McCarthy MC, Tarver RD et al. (1990) Traumatic rupture of the aorta. Indications for aortography. Am Surg 56:500–503

Eckert WG (1977) Crash injuries on the road. In: Tedeschi CG, Eckert WG, Tedeschi LG (eds) Forensic medicine. A study in trauma and environmental hazards, part 2. Saunders, Philadelphia, pp 853–862

Feczko JD, Lynch L, Pless JE et al (1992) An autopsy case review of 142 nonpenetrating (blunt) injuries of the aorta. J Trauma 33:846–849

Fishman JE (2000) Imaging of blunt aortic and great vessel trauma. J Thorac Imaging 15:97–103

Foord KD (1999) PACS workstation respecification: display, data flow, system integration, and environmental issues, derived from analysis of the Conquest Hospital pre-DICOM PACS experience. Eur Radiol 9:1161–1169

Frick EJ, Cipolle MD, Pasquale MD et al. (1997) Outcome of blunt thoracic aortic injury in a level I trauma center: an 8-year review. J Trauma 43:844–851

Garcia-Fernandez MA, Lopez-Perez JM, Perez-Castellano N et al. (1998) Role of transesophageal echocardiography in the assessment of patients with blunt chest trauma: correlation of echocardiographic findings with the electrocardiogram and creatine kinase monoclonal antibody measurements. Am Heart J 135:476–481

Guerrero-Lopez F, Vazquez-Mata G, Alcazar-Romero PP et al. (2000) Evaluation of the utility of computed tomography in the initial assessment of the critical care patient with chest trauma. Crit Care Med 28:1370–1375

Haydel MJ, Preston CA, Mills TJ, Luber S, Blaudeau E, DeBlieux PMC (2000) Indications for computed tomography in patients with minor head injury. N Engl J Med 343:100–105

Heystraten FM, Rosenbusch G, Kingma LM et al. (1986) Chronic posttraumatic aneurysm of the thoracic aorta: surgically correctable occult threat. AJR 146:303–308

Hunink MG, Bos JJ (1995) Triage of patients to angiography for detection of aortic rupture after blunt chest trauma: cost-effectiveness analysis of using CT. AJR 165:27–36

Junck KL, Berland LL, Bernreuter WK, McEachern M, Grandhi S, Lewey G (1998) PACS and CR implementation in a level I trauma center emergency department. J Digit Imaging 11 (Suppl 1):159–162

Karaaslan T, Meuli R, Androux R et al. (1995) Traumatic chest lesions in patients with severe head trauma: a comparative study with computed tomography and conventional chest roentgenograms. J Trauma 39:1081–1086

Katyal D, McLellan BA, Brenneman FD et al. (1997) Lateral impact motor vehicle collisions: significant cause of blunt traumatic rupture of the thoracic aorta. J Trauma 42: 769–772

Kundel HL, Polansky M, Dalinka MK et al. (2001) Reliability of soft-copy versus hard-copy interpretation of emergency department radiographs: a prototype study. AJR 177: 525–528

Lacqua MJ, Sahdev P (1994) Widened mediastinum in acute trauma: a complication of central venous catheterization. J Emerg Med 12:607–609

Leidner B, Adiels M, Aspelin P et al (1998) Standardized CT examination of the multitraumatized patient. Eur Radiol 8:1630–1638

Linsenmaier U, Krotz M, Hauser H et al. (2002) Whole-body computed tomography in polytrauma: techniques and management. Eur Radiol 12:1728–1740

Loo GT, Siegel JH, Dischinger PC et al. (1996) Airbag protection versus compartment intrusion effect determines the pattern of injuries in multiple trauma motor vehicle crashes. J Trauma 41:935–951

Mirvis SE (1997) Major vascular injury in trauma: influence of new technology. State of the art symposium: the acute trauma victim. Eur Radiol (Suppl 7):278

Mirvis SE, Shanmuganathan K (1995) Trauma radiology, part V. Imaging of acute cervical spine trauma. J Intensive Care Med 10:15–33

Nieman K, Rensing BJ, van Geuns RJ et al. (2002) Usefulness of multislice computed tomography for detecting obstructive coronary artery disease. Am J Cardiol 89:913–918

Nourjah P (1999) National hospital ambulatory medical care survey: 1997 emergency department summary. Advance Data from Vital and Health Statistics, National Center for Health Statistics, Hyattsville, Maryland 304; available from URL: http://www.cdc.gov/nchswww/nchshome.htm

Patel NH, Stephens KE Jr, Mirvis SE, Shanmuganathan K, Mann FA (1998) Imaging of acute thoracic aortic injury due to blunt trauma: a review. Radiology 209:335–348

Pathria MN, Petersilge CA (1991) Spinal trauma. Radiol Clin North Am 29:847–865

Peng R, Chang C, Gilmore D et al. (1998) Epidemiology of immediate and early trauma deaths at an urban Level I trauma center. Am Surg 64:950–954

Redfern RO, Horii SC, Feingold E, Kundel HL (2000) Radiology workflow and patient volume: effect of picture archiving and communication systems on technologists and radiologists. J Digit Imaging 13:97–100

Reiser M, Takahashi M, Modic M, Bruening R (2001) Multislice CT. Medical radiology. Springer, Berlin Heidelberg New York

Rizoli SB, Brenneman FD, Boulanger BR et al. (1994) Blunt diaphragmatic and thoracic aortic rupture: an emerging injury complex. Ann Thorac Surg 58:1404–1408

Rose JS, Levitt MA, Porter J et al. (2001) Does the presence of ultrasound really affect computed tomographic scan use? A prospective randomized trial of ultrasound in trauma. J Trauma 5:545–550

Sarant G, Chipman C (1982) Early management of cervical spine injuries. Postgrad Med J 71:164–176

Schnyder P, Wintermark M (2000) Radiology of blunt trauma of the chest. Medical radiology. Springer, Berlin Heidelberg New York

Shanmuganathan K, Mirvis SE (1999) Imaging diagnosis of nonaortic thoracic injury. Radiol Clin North Am 37: 533–551

Siegel JH, Mason-Gonzalez S, Dischinger P et al. (1993) Safety belt restraints and compartment intrusions in frontal and lateral motor vehicle crashes: mechanisms of injuries, complications, and acute care costs. J Trauma 34:736–759

Stengel D, Bauwens K, Schouli J et al. (2001) Systematic review and meta-analysis of emergency ultrasonography for blunt abdominal trauma. Br J Surg 88:901–912

Symbas PJ, Horsley WS, Symbas PN (1998) Rupture of the ascending aorta caused by blunt trauma. Ann Thorac Surg 66:113–117

Trupka A, Waydhas C, Hallfeldt KK et al. (1997) Value of thoracic computed tomography in the first assessment of severely injured patients with blunt chest trauma: results of a prospective study. J Trauma 43:405–412

Van Hise ML, Primack SL, Israel RS et al. (1998) CT in blunt chest trauma: indications and limitations. Radiographics 18:1071–1084

Verdun FR, Denys A, Pachoud M, Valley J-F, Schnyder P, Meuli R Detection of low-contrast lesions: an experimental comparison of single and multi-slice CT. Radiology (in press)

Vignon P, Rambaud G, Francois B et al. (1998) Quantification of traumatic hemomediastinum using transesophageal echocardiography: impact on patient management. Chest 113:1475–1480

Voggenreiter G, Aufmkolk M, Majetschak et al. (2000) Efficiency of chest computed tomography in critically ill patients with multiple traumas. Crit Care Med 28:1033–1039

Wicky S, Wintermark M, Denys A, Capasso P, Schnyder P (2000) Radiology of blunt chest trauma. Eur Radiol 10: 1524–1538

Williams JS, Graff JA, Uku JM et al. (1994) Aortic injury in vehicular trauma. Ann Thorac Surg 57:726–730

Wintermark M, Schnyder P (2001) Trauma of the chest. In: Taveras J, Ferrucci J (eds) Radiology: diagnosis, imaging, intervention. Lippincott, Williams and Wilkins, Philadelphia

Wintermark M, Wicky S, Schnyder P (2002) Imaging of acute traumatic injuries of the thoracic aorta. Eur Radiol 12: 432–442

Wintermark M, Mouhsine E, Theumann N et al. (2003) Multidetector-row CT for the depiction of thoraco-lumbar spine fractures in severe trauma patients. Radiology 227:681–689

Zinck SE, Primack SL (2000) Radiographic and CT findings in blunt chest trauma. J Thorac Imaging 15:87–96

29 CT-Guided Thoracic Interventions

R. Drosten, E. vanSonnenberg, S. Shankar

CONTENTS

R. Drosten, MD
Thoracic and Onco-Radiologist, Dana-Farber Cancer Institute, Brigham and Women's Hospital, and Harvard Medical School, 44 Binney Street, Boston, MA 02115-6084, USA
E. vanSonnenberg, MD
Chief of Radiology, Dana-Farber Cancer Institute, Visiting Professor of Radiology, Harvard Medical School, Interventional Radiologist, Brigham and Women's Hospital, Consulting Interventional Radiologist, Children's Hospital, 44 Binney Street, Boston, Massachusetts, 02115-6084, USA
S. Shankar, MD
Interventional and Onco-Radiologist, Brigham and Women's Hospital and Dana-Farber Cancer Institute, Instructor of Radiology, Harvard Medical School, 44 Binney Street, Boston, MA 02115-6084, USA

29.1 Introduction

Continuing improvements in computer hardware and software have reaffirmed computed tomography's (CT) position as an essential tool in the armamentarium of both the diagnostic and interventional radiologist. Major advances in data handling, storage capacity, and reliability of CT operating systems, coupled with the advent of multi-detector-row scanners contribute to a marked improvement in image quality and a decrease in scan times. Initially 4-channel, and now 16-channel, multi-detector-row CT scanners enable high quality studies to be performed, even on patients whose clinical conditions have made them notoriously difficult to produce high quality images. Improving quality of imaging equipment facilitates earlier diagnosis, better categorization, and improved monitoring of disease processes, allowing for better planning of potential interventions and effective management of complications.

In this chapter, we describe helical CT use in relation to current thoracic Interventional practice, with particular focus on transthoracic needle biopsy, percutaneous drainage, transcatheter infusion, tumor ablation, transbronchial stenting, and intercostal nerve block.

29.2 Interventions of the Lung – Transthoracic Needle Biopsy

Transthoracic needle biopsy (TNB) and the drainage of pleural, pulmonary parenchymal, and chest wall collections are the most commonly performed percutaneous interventional procedures of the thorax. CT and CT-fluoroscopic guided biopsy of pulmonary parenchymal, mediastinal, pleural, and pleural-based lesions are the gold standard imaging modality for these procedures. Pugatch et al. (1978) describe the utility of CT in differentiating between pleural and parenchymal lesions, and concludes that thoracic CT provided information not otherwise available in one third of the patients with complex combined pleural and parenchymal disease.

Indications for TNB

1. Pulmonary nodule
2. Mediastinal mass
3. Pleural or chest wall mass
4. Diffuse pleural thickening
5. Parenchymal process not responding to therapy
6. Parenchymal opacities in an immunocompromised host

Relative Contraindications for TNB

1. Lack of patient cooperation, e.g. intractable cough, inability to remain motionless, altered consciousness.
2. Bleeding diathesis; INR >1.3 or platelet count of <50000 per mm^3
3. Contralateral pneumonectomy
4. Mechanical ventilation
5. Hypervascular lesion, aneurysm
6. Severe COPD, FEV1<1 liter

29.2.1 Establishing a Diagnosis

Expectorated or bronchoscopically obtained sputum samples remain the initial diagnostic procedures of choice in acquiring a cellular sample in the presence of a central (endotracheal, endobronchial, peribronchial, and perihilar) lesion. More than 25% of cancers can be detected by the less invasive techniques of sputum collection and bronchoscopy. The techniques of conventional respiratory cytology and fine needle aspiration (FNA) biopsy cytology are complementary in the diagnosis of lung cancer (Johnston 1988).

TNB is an accurate tool for the diagnosis of intrathoracic malignancy, with a sensitivity of between 70 and 100% (Westcott 1980; Khouri et al. 1985; Stanley et al. 1987). TNB is the diagnostic procedure of choice in the assessment of peripheral lesions lacking an intimate relation to central bronchi (Gasparini et al. 1995; Chon et al. 1999). Richardson et al. (2002) analyzed current British transthoracic needle biopsy practice, providing data on 5444 biopsies and found that an average of 31 biopsies were performed per center per year. Procedures were performed on an outpatient basis in 71%. Complications included pneumothorax (20.5%), pneumothorax requiring chest drain (3.1%), hemoptysis (5.3%), and death (0.15%).

29.2.2 Biopsy Methods

Transthoracic needle biopsy (TNB) encompasses fine needle aspiration (FNA), coaxial fine needle biopsy, and core biopsy.

29.2.2.1 Fine Needle Biopsy

Fine needle biopsy (FNA) refers to biopsy performed with a needle diameter of less than or equal to 20-gauge. 22-gauge needles are commonly used. Evidence suggests that even finer caliber needles (25-gauge) may offer advantages in lesions surrounded by emphysematous parenchyma (vanSonnenberg et al. 2003), or in patients with bleeding dyscrasias. Lesion diameter is a critical factor in increasing the diagnostic accuracy. CT-guided needle biopsy is a feasible, useful, and safe technique for the histological diagnosis of small lung lesions, especially those larger than 8 mm in diameter (Yoshimura et al. 2002).

Advantages of single needle technique include ease of use, smaller pleural punctures, and the ability to sample various sites of the same lesion, or sample multiple lesions, with multiple individually targeted needle passes (Fig. 29.1).

Tandem technique entails the placement of a needle into the region of the target lesion (Fig. 29.2). Subsequent needle placements use the guiding needle to more efficiently and accurately access the target. This technique is more commonly utilized in the biopsy of parenchymal lesions that abut the pleura, pleural, or chest wall lesions. It is also facilitates fluoroscopy-guided procedures.

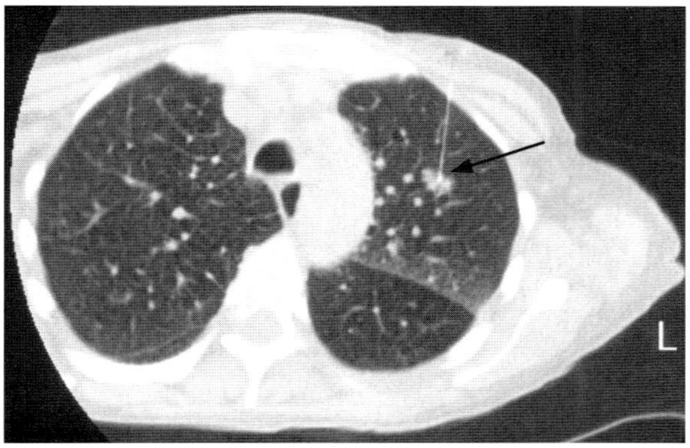

Fig. 29.1. CT guided 22-gauge fine needle biopsy of a primary non-small cell carcinoma of the left upper lobe

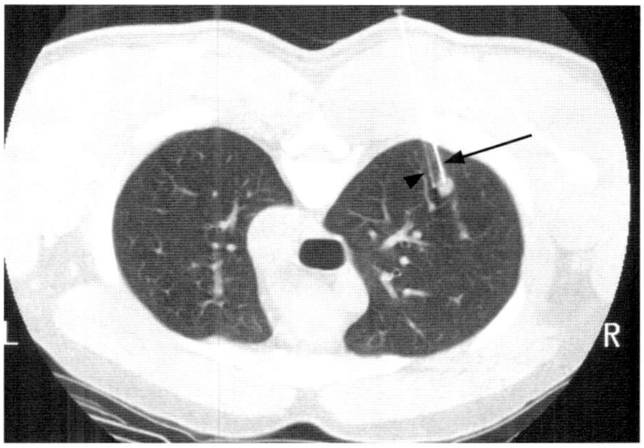

Fig. 29.2. CT-guided tandem technique. The initial needle is positioned adjacent to the target lesion. Subsequent needle placements use the guiding needle to accurately access the target lesion (*arrow*)

29.2.2.2
Coaxial (Transaxial) Biopsy

Coaxial (transaxial) biopsy involves the placement of a guiding needle tip adjacent to, or within, the target lesion, then passing a thinner biopsy needle through the wider guiding cannula into the substance of the target lesion (vanSonnenberg et al. 1983, 1984a). A 19-gauge outer cannula is commonly used, through which a 22-gauge FNA needle with a longer length shaft is passed. A 22-guage fine needle with a removable hub may be used as the initial needle, over which the outer 19-guage needle is placed.

Extrapleural coaxial technique entails the placement of an outer guiding cannula with its tip in the extrapleural soft tissues (Fig. 29.3). A fine needle is passed through the outer guiding cannula. If the target is an intraparenchymal lesion, only the inner fine needle will pass through the pleura, and thus a cytologic sample may be obtained.

Intraparenchymal coaxial technique entails the placement of an outer guiding cannula tip in the substance of the target lesion. A fine needle is passed through the outer guiding cannula. If the target is an intraparenchymal lesion, both the outer guiding cannula and inner fine needle will pass through the pleura. A cytologic sample is thus obtained. Once the inner fine needle has been removed, the larger caliber outer cannula can be used to acquire a larger histologic sample.

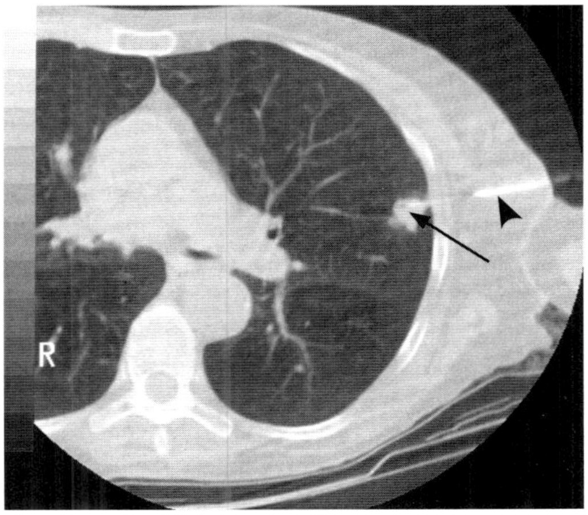

Fig. 29.3. Extrapleural coaxial technique. The outer guiding needle tip is in the extrapleural tissues (*arrowhead*), and only the inner fine needle perforates the pleura (*arrow*)

Advantages of Coaxial Systems Include

- The pleura will be traversed only once, with the outer cannula remaining in situ for subsequent FNA biopsies
- The outer cannula is less flexible, and is thus less likely to deviate from its course during placement, than a fine needle alone
- The outer cannula can be used to stabilize a lesion during biopsy
- The outer cannula can be used to acquire a histologic tissue sample as the final biopsy, before complete withdrawal of all needles

Disadvantages of Coaxial Systems Include

- The larger diameter outer cannula has an associated greater likelihood of pneumothorax

- "Dwell-time" (time that the cannula is left in situ) is longer, and therefore the likelihood of pneumothorax is greater
- Multiple FNA procedures must be performed sequentially, and both the outer cannula and the inner FNA needle may have to be removed, especially during the biopsy of deep pulmonary parenchymal lesions, while the cytopathologist assesses the samples obtained

For these reasons, coaxial systems are more commonly used in the biopsy of pulmonary parenchymal lesions abutting the pleura, pleural, and extra-pleural thoracic wall lesions.

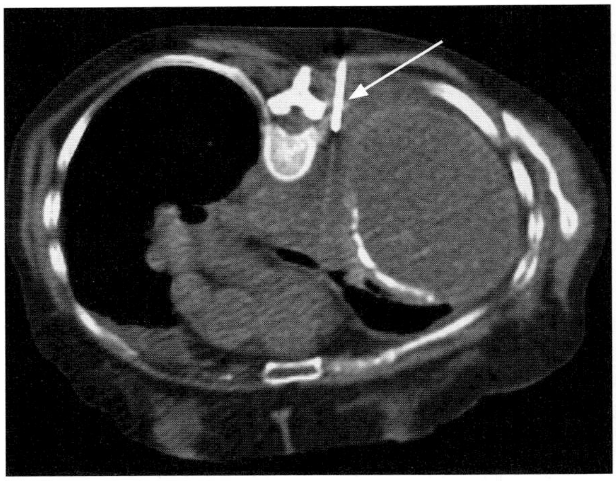

Fig. 29.4. CT-guided core biopsy of left pleural thickening (*arrow*). Diagnosis of B-cell lymphoma was made

29.2.2.3 Core Biopsy

Core biopsy with a cutting needle will best provide specimens suitable for histologic assessment in the setting of a non diagnostic FNA assessment made by an onsite cytologist (Haramati 1995). Core biopsy needles have a common mechanism whereby the biopsy system is positioned within the substance of a target lesion. A thinner needle with a tissue retaining recess is positioned within the lumen of the outer cannula and a manual or automatic triggering mechanism is activated. The outer cannula slides over the thinner inner needle guillotining a histologic specimen that is retained within the recess, and is protected by the outer cannula. Thus, the tissue sample is secured during withdrawal of the core biopsy needle. Fig. 29.4 demonstrates CT-guided core biopsy of left pleural thickening, resulting in a diagnosis of B-cell lymphoma.

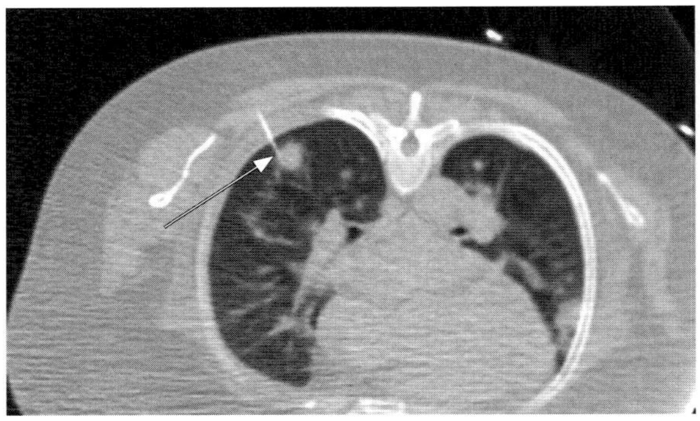

Fig. 29.5. CT-guided FNA of right upper lobe opacity (*arrow*). Note patient is prone. The biopsy diagnosis of organizing pneumonia was confirmed after VATS excision

29.2.2.4 Fine Needle vs. Core Biopsy

Benign Disease

By definition, a biopsy diagnostic for benign disease is one in which malignancy is excluded and a confident identification of a benign process is made (Fig. 29.5). Several large series report a yield of between 88–97% to exclude malignancy; however, the yield for specific benign diagnoses is only in the 16–68% (Westcott 1980; Khouri et al. 1985; Stanley et al. 1987) range.

Improving the likelihood of an accurate diagnosis of benign disease (Fig. 29.6) requires a combination of repeated sampling of multiple sites of focal lesions, including the use of cutting needles when necessary

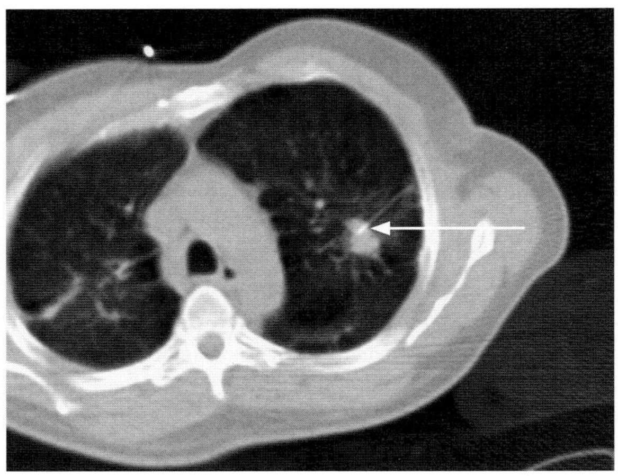

Fig. 29.6. Cytopathologic assessment of a CT-guided FNA of a speculated mass produced a diagnosis of benign chronic inflammation (*arrow*). The diagnosis was confirmed after the lesion was excised by video assisted thoracoscopic surgery (VATS), and was shown to contain hyaline, fibrosis and Aspergillus spores, in this patient with esophageal cancer

to obtain a representative sample, and expert cytopathology.

GRIEF et al. (1999) retrospectively studied the relative efficacy of CT-guided percutaneous core needle biopsy (PCNB) vs. fine needle aspiration (FNA) in the diagnosis of benign lung lesions. Both FNA and PCNB biopsies were carried out sequentially, at the same visit, in every patient. A specific benign diagnosis was made in 17% of cases by FNA and in 81% by PCNB. PCNB findings resulted in significant modification of the diagnosis established by FNA. The only significant complication encountered was pneumothorax (12%).

They concluded that radiologically guided PCNB is a safe procedure that can provide sufficient histologic material for a specific diagnosis of peripheral lung disease and may avoid more-invasive surgical procedures and that the histologic analysis provided by PCNB can increase diagnostic accuracy in benign pulmonary diseases compared with FNA (GRIEF et al. 1999) (Table 29.1).

WONG et al. (2002) assessed CT-guided transthoracic FNA in patients with hematologic malignancy, both before and after bone marrow transplant. FNA diagnosis provided a clinically useful diagnosis in 72% (51 of 71). The yield for lung cancer was 90% (9 of 10), for pulmonary lymphoma was 68% (21 of 31), and for infection was 67% (10 of 15). They concluded that transthoracic needle aspiration (TNA) of focal lung lesions has an excellent yield for detecting cancer and results were comparable to bronchoscopy to diagnose infections in patients with hematologic malignancy. The diagnosis of rheumatoid nodules (FILHO et al. 2002) and thoracic splenosis (SYED and ZAHAROPOULOS 2001) by CT-guided FNA of subpleural lung lesions has also been reported.

Malignant Disease

As PCNB offers no significant advantage over FNA in the evaluation of peripheral malignant lung lesions, FNA biopsy is recommended as the initial diagnostic procedure of choice in all cases of suspected malignancy (GREIF et al. 1998) (Fig. 29.7). Pneumothorax is the most significant complication (24%). The use of the percutaneous core needle biopsy technique is recommended when the diagnosis of malignancy by FNA is uncertain, or when a more specific characterization of the lesion is required.

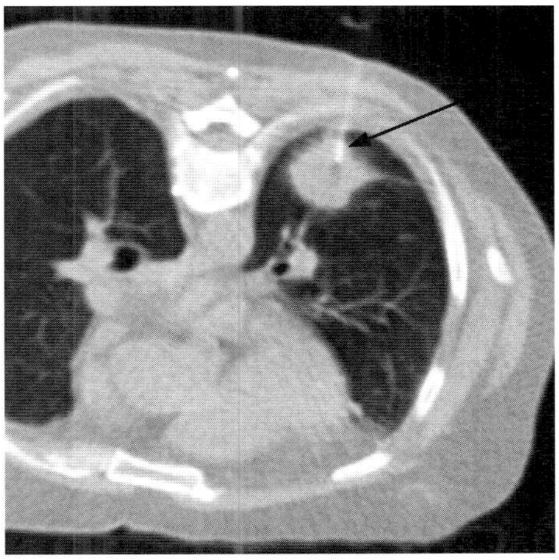

Fig. 29.7. CT-guided FNA of peripheral pulmonary mass (*arrow*). Diagnosis of non-small cell lung cancer was made

Comparison of CT-guided FNA biopsy of benign and malignant lesions (Table 29.2) demonstrates excellent results in the assessment of malignancy, but lower diagnostic yield in benign disease. These findings confirm the requirement of additional core biopsy sampling if a benign etiology is a diagnostic consideration, or if the initial FNA samples reviewed by the onsite cytologist are non-specific or non-diagnostic.

Table 29.2. Yield of FNA in malignancy vs. specific benign diagnosis

	Malignancy	Specific Benign Diagnosis
WESCOTT (1988)	385/400 (97%)	–
KHOURI et al. (1985)	460/486 (95%)	93/137 (68%)
STANLEY et al. (1987)	312/323 (97%)	54/113 (48%)

Table 29.1. Core biopsy for benign disease

Author	Needle gauge	Patient number	Sensitivity	Specificity
HARAMATI et al. (2001)	18G ASAP	15	80%	80%
NOPPEN et al. (1995)	20G Temno	9	100%	100%
KLEIN and ZARKA (1997)	20G ASAP	35	100%	100%*
ARAKAWA et al. (1996)	18G Biopsy	21	71%	52%
BOISELLE et al. (1997)	20G Quickcore	16	100%	69%*
LUCIDARME et al. (1998)	18 g ASAP	14	100%	71%

*Significant difference compared to FNA

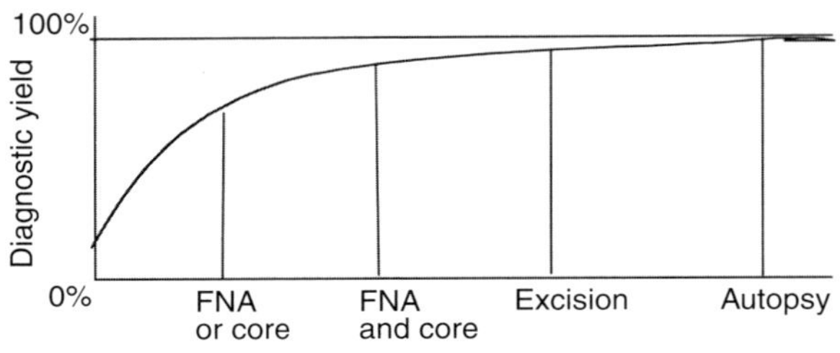

Graph 29.1. Relative yield of procedures in the diagnosis of both benign and malignant lesions to the thorax

The relative yield of procedures performed in the diagnosis of both benign and malignant lesions to the thorax is depicted in Graph 29.1. FNA with core biopsy provides a greater diagnostic yield than FNA alone. Excision biopsy obtained either by open surgery or by video assisted thoracoscopic surgery (VATS) has an insignificant benefit over FNA combined with core biopsy in the assessment of malignant disease, but it offers a greater yield in the assessment of benign pathology. Surgery is rarely indicated to diagnose benign pathology. Benign diagnoses often are made after a surgical procedure is performed when a malignant lesion is suspected. The treatment of benign lesions, particularly in indolent processes in immunocompromised hosts, by surgical excision is performed.

Layfield et al. (1996) assessed the effect of lesion size and location on CT-guided biopsy yield. Biopsy of peripheral lung lesions with diameters greater than 2 cm had a sensitivity of 93% and specificity of 100%. Sensitivity decreased to 60% and specificity dropped to 82% in the biopsy of lesions smaller than 1 cm, situated centrally in the lung bases.

Smolle-Juettner et al. (1996) addressed the clinical significance of CT-guided percutaneous fine-needle aspiration (FNA) cytology in patients with intrathoracic lesions. A significantly higher rate of correct FNA diagnoses was made in malignant lesions. The overall diagnostic accuracy of FNA was 77%, sensitivity 79% and specificity 91%. From a surgical point of view, reliance on the FNA diagnoses alone would have caused nine resectable lung cancers, three metastases, three other malignancies, and three tuberculomas to be missed. 18 pneumothoraces (9 requiring catheter drainage) occurred after FNA of 101 lesions. The authors concluded that the indication for FNA in otherwise resectable patients should be made carefully, keeping in mind the rate of diagnostic errors and of complications.

Core biopsy acquired specimens with a reported diagnostic cytological yield ranging between 60 and 75% (Herman et al. 1991) have had a significant impact on the non-surgical diagnosis of lymphoma. Specimens obtained by cutting needle biopsy provide diagnostic sample in patients with suspected lymphoma of the lung, mediastinum, and thoracic wall, in 83–95% of cases (Ben-Yehuda et al. 1996; Pappa et al. 1996).

Percutaneous needle biopsy is an excellent technique with a high accuracy rate in acquiring cellular material in order to assess bony metastases to the thorax (Treaba et al. 2002) (Fig. 29.8). The coaxial technique is effective in acquiring a cytologic sample in a bone eroded by metastasis. Bone trephine needles may be required to traverse an intact cortex in bones that are less prominently eroded.

The assessment of adrenal lesions is briefly discussed, as non-small cell lung neoplasm metastases have a predilection for the adrenal glands (Pagani 1984). The imaging appearance of an adrenal lesion is often characteristic and further imaging may not be necessary. Lesions with characteristic imaging appearances include adrenal adenoma, pheochromocytoma, myelolipoma, adrenal cyst, and some large adrenocortical carcinomas. However, small metastases, smaller primary adrenal carcinomas, lymphoma, granulomatous disease, and many adenomas may have indeterminate features and, depending on the clinical situation, follow-up imaging, or core biopsy may be necessary. Associated risks include infection and hemorrhage.

Gilliams et al. (1992) assessed the value of CT scanning and CT-guided percutaneous fine needle aspiration of adrenal masses in patients with biopsy-proven lung cancer. The preoperative CT scans of 546 preoperative biopsy-proven primary bronchial carci-

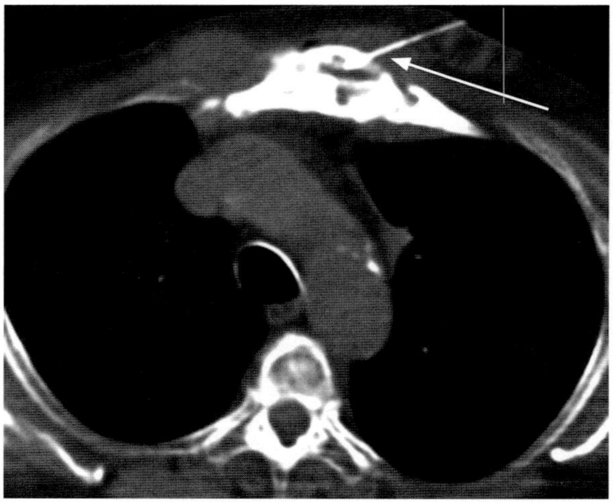

Fig. 29.8. CT-guided coaxial FNA of a breast cancer metastasis to the sternum (*arrow*)

nomas were reviewed. Twenty-two patients had solid adrenal tumors. Sixteen underwent percutaneous fine needle aspiration (FNA) and the CT appearance of these lesions was assessed. Well-defined, low attenuation lesions, that only involved part of the gland, were likely to be benign. Of these, four lesions were less than or equal to 2 cm in diameter. Low attenuation lesions with peripheral inhomogeneity were likely to be malignant. All measured more than 2 cm in diameter. They concluded that the CT appearances of most adrenal lesions were insufficiently distinctive to exclude malignancy, and that CT-guided biopsy was necessary to establish a diagnosis, in the right setting.

Singer et al. (1994) found that attenuation values (<10 Hounsfield units) and size (<2.5 cm) were the only useful criteria for differentiating adenomas from metastases on unenhanced CT scans. Lesions exceeding specific thresholds may still be benign and may require biopsy. Metastatic lesions may remain stable for up to 18 months and they advocate documenting lesion stability for a longer period of time.

Non-enhanced CT, contrast-enhanced CT, and chemical shift MRI are commonly utilized imaging modalities to differentiate between benign and malignant adrenal lesions (Lockhart et al. 2002). Adrenal adenomas are well-defined homogeneous low-density (due to the microscopic fat) lesions on non-enhanced CT. When low density criteria are not met, many may be characterized as adenomas by contrast wash out on CT, or a signal decrease using in-phase and out-of-phase MRI sequences. Other non-invasive modalities may incidentally discover adrenal lesions, but are not typically used in the work-up. NP-59 is an uncommonly used nuclear medicine technique that is very specific for adenoma when correlated with findings on other imaging studies.

29.2.3 Imaging Modalities and Transthoracic Needle Biopsy

29.2.3.1 CT vs. Fluoroscopy and Ultrasound

CT-Guided Transthoracic Needle Biopsy

CT is the guidance imaging modality of choice for transthoracic biopsy of pulmonary parenchymal lesions, mediastinal lesions, and lymph nodes.

The use of CT-guidance considerably expands the scope of thoracic lesions amenable to percutaneous biopsy (vanSonnenberg et al. 1988). There is an associated higher incidence of pneumothorax associated with the biopsy of difficult thoracic lesions.

Advantages of CT-Guided TNB over Ultrasound and Fluoroscopy

1. Better spatial resolution and image quality
2. Improved visualization of fissures, blood vessels, and bullae
3. More accurate assessment and planning of the access route
4. Ultrasound cannot image nodules surrounded by aerated lung
5. Even biplanar fluoroscopy units cannot match the image quality and spatial resolution of a CT image – most noticeable in the imaging of nodules with diameters of <2 cm
6. CT is better at imaging small nodules that may be invisible even on biplane fluoroscopy

Disadvantages of CT-Guided TNB vs. Ultrasound and Fluoroscopy

1. Lack of real-time visualization using sequential CT imaging. Ultrasound and fluoroscopy allow real-time visualization
2. Potential increase in procedure duration, as the needle may need to be repeatedly repositioned, and the area of interest rescanned
3. Associated potential for increases patient discomfort with increasing procedure duration
4. Increased radiation dose to the patient
5. A potentially higher incidence of pneumothorax and other complications
6. Greater expense compared with fluoroscopic or ultrasound guided biopsy.
7. The needle tract must be within the CT scanner imaging plane. As computer processing power and software continues to improve, the ability to scroll through real-time MIP stacks may obviate this limitation

Ultrasound-Guided TNB

Lesions in the lung apex, that abut the chest wall or the pleura, or that involve the anterior or posterior mediastinum, can be effectively accessed using ultrasound as the guidance modality (Doust et al. 1975; Sagar et al. 2000; Simeone et al. 1984). Ultrasound cannot image nodules surrounded by aerated lung, bulla, or pneumothorax. A post procedure chest radiograph should be routinely obtained to assess for pneumothorax and other clinically significant complications.

Fluoroscopy-Guided TNB

Transthoracic needle biopsy was first described using fluoroscopy for imaging (Nodenstrom 1967). Biplanar or C-arm fluoroscopy can still be used as the guiding imaging modality (Fig. 29.9a, b). A pre-procedure CT scan enables assessment for interval change, and aids planning of the fluoroscopic biopsy. Obtaining a pre-procedure CT is of particular benefit in the presence of bullous disease, when small central lesions abut major vessels, or when hypervascular metastases are a differential diagnosis. Lesions seen on only one plane by radiography or fluoroscopy can be localized using CT.

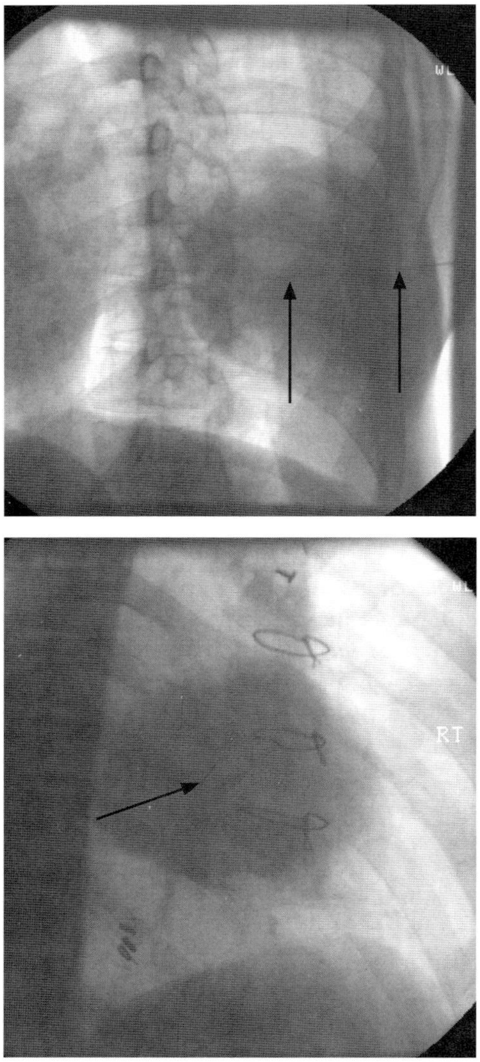

a

b

Fig. 29.9a, b. Fluoroscopy-guided FNA of non-small cell lung cancer (*arrows*)

Advantages of Ultrasound and Fluoroscopy over CT-Guided Biopsy

1. Ultrasound has multiplanar capability.
2. Depending on imaging duration, CT may expose the patient to a larger dose of ionizing radiation than fluoroscopy. Ultrasound produces no ionizing radiation.
3. Ultrasound and fluoroscopy are usually less expensive than CT.
4. Ultrasound is a portable imaging modality and procedures can be performed at the bedside or as an office biopsy. CT and fluoroscopy have an inherent lack of portability.

29.2.3.2 CT and CT-Fluoroscopy

New advances in multi-detector CT technology, faster data processing times, improved image quality and the advent of the 16-channel CT scanners and CT-fluoroscopy, facilitates efficient initial patient assessment, visualization during CT-guided biopsy, and the assessment and management of post procedure complications (Fig. 29.10a, b).

Multi-detector spiral CT scanners that are capable of generating hundreds of images in a single breath-hold place considerable strain on daily clinical practice. Workstations will soon have the capability to produce seamless real-time transition between axial, coronal, and sagittal images, produce instantaneous sliding maximum intensity projection and volumetrically rendered images, allow instantaneous transition between thick and thin sections. Nearly instantaneous co-registration between studies of different dates, allow identification and comparison of lesions.

Advantages of CT-Fluoroscopic-Guided Transthoracic Biopsy

1. Real-time visualization of the target lesion and the biopsy needle.
2. Allows the radiologist to assess patient compliance prior to needle insertion.
3. Fewer needle passes and fewer pleural perforations may be required.
4. Allows for decreased procedure times and resultant better patient tolerance of the procedure.
5. A needle tract that is not in the plane of imaging can be assessed efficiently without the time delay associated with non-fluoroscopic CT-guided biopsy.

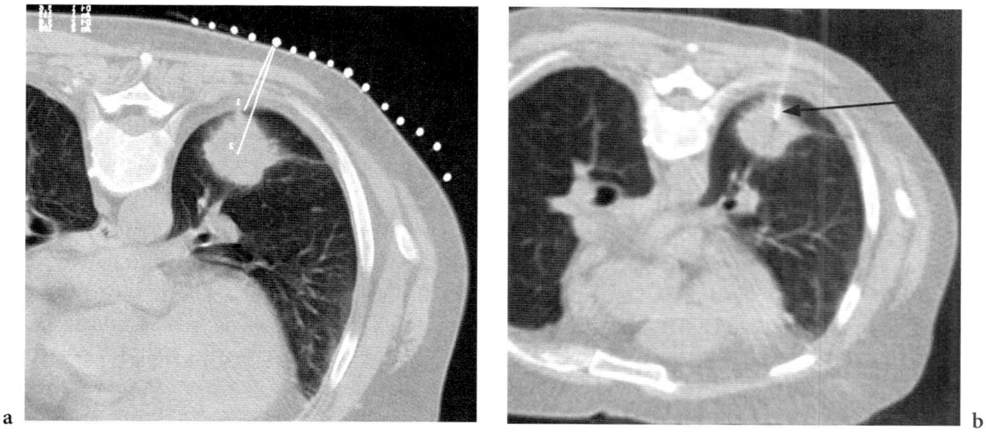

Fig. 29.10. CT-fluoroscopic guided biopsy of a lung lesion. a – CT planning. b – CT-fluoroscopic guided biopsy of non-small cell lung cancer (*arrow*)

Disadvantages of CT-Fluoroscopic-Guided TNB

Disadvantages of CT-fluoroscopic guided TNB include the use of ionizing radiation and a higher procedure cost than ultrasound. While patient-related radiation exposure is similar, operator-related radiation exposure remains a distinct disadvantage associated with CT-fluoroscopy (Froelich et al. 2002).

29.2.3.3 Positron Emission Tomography (FDG-PET) and CT-PET Imaging

FDG-PET has already established itself as an effective modality in the evaluation of pulmonary nodules with a reported sensitivity as high as 96%, and a specificity and accuracy ranging from 88% to 94% (Albes et al. 2002; Coleman 2001; Haberkorn and Schoenberg 2001; Keith et al. 2002; Salminen and MacManus 2001; Wong et al. 2001). 2-[fluorine-18]-fluoro-2-deoxy-D-glucose (FDG) is the most commonly utilized glucose analogue. The ability to provide functional information and to perform whole body imaging is an important benefit of FDG-PET imaging. Nodules, post therapy scars, masses, and mediastinal lesions are increasingly evaluated using PET (Fig. 29.11a, b). Current limitations of PET include a minimum 7 mm nodule diameter imaging sensitivity on high quality well calibrated scanners, a tendency to obtain false negative studies in patients with bronchoalveolar cell carcinoma (Yap et al. 2002), and an incidence of false positives in assessing inflammatory processes. Nonetheless, the applications for FDG-PET imaging continue to increase dramatically.

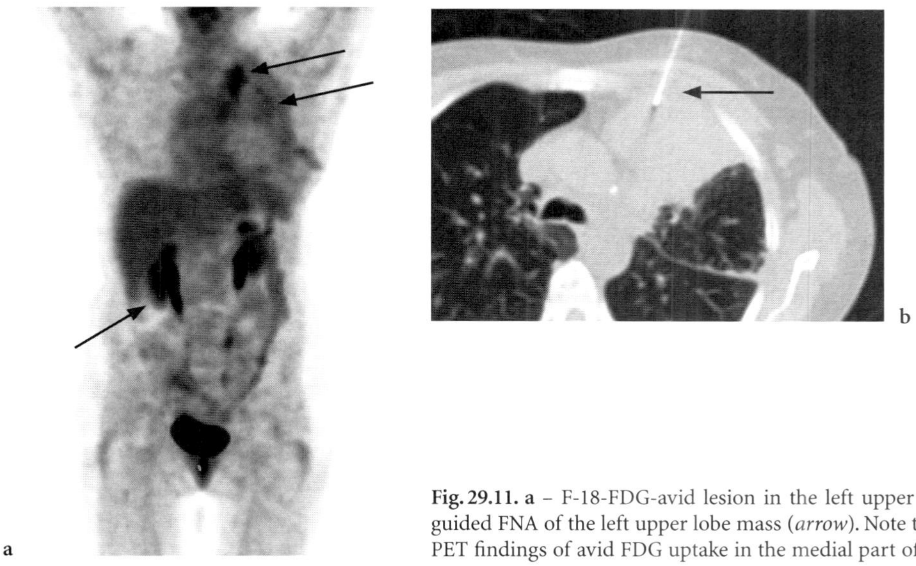

Fig. 29.11. a – F-18-FDG-avid lesion in the left upper lobe on PET (*arrows*). b – CT-guided FNA of the left upper lobe mass (*arrow*). Note that FNA biopsy is guided by the PET findings of avid FDG uptake in the medial part of the large left upper lobe lesion

High hopes exist for the future value of the exciting and rapidly evolving field of CT-PET imaging. Sequentially acquired multi-detector-row CT and PET studies are fused, offering a quantum improvement in both sensitivity and specificity of lesion imaging. CT-PET has been shown to be both cost effective (Gambhir et al. 1996), valuable in thoracic tumor staging (D'Amico et al. 2002; Magnani et al. 1999; Vansteenkiste et al. 1998), and beneficial in radiotherapy treatment planning (Erdi et al. 2002). It is envisioned that CT-PET-guided TNB of thoracic lesions will closely follow on the heels of the initial diagnostic use of CT-PET.

29.2.3.4 *Bronchoscopy-Guided Transthoracic Needle Biopsy*

Bronchoscopy with bushings, washings, endobronchial, or transbronchial biopsy is the diagnostic procedure of choice in the setting of patients with clinical symptoms (hemoptysis), or radiologic findings that indicate central airway involvement (Naidich et al. 1988).

Bronchoscopy is usually limited to the assessment of central, peribronchial, or endobronchial lesions. Chechani (1996) showed that a skilled bronchoscopist can establish the diagnosis in up to 73% of patients with solitary pulmonary nodules. The yield for bronchoscopically diagnosed lesions larger than 3 cm approaches 80% (Chechani 1996), and the yield for lesions smaller than 2 cm is as low as 28% (Radke et al. 1979). Biopsy of apical and basal lesions produces yields that are lower than those of perihilar lesions, and vary significantly with the experience of the bronchoscopist (Chechani 1996).

Kardos et al. (1999) demonstrated a greater diagnostic value of CT-guided core biopsy (86% sensitivity) relative to fluoroscopic-guided biopsy (15%) or bronchoscopic sampling (12.5%) in the assessment of pulmonary nodules.

CT-guided bronchoscopy can increase the diagnostic yield in selected cases of peribronchial lesions that do not have an endobronchial component. Kobayashi et al. (1997) describe CT-guided bronchoscopic placement of barium sulfate suspension in the region of fluoroscopically invisible peripheral pulmonary nodules, facilitating thoracoscopic resection. Transbronchial cyst aspiration may be both diagnostic and therapeutic and the transbronchial biopsy of subcarinal lymph nodes can provide diagnostic material.

29.2.4 Planning the CT-Guided TNB

The majority of transthoracic needle biopsies are performed as outpatient procedures. The patient is provided with information describing the time and venue of the procedure, is advised to discontinue the use of aspirin (vanSonnenberg and Wittich 1998) and/or nonsteroidal anti-inflammatory agents for at least 72 hours, and is required to fast for 10 hours prior to the procedure. Recent blood tests – full blood count (CBC), INR, coagulation profile, platelet count, blood urea, and serum creatinine – are obtained. Any abnormal results should be corrected before the elective biopsy procedure is performed.

On the day of the biopsy, the patient presents two hours prior to the scheduled time of the procedure. The benefits of the procedure, possible alternatives, possible complications and their management are discussed and questions are answered. Informed consent is documented.

The presence of an onsite cytopathologist and immediate cytologic assessment of the biopsy samples obtained ensures that the aspirate material is handled optimally, and that the incidence of unsatisfactory and false negative lung FNA is thus reduced. The cytopathologist requires pertinent clinical information and an indication of the likely radiologic diagnosis. Preparation of the biopsy samples with routine fixatives (alcohol for a smear slide, and formalin for cell block preparation), flow cytometry, aerobic and anaerobic sterile culture media and glutaraldehyde for electron microscopy and assessment is tailored according to the differential diagnosis.

29.2.5 Preparing for the CT-Guided Biopsy

IV access is secured. A blood pressure monitor, electrocardiogram leads, and a pulse oximeter are applied. The biopsy room should be equipped with oxygen, suction, oral and nasal airways, an Ambu-bag, a pleural evacuation device, and a resuscitation (crash) cart. The patient is placed on the CT table in a position that takes patient comfort and ease of access to the target lesion into account. A limited CT is obtained through the region of interest to assess for any interval change, and the access route is planned. Technical considerations include planning a route that will avoid neurovascular bundles (supraclavicular, axillary, inferior to each rib, paraspinal), vital structures, the esophagus, crossing fissures, bronchi, larger intrapulmonary vessels, and bullae, when possible. The skin is prepared using aseptic technique, draped, and subcutaneous and intercostal local anesthesia is administered. The patient's ability to cooperate with breathing instructions, and the range of nodule movement during respiration, is assessed.

29.2.6 Performing the CT-Guided Biopsy

The biopsy needle is inserted using CT-guidance. Effective hand guided biopsy requires experience. This is particularly true in accessing out-of-plane lesions. Stereotactic guidance may decrease radiation exposure, biopsy time, and trauma from multiple needle punctures, however, stereotactic systems are more expensive and their use requires practice (Onik et al. 1988).

The biopsy needle is positioned with its tip just outside the pleural space, in the intercostal soft tissues, above the rib, to avoid the neurovascular bundle. The needle is advanced during suspended respiration – preferably after end expiration – and visualized under repeated sequential CT, or real-time CT-fluoroscopic guidance. Great care is taken to avoid performing side-to-side, or translational, movement of the needle, with its associated increased pneumothorax complication rate. If the initial needle insertion is misdirected, it is preferable to withdraw the needle tip until it is outside the pleural space, in the subcutaneous tissues, and then re-insert the needle under CT-guidance.

The needle tip is advanced into the target lesion, the internal stylet is removed, and a syringe is attached to the needle hub. 5–10 cc of suction are applied, and a series of up and down and rotary maneuvers are performed, carefully avoiding lateral movement. Capillary technique (identical needle movement, but without syringe suction) can be performed during the biopsy of highly vascular lesions, with the goal of minimizing aspirated blood dilution of the cellular sample. The cell sample acquired by using capillary technique may be inferior to that achieved with aspiration technique (Hopper et al. 1996). The needle and syringe are removed as a unit and handed to the cytopathologist.

If a core biopsy is performed, the histologic sample is placed in formalin, either by using a needle to brush it into the container, or rinsed into formalin using a saline filled syringe and 25-gauge needle to produce a high velocity stream (Wachsberg 1993).

Coaxial technique may be useful in obtaining cellular material from chest wall, pleura, lung, or mediastinal lesions (vanSonnenberg et al. 1983). The 19-gauge guiding outer cannula (intraparenchymal coaxial technique) remains in situ while multiple sequential 22-gauge FNA procedures are performed. A larger sample can be obtained with the outer 19-gauge needle once the inner needle has been removed, as the last component of the biopsy procedure. It is recommended that all needles be withdrawn once samples have been obtained in the biopsy of lesions surrounded by aerated lung. The outer guiding cannula may remain in situ, while the cytologist assesses the sample acquired, in the biopsy of chest wall, pleura, or mediastinal lesions, or in the biopsy of a lung lesion directly abutting the pleura.

Innovative lung protective techniques for CT-guided biopsy access are valuable, and occasionally essential, adjuncts for biopsy in selected cases.

Iatrogenic pneumothorax entails creating a pneumothorax in a controlled fashion, to displace lung from the planned path of the biopsy needle. The technique is performed under CT-guidance and has its greatest utility in the biopsy of mediastinal lesions, especially in patients with emphysema.

Salinoma technique refers to the injection of saline into the intrathoracic extrapleural tissues under CT-guidance to create a "salinoma window" (Fig. 29.12a–d). This produces an iatrogenic route through which the biopsy needle passes, without having to traverse aerated lung, thus decreasing or eliminating the possibility of pneumothorax. This technique is especially useful in patients with emphysema. Pneumothorax was detected in only 10% of patients when using a "protective" technique (Goodacre et al. 2002).

Iatrogenic pneumothorax and the salinoma technique are particularly useful in the biopsy of deep mediastinal lesions that are difficult to access by mediastinoscopy (subcarinal and aorticopulmonary window), and those not even possible to access by mediastinoscopy – paraesophageal, and pulmonary ligament, parasternal, and para-aortic stations.

29.2.7 Complications and Complication Management

The most common complications of TNB are pneumothorax and hemorrhage. The incidence of pneumothorax varies from 0% (Gleeson et al. 1990) in chest wall and pleural biopsies, to 60% in peripheral intraparenchymal lesions, and close to 100% in small central lesions surrounded by emphysematous bulla (Fink et al. 1982). There is a higher incidence of pneumothorax in the biopsy of difficult thoracic lesions (vanSonnenberg et al. 1988).

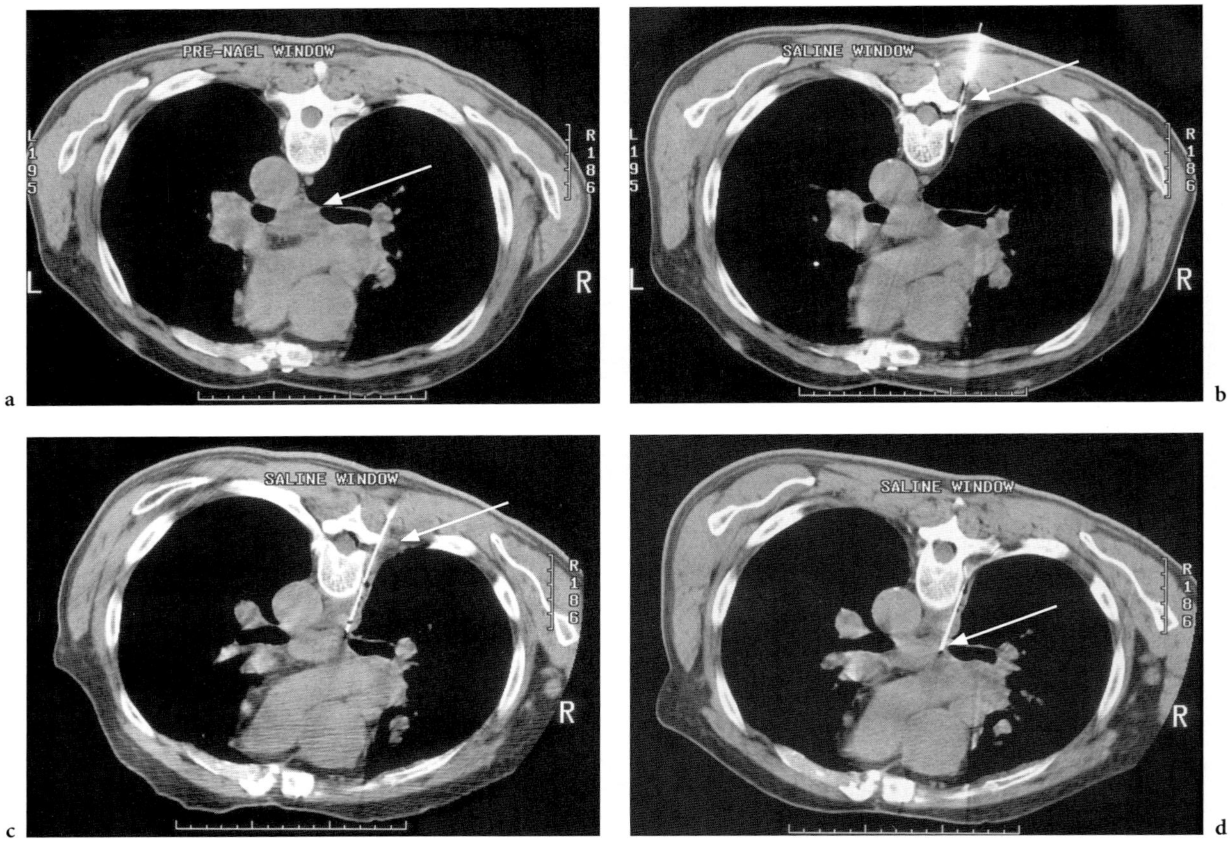

Fig. 29.12. Salinoma window technique. **a** – Subcarinal lesion before biopsy (*arrow*). **b** – Early saline window (*arrow*). **c** – Completed saline window (*arrow*). **d** – Trans-salinoma FNA biopsy of subcarinal mass without perforating the pleura (*arrow*)

Phillips et al. (1997) comment that the diagnosis and treatment of pneumothorax in patients with complex cystic lung disease may be difficult when relying on plain chest radiography alone. CT enables rapid and accurate assessment of complications, optimally guides drainage catheter placement, and demonstrates the response to initial aspiration.

A small pneumothorax can be managed conservatively. Supplemental nasal oxygen is administered to promote pneumothorax resorption. An immediate post procedure baseline chest radiograph is obtained, and is used to compare pneumothorax size on subsequent plain films. The patient is transferred to a post procedure observation unit, and a chest radiograph is obtained 2–4 hours post biopsy. If the patient is clinically stable, the pneumothorax is small, and has not enlarged, the patient can be discharged with post procedure instructions (Dennie et al. 2001).

Post procedure instructions include bed rest and limited physical activity for a 12-hour period. The emergency contact details of the radiologist who performed the procedure are provided, and the patient is advised to present to an emergency department if any symptoms or signs develop. The percentage of patients who require chest tube placement to manage their pneumothorax ranges from 0% to 20% (Westcott 1980; Protopapas et al. 1996). 98% of all pneumothoraces, and 100% of pneumothoraces that require chest tube drainage, are detected within 1 hour of biopsy (Perlmutt et al. 1986).

Indications for Chest Tube Placement in Pneumothorax Management

1. Tension pneumothorax,
2. Large (>33%) pneumothorax,
3. Increasing pneumothorax size on subsequent imaging,
4. Symptomatic, low oxygen saturation, or other significant cardio-respiratory conditions.
5. Ventilator dependent,
6. As part of an "iatrogenic pneumothorax" procedure.

The risk of pneumothorax increases significantly with smaller size lesions and increased lesion depth. The percutaneous manual aspiration of an iatrogenic pneumothorax, performed immediately after the biopsy, may prevent progressive pneumothorax and subsequent chest tube placement (Yamagami et al. 2002).

A tension, large, or symptomatic pneumothorax can be treated on the CT table by placement of a small-bore catheter and one-way valve. Casola et al. (1988) described the successful use of small catheters (7, 8.2, and 9.4 F) to decompress 30 pneumothoraces (15 under tension) resulting from percutaneous lung biopsy. The catheters were inserted under CT or fluoroscopic guidance by radiologists, in the radiology department.

If the initial pneumothorax management attempt is unsuccessful, a chest tube can be placed. Immediate evaluation using CT, or CT-fluoroscopy, can be performed after placement of the pneumothorax drainage device. An immediate post procedure chest radiograph should be obtained to assess for pneumothorax size, and to use as a baseline to compare with the 2-hour post procedure radiograph (Moore 1997).

Factors Associated with a Higher Incidence of Pneumothorax and CT-Guided Chest Tube Placement Include
(Miller et al. 1988; Vitulo et al. 1996; Saji et al. 2002)

1. Emphysema or obstructive airways disease,
2. Cavitary lesions,
3. Advanced patient age,
4. Intractable coughing,
5. Increased lesion depth,
6. Wider the trajectory angle is from the perpendicular,
7. Small lesion size,
8. Larger biopsy needle outer diameter,
9. Cutting needles or biopsy guns,
10. Repeated traversing of the pleura,
11. Longer needle dwell time,
12. Longer total procedure time,
13. Increased predicted forced vital capacity (FVC).

Complications of needle-aspiration lung biopsy can be limited by optimizing biopsy technique.

Hemorrhage is well visualized using CT, and is usually self-limited (Fig. 29.13). Larger biopsy needle size is associated with an increase in the incidence of hemorrhage; the use of 25-gauge needles may offer an advantage. Miller et al. (1988) reported one death due to hemorrhage following transthoracic fine needle biopsy.

A patient with hemoptysis will understandably be concerned, and should be reassured that hemoptysis is usually non-hemodynamically significant, and self-limited. The patient is positioned biopsy-site down to limit transbronchial blood aspiration. Vital signs are monitored, and IV access is secured. Emergency life support (ATLS/ACLS) measures are instituted in the event of a hemodynamically significant or life threatening hemorrhage, and the patient is transferred to a high-care unit for continued management.

Systemic air embolization is a rare complication of TNB. Air embolism most likely occurs when air that enter the pulmonary vein, either directly from the needle that opens to the atmosphere or from a broncho-venous or alveolo-venous fistula induced during placement of the needle. Factors that increase airway pressure result in a greater risk for air embolism. These include coughing and positive pressure ventilation. Biopsy guns may also increase the risk for air embolism. Complications of air embolism include arrhythmia, myocardial infarction, stroke, or death. As little as 0.5 ml of air is sufficient to induce coronary artery ischemia and fatal arrhythmias (Moore 1997). Treatment consists of placing the patient in a left lateral decubitus position (to prevent air in the left atrium from embolizing systemically) and/or Trendelenburg position (to limit the likelihood of endovascular and intra-atrial air from passing into the cerebral circulation). Ventilatory support with 100% oxygen should be administered to promote resorption of air bubbles.

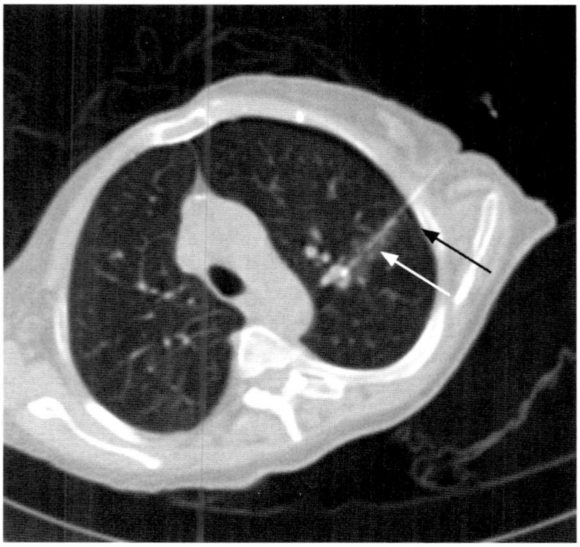

Fig. 29.13. Small self-limiting hemorrhage (*white arrow*) and pneumothorax complicating FNA of a left upper lobe lesion (*black arrow*).

Transfer to a hyperbaric chamber may be necessary (Klein and Zarka 1997).

Other, fortunately rare, complications of TNB include malignant seeding of the biopsy tract, pericarditis, and lung torsion (Sawabata et al. 2000; Sing et al. 1996; Paik et al. 1994; Moloo et al. 1985).

29.2.8 Post-biopsy Procedure

Immediate post procedure expiratory CT-fluoroscopy or single slice CT through the upper lobes and at the level of the hila is performed to assess for post-biopsy pneumothorax (Perlmutt et al. 1986).

If no complications are detected, the patient is moved onto a stretcher, with the biopsy site dependent. This position reduces the incidence of air leak and post biopsy pneumothorax, and also prevents transbronchial spread of biopsy-induced hemorrhage (Moore et al. 1991). The patient is advised not to cough or talk excessively, and is transferred to a post procedure observation unit for monitoring vital signs and clinical symptoms.

90% of pneumothoraces develop within one hour of a TNB procedure (Perlmutt et al. 1986). A chest radiograph is obtained at 2–4 hours post biopsy in our unit. If the delayed chest radiograph is normal, the patient can be discharged with post procedure orders (see below).

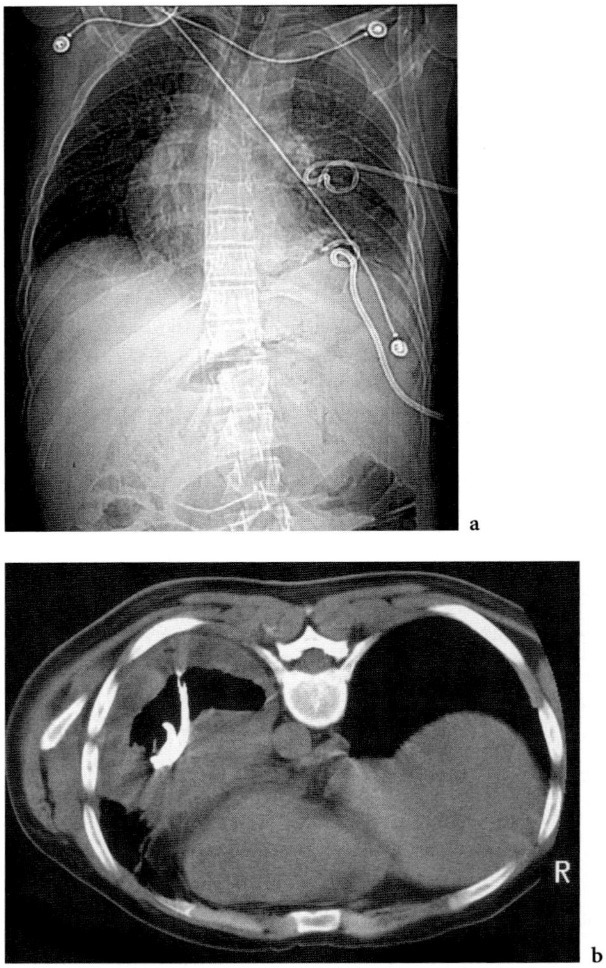

Fig. 29.14a, b. CT-guided percutaneous drainage of a left lower lobe abscess in a patient who remained febrile despite antibiotic therapy

29.3 Interventions of the Lung

29.3.1 Percutaneous Lung Abscess Drainage

CT-guided percutaneous drainage is performed for lung abscesses that are refractory to medical therapy, possibly complicated by empyema, or in immunocompromised patients. Percutaneous drainage will prevent a major operation in most patients (vanSonnenberg et al. 1991a, 1992; Klein et al. 1995)(Fig. 29.14). A catheter route through the abscess-pleural syndesis or contiguous abnormally thickened pleura is preferred. CT is the most useful imaging modality for planning the access route (vanSonnenberg et al. 1991b, 1992) (Fig. 29.15). Reported complications are usually associated with traversing lung. These include pneumothorax, bronchopleural fistula, empyema, and hemorrhage (vanSonnenberg et al. 1991b). VanSonnenberg et al. (1991a) reported an overall success rate of 84%, and associated avoidance of surgery in these patients (vanSonnenberg et al. 1991a,b).

29.3.2 Transcatheter Infusion – Transcavitary Fungal Infusion

Percutaneous infusion of antifungal or other medications directly into a cavity is a natural extension of the fine needle biopsy procedure (Maesaki et al. 1993; Tabeta and Moriya 1995; Yokoyama et al. 1989). Aspergilloma are particularly suited to this approach, as they are usually solitary, have thick

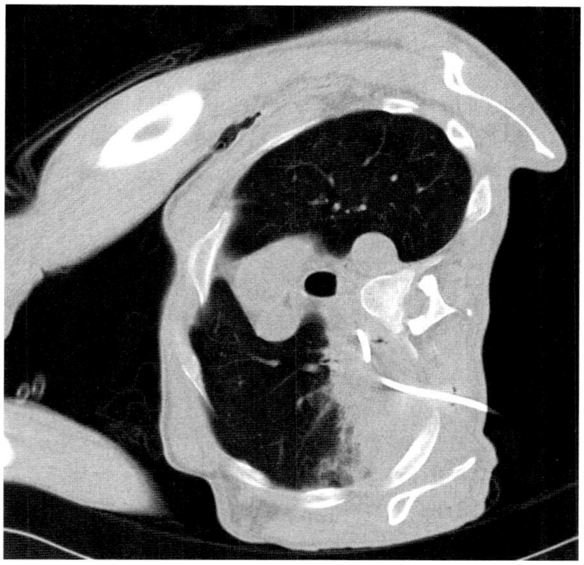

Fig. 29.15. CT-guided percutaneous drainage of a left upper lobe abscess. The drainage is performed with the abscess dependent to minimize the risk of aspiration

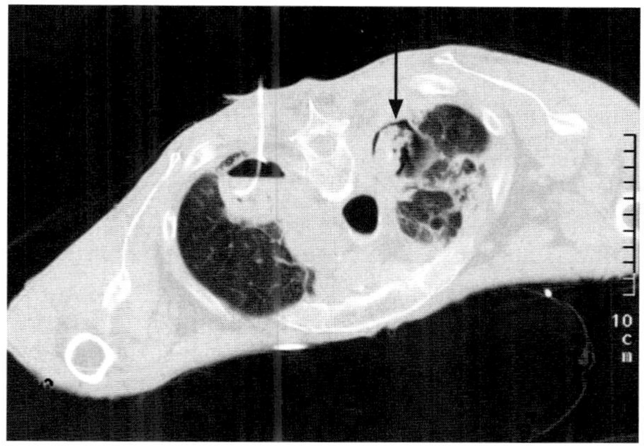

Fig. 29.16. CT-guided percutaneous infusion of antifungal medication into a mycetoma containing left upper lobe cavity. Note contralateral aspergilloma (*arrow*) that was treated at a later date

walls, and do not usually communicate with a bronchus (Fig. 29.16). Instillation of antifungal medication (amphotericin B, fluconazole) for a period of up to 6 weeks may be required to achieve a therapeutic benefit.

29.3.3 Tunneled Hemodialysis Catheter Placement

Ultrasound is the most commonly used guidance imaging modality in the placement of hemodialysis catheters. Catheters placed by radiologists do not have a higher rate of complications or failure than catheters placed by surgeons (Lund et al. 1996). The radiologic placement of tunneled central venous catheters is a safe and effective alternative to surgery (Docktor et al. 1999).

29.4 Interventions of the Pleura

The most common clinical manifestation of pleural pathology is the formation of pleural effusions, regardless of whether the etiology is primary or secondary pleural disease (Vix 1977; Rigler 1931). The parietal and visceral pleura are membranes that are subject to a steady flux of fluid each day. These membranes are highly effective in keeping the pleural space essentially dry and free of protein and particulate matter by means of hydrostatic and oncotic pressure gradients, as well as specialized histologic features. Derangement of any of these features will result in a pleural effusion (Black 1972; Miserocchi and Agostoni 1971; Nebut et al. 1983). Lewandowski et al. (1981) described features that differentiate between pericardial and pleural effusions, and described sonographic demonstration of the right pleural space (Lewandowski and Winsberg 1982). They found that large pericardial effusions are situated anterior to the descending aorta both at the level of the left atrium and the left ventricle, whereas large posterior paramediastinal pleural effusions lie posterior, lateral, or posterolateral to the descending aorta. The interface sign can help distinguish pleural and intra-abdominal fluid readily and accurately (Teplick et al. 1982).

Plain radiography, ultrasound, CT, and MRI permit the in vivo visualization and characterization of pleural effusions. These modalities have enhanced our understanding of the factors that affect the distribution of fluid within the thorax, and are invaluable as a guide for clinical diagnostic and therapeutic measures. Cross sectional imaging, in particular CT, plays an increasingly important role in determining the timing and planning for interventional and surgical procedures in the thorax.

29.4.1 Diagnostic Thoracentesis

Thoracentesis, also known as pleuracentesis, involves the removal of fluid or air through a needle or tube. Diagnostic thoracentesis, in the presence of a pleural effusion, should precede most pleural interventions. Thoracentesis is a low risk bedside procedure in the presence of a pleural effusion diagnosed on clinical examination. In the setting of smaller effusions, or if technical concerns exist (pleural adhesions/loculations, ideal positioning not possible due to patient clinical condition, etc.), access may be performed with radiologic guidance. A chest radiograph will confirm the size and location of the effusion. A decubitus radiograph may demonstrate small effusions not detectable on erect imaging, differentiate between pleural effusion and pleural thickening, and determine whether the effusion is loculated or free to move within the pleural space. Decubitus imaging provides no additional diagnostic information in the presence of a large pleural effusion that causes complete opacification of a hemithorax.

Some clinical services teach that a diagnostic thoracentesis should be performed if clinical symptom resolution is delayed. Given that parapneumonic effusions occur in 35–40% of community acquired pneumonias, and the paracentesis yield in this group is low, it is recommended that thoracentesis of parapneumonic effusions be performed only when the effusion measures more then 1 cm on the decubitus radiograph, or if the effusion is loculated (Klein et al. 1995).

Loculated effusions are likely to be exudative, and the yield of thoracenteses in this group is higher. 74% of septate loculations contained exudative fluid (Hirsch et al. 1981). Anechoic collections that are apparently simple effusions by ultrasound criteria produce exudative and transudative fluid with an approximately equal frequency.

Ultrasound is an excellent imaging modality to assess small pleural effusions, or effusions complicated by adhesions and loculations. Ultrasound can guide targeted transthoracic drainage of complicated loculated effusions (Simeone et al. 1984; vanSonnenberg et al. 1998). An ultrasound performed prior to a bedside thoracentesis procedure, with the access site marked on the patient's skin, provides guidance information on effusion dimensions and character, as well as safe position and depth of needle penetration.

Ultrasound guided thoracentesis is an efficiently performed, inexpensive procedure with a low complication rate in experienced hands (O'Moore et al. 1987). Percutaneous catheter drainage of thoracic empyemas with imaging guidance ensures accurate catheter placement with a high success and a low complication rate and that pre-procedural US can predict the likelihood of success of image-guided percutaneous catheter drainage (Shankar et al. 2000).

The patient is placed in a comfortable position, preferably seated. A pre-procedure ultrasound of a pleural effusion should characterize its anatomic site, relationship to surrounding structures, the effusion dimensions, character, and the presence of septa, adhesions, and loculations. Vital structures in the vicinity of the planned access route should be avoided. Assessment of the patient's respiration, including the range of diaphragmatic motion during quiet respiration, and patient's ability to control respiration during arrested deep inspiration and expiration, should be made.

Access is performed using aseptic technique. Local anesthesia is used to improve patient comfort. A variety of needles is available for thoracentesis. The smallest diameter needle allowing for adequate aspiration should be used. A 22-gauge spinal needle usually will suffice. Use of a larger diameter needles should be considered in echogenic, complicated effusions.

All interventions of the thorax should be performed via an access route passing above the rib below, rather than below the rib above, so as to avoid the neurovascular bundle that is situated in the neurovascular groove on the undersurface of each rib.

CT-guidance is not the initial imaging modality of choice for an isolated thoracentesis procedure. CT is primarily used to guide thoracentesis when thoracentesis is performed as part of a CT-guided TNB of the lung, mediastinum or pleura. The ability to assess differential density and post intravenous contrast enhancement characteristics of multiloculated pleural collections makes CT useful in guiding targeted transthoracic sampling or drainage of specific loculations in complicated collections. CT imaging is recommended in the presence of a pneumothorax in the region of potential percutaneous access, where the intervening air limits the utility of ultrasound.

Regardless of the reason for thoracentesis, fluid should be sent for cytologic assessment. Light et al. (2001) found that in approximately 50% of 436 patients undergoing thoracentesis the effusions were due to neoplasm. Multiple thoracentesis procedures increase the cytologic yield, which approaches 90% when three or more aspiration procedures are performed (Colins et al. 1972).

29.4.2 Therapeutic Thoracentesis

Therapeutic thoracentesis follows diagnostic thoracentesis, and is readily accomplished using trocar technique and a 5 to 9 French catheter (vanSonnenberg et al. 1992). The pleural collection is aspirated and the catheter is either immediately removed, or left in situ, and connected to a collection device or negative suction to allow for ongoing drainage (Fig. 29.17). An expiratory post procedure chest radiograph is obtained to assess for pneumothorax. If the patient experiences pain, severe cough, or shortness of breath, a chest radiograph can be obtained with the catheter in position, allowing for immediate management of a pneumothorax and other complications.

It is prudent not to withdraw more than 1000 ml of pleural fluid at a sitting. If the removal of more than one liter is planned, it is recommended that a period of 15 minutes should elapse between the removal of the first, and subsequent, one-liter volumes. This limits the likelihood of re-expansion pulmonary edema, a rare complication (Waqaruddin and Bernstein 1975).

29.4.3 Thoracostomy for Pneumothorax

Thoracostomy entails the placement of a tube in the pleural space through a small skin incision.

Percutaneous catheter drainage is commonly used to manage spontaneous or traumatic pneumothorax involving greater that 33% collapse, or enlargement over time, particularly if associated with respiratory distress or a gas exchange abnormality; for massive or recurrent benign pleural effusions not responding to thoracentesis; for hemothorax; and for malignant effusions (before intrapleural chemotherapy and/or sclerosing agents are used and briefly afterward, to drain the weeping pleura). Casola et al. (1988) describe the effective drainage of pneumothorax using small (7, 8.2, and 9.4 F) catheters. CT-guided percutaneous catheter drainage in mechanically ventilated patients with acute respiratory distress syndrome provides effective treatment for loculated thoracic air collections and obviates surgical intervention in these critically ill, high-surgical-risk patients.

29.4.4 Thoracostomy for Complicated Effusions and Empyema

Serial thoracentesis may be employed in lieu of thoracostomy if an effusion is small enough and if chest tube drainage is technically difficult, or potentially hazardous to the patient. Serial thoracentesis is also indicated in the setting of an uncomplicated parapneumonic effusion, in which fever and leucocytosis persist, and a loculated process is suspected (Sherman et al. 1977).

Empyema is defined as the presence within the pleural space of gross pus, organisms on Gram stain, pH below 7.0, and glucose level below 40 mg per dl (2.2 mmol per liter). Complicated effusions and empyema should be treated by tube thoracostomy to decrease the likelihood of complicating fibrothorax (Light 2001). The presence of empyema requires hospital admission and continuous drainage (Fig. 29.18).

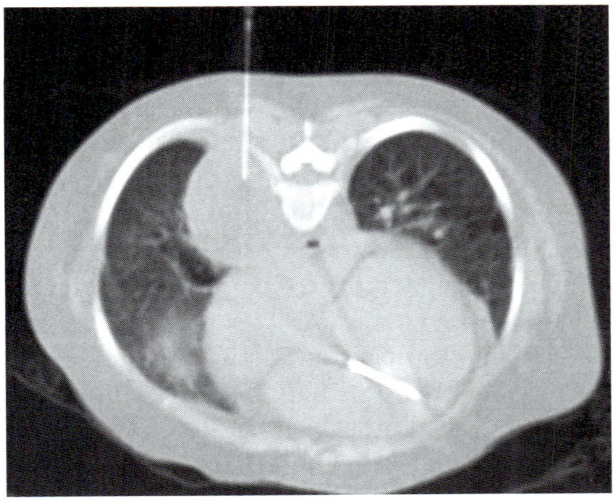

Fig. 29.17. CT-guided percutaneous aspiration of a loculated effusion in a patient with tetralogy of Fallot

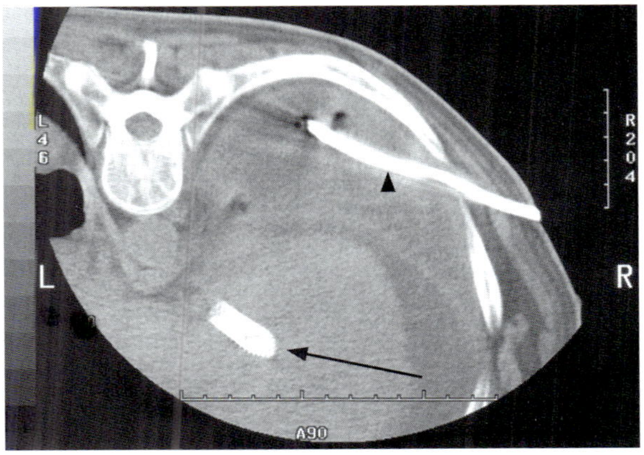

Fig. 29.18. CT-guided percutaneous 12-French pigtail catheter drainage of empyema. Note is made of a metallic stent in the liver

Differentiating between subphrenic abscess and pleural effusion can be difficult on CT (ALEXANDER et al. 1983). STARK et al. (1983) compared conventional chest radiographs and CT scans in differentiating lung abscess from empyema. CT more accurately defined the extent of disease. The most reliable CT features in differentiating lung abscess from empyema were wall characteristics, pleural separation, and the presence of lung compression. Conventional radiographic features such as size, shape, and the angle of the lesion with the chest wall were less helpful, although also best assessed by CT. Catheter placement under ultrasound guidance is easily performed in the presence of large or free flowing empyemas (VANSONNENBERG et al. 1992).

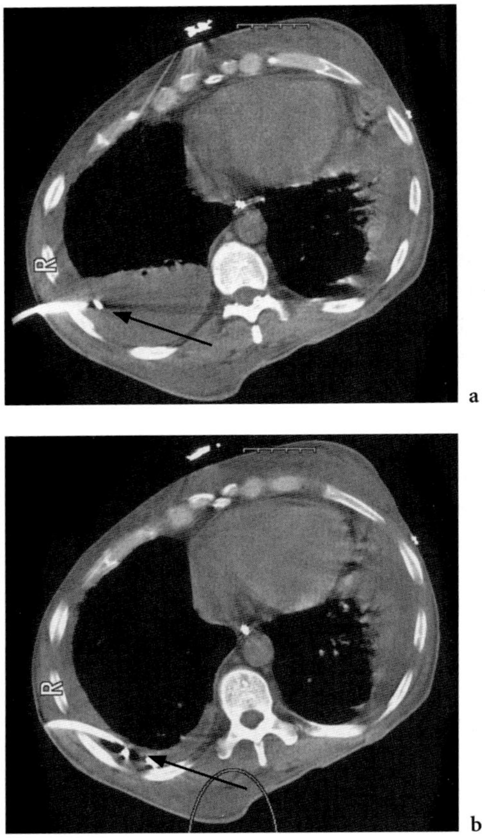

Fig. 29.19. Pre- and post-drainage of empyema secondary to underlying pneumonia. **a** – Percutaneous catheter in a loculated empyema (*arrow*). **b** – Post empyema drainage (*arrow*)

Empyemas may develop in the following sequence:

Stage 1, exudative stage; An infected process contiguous to the pleura may produce a transudate that becomes secondarily infected, contains polymorphonuclear leucocytes on microscopic examination, and have a normal pH and glucose concentration.

Stage 2, fibrinopurulent stage; The sterile exudative pleural effusion becomes secondarily infected, the effusion becomes more viscous, the pH and glucose concentrations fall, and loculations may develop.

Stage 3, inelastic pleural thickening; Fibrin is deposited and a pleural peel develops (SILVERMAN et al. 1989).

Patients with transudative, and stage 1 exudative, pleural effusions usually respond well to conservative management and do not require percutaneous drainage.

Early stage 2 pleural effusions are usually successfully managed by percutaneous catheter drainage (LIGHT 2001) (Fig. 29.19a, b). The management of any drainage catheter should be the responsibility of the radiologist or physician who placed it. The timing of the tube thoracostomy procedure is important. Once an infectious process becomes organized, open drainage or decortication may be required (SHERMAN et al. 1977).

Late stage 2 and early stage 3 effusions account for many drainage failures. Reversible failures are attributed to tube clogging, kinking, improper tube position, or the presence of loculations (STARK et al. 1983). Streptokinase, TPA or urokinase have been shown to improve results when attempting drainage of extremely viscous fluid (BOUROS et al. 1996, 1999; LAISAAR et al. 1996; ROBINSON et al. 1994). However BALCI et al. (2002) showed that continued conservative therapy risks morbidity and mortality in the treatment of multiloculated thoracic empyema in children and that thoracotomy-decortication must remain the preferred method of treatment in this group. Imaging is performed to diagnose preventable causes of drainage failure.

Traditional teaching is that stage 3 pleural peel requires thoracotomy and surgical decortication. NEFF et al. (1990) used computed tomography (CT) to examine the resolution of pleural abnormalities following radiologic catheter drainage of empyemas. They demonstrated that the pleural surfaces have a remarkable capacity for healing after empyema drainage, and that the pleural peel resolves in most cases. Their results suggest that decortication need not be performed routinely when empyemas are encountered; rather, patients should be treated on an individualized basis and studied with serial CT to determine the necessity of decortication.

In the presence of a large pleural collection, thoracostomy can be performed as a bedside procedure without imaging guidance, or with prior ultrasound assessment and access site marking of the skin. Ultrasound, CT, or CT-fluoroscopic guidance is indicated in the presence of smaller collections, as part of an imaging-guided biopsy procedure, or when access of specific loculations is planned. vanSonnenberg et al. (1984b) described the benefits of CT- and ultrasound-guided catheters in the management of empyemas in 1984. 88.2% of patients were treated successfully, averting surgery or further drainage, and bacteremia in 1 patient was the only complication.

Catheter choice is dictated by fluid characteristics at thoracentesis (vanSonnenberg et al. 1998). Viscous collections require larger drainage tubes (16–36F), and are more likely to become blocked before complete evacuation is attained. The trocar technique is commonly used to access the pleural space. Catheters are held on a stylet-cannula assembly for trocar insertion. The Seldinger technique requires guide wire exchanges and has an accompanying theoretical possibility of air introduction during the necessary tract dilatation phase of the procedure. Disruption of effusion septa and loculations can occur during pigtail placement.

A post procedure chest radiograph is obtained after catheter placement, to ensure that no pneumothorax has developed. The drainage catheter is tethered to the skin and connected to a Pleurevac catheter, two-piece ostomy system (e.g. Hollister, Libertyville, IL), or is connected to an underwater seal pleural drainage system. A repeat CT can be performed to ensure that no loculated collections remain.

CT-guidance has facilitated the placement of drainage catheters from its inception. Stavas et al. (1987) described improved percutaneous catheter drainage of pleural collections with CT-guidance as compared with the then more commonly used "blind" techniques. CT is invaluable in the presence of air-containing collections that limit ultrasound transmission within the pleural space, collections close to vital structures, and dependent collections in patients with limited mobility.

Catheter placement may be performed using ultrasound-guidance (vanSonnenberg et al. 1998). Imaging-guided percutaneous catheter drainage of thoracic empyemas ensures accurate catheter placement an associated low complication rate (Shankar et al. 2000). Pre-procedural ultrasound can predict the likelihood of success of image-guided percutaneous catheter drainage.

Open drainage is indicated in the setting of persistent fever and leucocytosis not responding to closed drainage. Open drainage may require partial rib resection and manual removal of the exudate and disruption of loculations (Sherman et al. 1977; Andrews and Parker 1962).

29.4.5 Pleural Sclerosis, Pleurodesis

Pleurodesis can provide palliation and relief of symptoms in patients with recurrent, often malignant, pleural effusions. Pleurodesis is usually performed under ultrasound or CT-guidance (vanSonnenberg et al. 1998). The pleural effusion is drained via a percutaneously placed catheter. Once the rate of pleural fluid production falls below 100 ml per day (below 10 ml per day is preferable), a sclerosing agent (talc, tetracycline, bleomycin) is instilled. The tube is clamped for 15–30 minutes and patient position is repeatedly altered to allow for diffuse sclerosant dispersal. The procedure may need to be repeated several times. Doxycycline is an inexpensive, safe, and commonly used sclerosing agent.

Complications include fever and pain. Talc is often painful, and bleomycin is better tolerated. Administration of narcotic analgesia and injection of local anesthesia into the pleural space prior to instillation of the sclerosing agent is recommended. Best expected pleural effusion control results approach 70% (Ruckdeschel 1988).

29.4.6 Pleural Biopsy

Pleural biopsy has fewer complications if performed in the presence of pleural fluid, but can be performed if only pleural thickening is present (Light 2001). Pleural biopsy should be considered when noninvasive diagnostic procedures such as sputa expectoration, bronchial washings, and minimally invasive procedures like bronchoscopy and thoracentesis fluid analysis, are non-diagnostic (Johnston 1988), and when tuberculosis or malignancy is suspected (Sahebajami and Loudon 1977) (Fig. 29.20).

Pleural biopsy can be performed as a bedside procedure without imaging guidance, or with prior ultrasound assessment and access site marking of the skin, in the presence of a large pleural effusion. Pleural biopsy needle (e.g. using an 18–22 gauge Wescott or Cope needle) placement is readily performed using real-time ultrasound guidance in the presence of smaller effusions. Fiberoptic bronchoscopy may

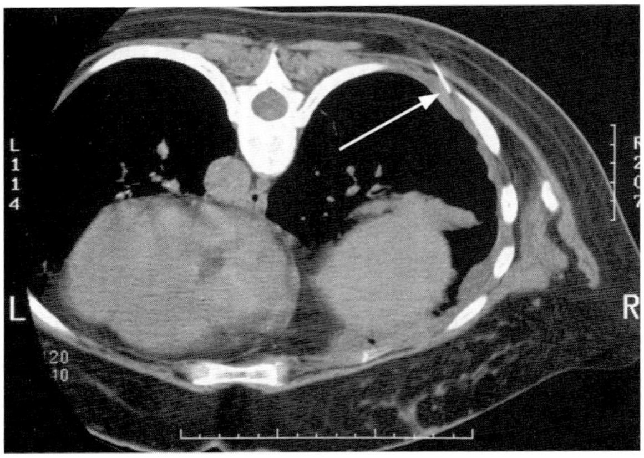

Fig. 29.20. CT-guided core biopsy of left pleural thickening (*arrow*)

be useful as an adjunctive procedure in a high-risk population when the effusion is of unknown etiology, as the effusion may be secondary to occult bronchogenic carcinoma (Light 2001). However, the yield from bronchoscopy in this setting is too low to justify its routine use (Feinsilver et al. 1986).

CT may be used to guide pleural biopsy, especially if a soft tissue target exists. CT-guided core needle biopsy provides a correct histologic diagnosis in the assessment of diffuse pleural thickening in 87% of patients (Scott et al. 1995).

29.4.7 Complication Management Post-pleural Intervention

The incidence of pneumothorax complicating transthoracic needle biopsy of the pleura and chest wall is very low. Silverman et al. (1988) describe a series of 970 thoracic pleural aspirations that were complicated by pneumothorax in 2%. 1% required catheter therapy due to patient symptoms, or to size of the pneumothorax.

The management of post pleural biopsy pneumothorax is identical to the management of pneumothorax complicating TNB of pulmonary parenchymal lesions. A baseline chest radiograph is acquired directly after completion of the procedure, the patient is monitored in a post procedure observation area, is administered supplemental oxygen, and a second radiograph is obtained 2 hours after the first. If the patient experiences no significant symptoms and vital signs and pneumothorax size remain stable, the patient can be discharged with post procedure instructions that include a description of potential complications, and the contact details of support medical care. In the majority of instances, a lack of patient symptoms, stable vital signs, and a less than 25% pneumothorax, allows for conservative management. Pneumothoraces of up to 33% in stable patients without symptoms have been treated conservatively with success.

Active management (see Thoracostomy) is indicated in the setting of tension pneumothorax, pneumothoraces larger than 20% on the initial post procedure radiograph, progressive enlargement of the pneumothorax on the follow-up radiograph, disease of the contralateral lung, or significant clinical features of respiratory compromise (Deslauriers 1994).

Pneumothorax drainage entails inserting a tube through the anterior 2nd or 3rd intercostal space in the midclavicular line, directed toward the apex of the lung, for the drainage of. Placement of a 7 to 9 F catheter, using trocar technique and CT-fluoroscopic guidance, attachment of a 3-way valve and flexible tubing, followed by aspiration under intermittent visualization, is often the only active management required. A posteriorly directed tube is inserted through the 5th or 6th intercostal space in the midaxillary line for the drainage of pleural effusions. Tubes for loculated effusions or empyemas are positioned as required.

A pneumothorax set containing a one-way flutter valve (Pleurevac, Heimlich, Bard-Parker, Rutherford, NJ) can be attached to an 11 to 14F diameter, 10 to 30 cm long connecting tube (Cook, Bloomington, IN), which is attached to the pleural catheter. O'Laoide et al. (1994) describe effective pneumothorax treatment with a self-contained pneumothorax treatment device. Continuous negative suction can be applied in the absence of improvement in pneumothorax size after a period of observation.

29.5 Interventions of the Mediastinum and Pericardium

29.5.1 Transthoracic Biopsy of Mediastinal Lesions

CT-guided TNB of mediastinal lesions is effective in the diagnosis of mediastinal and hilar lymph node metastases (vanSonnenberg et al. 1992; Protopapas and Westcott 1996; D'Agostino et al. 1993) (Fig. 29.21).

Zwischenberger et al. (2002) retrospectively assessed 89 patients with mediastinal lymph nodes (N2 or N3) with a short-axis diameter greater than

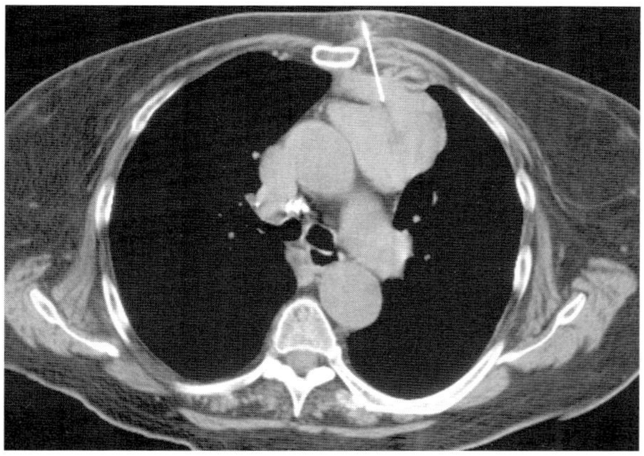

Fig. 29.21. CT-guided percutaneous biopsy of anterior mediastinal mass. 25-gauge fine needle biopsy produced abundant lymphocytes on cytologic assessment, and a core biopsy performed during the same procedure confirmed non-Hodgkin's lymphoma

15 mm, as part of lung cancer staging. Samples were obtained by CT-guided transthoracic needle biopsy and core biopsy. Mediastinoscopy was performed only when FNA failed to yield a diagnosis. Transthoracic needle biopsy of nodal stations judged readily accessible by mediastinoscopy (paratracheal and highest mediastinal) (Fig. 29.22), those more difficult to access via mediastinoscopy (subcarinal and aorticopulmonary window) and those not possible to access by mediastinoscopy (paraesophageal and pulmonary ligament, parasternal, and para-aortic stations) were assessed. TNB was diagnostic in 78% of patients for cancer cell type, sarcoidosis, and caseating granulomas with or without tuberculosis.

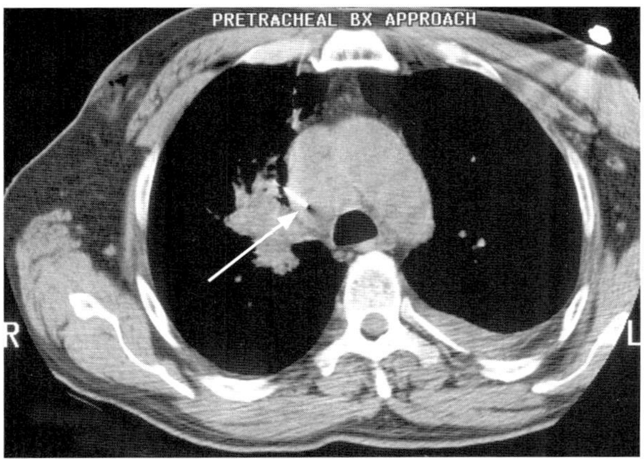

Fig. 29.22. CT-guided percutaneous FNA of a pretracheal mediastinal lesion in a patient with adenocarcinoma of the lung (*arrow*). This deep mediastinal biopsy upstaged the malignancy and associated management

Transthoracic FNA, with or without core biopsy, failed to yield a diagnosis in 22% patients, and all then underwent mediastinoscopy, with 55% of these procedures diagnostic for cancer, and 45% producing a benign diagnosis. They concluded that TNB of mediastinal masses should precede mediastinoscopy in the staging of lung cancer or workup of mediastinal masses.

The transsternal approach (Fig. 29.23a–c) utilizing a coaxial system for biopsy of anterior mediastinal lesions is a safe and well-tolerated procedure (D'Agostino et al. 1993). This technique obviates traversing the lung, and thus prevents pneumothorax.

Transtracheal biopsy of mediastinal lesions has been performed without complication (Fig. 29.24).

Innovative lung protective techniques that may aid CT-guided biopsy access include iatrogenic pneumothorax and the salinoma technique, and were described previously.

29.5.2 Endoscopic Transesophageal Ultrasound-Guided FNA of Mediastinal Masses

Over the past two decades, endoscopic ultrasonography (EUS) has undergone a transition from being a novel imaging technique to becoming increasingly useful clinically. It has been used predominantly in the detection and staging of gastrointestinal cancers.

EUS-guided fine-needle aspiration (FNA) continues to develop into a useful diagnostic tool in the management of lung cancer and other mediastinal diseases. New applications for EUS-FNA are emerging, including the possible application of EUS-guided therapy (Pfau and Chak 2002) of mediastinal lesions. Rosenberg et al. (2002) showed that patients with NSCLC and suspicious lymphadenopathy may benefit from EUS/FNA of enlarged posterior mediastinal lymph nodes, even with negative findings on PET-imaging. Catalano et al. (2002) assessed endoscopic ultrasound-guided fine needle aspiration (EUS-FNA) in the diagnosis of mediastinal masses of unknown origin and conclude that EUS-FNA can establish the diagnosis in the majority of cases (infectious 60%, benign/inflammatory 78%, and malignant 92%) presenting with idiopathic mediastinal masses, particularly in those with malignant disease.

The emergence of transesophageal EUS-FNA of the mediastinum provides the ability to alter subsequent workup and therapy, obviating the need for more invasive diagnostic studies such as thoracotomy.

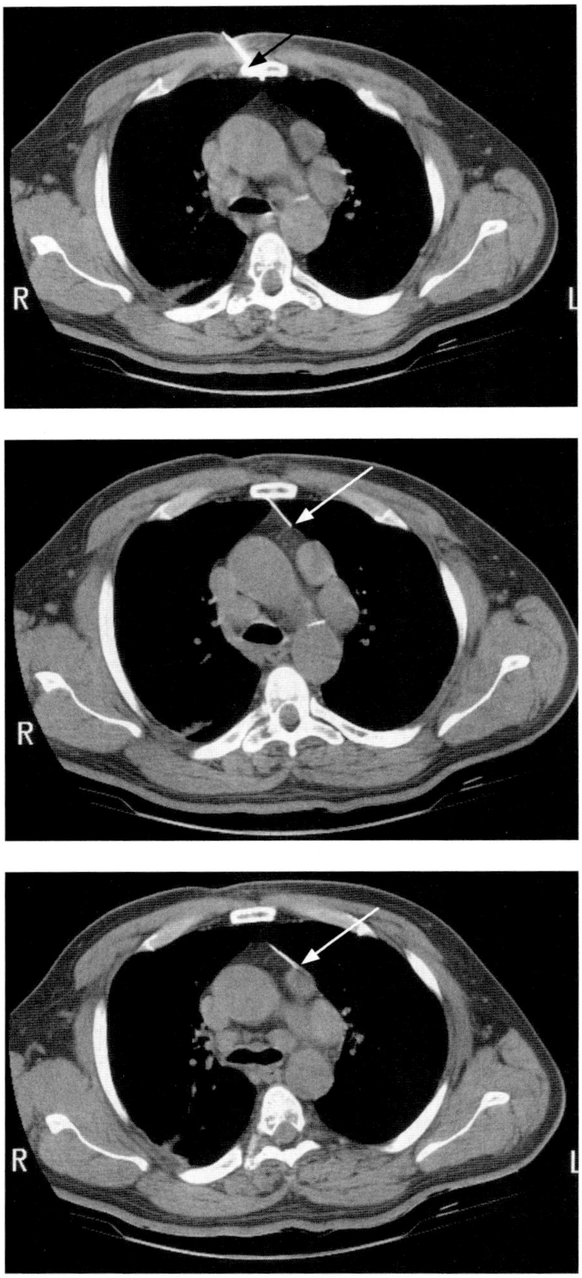

a

b

c

Fig. 29.23. Transsternal biopsy of an aortopulmonary window mass. **a** – The outer cannula of the coaxial system traverses the sternum (*arrow*). **b** – Inner fine needle en route to the lymph node (*arrow*). **c** – Needle in substance of target lesion (*arrow*)

29.5.3 Percutaneous Drainage of Mediastinal Abscess or Cyst

Percutaneous drainage of a mediastinal abscess or cyst is a similar procedure to the drainage of lung

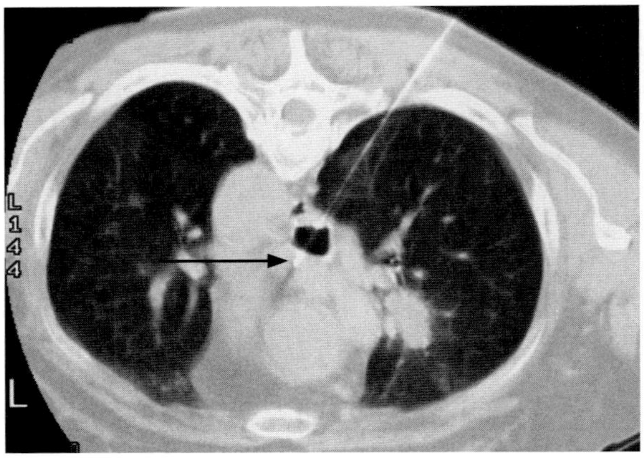

Fig. 29.24. Transtracheal biopsy of mass interposed between the trachea and the ascending thoracic aorta (*arrow*)

abscess or pleural effusion (Fig. 29.25a, b). Salinoma technique and iatrogenic pneumothorax are innovative techniques that may facilitate drainage in selected cases.

29.5.4 Percutaneous Drainage of Pericardial Effusion, Pericardial Empyema, and Hemopericardium

Percutaneous drainage of a pericardial effusion or empyema and hemopericardium is best performed using CT or ultrasound-guidance. A small-bore catheter is placed in the pericardial space via a percutaneous route directed from beneath the costal angle/xiphoid process of the sternum.

29.5.5 Tracheobronchial Stents

Tracheobronchial stenting, using metallic stents, is performed radiologically via fluoroscopic guidance through an endotracheal tube. Axial, helical, and multi-detector CT with 3D reconstruction provides valuable information for planning the procedure. The precise site of the stricture, the length of the strictures, the juxtaposition to bronchial branch points, and strictures are demonstrated. This information is used to extrapolate the dimension and length of metal stents to be inserted.

Zwischenberger et al. (1997) confirm the benefit of CT assessment prior to stent placement and describe an airway imaging protocol to guide selective endobronchial metallic stent placement

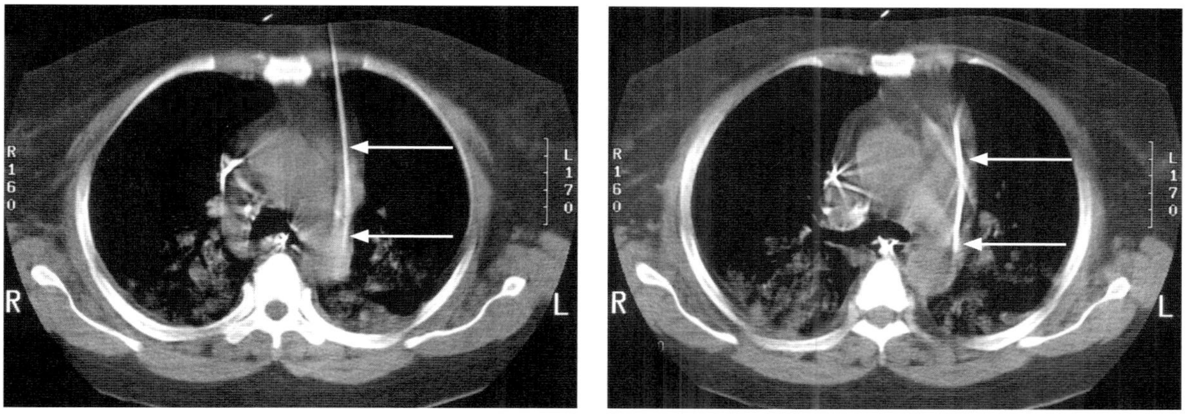

a b

Fig. 29.25a, b. CT-guided percutaneous pigtail catheter drainage of a mediastinal collection in a renal transplant patient (*arrows*)

that combines helical computed tomography with three-dimensional reconstruction, bronchography, and bronchoscopy and allows accurate assessment of malignant airway obstruction. Patient selection to favor effective palliation and cost effectiveness has yet to be defined.

Post procedure, CT is again utilized to access the effects of stent insertion. Thus, bronchial patency, lung re-expansion, and stent placement are all assessed. 3D reconstruction is particularly valuable (Khiari et al. 1996).

29.6 Tumor Ablation and Sclerosis

Microwave, laser, and radiofrequency waves can all produce hyperthermic coagulative necrosis. Hyperthermic coagulative necrosis and cryotherapy procedures can be performed percutaneously.

29.6.1 Radiofrequency Ablation

Radiofrequency ablation (RFA) involves the local application of radiofrequency (RF) thermal energy to a lesion. A high frequency alternating current moves from the electrode tip into the surrounding tissue. The ions move within the tissue in an attempt to follow the changing direction of the alternating current, which results in heating of the tissue. As the temperature rises beyond 600∞C, cells begin to die, with a resultant zone of necrosis that surrounds the electrode (Dupuy and Goldberg 2001; Dupuy et al. 2000). The splayed tines of the umbrella probe increase the volume of necrosis produced per burn (Fig. 29.26).

Lesions that are located near large vessels may be inadequately treated because of the heat sink effect of rapid blood flow (Goldberg et al. 1998). This phenomenon can result in a theoretical site of refuge for incompletely treated neoplastic cells, and a resultant increase in local recurrence rates (Michaels et al. 2001).

RFA has been used in patients who do not meet the criteria for tumor resectability, but who were candidates for control of tumor when cure is not possible.

Commonly used needle electrodes are 15 to 25 cm long, 15-gauge, with an insulated cannula that con-

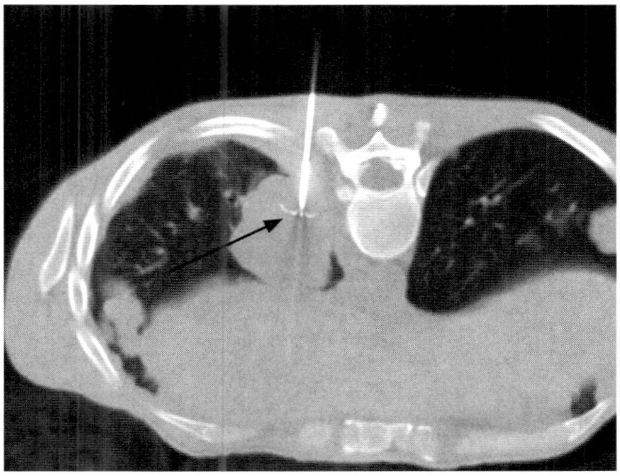

Fig. 29.26. CT-guided RF ablation of an adenoid cystic carcinoma metastasis to the lung in a young man. Note umbrella array of RF probe tines that increases the volume of necrosis per burn (*arrow*)

tain 10 individual hook-shaped electrode arms or tines. Once deployed, the array of tines extends out to a diameter of between 2.0 and 4.0 cm. The needle electrode is attached to a radiofrequency generator.

Technique

A needle electrode is advanced into the tumor via a percutaneous route using CT guidance.

Tumors less than 3 cm in their greatest diameter can be completely ablated by treatment with an electrode that causes necrosis of a diameter of 3.5 cm. Tumors larger than 3 cm require more than one deployment of the needle electrode. Typically, the array is first placed at the interface most distant from the skin access site, between the tumor and nonmalignant lung parenchyma, and then repositioned for repeat deployments anteriorly at 2.0 to 2.5 cm intervals within the tissue. The needle electrode is used to produce a thermal lesion that incorporates not only the tumor but also non-neoplastic lung parenchyma in a zone 1 cm wide surrounding the tumor (Dupuy et al. 2000) for cure.

Radiofrequency therapy can be administered to palliate pain and is aided by performing intercostal nerve ablation as the final component of the RF ablation procedure. RF is used to ablate metastatic rib lesions, and may be offer pain relief in the setting of a pathologic rib fracture (Fig. 29.27). Patients can be monitored, using ultrasound or CT, to determine if additional therapy is necessary.

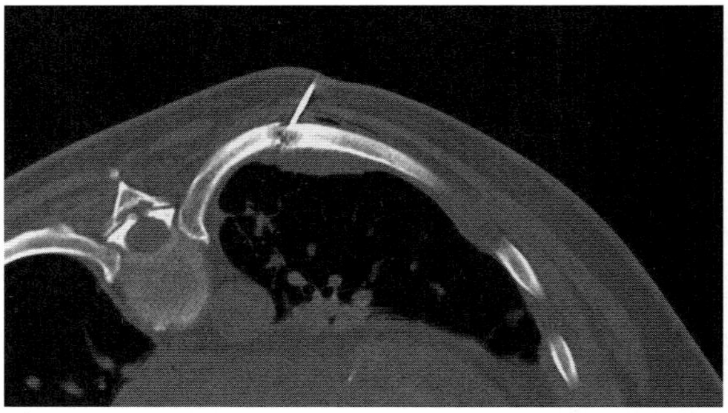

Fig. 29.27. CT-guided percutaneous radiofrequency ablation of a rib metastasis with an associated pathologic fracture causing significant pain

Complications that may occur during the procedure include a reported 20–40% pneumothorax incidence, with a higher than the average incidence of pneumothorax requiring chest tube drainage (Fig. 28a, b). Factors related to the increased pneumothorax rate in the RF ablation population include the use of 14 to17-gauge RF needles, and the incidence of emphysema in patients likely to be offered RF ablation. Initial management of the pneumothorax is by needle aspiration with a 60 ml syringe. If not successful, a 7-French small-bore catheter can be inserted into the area of maximal pneumothorax. Once the pneumothorax is controlled and the patient's vital signs are stable, the ablation procedure can be completed (Shankar et al. 2003).

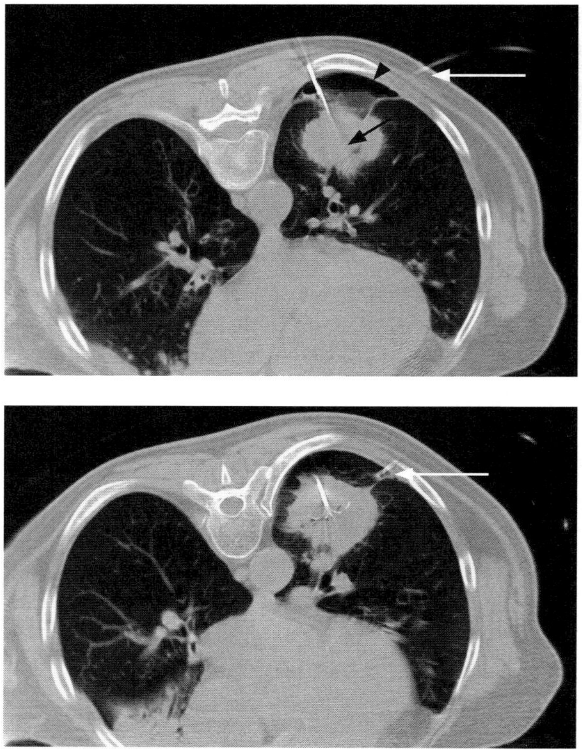

a

b

Fig. 29.28. CT-guided catheter drainage of an iatrogenic pneumothorax during a radiofrequency ablation procedure. **a** – Pneumothorax (*arrowheads*), with RF needle (*black arrow*) and percutaneous catheter in situ (*white arrow*). **b** – Treated pneumothorax (Shankar et al. 2003)

Real-time image guidance using CT-fluoroscopy minimizes the risk of iatrogenic damage to anatomical structures. A single case report of massive hemorrhage during radiofrequency ablation of a pulmonary neoplasm has been described (Vaughn et al. 2002).

RFA is a useful local treatment option, particularly in those patients who are not surgical candidates, either for reasons related to the extent of their disease, or secondary to co-morbid diseases and medical conditions (Dupuy and Goldberg 2001). Recent refinements in ablation technology enable large tumor volumes to be treated by percutaneous, laparoscopic, or open surgical image-guided needle probe placement. Local disease control could result in enhanced operability, improved morbidity, and possibly improved mortality in selected cases.

Despite the proliferation of sites offering RF technology, the indications for RF ablation in oncology are still ill defined. More rigorous scientific review, long-term follow-up, and randomized prospective trials are needed to help define the role of RFA in thoracic oncology (Wood et al. 2002; Putnam 2002).

29.6.2 Cryotherapy

Cryo-ablation entails the rapid cooling of the target tissue to produce intracellular freezing. Cell death depends upon the interaction of ice crystals, the solution surrounding the ice crystals, and the cells. Bronchoscopic cryotherapy was first used to treat carcinomatous bronchial obstruction in 1968 (Homasson et al. 1986). Seven years later, a case series of 28 patients with metastases to the lung at the Mayo Clinic showed that cryotherapy was a viable palliative modality. Nevertheless, the technique was not widely adopted. Cryotherapy was reintroduced in Europe during the mid-1980's (Homasson et al. 1986; Maiwand 1986) and is now used in a variety of specialties, but its use is still infrequent in the thorax.

Difficulty in determining the true margin of the lesion, which often extends beyond the leading edge, and the lack of specificity of tissue damage, applies to ethanol injection, RFA, and cryotherapy. Although the borders of the ice-ball are well seen on CT and MRI, a gradient of effect ranges from cell survival to cell death that is not visible using currently available by imaging. Evaluation with PET may prove helpful in this situation.

29.7 Intercostal Nerve Block

An anesthesiologist using anatomical landmarks for guidance typically performs the intercostal nerve block. Interventional radiologists performing thoracic or upper abdominal procedures may also perform intercostal nerve blocks for temporary or more prolonged pain relief. Zylocaine or Marcaine is typically injected in the tissues along the lower surface of the rib where the neurovascular bundle courses, within a few centimeters of the posterior medial origin of the rib.

Intercostal nerve block has been performed as part of radiofrequency ablation procedures in the management of pain in both symptomatic pulmonary parenchymal lesions abutting the pleura (Fig. 29.29), and to metastatic rib lesions, with or without associated pathologic fracture.

29.8 Brachytherapy

Radiation seeds are implanted into the substance of a lesion to produce a local radiation dose that is higher than that which is safely possible using external bean radiation therapy (Nori et al. 1987). Intraoperative lung and/or endobronchial brachytherapy management of non-small-cell lung cancer offers curative potential in patients with well-defined, small to moderate in size, accessible localized tumors that are technically inoperable (Hilaris and Mastoroas 1998; Raben and Mychalczak 1997). Bronchoscopically placed radiation seeds are also used in the palliation of central endobronchial masses, usually in an attempt to delay, or reverse, bronchial occlusion by tumor. The procedure can often be performed on an outpatient basis.

CT-guided percutaneous placement of brachytherapy seeds using (often multiple) 16-gauge needles (vanSonnenberg et al. 1992) may be performed in the local management of recurrent or refractory tumor that involves, or abuts, the pleura.

Brachytherapy complications include hemoptysis and radiation bronchitis. The onset of hemoptysis is

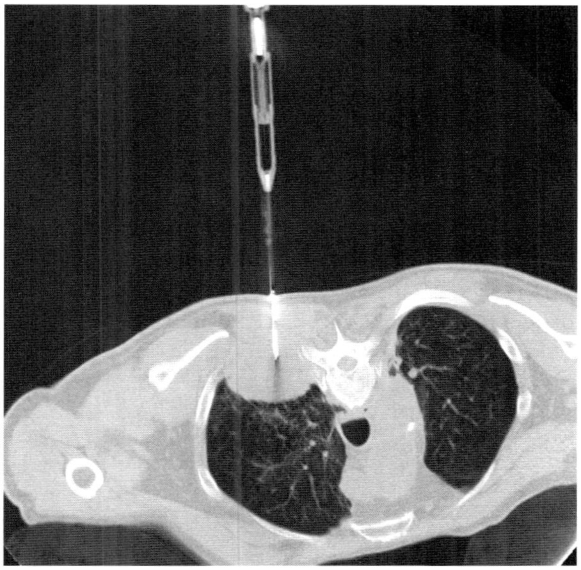

Fig. 29.29. CT-guided RF ablation to right upper lobe lung carcinoma eroding an underlying rib

secondary to disease progression, with the bleeding being facilitated by brachytherapy (Hennequin et al. 1998). Risk factors for massive hemoptysis after endobronchial brachytherapy in patients with tracheobronchial malignancies include direct contact between the endobronchial brachytherapy applicator and the tracheobronchial walls in the vicinity of the great vessels. A specific spacer should be employed to maintain a safe distance between the applicator and the bronchial wall and prevent massive hemoptysis (Hara et al. 2001).

In contrast, radiation bronchitis occurs more frequently in patients with controlled disease, and is significantly influenced by tumor location and technical factors (dose and volumes treated).

29.9 Summary

New advances in multi-detector CT technology, faster data processing times, better image quality and the advent of the 16-channel CT scanners and CT-fluoroscopy, facilitates efficient initial patient assessment, visualization during CT-guided thoracic interventions, and the assessment and management of post procedure complications.

Multi-detector spiral CT scanners are capable of generating hundreds of images in a single breath-hold, thus placing considerable strain on daily clinical practice. Workstations facilitate routine interpretation of CT images and will soon have the capability to produce seamless real-time transition between axial, coronal, and sagittal images, produce instantaneous sliding maximum intensity projection and volumetrically rendered images, allow instantaneous transition between thick and thin sections, and allow nearly instantaneous co-registration between studies of different dates allowing for efficient identification and comparison of thoracic pathology. High hopes exist for the future value of the exciting and rapidly evolving field of CT-PET imaging. It is envisioned that CT-PET-guided TNB of thoracic lesions will closely follow on the heels of the initial diagnostic use of CT-PET.

References

Albes JM, Dohmen BM, Schott U, Schulen E, Wehrmann M, Ziemer G (2002) Value of positron emission tomography for lung cancer staging. Eur J Surg Oncol 28:55–62

Alexander ES, Proto AV, Clark RA (1983) CT differentiation of subphrenic abscess and pleural effusion. AJR Am J Roentgenol 140:47–51

Andrews N, Parker E (1962) Management of non-tuberculous empyema. Am Rev Respir Dis 85:935–936

Arakawa H, Nakajima Y, Kurihara Y, Niimi H, Ishikawa T (1996) CT-guided transthoracic needle biopsy: a comparison between automated biopsy gun and fine needle aspiration. Clin Radiol 51:503–506

Balci AE, Eren S, Ulku R, Eren MN (2002) Management of multiloculated empyema thoracis in children: thoracotomy versus fibrinolytic treatment. Eur J Cardiothorac Surg 22:595–598

Ben-Yehuda D, Polliack A, Okon E et al (1996) Image-guided core-needle biopsy in malignant lymphoma: experience with 100 patients that suggests the technique is reliable. J Clin Oncol 14:2431–2434

Black LF (1972) The pleural space and pleural fluid. Mayo Clin Proc 47:493–506

Boiselle PM, Shepard JA, Mark EJ et al (1997) Routine addition of an automated biopsy device to fine-needle aspiration of the lung: a prospective assessment. AJR Am J Roentgenol 169:661–666

Bouros D, Schiza S, Tzanakis N, Drositis J, Siafakas N (1996) Intrapleural urokinase in the treatment of complicated parapneumonic pleural effusions and empyema. Eur Respir J 9:1656–1659

Bouros D, Schiza S, Tzanakis N, Chalkiadakis G, Drositis J, Siafakas N (1999) Intrapleural urokinase versus normal saline in the treatment of complicated parapneumonic effusions and empyema. A randomized, double-blind study. Am J Respir Crit Care Med 159:37–42

Casola G, vanSonnenberg E, Keightley A, Ho M, Withers C, Lee AS (1988) Pneumothorax: radiologic treatment with small catheters. Radiology 166:89–91

Catalano MF, Rosenblatt ML, Chak A, Sivak MV Jr, Scheiman J, Gress F (2002) Endoscopic ultrasound-guided fine needle aspiration in the diagnosis of mediastinal masses of unknown origin. Am J Gastroenterol 97:2559–2565

Chechani V (1996) Bronchoscopic diagnosis of solitary pulmonary nodules and lung masses in the absence of endobronchial abnormality. Chest 109:620–625

Chon KS, vanSonnenberg E, D'Agostino HB, O'Laoide RM, Colt HG, Hart E (1999) CT-guided catheter drainage of loculated thoracic air collections in mechanically ventilated patients with acute respiratory distress syndrome. AJR Am J Roentgenol 173:1345–1350

Coleman RE (2001) PET in lung cancer staging. Q J Nucl Med 45:231–234

Colins JD, Burwell D, Furmanski S, Lorber P, Steckel RJ (1972) Minimal detectable pleural effusions. A roentgen pathology model. Radiology 105:51–53

D'Agostino HB, Sanchez RB, Laoide RM et al (1993) Anterior mediastinal lesions: transsternal biopsy with CT guidance (work in progress). Radiology 189:703–705

D'Amico TA, Wong TZ, Harpole DH, Brown SD, Coleman RE (2002) Impact of computed tomography-positron emission tomography fusion in staging patients with thoracic malignancies. Ann Thorac Surg 74:160–163; discussion 163

Dennie CJ, Matzinger FR, Marriner JR, Maziak DE (2001) Transthoracic needle biopsy of the lung: results of early discharge in 506 outpatients. Radiology 219:247–251

Deslauriers J (1994) The management of spontaneous pneumothorax. Can J Surg 37:182

Docktor BL, Sadler DJ, Gray RR, Saliken JC, So CB (1999) Radiologic placement of tunneled central catheters: rates of success and of immediate complications in a large series. AJR Am J Roentgenol 173:457–460
Doust BD, Baum JK, Maklad NF, Doust VL (1975) Ultrasonic evaluation of pleural opacities. Radiology 114:135–140
Dupuy DE, Goldberg SN (2001) Image-guided radiofrequency tumor ablation: challenges and opportunities, part II. J Vasc Interv Radiol 12:1135–1148
Dupuy DE, Zagoria RJ, Akerley W, Mayo-Smith WW, Kavanagh PV, Safran H (2000) Percutaneous radiofrequency ablation of malignancies in the lung. AJR Am J Roentgenol 174: 57–59
Erdi YE, Rosenzweig K, Erdi AK et al (2002) Radiotherapy treatment planning for patients with non-small cell lung cancer using positron emission tomography (PET). Radiother Oncol 62:51–60
Feinsilver SH, Barrows AA, Braman SS (1986) Fiberoptic bronchoscopy and pleural effusion of unknown origin. Chest 90:516–519
Filho JS, Soares MF, Wal R, Christmann RB, Liu CB, Schmitt FC (2002) Fine-needle aspiration cytology of pulmonary rheumatoid nodule: case report and review of the major cytologic features. Diagn Cytopathol 26:150–153
Fink I, Gamsu G, Harter LP (1982) CT-guided aspiration biopsy of the thorax. J Comput Assist Tomogr 6:958–962
Froelich JJ, Ishaque N, Regn J, Saar B, Walthers EM, Klose KJ (2002) Guidance of percutaneous pulmonary biopsies with real-time CT fluoroscopy. Eur J Radiol 42:74–79
Gambhir SS, Hoh CK, Phelps ME, Madar I, Maddahi J (1996) Decision tree sensitivity analysis for cost-effectiveness of FDG-PET in the staging and management of non-small-cell lung carcinoma. J Nucl Med 37:1428–1436
Gasparini S, Ferretti M, Secchi EB, Baldelli S, Zuccatosta L, Gusella P (1995) Integration of transbronchial and percutaneous approach in the diagnosis of peripheral pulmonary nodules or masses. Experience with 1,027 consecutive cases. Chest 108:131–137
Gillams A, Roberts CM, Shaw P, Spiro SG, Goldstraw P (1992) The value of CT scanning and percutaneous fine needle aspiration of adrenal masses in biopsy-proven lung cancer. Clin Radiol 46:18–22
Gleeson F, Lomas DJ, Flower CD, Stewart S (1990) Powered cutting needle biopsy of the pleura and chest wall. Clin Radiol 41:199–200
Goldberg SN, Hahn PF, Tanabe KK et al (1998) Percutaneous radiofrequency tissue ablation: does perfusion-mediated tissue cooling limit coagulation necrosis? J Vasc Interv Radiol 9:101–111
Goodacre BW, Savage C, Zwischenberger JB, Wittich GR, vanSonnenberg E (2002) Salinoma window technique for mediastinal lymph node biopsy. Ann Thorac Surg 74: 276–277
Greif J, Marmor S, Schwarz Y, Staroselsky AN (1999) Percutaneous core needle biopsy vs. fine needle aspiration in diagnosing benign lung lesions. Acta Cytol 43:756–760
Greif J, Marmur S, Schwarz Y, Man A, Staroselsky AN (1998) Percutaneous core cutting needle biopsy compared with fine-needle aspiration in the diagnosis of peripheral lung malignant lesions: results in 156 patients. Cancer 84: 144–147
Haberkorn U, Schoenberg SO (2001; Imaging of lung cancer with CT, MRT and PET. Lung Cancer 34 [Suppl 3]:S13–S23
Hara R, Itami J, Aruga T et al (2001) Risk factors for massive hemoptysis after endobronchial brachytherapy in patients with tracheobronchial malignancies. Cancer 92:2623–2627
Haramati LB (1995) CT-guided automated needle biopsy of the chest. AJR Am J Roentgenol 165:53–55
Haramati LB, Lee G, Singh A, Molina PL, White CS (2001) Newly diagnosed pulmonary sarcoidosis in HIV-infected patients. Radiology 218:242–246
Hennequin C, Tredaniel J, Chevret S et al (1998) Predictive factors for late toxicity after endobronchial brachytherapy: a multivariate analysis. Int J Radiat Oncol Biol Phys 42: 21–27
Herman SJ, Holub RV, Weisbrod GL, Chamberlain DW (1991) Anterior mediastinal masses: utility of transthoracic needle biopsy. Radiology 180:167–170
Hilaris BS, Mastoras DA (1998) Contemporary brachytherapy approaches in non-small-cell lung cancer. J Surg Oncol 69: 258–264
Hirsch JH, Rogers JV, Mack LA (1981) Real-time sonography of pleural opacities. AJR Am J Roentgenol 136:297–301
Homasson JP, Renault P, Angebault M, Bonniot JP, Bell NJ (1986) Bronchoscopic cryotherapy for airway strictures caused by tumors. Chest 90:159–164
Hopper KD, Grenko RT, Fisher AI, TenHave TR (1996) Capillary versus aspiration biopsy: effect of needle size and length on the cytopathological specimen quality. Cardiovasc Intervent Radiol 19:341–344
Johnston WW (1988) Fine needle aspiration biopsy versus sputum and bronchial material in the diagnosis of lung cancer. A comparative study of 168 patients. Acta Cytol 32:641–646
Kardos L, Nagy E, Morvay Z et al (1999) Value of CT-guided biopsy compared to fluoroscopy-guided transthoracic biopsy and bronchoscopic sampling in the diagnosis of pulmonary nodules. Orv Hetil 140:931–933
Keith CJ, Miles KA, Griffiths MR, Wong D, Pitman AG, Hicks RJ (2002) Solitary pulmonary nodules: accuracy and cost-effectiveness of sodium iodide FDG-PET using Australian data. Eur J Nucl Med Mol Imaging 29:1016–1023
Khiari A, Navarro F, Fabre JM et al (1996) Value of percutaneous hepatic biopsy in the diagnosis of presumed benign tumors of the liver. Ann Chir 50:532–537
Khouri NF, Stitik FP, Erozan YS et al (1985) Transthoracic needle aspiration biopsy of benign and malignant lung lesions. AJR Am J Roentgenol 144:281–288
Klein JS, Zarka MA (1997) Transthoracic needle biopsy: an overview. J Thorac Imaging 12:232–249
Klein JS, Schultz S, Heffner JE (1995) Interventional radiology of the chest: image-guided percutaneous drainage of pleural effusions, lung abscess, and pneumothorax. AJR Am J Roentgenol 164:581–588
Kobayashi T, Kaneko M, Kondo H et al (1997) CT-guided bronchoscopic barium marking for resection of a fluoroscopically invisible peripheral pulmonary lesion. Jpn J Clin Oncol 27:204–205
Laisaar T, Puttsepp E, Laisaar V (1996) Early administration of intrapleural streptokinase in the treatment of multiloculated pleural effusions and pleural empyemas. Thorac Cardiovasc Surg 44:252–256
Layfield LJ, Coogan A, Johnston WW, Patz EF (1996) Transthoracic fine needle aspiration biopsy. Sensitivity in relation to guidance technique and lesion size and location. Acta Cytol 40:687–690

Lewandowski BJ, Jaffer NM, Winsberg F (1981) Relationship between the pericardial and pleural spaces in cross-sectional imaging. J Clin Ultrasound 9:271–274

Lewandowski BJ, Winsberg F (1982) Sonographic demonstration of the right paramediastinal pleural space. Radiology 145:127–131

Light R (2001) Pleural diseases. 108–135, 358–378, 391–399

Lockhart ME, Smith JK, Kenney PJ (2002) Imaging of adrenal masses. Eur J Radiol 41:95–112

Lucidarme O, Howarth N, Finet JF, Grenier PA (1998) Intrapulmonary lesions: percutaneous automated biopsy with a detachable, 18-gauge, coaxial cutting needle. Radiology 207:759–765

Lund GB, Trerotola SO, Scheel PF Jr et al (1996) Outcome of tunneled hemodialysis catheters placed by radiologists. Radiology 198:467–472

Maesaki S, Kohno S, Tanaka K et al (1993) A case of pulmonary aspergilloma successfully treated with combination therapy of intracavitary injection of amphotericin B and intravenous administration of urinastatin. Nihon Kyobu Shikkan Gakkai Zasshi 31:1327–1331

Magnani P, Carretta A, Rizzo G et al (1999) FDG/PET and spiral CT image fusion for medistinal lymph node assessment of non-small cell lung cancer patients. J Cardiovasc Surg (Torino) 40:741–748

Maiwand MO (1986) Cryotherapy for advanced carcinoma of the trachea and bronchi. Br Med J (Clin Res) 293:181–182

Michaels M, Silverman M, Libertino J (2001) Absence of total tumor necrosis in radiofrequency ablated renal tumors (abstract). J Urol 165:21a

Miller KS, Fish GB, Stanley JH, Schabel SI (1988) Prediction of pneumothorax rate in percutaneous needle aspiration of the lung. Chest 93:742–745

Miserocchi G, Agostoni E (1971) Contents of the pleural space. J Appl Physiol 30:208–213

Moloo Z, Finley RJ, Lefcoe MS, Turner-Smith L, Craig ID (1985) Possible spread of bronchogenic carcinoma to the chest wall after a transthoracic fine needle aspiration biopsy. A case report. Acta Cytol 29:167–169

Moore E (1997) Needle-aspiration lung biopsy: a comprehensive approach to complication reduction. J Thorac Imaging 12:259–271

Moore E, LeBlanc J, Montesi S (1991) Effects of patient positioning after needle aspiration lung biopsy. Radiology 181: 385–387

Naidich DP, Sussman R, Kutcher WL, Aranda CP, Garay SM, Ettenger NA (1988) Solitary pulmonary nodules. CT-bronchoscopic correlation. Chest 93:595–598

Nebut M, Hirsch A, Chretien J (1983) Embryology and anatomy of the pleura. 1–9

Neff CC, vanSonnenberg E, Lawson DW, Patton AS (1990; CT follow-up of empyemas: pleural peels resolve after percutaneous catheter drainage. Radiology 176:195–197

Nodenstrom B (1967) Transthoracic needle biopsy. N Engl J Med 276:1081–1082

Noppen MM, de Mey J, Meysman M, Opdebeeck B, Vincken WG, Osteaux M (1995) Percutaneous needle biopsy of localized pulmonary, mediastinal, and pleural diseased tissue with an automatic disposable guillotine soft-tissue needle. Preliminary results. Chest 107:1615–1620

Nori D, Hilaris BS, Martini N (1987) Intraluminal irradiation in bronchogenic carcinoma. Surg Clin North Am 67: 1093–102

O'Laoide R, Fundell LJ, vanSonnenberg E, D'Agostino H, Oglevie SB, Rosenkrantz H (1994) Treatment of postbiopsy pneumothorax with a self-contained pneumothorax treatment device. Radiology 193:393–395

O'Moore PV, Mueller PR, Simeone JF et al (1987) Sonographic guidance in diagnostic and therapeutic interventions in the pleural space. AJR Am J Roentgenol 149:1–5

Onik G, Cosman ER, Wells TH Jr et al (1988) CT-guided aspirations for the body: comparison of hand guidance with stereotaxis. Radiology 166:389–394

Pagani JJ (1984) Non-small cell lung carcinoma adrenal metastases. Computed tomography and percutaneous needle biopsy in their diagnosis. Cancer 53:1058–1060

Paik HC, Lee DY, Lee HK, Kim SJ, Lee KB (1994) Chest wall implantation of carcinoma after fine needle aspiration biopsy. Yonsei Med J 35:349–354

Pappa VI, Hussain HK, Reznek RH et al (1996) Role of image-guided core-needle biopsy in the management of patients with lymphoma. J Clin Oncol 14:2427–2430

Perlmutt LM, Braun SD, Newman GE, Oke EJ, Dunnick NR (1986) Timing of chest film follow-up after transthoracic needle aspiration. AJR Am J Roentgenol 146:1049–1050

Pfau PR, Chak A (2002) Endoscopic ultrasonography. Endoscopy 34:21–28

Phillips GD, Trotman-Dickenson B, Hodson ME, Geddes DM (1997) Role of CT in the management of pneumothorax in patients with complex cystic lung disease. Chest 112: 275–278

Protopapas Z, Westcott JL (1996) Transthoracic needle biopsy of mediastinal lymph nodes for staging lung and other cancers. Radiology 199:489–496

Protopapas Z, White C, Miller B (1996) Transthoracic needle biopsy practices: results of a nationwide survey. Radiology 201:270

Pugatch RD, Faling LJ, Robbins AH, Snider GL (1978) Differentiation of pleural and pulmonary lesions using computed tomography. J Comput Assist Tomogr 2:601–606

Putnam JB Jr (2002) New and evolving treatment methods for pulmonary metastases. Semin Thorac Cardiovasc Surg 14: 49–56

Raben A, Mychalczak B (1997) Brachytherapy for non-small cell lung cancer and selected neoplasms of the chest. Chest 112:276S–286S

Radke JR, Conway WA, Eyler WR, Kvale PA (1979) Diagnostic accuracy in peripheral lung lesions. Factors predicting success with flexible fiberoptic bronchoscopy. Chest 76: 176–179

Richardson C, Pointon K, Manhire A, Macfarlane J (2002) Percutaneous lung biopsies: a survey of UK practice based on 5444 biopsies. Br J Radiol 75:731–735

Rigler L (1931) Roentologic observations on the movement of pleural effusions. AJR 25:220–229

Robinson LA, Moulton AL, Fleming WH, Alonso A, Galbraith TA (1994) Intrapleural fibrinolytic treatment of multiloculated thoracic empyemas. Ann Thorac Surg 57:803–813; discussion 813–814

Rosenberg JM, Perricone A, Savides TJ (2002) Endoscopic ultrasound/fine-needle aspiration diagnosis of a malignant subcarinal lymph node in a patient with lung cancer and a negative positron emission tomography scan. Chest 122:1091–1093

Ruckdeschel JC (1988) Management of malignant pleural effusion: an overview. Semin Oncol 15:24–28

Sagar P, Gulati M, Gupta SK et al (2000) Ultrasound-guided transthoracic co-axial biopsy of thoracic mass lesions. Acta Radiol 41:529–532
Sahebajami H, Loudon R (1977) Pleural effusions: pathophysiology and clinical features. Semin Roentgenol 269–275
Saji H, Nakamura H, Tsuchida T et al (2002) The incidence and the risk of pneumothorax and chest tube placement after percutaneous CT-guided lung biopsy: the angle of the needle trajectory is a novel predictor. Chest 121:1521–1526
Salminen E, MacManus M (2001) Impact of FDG-labelled positron emission tomography imaging on the management of non-small-cell lung cancer. Ann Med 33:404–9
Sawabata N, Ohta M, Maeda H (2000) Fine-needle aspiration cytologic technique for lung cancer has a high potential of malignant cell spread through the tract. Chest 118:936–939
Scott EM, Marshall TJ, Flower CD, Stewart S (1995) Diffuse pleural thickening: percutaneous CT-guided cutting needle biopsy. Radiology 194:867–870
Shankar S, Gulati M, Kang M, Gupta S, Suri S (2000) Image-guided percutaneous drainage of thoracic empyema: can sonography predict the outcome? Eur Radiol 10:495–499
Shankar S, vanSonnenberg E, Silverman SG, Tuncali K, Morrison PR (2003) Management of pneumothorax during percutaneous radiofrequency ablation of a lung tumor: technical note. J Thorac Imaging 18:106–109
Sherman MM, Subramanian V, Berger RL (1977) Managment of thoracic empyema. Am J Surg 133:474–479
Silverman SG, Saini S, Mueller PR (1989) Pleural interventions. Indications, techniques, and clinical applications. Radiol Clin North Am 27:1257–1266
Simeone JF, Mueller PR, vanSonnenberg E (1984) The uses of diagnostic ultrasound in the thorax. Clin Chest Med 5:281–290
Sing RF, Kefalides PT, Mette SA, Fallahnejad M (1996) Chest wall metastasis after percutaneous fine-needle aspiration biopsy. J Am Osteopath Assoc 96:546–547
Singer AA, Obuchowski NA, Einstein DM, Paushter DM (1994) Metastasis or adenoma? Computed tomographic evaluation of the adrenal mass. Cleve Clin J Med 61:200–205
Smolle-Juettner FM, Woltsche M, Roeger G, Gabor S, Fladerer H, Popper H (1996) Is preoperative percutaneous fine-needle aspiration cytology of intrathoracic lesions advisable in resectable patients? Eur J Cardiothorac Surg 10: 1047–1050; discussion 1051
Stanley J, Fish G, Andrioe J (1987) Lung lesions: cytological diagnosis by fine-needle biopsy. Radiology 162:389–391
Stark DD, Federle MP, Goodman PC, Podrasky AE, Webb WR (1983) Differentiating lung abscess and empyema: radiography and computed tomography. AJR Am J Roentgenol 141:163–167
Stark DD, Federle MP, Goodman PC (1983) CT and radiographic assessment of tube thoracostomy. AJR Am J Roentgenol 141:253–258
Stavas J, vanSonnenberg E, Casola G, Wittich GR (1987) Percutaneous drainage of infected and noninfected thoracic fluid collections. J Thorac Imaging 2:80–87
Syed S, Zaharopoulos P (2001) Thoracic splenosis diagnosed by fine-needle aspiration cytology: a case report. Diagn Cytopathol 25:321–324
Tabeta H, Moriya T (1995) A case of chronic necrotizing pulmonary aspergillosis in which intravenous infusion of amphotericin B was effective. Nihon Kyobu Shikkan Gakkai Zasshi 33:342–347
Teplick JG, Teplick SK, Goodman L, Haskin ME (1982) The interface sign: a computed tomographic sign for distinguishing pleural and intra-abdominal fluid. Radiology 144:359–362
Treaba D, Assad L, Govil H et al (2002) Diagnostic role of fine-needle aspiration of bone lesions in patients with a previous history of malignancy. Diagn Cytopathol 26:380–383
vanSonnenberg E, Wittich G (1998) Hemoptysis during lung biopsy after aspirin. AJR Am J Roentgenol 171:261
vanSonnenberg E, Lin AS, Deutsch AL, Mattrey RF (1983) Percutaneous biopsy of difficult mediastinal, hilar, and pulmonary lesions by computed tomographic guidance and a modified coaxial technique. Radiology 148: 300–302
vanSonnenberg E, Lin AS, Casola G, Nakamoto SK, Wing VW, Cubberly DA (1984a) Removable hub needle system for coaxial biopsy of small and difficult lesions. Radiology 152 226
vanSonnenberg E, Nakamoto SK, Mueller PR et al (1984b) CT- and ultrasound-guided catheter drainage of empyemas after chest-tube failure. Radiology 151:349–353
vanSonnenberg E, Casola G, Ho M et al (1988) Difficult thoracic lesions: CT-guided biopsy experience in 150 cases. Radiology 167:457–461
vanSonnenberg E, D'Agostino HB, Casola G, Wittich GR, Varney RR, Harker C (1991a) Lung abscess: CT-guided drainage. Radiology 178:347–351
vanSonnenberg E, D'Agostino HB, Casola G, Halasz NA, Sanchez RB, Goodacre BW (1991b) Percutaneous abscess drainage: current concepts. Radiology 181:617–626
vanSonnenberg E, Casola G, D'Agostino HB, Goodacre B, Sanchez R (1992) Interventional radiology in the chest. Chest 102:608–612
vanSonnenberg E, Wittich GR, Goodacre BW, Zwischenberger JB (1998) Percutaneous drainage of thoracic collections. J Thorac Imaging 13:74–82
vanSonnenberg E, Goodacre BW, Wittich GR, Logrono R, Kennedy P, Zwischenberger JB (2003) Image-guided 25-gauge needle biopsy for thoracic lesions: diagnostic feasibility and safety. Radiology 227
Vansteenkiste JF, Stroobants SG, de Leyn PR et al (1998) Lymph node staging in non-small-cell lung cancer with FDG-PET scan: a prospective study on 690 lymph node stations from 68 patients. J Clin Oncol 16:2142–9
Vaughn C, Mychaskiw G II, Sewell P (2002) Massive hemorrhage during radiofrequency ablation of a pulmonary neoplasm. Anesth Analg 94:1149–1151; table of contents
Vitulo P, Dore R, Cerveri I, Tinelli C, Cremaschi P (1996) The role of functional respiratory tests in predicting pneumothorax during lung needle biopsy. Chest 109:612–615
Vix VA (1977) Roentgenographic manifestations of pleural disease. Semin Roentgenol 12:277–286
Wachsberg RH (1993) The sticky biopsy specimen: a saline solution. AJR Am J Roentgenol 161:1336–1337
Waqaruddin M, Bernstein A (1975) Re-expansion pulmonary oedema. Thorax 30:54–60
Westcott JL (1980) Direct percutaneous needle aspiration of localized pulmonary lesions: result in 422 patients. Radiology 137:31–35
Wong CY, Nunez R, Bohdiewicz P et al (2001) Patterns of abnormal FDG uptake by various histological types of non-small cell lung cancer at initial staging by PET. Eur J Nucl Med 28:1702–1705

Wong PW, Stefanec T, Brown K, White DA (2002) Role of fine-needle aspirates of focal lung lesions in patients with hematologic malignancies. Chest 121:527–532

Wood BJ, Ramkaransingh JR, Fojo T, Walther MM, Libutti SK (2002) Percutaneous tumor ablation with radiofrequency. Cancer 94:443–451

Yamagami T, Nakamura T, Iida S, Kato T, Nishimura T (2002) Management of pneumothorax after percutaneous CT-guided lung biopsy. Chest 121:1159–1164

Yap CS, Schiepers C, Fishbein MC, Phelps ME, Czernin J (2002) FDG-PET imaging in lung cancer: how sensitive is it for bronchioloalveolar carcinoma? Eur J Nucl Med Mol Imaging 29:1166–1173

Yokoyama S, Taniguchi H, Kondo Y, Matsumoto K, Okada A (1989) A case of bronchopulmonary aspergillosis recurring in a residual tuberculous cavity. Kekkaku 64:579–584

Yoshimura N, Takeda K, Tada H et al (2002) The factors determining diagnostic accuracy in CT-guided percutaneous needle biopsy of small pulmonary nodules. Nihon Kokyuki Gakkai Zasshi 40:101–105

Zwischenberger JB, Savage C, Alpard SK, Anderson CM, Marroquin S, Goodacre BW (2002) Mediastinal transthoracic needle and core lymph node biopsy: should it replace mediastinoscopy? Chest 121:1165–1170

Zwischenberger JB, Wittich GR, vanSonnenberg E et al (1997) Airway simulation to guide stent placement for tracheobronchial obstruction in lung cancer. Ann Thorac Surg 64: 1619–1625

30 Medical Legal Aspects of Multidetector CT

E. J. Potchen

CONTENTS

What are the medical-legal ramifications of multi-detector CT? Are there any unique features of this technology that distinguish it from the other legal implications of the practice of medicine? This chapter seeks to review the basis of medical-legal responsibility when advocating and implementing multi-detector CT in the diagnosis of thoracic lesions. An example drawn from personal experience will be presented as a framework for analysis. This case exemplifies some legal issues that can embroil the practice of radiology.

Medical malpractice litigation dominates the medical-legal ramifications of diagnostic imaging. Typically, radiologists are concerned about being sued for a failure to diagnose something that is subsequently demonstrated to have been present on the image, but it was either not observed or not correctly interpreted by the person who reports the film. In "screening" procedures, the patient is considered to be "normal" prior to the procedure. In such a situation a false positive result can potentially injure the patient as much as a false negative result. The follow-up biopsy of a suspicious lesion may injure the patient even though no significant disease was found to be present. In advocacy of screening procedures, physicians have to be especially vigilant about the ramifications of false positive results in view of the possibility of injury to a patient who, but for the diagnostic procedure, would have remained healthy.

E. J. Potchen, MD
Department of Radiology, Michigan State University, 160 Radiology Building, East Lansing, MI 48824, USA

In the legal context, the advocacy of new technology carries an additional burden of proving that any change is worth the risk. Standards that would apply to newly advocated technologies have not yet been set. Thus, reasonably prudent behavior should govern what is to be considered the standard of care.

30.1 A Case of Lung Cancer Where Malpractice Litigation Was Based upon the Interpretation of Multidetector CT Images

The problem of identifying early lung cancer on multi-detector CT is well exemplified in a case where the CT was done to evaluate an abdominal problem. This eventually resulted in malpractice litigation for failure to classify properly an abnormality seen in the lung on the abdominal CT. The patient presented with acute abdominal pain and was ultimately diagnosed as having acute diverticulitis with subsequent peritonitis. The patient was in severe pain from her abdominal problem and an abdominal CT was performed (Fig. 30.1). The report associated with those images is as follows:

"Correlation is made with an abdominal ultrasound dated 4/22/97. Study performed with 110 cc of Hypague-60 contrast. Limited study through the lung bases demonstrates a 1.8 cm mass in the lingula of the left lung containing central calcification most consistent with a granuloma. The lung bases are otherwise clear with no evidence of pleural fluid. The pre-contrast study demonstrates focal area of amorphous low density in the pelvis which may represent multiple adherent unopacified bowel loops versus fluid around the bowel in the region of the sigmoid colon. There are also perirectal inflammatory changes in the mesentery. Though the contrast-enhanced study is obtained relatively delayed because of mechanical failure, this region is persistent and may represent sigmoid colonic diverticulitis. The inflammatory changes around the rectosigmoid

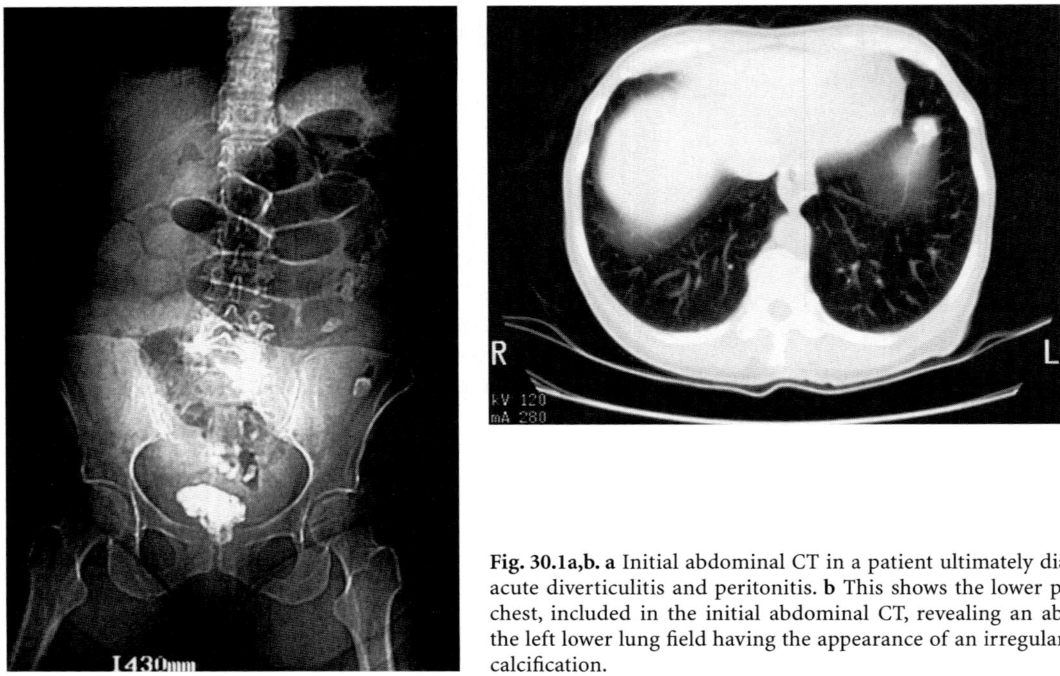

a b

Fig. 30.1a,b. a Initial abdominal CT in a patient ultimately diagnosed with acute diverticulitis and peritonitis. **b** This shows the lower portion of the chest, included in the initial abdominal CT, revealing an abnormality in the left lower lung field having the appearance of an irregular nodule with calcification.

region are again noted. There is a cyst in the mid pole of the right kidney and no free fluid in the upper abdomen. No free air is identified. There appears to be a calcification in the region of the right ureter with mild distention of the right renal collecting system and streak opacification of the right kidney following contrast. This calcification, possibly interureteral, may be partially occlusive."

Impression: (1) "There is perirectal and pericolonic mesenteric stranding possibly associated with fluid around the sigmoid colon. These findings may be related to diverticulitis. (2) Partially occlusive right ureteral calculus with mild right-sided hydronephrosis and streaky opacification of the right kidney. (3) Status-post hysterectomy. (4) 1.85 cm granuloma in the left lung. (5) Right-sided renal cyst."

On the basis of this CT image, the radiologist reported the presence of a 1.85 cm granuloma in the left lung. The referring surgeon therefore considered this to be a benign process.

A subsequent CT study performed two days later, with contrast, stated that there were some non-specific increased markings in the lung bases. Again, the CT primarily emphasized the abnormality in the abdomen for which the examination was performed. More than one year later, the patient presented with chest symptoms, and evidence of malignancy was found on CT. The case ultimately went to litigation. In this case, the lung abnormality was detected, but the interpretation of the abnormality was in question. The radiologists were not accused of a failure to detect the lesion; rather, the plaintiff complained of a failure by the radiologist to interpret correctly what was observed. The radiologist, who identified the abnormality, was not held responsible for malpractice, whereas the second radiologist, who did not comment on the abnormality, was found guilty. In the opinion of an expert called to testify, the first radiologist did what a reasonably prudent radiologist would do under the same or similar circumstances. Another expert considered the radiologist's action to be a breach of the standard of care, in that he believed the report should have been constructed to alert the surgeon that this abnormality might have been due to a lung cancer rather than a granuloma. The trial testimony revolved around whether the diagnostic impression of granuloma was a breach of the standard of care. Was the calcification central or eccentric? Was the pattern of the density consistent with a granuloma? In court, references taken from journal articles (Siegelmann et al. 1986) were used in an attempt to teach the jury whether or not a reasonably prudent person would have concluded that this was a granuloma (Fig. 30.2).

The jury was presented a detailed tutorial regarding the attributes used by radiologists to distinguish a granuloma from a malignancy when interpreting

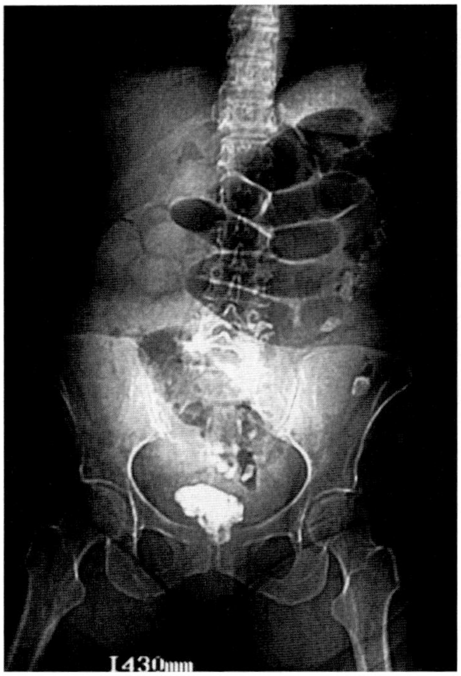

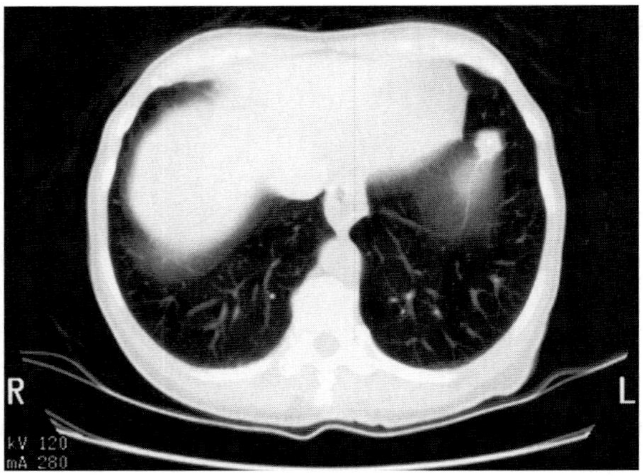

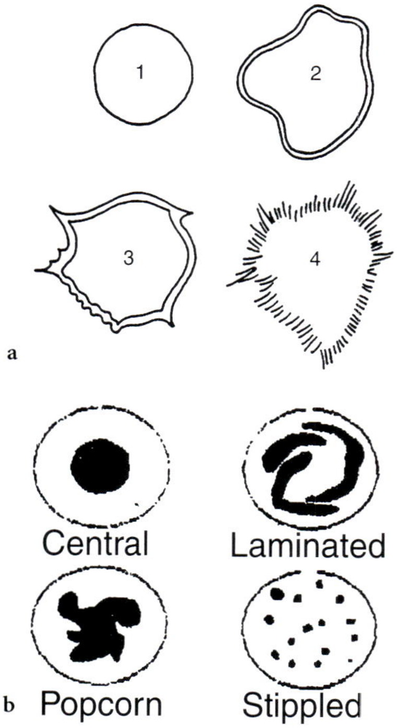

Fig. 30.2a,b. a Figure taken from a radiologic text used in Court, by the Plaintiff, in an attempt to have the expert witness define specifically the nature and character of the nodular lesion seen in the lung. **b** Figure taken from a radiologic test used in Court, by the Plaintiff, in an effort to have the radiologic expert witness define the nature of the calcifications seen in the CT studyure 2b Figure taken from a radiologic test used in Court, by the Plaintiff, in an effort to have the radiologic expert witness define the nature of the calcifications seen in the CT study.

multi-slice CT images. They were instructed on the patterns of calcification and the subtleties of edge analysis that are applied in ascertaining whether the lesion was smooth, rounded, lobular, or spiculated. The details that are presented in jury instruction in such cases astound most radiologists who are being defended for potential malpractice litigation.

In this instance, the plaintiff was seeking damages in excess of $5 million. Prior to litigation, the defendant had offered some $1 million in settlement, which was refused by the plaintiff. During the course of litigation there was concern early in the trial that the evidence was not sufficiently compelling for an acquittal of the defendant. The defendant's counsel agreed to increase the settlement. These offers were refused by the plaintiff. This is not unusual for cases where the plaintiff is confident that he/she will be victorious in the jury decision. However, in this case, the last part of the testimony read to the jury was from the notes in the file of the defendant's expert.

Notes for File: "The Patient presents with acute diverticulitis and a pericolonic abscess. A CT of the abdomen was performed, which clearly shows a substantial abnormality in the pelvis. There is an incidental peripheral note made of what may be a granuloma in the lingula of the left lung. The conclusion of the radiologist is that it was a granuloma. That is what a reasonably prudent physician may do under the same or similar circumstances. In this case, however, it appears to have been in error. Apparently, this turned out to be a carcinoma. I believe that one would not expect the surgeon to do anymore about this case once the definitive statement of granuloma is made, and that statement may be slightly over reaching compared to what I would have said. However, in my opinion, it is not inconsistent with what a reasonably well qualified physician may have done under the same circumstances."

This testimony conveyed sufficient uncertainty for the jury to diminish the award below what had been offered to the plaintiff. The modulation in the magnitude of the award was, in part, due to the jury's awareness that a normally prudent radiologist may well have concluded this to be a granuloma. This case raises many issues that are extremely common when reviewing multi-detector CTs of the chest.

30.2 The Problem of Thoracic CTs

For those who advocate screening CTs, the problem of miscast granulomas is even more acute. The frequency with which granulomas are identified in the midwest of the United States is so high that it calls into question the use of CT screening as a routine procedure (Swensen 2002). Diagnostic decisions are, in part, based on ambient frequency of disease. The utility of the features used to distinguish granulomas from carcinoma is, in part, dependent on the ambient frequency of the disease. Since most granulomas that are found on screening are benign, it is extremely difficult to ascertain which of these lesions is a carcinoma. This case well exemplifies that problem.

A cautious observer may well increase false positive diagnoses in the face of frequent granulomas and a threat of malpractice litigation. False positive interpretation on screening thoracic CTs may lead to unnecessary further diagnostic interventions, such as needle or surgical biopsies. These, too, carry a risk. The radiologist, who is concerned about the legal liability in missing a cancer and who compensates by increased false positive interpretations of benign disease, may be liable if the patient were to be injured in a subsequent diagnostic procedure. While it is reasonable to be concerned about this possibility, there is no ready reference to a case where such a false positive interpretation resulted in an award to the plaintiff for medical malpractice based on an "overcall." By far, the most common complaint is "failure to diagnose" when the disease is present. Thus, if one seeks to diminish malpractice risk, it is reasonable to practice defensive medicine by erring on the side of the false positive. The economic consequences of this phenomenon are formidable.

In this case, the question as to whether or not the carcinoma arose in or near the granuloma was contested in court. However, since a carcinoma eventually occurred in this region of the patient's lung, the plaintiff's position presumed that the abnormality detected on the initial CT was the cancer. The cancer was neither clinically apparent nor diagnosed for more than one year after the contested CT examinations were performed. At that time the patient had symptoms that required a thoracic CT exam, and a malignancy was identified.

This case raises many questions that may not be appreciated by most physicians. Why is the physician liable if he/she cannot prove the cancer was present on the original CT exam? Why is the radiologist liable at all? Through a further understanding of the duties of a professional, the reader might better appreciate the answers to these questions. Often, physicians, who are disturbed about the state of medical malpractice liability, do not seem to recognize the ambiguities everyone deals with in making decisions. In reality, these are no different for a radiologist trying to decide at the border lands of interpretation and the jury trying to decide who, if anyone, to hold responsible when someone is injured.

30.3 The Legal Basis for Professional Liability

Physicians are liable for their acts in the practice of medicine, because professionals assume a public trust which includes acting responsibly. What does it mean to act responsibly? The law considers that a responsible person would do what reasonably prudent people do under the same or similar circumstances.

All meaningful decisions are made under conditions of uncertainty. All decisions under uncertainty have an error rate. Errors will occur when making decisions in ambiguous circumstances. Errors, per se, are not malpractice.

Radiologists, when interpreting a film, provide information. Information is defined as a reduction in uncertainty, i.e., a reduction in randomness. Radiologists are in the business of uncertainty reduction. The very process of medical diagnosis results in some errors and many diagnostic errors occur that are not medical malpractice. Diagnostic errors are an everyday occurrence. Most of these errors do not reach the threshold of being outside of the standard of care.

30.4 The Use of Errors

Japanese insight into quality assurance sees "error as opportunity." In the United States we have been "mistake phobic." It is this fear of making mistakes that, in part, has occasioned a considerable increase in the amount of tests done in the United States when compared to other countries. Defensive medicine, as practiced in the United States, is related to a culture where people are so afraid to risk an error that they do things that are not only unnecessary, but sometimes are potentially hazardous. Diagnostic decisions rooted in defensive practices result in a marked increase in false positive interpretations. A screening CT with a questionable abnormality may result in follow-up studies, some of which may be risky. If the CT had not been performed, the biopsy would never have occurred. Or in legal terms, "but for" the CT, the patient would not have been subjected to the risk of a biopsy.

Radiologists, who are prone to have a high number of false positive results, will suggest more biopsies. Moreover, the biopsy is more likely to be normal when radiologists, who read the films, are adverse to risk. Those who practice radiology and are highly sensitive to the threat of malpractice litigation may suggest a biopsy with a significantly greater frequency than the average radiologist. The number of biopsies suggested per thoracic CT varies widely among radiologists. While this defensive practice may not result in malpractice litigation, this behavior is frequently unwarranted and diminishes the fidelity of the examination procedure.

A reasonable sensitivity to the risk of malpractice litigation is prudent behavior. However, where the frequency of disease is low with a screening procedure, over-reading the results may lead to more patients being harmed by the procedure than those benefiting from it.

Because of the risk of injury from excessive biopsies, most radiologists recommend close observation of suspicious nodules rather than recommend biopsy of nodular lesions of low suspicion for malignancy. They seek to observe the lesion over time to see if it changes in character, size, or configuration. This type of rational delay in those patients, who are eventually found to have cancer, is readily defensible in court. FDG positron emission tomography (PET) scanning is another approach to ambiguous nodules. PET may clarify whether a pulmonary nodule is likely to be malignant. Each of these decisions carries a risk of being the basis of malpractice litigation.

Malpractice litigation usually occurs when one party thinks something went wrong. They think an error was made. When performing images of any type, one has to be aware of what could possibly go wrong.

As in other radiologic procedures, multi-slice CT has many sources of potential error. There can be mistakes made in obtaining the image, in observing the image, in interpreting the image, and in reporting what is interpreted. Malpractice litigation often occurs when reports are either unclear, confusing, or ambiguous. Not only do these reports not make a substantial contribution to the care of the patient, they alone can lead to malpractice litigation. The technical aspects of obtaining the diagnostic image are infrequently the cause of malpractice litigation. The most likely source of malpractice litigation, when using multi-slice CT, is a failure to observe an abnormality that is subsequently seen by someone else. For the case to become the subject of a malpractice suit, the patient or the patient's family must suspect that a mistake has been made.

The control of professional behavior has traditionally been held by the profession. Through the system of tort litigation, however, the public plays a role in controlling professional behavior. There are three ways the legal system impacts on the control of professional behavior: tort litigation, legislation, and rule making. In the United States, tort litigation is a far more common means of public control than is legislation or rule making. In civil law, a tort is defined as a wrong doing for which damages can be sought by the injured party. Errors in patient care are not necessarily negligence. Errors can be tolerated by the legal system as long as they are within the bounds of what a reasonably prudent person would do under the same or similar circumstances. Physicians are not held to a standard of perfection.

In some instances, where the mismanagement of a patient's care is so egregious, the courts may find *res ipsa loquitor*, which means "the facts speak for themselves." These are found in such cases as removing the wrong limb in an orthopedic surgical procedure or the wrong kidney in a urological surgical procedure. However, *res ipsa loquitor* cases are not often found in diagnostic medicine. Almost never have the facts alone been sufficient to say that without further prove this is such an egregious mistake that a reasonably prudent person would not do it. Some expert must convince the "trier of fact" (the judge or jury) that what was done was outside the standard of care.

In order for medical malpractice litigation to be successful, the elements of negligence must be met. The elements of negligence are fourfold: (1) A *duty* to practice to the standard of care. This duty must be (2) *breached*. For example, the professional duty is breached when a physician does not practice to the standard of care. This breach of the standard of care must be the (3) *proximate cause* of a (4) *substantial injury*.

The requirement for proximate cause is often not understood by physicians being sued for medical malpractice. The legal thresholds of a causal relationship between an act and an injury begin with the "but for" doctrine. This means that but for the action of the physician, the patient would not have sustained an injury. While this is a necessary component of cause, it is insufficient. The legal term for the threshold required for a successful malpractice action by a plaintiff is "proximate cause." Not only would the injury not have occurred "but for" the actions of the physician, but there were no intervening causes between what the physician did and what happened to the patient. The negligent act must be the "proximate" cause of the injury. Often in malpractice litigation, even when the physicians are found to be in breach of a standard of care, they are not found guilty of negligence, because what they did was not the proximate cause of the injury sustained by the patient. All four elements (duty, breach, proximate cause and substantial injury) are necessary before medical malpractice can be established.

In some cases, even though there is an obvious breach of a duty, the patient is so ill at the time of the radiologic procedure, that even if the diagnosis had been made at the time the radiologist missed the lesion, it would have had little or no effect on what eventually happened to the patient. In this instance, even an egregious error may not be considered to be the proximate cause of "a substantial injury." For example, in some cases of lung cancer the disease is so far advanced at the time of the initial imaging procedure that the injury would have occurred even had the radiologist been correct in the interpretation.

What is considered a breach in the standard of care? A breach requires an act that a responsible person would not do. What is a responsible person? An external standard is applied to the situation, i.e., others have to conclude that the act done was what a responsible person would do. The words used in evidence are "what a reasonably prudent person would do under the same or similar circumstances." The standard of care is not based on what an individual physician presumes is wrong or right in a specific case; rather, it relates to the contest of experts where the opposing experts assert that in their opinion the reasonably prudent physician would or would not have done this. It has to be believed by an independent trier of fact, either a judge or a jury. Thus, one cannot get up and say that he/she acts responsibly, because he/she is a responsible person. Others must reach the same conclusion to avoid the risk of medical malpractice litigation. Responsibility is defined as the art of doing what is right. And these facts are determined by an independent, unbiased party.

30.5 The Nature of Medical Malpractice

Reviews of American medical practice suggest that the number of malpractice cases filed is considerably fewer than the number of malpractice events that have occurred. There are far fewer malpractice claims filed in court than malpractice incidents which take place in the American health care system.

The median period between the occurrence of the malpractice incident and a payment for the injury is three years. In some 40 million patients hospitalized each year in the U.S., it is estimated that 1.5 million suffer some kind of disabling injury on the basis of this medical encounter. Of these, approximately 400,000 involve negligence on the part of some provider. More than 100,000 involve fatal and serious permanent injuries. However, less than 50,000 malpractice suites are filed every year, fewer than half of the claimants receive any payments, and a sizable number of the remainder collect very little money because of the "tenuous quality of the claims." (Weller 1995)

Twice the proportion (11% v. 5%) of malpractice suits go to trial than do other types of personal injury suits. This is, in part, because the public, as a whole, has confidence in physicians, and many people realize that physicians, too, are human. If physicians believe this and act in a caring manner, malpractice litigation can often be avoided by the patient who believes that the physician did his or her best in any given situation. Indeed, the best protection against malpractice litigation, in addition to diminishing errors, is to have a favorable relationship with a patient.

Most patients realize that medicine is imperfect. Physicians should also realize that. The arrogance of medicine does more to initiate malpractice litigation than any other single element. In fact, if one starts to trace the initial consideration of malpractice litigation from patients, the findings will point to the physician who did not respect the patient's concerns to the level that the patient felt was appropriate.

The citizens and lawyers of the U.S. are not wantonly litigious. A nationwide RAND Institute survey found that of every 100 citizens who reported they were injured, only 19 considered legal action. Only seven of those consulted a lawyer, and only two of them found a lawyer willing to file a suit. In this instance, only one of those 100 collected any tort damage, whether by settlement or by verdict (Weller 1995).

The frequency with which lung lesions are missed on chest x-ray has been well documented (Muhm et al. 1983). With the use of CT there may be fewer missed lesions, but there are more likely to be more false positive interpretations. While litigation for false positive diagnosis is by no means as common as litigation for a diagnosis where the lesion is subsequently found, the fact is that thoracic multislice CT studies produce many more false positive results, which occasionally injure the patient. This suggests that an over-abundance of false positive interpretations may become an increasing problem for the medical legal system. In the NSCLC Study (US Public Health Service 1981; Potchen and Austin 1993), the correct diagnosis for 19% of 259 patients with non-small cell lung cancer, which presented as a nodular lesion in the chest radiograph, were initially missed. They were only discovered on a later study. This miss rate was not dependent on location. Superimposing structures were more often present in the group of missed lesions, and, therefore, it is likely that CT will pick up many of these lesions not identified on plain chest films. The defense when a lesion is missed on CT is similar to the defense that one could bring for chest x-rays. The distinction between an acceptable missed lesion that a reasonably prudent person would miss relates to its conspicuity. Conspicuity determines the ability to discern a lesion. It is measured by observing the difference in the rate of change in density and contrast between the lesion and the surround. Quite similarly, that is one of the many features that will raise the specter of potential abnormality on a screening CT. Lack of conspicuity has been an effective defense in malpractice for missed lung cancers in standard chest x-rays.

References

Muhm J, Miller WE, Fontana RS, Sanderson DR, Uhlenhopp MA (1983) Lung cancer detected during a screening program using four-month chest radiographs. Radiology 148: 609–615

Potchen EJ, Austin JHM (1993) Problems and pitfalls in the diagnosis of early lung cancer. In: Potchen EJ, Granger RG, Greene R (eds) Pulmonary radiology. The Fleischner Society. Saunders, Philadelphia

Siegelman SS, Khouri NF, Leo FP, Fishman EK, Braverman RM, Zerhouni EA (1986) Solitary pulmonary nodules: CT assessment. Radiology 160:307–312

Swensen S (2002) High false-positive rate seen with CT scans for lung. Am J Roentgenol 179:833–842

US Public Health Service (1981) Surveillance, epidemiology and end results: incidence and mortality data, 1973–1977. Natl Cancer Inst Monogr 57

Weller PC (1995) Fixing the tail: the place of malpractice in health care reform. Rudgers Law Review, Spring, p 1157

31 Future Technical Developments for CT of the Thorax

W. A. Kalender and M. Kachelriess

CONTENTS

31.1 Introduction

What will the future bring? It is unnecessary to state that any prediction may prove to be wrong in the years to come, or, in the worst case, as soon as the book is printed. (This may be a reason why a wise editor transfers the respective task to make predictions to a potential author who is not wise enough to deny the task.) Predictions, or better yet, the discussion of future developments can be based on what technology and physics will provide, or it can be based on what the clinical demands are or will likely be. The question is: Will future developments be technology driven or application driven?

The initial development of spiral CT was application driven. The original project was initiated by the desire to detect pulmonary nodules reliably (Kalender et al. 1990; Vock et al. 1990). While it was easy to show early on that spiral CT allowed to provide the necessary performance in principle (Fig. 31.1a), it also became apparent immediately that the available technology, in particular the available X-ray power, was insufficient to image complete organs of large size, such as the lungs, fast enough and with high spatial resolution. The general goal of imaging complete organs in time intervals shorter than a breath-hold period and at high isotropic resolution was not limited to the thorax, of course. In particular, all applications involving contrast medium administration and CT angiography in particular demanded faster scanning.

The necessary and successful strategy in the 1990s was to provide multi-row detectors so that several slices could be measured simultaneously. The state of the art which has been reached after 14 years of spiral CT and which is documented in this textbook is represented by scanners which allow to acquire 16 slices of less than 1 mm each with a scanner rotation time of 0.5 s or less per 360° (Fig. 31.1b). It has been described in an excellent manner in the preceding chapters, both with respect to physics and technology and with respect to clinical applications. Isotropic sub-millimeter spatial resolution and effective scan times as low as 100 ms are essential features which are routinely available. Apparently, CT has reached a very high level of performance, and it may seem that the present multi-slice scanners already fulfill all clinical demands.

Is there still a need for further technical developments in CT? Will future developments be driven by technology or by applications? Economic reason tells us that developments have to be application driven. From the preceding chapters we learned, however, that only phase-selective imaging of the heart and the coronary arteries may demand further improvements in technology.

At the same time we observe many research activities in the field of experimental CT imaging with area detectors and circular or spiral cone-beam scan trajectories. The underlying mathematical concepts form a completely new field of science (e.g., see Huesman 2002; Wang et al. 2000). Moreover, there are many promising and exciting results already. The CT imaging based on flat-panel detector technology is a hot topic as is pointed out in Chap. 3; respective images show impressive anatomical detail of the order of 100–300 µm (Fig. 31.2a). High-resolution imaging of biopsies, specimens, and small animals has become known as "micro-CT" (Karolczak et al. 2001; Siewerdsen and Jaffray 2000). Based on small focus or "micro-focus" X-ray tubes and area detectors with small pixel pitch, it allows, for example, to image anatomy in experimental animals such as gene-manipulated mice

W. A. Kalender, PhD
Professor, Institute of Medical Physics, Universität Erlangen-Nürnberg, Krankenhausstrasse 12, 91054 Erlangen, Germany
M. Kachelriess, PhD
Institute of Medical Physics, Universität Erlangen-Nürnberg, Krankenhausstrasse 12, 91054 Erlangen, Germany

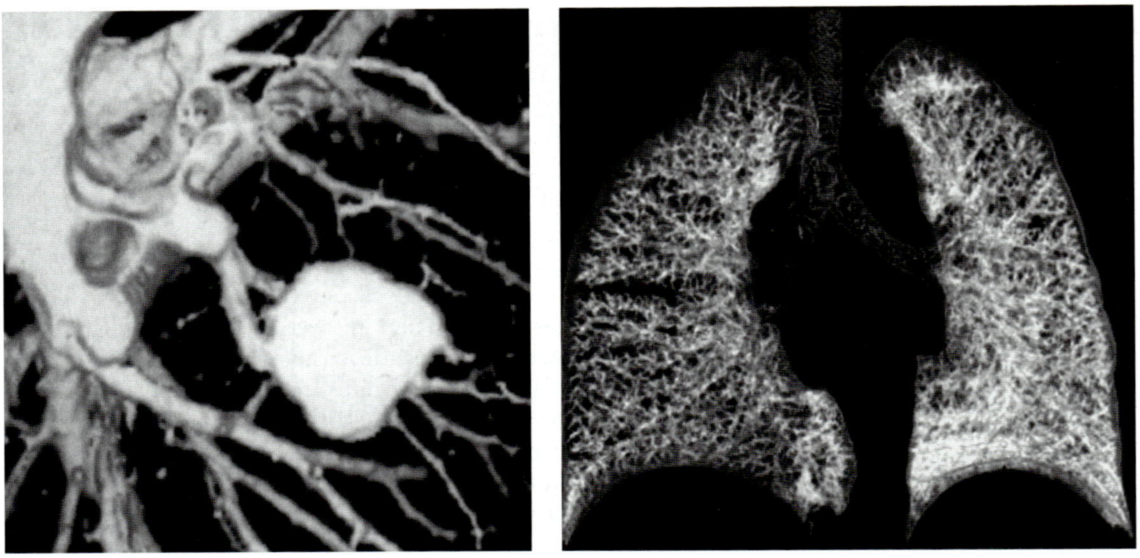

a b

Fig. 31.1a, b. Spiral CT has made tremendous progress within approximately one decade. a The first scans of the thorax in 1989 were taken with single-row scanners at 10-mm collimation. b In 2001, 16-slice scanning at sub-millimeter collimation and with isotropic spatial resolution became available

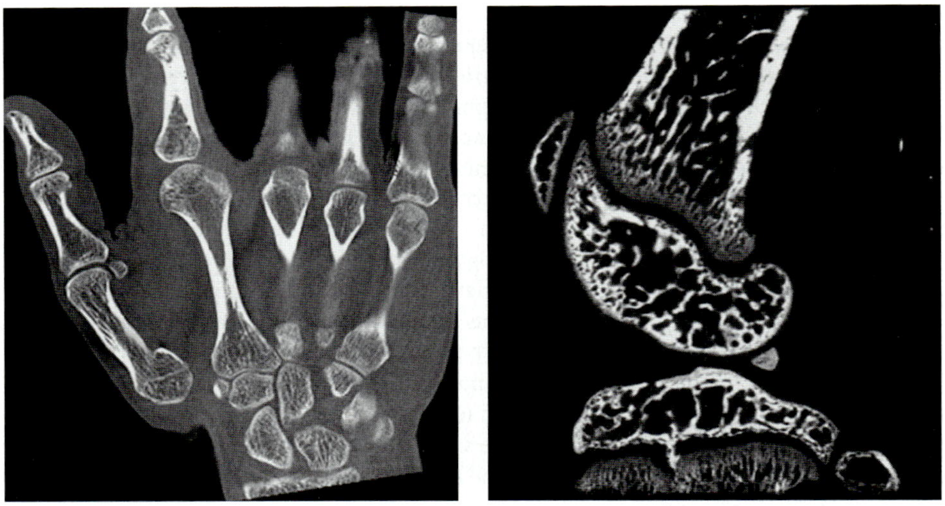

a b

Fig. 31.2a, b. High-resolution cone-beam CT using flat-panel detectors provides impressive anatomical detail and indicates the potential for further improvements in CT. a Image of a human hand at approximately 200-µm isotropic resolution. (Courtesy of Siemens Medical Solutions). b Image of a mouse knee at approximately 20-µm isotropic resolution

at levels of 10–100 µm (Fig. 31.2b). Although there are many drawbacks and limitations to be considered with respect to potential clinical use, these activities stimulate appetite. Expectations are boosted further by marketing-driven hyperpositive statements from some of the manufacturers. In all, this may cause future developments to be driven by advances in technology rather than by clinical demand.

In 2002 the question frequently asked was: "Will the slice race continue?" All manufacturers try to live up to customer demands and expectations, and consequently they investigate solutions for detectors with higher numbers of slices or area detectors which allow covering the organ or region of interest in a single view.

This final chapter initially focuses on respective possible or likely developments in technology. It continues with considerations of image quality and dose to point out which basic physics constraints have to be kept in mind. It comes back to application-related aspects in the Conclusion section.

31.1 Technical Developments

Technical developments can be divided into those related to scanner mechanics, X-ray system, detector, etc., the "hardware" as the first category, and into image reconstruction, data handling, dedicated evaluation software, and other algorithms, with the "software" as the second category. We discuss hardware-related aspects first.

It is obvious that the rotation frequency of mechanical gantries can be increased further. There are many technical instruments of similar size and mass which rotate much faster; however, there are two problems related to CT: the number and the complexity of subsystems such as integrated circuit boards, rotating X-ray tube anodes, etc., which would demand very specific adaptations to cope with the increasing centrifugal forces. This means increased or prohibitive cost and, in the worst case, susceptibility to failure. Another important aspect is that it will be difficult to provide the necessary number of X-ray photons in shorter and shorter rotation times. Electron-beam CT is capable of performing scans within 100 ms or less; however, for high image quality and good low-contrast resolution single sweeps have to be added up resulting in high effective scan times. This was the reason why CT adopted multi-row detector technology and multi-slice scanning when the demand for higher-volume scan speed arose (Kalender 2003). Further reduction of rotation times seems to be indicated only for cardiac applications, and this is technically feasible. Rotation times of 0.2 or 0.3 s are the goal and would allow for effective scan times of below 100 ms using state-of-the-art algorithms for phase-selective cardiac reconstructions (Kachelriess and Kalender 1998; Kachelriess et al. 2000a, b). Fast "conventional "scanners dedicated to cardiac applications are likely to become available in the future.

To provide detectors beyond the current state of the art of 16 simultaneously acquired slices is certainly possible, and they will become available in the near future. The design of multi-row detectors (an example is shown in Fig. 31.3a) can be extended; a prototype of a 256-row true CT detector (Fig. 31.3b) has already gone into operation. The related technical challenge is, to a lesser extent, the detector itself, but rather the electronics involved and the cost associated with it. In any case, CT detectors in larger formats with performance characteristics equivalent to the present prime clinical systems will become available. Only the point in time and the cost are unknown.

In addition, other types of detectors, primarily flat-panel detectors designed for conventional X-ray imaging, are under investigation. Amorphous silicon (aSi) flat-panel detectors (FPD; Fig. 31.3c) and image-intensifier systems (Fig. 31.3d) are in clinical use already for special applications such as for 3D angiography or intra-operative imaging of high-contrast structures. Smaller-format solutions, such as charge-coupled devices (CCD) coupled optically to a phosphor screen, are in use for small-animal imaging (Fig. 31.3e) but do not easily lend themselves to an extension for clinical use comparable to the present standard CT image quality level; however, beyond the available sizes there is another essential problem associated with these "non-CT"-type detectors: their characteristics, mostly the dynamic range, dose efficiency, and temporal response will be limiting their performance with respect to low-contrast imaging.

To make up for low absorption efficiency by higher exposure, and thereby higher patient dose, is not acceptable and will not be permitted due to regulations on the general use of CT. The definition and enforcement of reference dose levels for most standard CT applications, for example, will prevent the introduction of detectors with reduced dose efficiency (Die neue Röntgenverordnung 2002; European Commission's Study Group 1998). Limitations in dynamic range and poor temporal resolution of present flat-panel detectors additionally imply limitations with respect to image quality. With the hope that researchers and industrial developers prove us wrong, we predict that flat-panel detector technology will not be able to replace dedicated CT-detector technology. Such detectors, will, however, establish themselves for special applications such as intra-operative imaging.

With respect to other hardware components, it is easy to predict that CT will benefit from the general technical development. Performance increases for computing power following Moore's law are likely. The same applies to other components such as data rendering and display technology. Improvements with respect to X-ray power, an old and mature technology, will not be dramatic. Tremendous improvements have been provided since the introduction of spiral CT. But the physical and technical potential for further improvements is limited, and so is the motivation. The advent of multi-slice acquisition meant that the demand for long scan times diminished. It is not higher average power, but – if at all – higher peak power ratings that are demanded, in particular for cardiac CT with its short scan times.

Some software developments, e.g., new approaches to image reconstruction and to computer-aided diag-

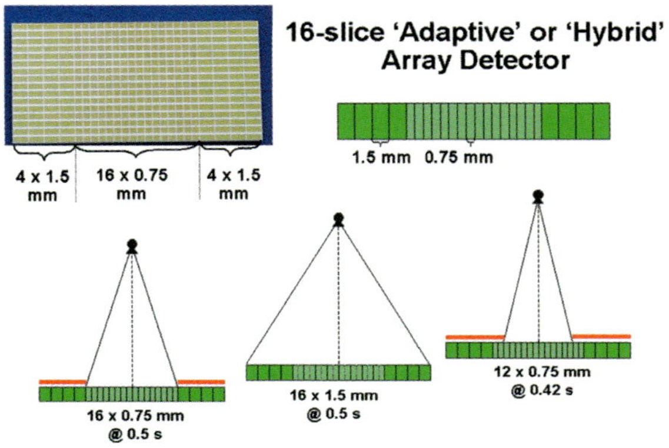

a

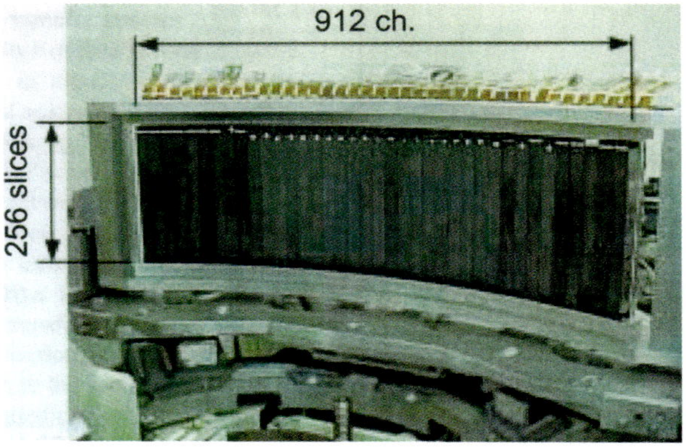

b

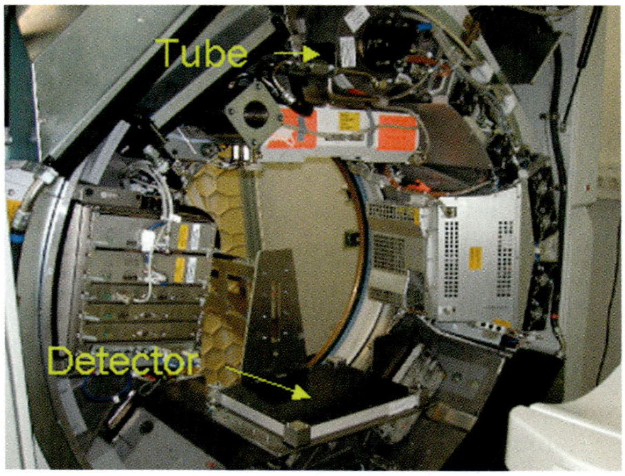

c

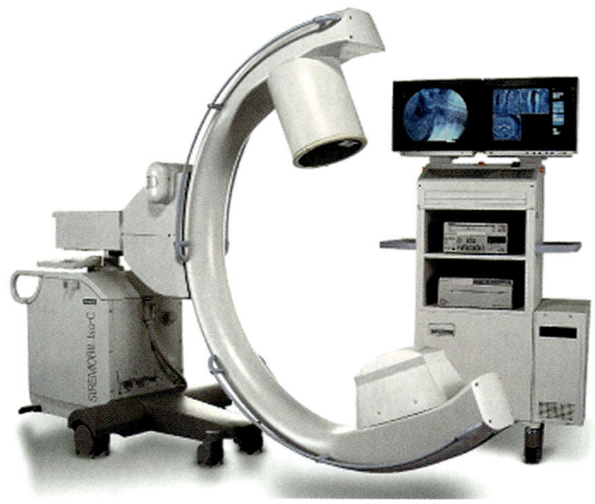

d

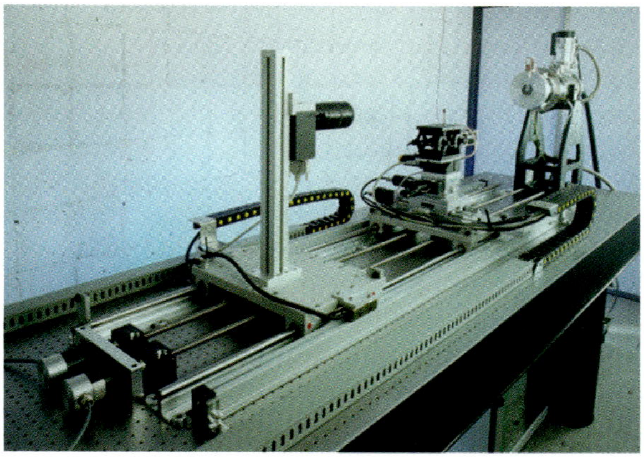

e

Fig. 31.3a–e. Area detectors for CT data acquisition. **a** Typical detector array used in clinical CT at present. It allows acquisition of data for 16 slices of 0.75 mm simultaneously or alternatively 16 slices of 1.5-mm thickness each. **b** New concept for a 256-slice CT detector. (Courtesy of Toshiba Medical Systems). **c** Radiographic flat-panel detector integrated into a CT gantry. (Courtesy of Siemens Medical Solutions). **d** Image intensifier on a mobile C-arm used for intra-operative CT imaging of skeletal structures. (Courtesy of Siemens Medical Solutions). **e** Experimental setup for micro-CT using a charge-coupled devices coupled optically to a phosphor screen

nosis, have been discussed in previous chapters. An important question for future developments is the question of whether reconstruction algorithms will be available that provide the established high level of image quality for scanners with slice numbers far beyond 16. Respective concepts for algorithms have been published and evaluated, and the necessary optimized implementations will certainly become available. An excellent review of the present concepts is given in Chap. 1. The interested reader is also referred to specific literature (e.g., Wang et al. 2000; Huesman 2002; Kalender 2003).

By now, many results have been obtained for cone-beam CT (CBCT) by simulations (Fig. 31.4a) and in small-animal imaging (Fig. 31.4b). They indicate that image quality at a level comparable to the present 16-slice scanners will be possible for clinical CBCT scanners at 256 slices and beyond. The question which remains relates to the necessary reconstruction times which are prohibitively long for some of the reconstruction approaches. Nevertheless, we can expect that solutions adequate for routine clinical use will be available for CBCT. The situation which arose with the introduction of spiral CT will persist, however: data acquisition will be faster than image reconstruction. [We refer to multi-slice spiral CT (MSCT) as long as the assumption is acceptable that the different slice fans are strictly in parallel. This is the case up to four slices. Whenever the cone-beam geometry is taken into account explicitly during image reconstruction, we refer to CBCT.]

31.2 Image Quality and Dose

Image quality and dose in CT are very closely related. Most of the facts are well known. In particular, the dependence of noise on dose for otherwise unchanged parameters of scanning and image reconstruction holds true for conventional CT, for MSCT, and for the various forms of CBCT under discussion; however, there are aspects, such as the relationship between spatial resolution, i.e., the size of the resolution volume element, and dose, which are not general knowledge at present. A review of the situation has been given recently (Fuchs and Kalender 2003; Kalender 2003) and is also addressed in Chap. 3. We only briefly restate the important findings and comment specifically on the situation which results in increases in spatial resolution that can be provided with future CBCT systems (Fig. 31.2).

Patient dose in CT is one of the most important topics regarding the future as the general acceptance of CT is often linked to dose issues and potential associated risks. It will be essential in the future to provide the information about the actual patient dose values for any given CT examination. Such efforts have started recently (Kalender et al. 1999; Nagel 2000). Information will help to counteract some of the irrational fears. It is the conviction of the present authors that CT is in fact a low-dose modality. Using state-of-the-art approaches, as already described in

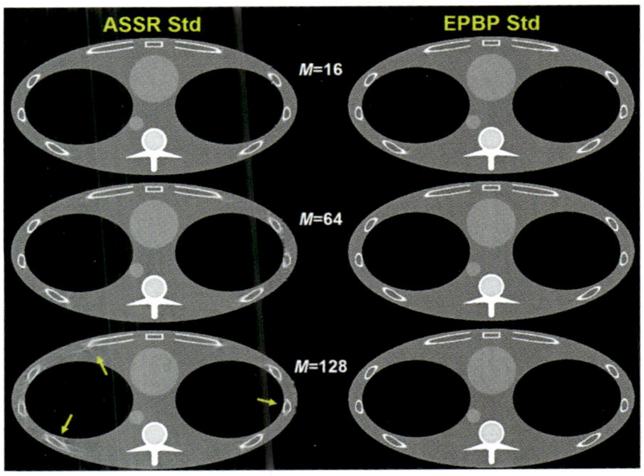

a

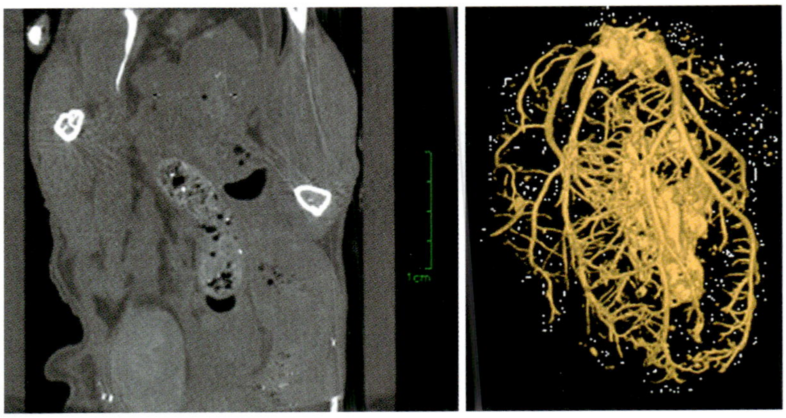

b

Fig. 31.4. Cone-beam CT reconstruction algorithms and image quality have been assessed with very promising results in **a** simulations and in **b** practical applications such as small animal imaging. Dose-efficient algorithms are available which provide adequate image quality even for large slice numbers chapter 3, it can be assured that the effective dose to the patient will be kept low, typically at 0.1–20 mSv, and definitely far below the 200-mSv value which is considered as the limit of the "low-dose region" (Kalender 2003).

The necessary concepts for dose management are described in detail in Chap. 3. In general, patient dose increases linearly with the tube current–time product, the "mAs product," for unmodulated tube current and for all other parameters kept unchanged; noise varies inversely with the square root of the mAs product. This holds true for scanning in sequential and in spiral mode, and for single-slice, multi-slice, and cone-beam CT. The mAs product and thereby the noise level are chosen according to the diagnostic needs. Modulation of the tube current during each rotation and along the z-axis according to the attenuation allows reduction of dose and tube load efficiently without a loss in image quality. The development of highest relevance for the future of CT is an automated exposure control (AEC) which will make sure that a given level of image quality which has to be defined or selected by the user will be provided in an automatic fashion (Fig. 31.5). Respective technical concepts and implementations are available by now as is pointed out in Chap. 3. These developments will become the state of the art in the future. They will ensure that, with image quality kept at a specified level, patient dose levels will decrease.

What are specific aspects relevant to CBCT? Irrespective of the aforementioned considerations, dose will depend on the detector's geometric and absorption efficiency. The present CT detectors operate at high levels of typically 80% or better with respect to both parameters. The absorption efficiency of flat-panel detectors is significantly lower, however, as has been pointed out already. With respect to geometric efficiency, we have to consider that several of the scan and reconstruction approaches proposed at present do not make full use of all rays measured. This problem is not well known and not transparent to the user. Often, data measured in the periphery of the area detector cone are not used in the reconstruction process. There are concepts and proven approaches by now, however, which allow full use of the data (Fig. 31.4a, right; Kachelriess and Kalender 2002); therefore, if the problem of absorption efficiency is solved, detector and dose efficiency will not pose a principle problem in the future.

There are constraints set by physics, however, which will remain unaltered and which set limits. Image noise increases with the fourth power of the spatial resolution element, e.g., measured as the sampling distance (Fig. 31.6). Intuitively, this fact can be understood when looking at images reconstructed with different convolution kernels: image noise is reduced strongly when going from a sharp to a smooth convolution kernel. The mathematical background was elaborated in the early days of CT. It has been clarified both theoretically and experimentally again lately in view of the new situation with high-resolution flat-panel detectors (Fuchs and Kalender 2003).

When going from a typical multi-row CT detector offering approximately 0.5- to 0.8-mm sampling

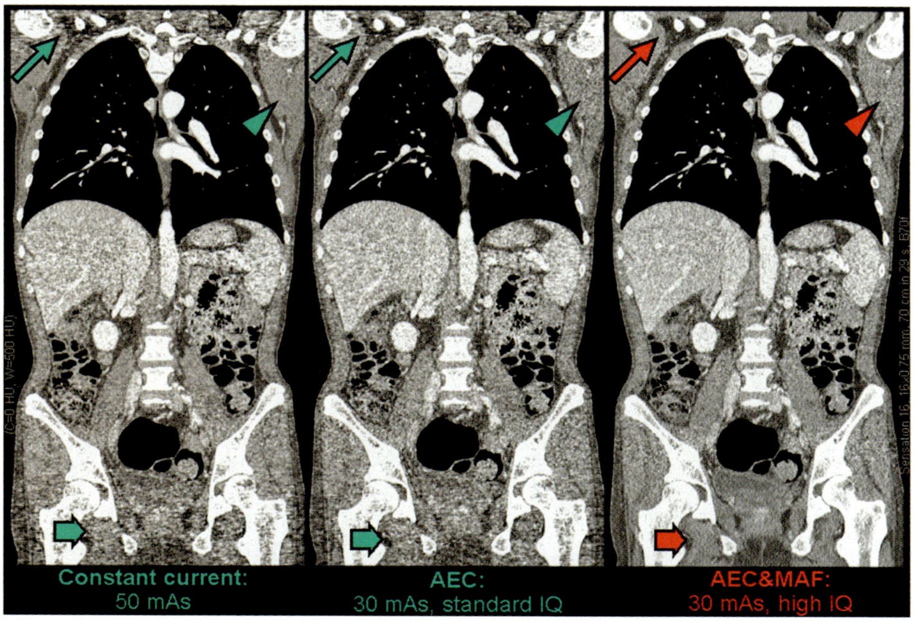

Fig. 31.5. Automatic exposure control in CT. In standard scanning with constant tube current (*left*) image quality varies with anatomical level. Modulation of the tube current with projection angle and z-position allows to reduce mAs significantly without a loss in image quality (*middle*). Adaptive filtering which does not impair resolution leads to improved image quality at reduced mAs (*right*)

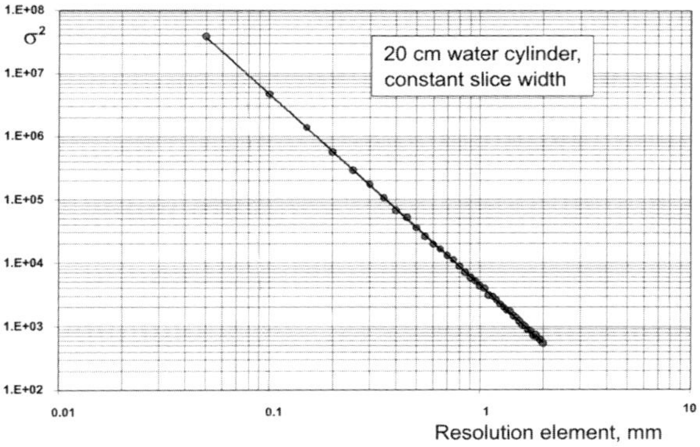

Fig. 31.6. Fundamental relationships between noise and spatial resolution. Image noise is inversely related to the fourth power of isotropic 3D spatial resolution. (From FUCHS and KALENDER 2003)

distance at the center of rotation to a flat-panel array the sampling distance is reduced typically by factors of 3 to 5. It is exactly this feature which is marketed by manufacturers presently as the promise of "CT of the future"; "100-μm resolution" are quoted even in direct reference to cardiac applications. Clearly, we do not expect that this will be the future of clinical CT. Scanners operating at such levels of resolution can be set to use in research situations with small objects such as biopsies or small animals. This is the case already at present. Here the implication of the increase in spatial resolution on dose is tolerable as the object diameter and thereby attenuation decreases by orders of magnitude. The scan of a mouse shown in Fig. 31.4b is associated with an effective dose of typically 200 mSv.

In clinical CT, such as, for example, in CT of the thorax, reduction of the sampling distance by a factor of 4 and a respective increase in spatial resolution would mean an increase in dose of 256 if we expect the same noise level as for the standard scan. This is not acceptable! We are in the comfortable situation presently that typical values of the effective dose in CT are of the order of or up to tenfold the natural background radiation levels (KALENDER 2003). To postulate significant increases in spatial resolution with otherwise unchanged parameters would demand higher X-ray power and would incur significantly increased radiation levels well into the order of magnitude where even deterministic radiation effects can be expected. Confirmation that this is not just a theoretical scenario can be obtained from small-animal imaging: according to reports from the U.S., mice have died due to scanning at very high resolution in inefficient micro-CT scanners. The simple but fundamental message of Fig. 31.6 cannot be ignored. If strongly increased spatial resolution is desired, strongly increased noise levels have to be accepted. This means that low-contrast resolution or soft tissue discrimination will suffer or remain limited.

31.3 Conclusion

Computed tomography in general and, similarly, CT of the thorax, have reached a very high level of performance. The technology can be considered mature, the dose levels are acceptable, and most clinicians are content at present. There is no doubt that there will be further improvements: scan speed will be increased, the size of detector arrays will be enlarged, reconstruction approaches and speed will be improved, and all this will make CT scanning easier both for the radiology staff and for the patients. The rate of progress driven by technology will not be as overwhelming as it was in the past years. Patient dose considerations will set the limit in many respects.

Applications of CT in the thorax will be improved also. Dynamic CT, e.g., for the determination of ventilation and perfusion of the lung, myocardial perfusion measurements, and cardiac CT in general, are to be named. Moreover, cardiac CT appears to be the one and only candidate which may initiate significant application-driven developments. The use of detector arrays wide enough to cover the complete heart offers fundamentally new capabilities. Imaging of the complete heart will thereby be reduced from now typically 10–30 s to the order of 1 s or less.

Acknowledgements. The figures in this chapter, unless labeled otherwise in the legend, have been taken from the textbook, "Computed Tomography" (KALENDER 2003), with permission of the publisher.

References

Die neue Röntgenverordnung (2002) 9th edn. Hoffmann, Berlin
European Commission's Study Group (1998) Quality criteria for computed tomography. EUR 16262
Fuchs T, Kalender WA (2003) On the correlation of pixel noise, spatial resolution and dose in computed tomography: theoretical prediction and verification by simulation and measurement. Physica Medica (in press)
Huesman RH (ed) (2002) Sixth international meeting on fully three-dimensional reconstruction in radiology and nuclear medicine. Phys Med Biol 47 (and http://cfi.lbl.gov/3D-2001/3D_Prog.html)

Kachelriess M, Kalender WA (1998) Electrocardiogram-correlated image reconstruction from subsecond spiral CT scans of the heart. Med Phys 25:2417–2431

Kachelriess M, Kalender WA (2002) Extended parallel backprojection for cardiac cone-beam CT for up to 128 slices. Radiology 225:310

Kachelriess M, Ulzheimer S, Kalender WA (2000a) ECG-correlated image reconstruction from subsecond multi-slice spiral CT scans of the heart. Med Phys 27:1881–1902

Kachelriess M, Ulzheimer S, Kalender WA (2000b) ECG-correlated imaging of the heart with subsecond multi-slice spiral CT. IEEE Trans Med Imaging (special issue) 19:888–901

Kalender WA (2003) Computed tomography. Wiley, New York

Kalender WA, Seissler W, Klotz E et al. (1990) Spiral volumetric CT with single-breath-hold technique, continuous transport, and continuous scanner rotation. Radiology 176:181–183

Kalender WA, Schmidt B, Zankl M et al. (1999) A PC program for estimating organ dose and effective dose values in computed tomography. Eur Radiol 9:555–562

Karolczak M, Schaller S, Engelke K et al. (2001) Implementation of a cone-beam reconstruction algorithm for the single circle source orbit with embedded misalignment correction using homogenous coordinates. Med Phys 26: 2050–2069

Nagel HD (ed) (2000) Radiation exposure in computed tomography. Fundamentals, influencing parameters, dose assessment, optimisation, scanner data, terminology. COCIR European Coordination Committee of the Radiological and Electromedical Industries, Frankfurt, Germany

Siewerdsen JH, Jaffray DA (2000) Optimization of X-ray imaging geometry (with specific application to flat-panel conebeam computed tomography). Med Phys 27:1903–1914

Vock P, Soucek M, Daepp M et al. (1990) Lung: spiral volumetric CT with single-breath-hold technique. Radiology 176:864–867

Wang G, Crawford CR, Kalender WA (eds) (2000) Special issue on multirow detector and cone-beam spiral/helical CT. IEEE Trans Med Imaging 19

Subject Index

List of Contributors

John Aldrich, PhD
Department of Radiology
Vancouver General Hospital
University of British Columbia and Vancouver
Hospital and Health Sciences Centre
855 West 12th Avenue
Vancouver, BC V5Z 1M9
Canada

Christoph R. Becker, MD
Department of Radiology
University Hospital Grosshadern
University of Munich
Marchioninistr. 15
81377 Munich
Germany

Catherine Beigelman-Aubry, MD
Service de Radiologie
Hopital de la Pitié-Salpêtrière
47-83, boulevard de l'Hopital
75651 Paris cedex 13
France

Phillip M. Boiselle, MD
Director of Thoracic Imaging
Beth Israel Deaconess Medical Center
Assistant Professor of Radiology, Harvard Medical School
Department of Radiology
330 Brookline Ave
Boston, MA 02215
USA

Philip Costello, MD
Department of Radiology
Harvard Medical School
Brigham and Women's Hospital
75 Francis Street
Boston, MA 02115
USA

Marco Das, MD
Department of Radiology
University Hospital
RWTH Aachen
Pauwelsstrasse 30
52074 Aachen
Germany

Ralph Drosten, MD
Thoracic and Onco-radiologist
Brigham and Women's Hospital
Dana-Farber Cancer Institute and
Harvard Medical School
Boston, MA 02115
USA

Catalin Fetita, PhD
Department ARTEMIS
Institut National des Télécommunications
9, rue Charles Fourier
91011 Evry cedex
France

Roman Fischbach, MD
Department of Clinical Radiology
University of Muenster
Albert-Schweitzer-Str. 33
48149 Muenster
Germany

Elliot K. Fishman, MD, FACR
The Russell H. Morgan Department of Radiology
and Radiological Science
Johns Hopkins University School of Medicine
601 North Caroline Street/Room 3254
Baltimore, MD 21287-0801
USA

Dominik Fleischmann, MD
Associate Professor of Radiology
Department of Angiography and Interventional Radiology
University of Vienna
Waehringer Guertel 18-20
1090 Vienna
Austria
and
Assistant Professor of Radiology
Divisions of Thoracic and Cardiovascular Imaging
Department of Radiology
Stanford University Medical Center
Stanford CA
USA

Thomas G. Flohr, PhD
CT Division
Siemens Medical Solutions
Siemensstr. 1
91301 Forchheim
Germany

Luciano Gattinoni, MD, FRCP
Professor of Anesthesiology
Istituto di Anestesia e Rianimazione
Università degli Studi di Milano
Ospedale Maggiore di Milano Italy I.R.C.C.S.
Milano
Italy

Benoît Ghaye, MD
Department of Medical Imaging
University Hospital of Liège
Sart Tilman B 35Liège
4000 Liège
Belgium

Lawrence R. Goodman, MD, FACR
Professor of Diagnostic Radiology and Pulmonary Medicine
Director, Thoracic Radiology
Department of Radiology
Medical College of Wisconsin
9200 West Wisconsin Ave
Milwaukee, WI 53226
USA

Philippe A. Grenier, MD
Professor, Service de Radiologie
Hopital de la Pitié-Salpêtrière
47–83, boulevard de l'Hopital
75651 Paris cedex 13
France

Claudia I. Henschke, PhD, MD
Professor, Department of Radiology
New York Presbyterian Hospital
Weill Medical College of Cornell University
525 East 68 Street
New York, NY 10021
USA

Christian J. Herold, MD
Professor of Radiology
Director, Medical Diagnostic Division
Department of Radiology
University of Vienna Medical School
General Hospital
Waehringer Guertel 18–20
1090 Vienna
Austria

Peter Herzog, MD
Institute of Clinical Radiology
Ludwig-Maximilians University of Munich
University Hospital Grosshadern
Marchioninistr. 15
81377 Munich
Germany

Andetta R. Hunsaker, MD
Assistant Professor of Radiology
Department of Radiology
Harvard Medical School
Brigham and Women's Hospital
75 Francis Street
Boston, MA 02115
USA

Francine L. Jacobson, MD, MPH
Department of Radiology
Brigham and Women's Hospital
Harvard Medical School
75 Francis Street
Boston, MA 02115
USA

Marc Kachelriess, PhD
Institute of Medical Physics (IMP)
University Erlangen-Nürnberg
Krankenhausstr. 12
91054 Erlangen
Germany

Willi A. Kalender, PhD
Professor, Institute of Medical Physics (IMP)
University Erlangen-Nürnberg
Krankenhausstr. 12
91054 Erlangen
Germany

Hans-Ulrich Kauczor, MD
Professor, Department of Radiology
Deutsches Krebsforschungszentrum (DKFZ)
Im Neuenheimer Feld 280
69120 Heidelberg
Germany

Jane P. Ko, MD
Assistant Professor of Radiology
New York University Medical Center
560 1st Avenue
New York, NY 10016
USA

William Kostis, PhD
Department of Radiology
New York Presbyterian Hospital
Weill Medical College of
Cornell University
525 East 68 Street
New York, NY 10021
USA

Leo P. Lawler, MB, FRCR
Assistant Professor
The Russell H. Morgan Department of Radiology
and Radiological Science
Johns Hopkins University
School of Medicine
601 North Caroline Street/Room 3254
Baltimore, MD 21287-0801
USA

Ann N. Leung, MD
Stanford University Medical Center
Department of Radiology
300 Pasteur Drive, Rm-S072
Stanford, CA 94305
USA

Reinhard Loose, MD, PhD
Institute for Diagnostic and Interventional Radiology
Hospital Nuremberg-North
Prof.-Ernst-Nathan-Str. 1
90419 Nuremberg
Germany

Jens M. Martensen, MD
Department of Radiology
Brigham and Women's Hospital
Harvard Medical School
75 Francis Street
Boston, MA 02115
USA

Yves Martin-Bouyer, MD
Service de Radiologie
Clinique du Val d'Or
16, rue Pasteur
92210 St Cloud
France

John R. Mayo, MD
Department of Radiology
University of British Columbia and Vancouver
Hospital and Health Sciences Centre
855 West 12th Avenue
Vancouver, BC V5Z 1M9
Canada

David P. Naidich, MD
Professor of Radiology and Medicine
Co-Director, Section Thoracic Imaging
New York University Medical Center
560 1st Avenue
New York, NY 10016
USA

A. Nchimi, MD
Department of Medical Imaging
Clinique Saint Joseph
4000 Liège
Belgium

Matthias U. Niethammer, MSc
Siemens Medical Solutions
Computed Tomography
Siemensstrasse 1
91301 Forchheim
Germany

Bernd M. Ohnesorge, PhD
CT Division
Siemens Medical Solutions
Siemensstr. 1
91301 Forchheim
Germany

Manfred Oldendorf, MD
Institute for Diagnostic and Interventional Radiology
Hospital Nuremberg-North
Prof.-Ernst-Nathan-Str. 1
90419 Nuremberg
Germany

Bernhard L. Partik, MD
Associate Professor of Radiology
Department of Radiology
University of Vienna Medical School
General Hospital
Waehringer Guertel 18-20
1090 Vienna
Austria

E. James Potchen, MD
University Distinguished Professor and
Chairman Department of Radiology
Michigan State University
160 Radiology Building
East Lansing, MI 48824
USA

Maximilian F. Reiser, MD
Professor and Chairman Institute of Clinical Radiology
Ludwig-Maximilians University of Munich
University Hospital Grosshadern
Marchioninistrasse 15
81377 München
Germany

Geoffrey D. Rubin, MD
Department of Radiology
Stanford University School of Medicine
Room S-072B
Stanford CA 94305-5105
USA

Stefan Schaller, PhD
CT Division
Siemens Medical Solutions
Siemensstr. 1
91301 Forchheim
Germany

Pierre Schnyder, MD
Professor, Department of Diagnostic
and Interventional Radiology
University Hospital (CHUV)
1011 Lausanne
Switzerland

U. Joseph Schoepf, MD
Department of Radiology
Brigham and Women's Hospital
Harvard Medical School
75 Francis Street
Boston, MA 02115
USA

Dorith Shaham, MD
Lecturer in Radiology
Hadassah University Hospital
Kiryat Hadassah
Jerusalem 91120
Israel

Sridhar Shankar, MD
Interventional and Onco-radiologist
Brigham and Women's Hospital and
Dana-Farber Cancer Institute
Instructor of Radiology
Harvard Medical School
Boston, MA 02115
USA

Marilyn J. Siegel, MD
Professor of Radiology and Pediatrics
Mallinckrodt Institute of Radiology
Washington University School of Medicine
510 South Kingshighway Blvd.
St. Louis, MO 63110
USA

Hans C. Steinert, MD
Senior staff Nuclear Medicine
Department of Medical Radiology
University Hospital
Raemistr. 100
8091 Zurich
Switzerland

Eric vanSonnenberg, MD
Chief of Radiology
Dana-Farber Cancer Institute
Interventional Radiology
Brigham and Women's Hospital
Visiting Professor of Radiology
Harvard Medical School
44 Binney St.
Boston, MA 02115
USA

Madeline Vazquez, MD
Associate Professor of Clinical Pathology
Weill Medical College of Cornell University
525 East 68 Street
New York, NY 10021
USA

Johny Verschakelen, MD, PhD
Professor, Department of Radiology
U.Z. Gasthuisberg
Herestraat 49
3000 Leuven
Belgium

Gustav K. von Schulthess, MD, PhD
Professor and Director, Nuclear Medicine
University Hospital
Raemistr. 100
8091 Zurich
Switzerland

Joachim Ernst Wildberger, MD
Department of Diagnostic Radiology
University Hospital
RWTH Aachen
Pauwelsstrasse 30
52074 Aachen
Germany

Max Wintermark, MD
Department of Diagnostic and Interventional Radiology
University Hospital (CHUV)
1011 Lausanne
Switzerland

Susan A. Wood, PhD
Vice President, CT Products
R2 Technology, Inc.
1195 West Freemont Avenue
Sunnyvale, CA 94087
USA

David Yankelevitz, MD
Professor, Department of Radiology
New York Presbyterian Hospital
Weill Medical College of Cornell University
525 East 68 Street
New York, NY 10021
USA

MEDICAL RADIOLOGY Diagnostic Imaging and Radiation Oncology

Titles in the series already published

DIAGNOSTIC IMAGING

Innovations in Diagnostic Imaging
Edited by J. H. Anderson

Radiology of the Upper Urinary Tract
Edited by E. K. Lang

The Thymus – Diagnostic Imaging, Functions, and Pathologic Anatomy
Edited by E. Walter, E. Willich, and W. R. Webb

Interventional Neuroradiology
Edited by A. Valavanis

Radiology of the Pancreas
Edited by A. L. Baert, co-edited by G. Delorme

Radiology of the Lower Urinary Tract
Edited by E. K. Lang

Magnetic Resonance Angiography
Edited by I. P. Arlart, G. M. Bongartz, and G. Marchal

Contrast-Enhanced MRI of the Breast
S. Heywang-Köbrunner and R. Beck

Spiral CT of the Chest
Edited by M. Rémy-Jardin and J. Rémy

Radiological Diagnosis of Breast Diseases
Edited by M. Friedrich and E.A. Sickles

Radiology of the Trauma
Edited by M. Heller and A. Fink

Biliary Tract Radiology
Edited by P. Rossi

Radiological Imaging of Sports Injuries
Edited by C. Masciocchi

Modern Imaging of the Alimentary Tube
Edited by A. R. Margulis

Diagnosis and Therapy of Spinal Tumors
Edited by P. R. Algra, J. Valk, and J. J. Heimans

Interventional Magnetic Resonance Imaging
Edited by J. F. Debatin and G. Adam

Abdominal and Pelvic MRI
Edited by A. Heuck and M. Reiser

Orthopedic Imaging
Techniques and Applications
Edited by A. M. Davies and H. Pettersson

Radiology of the Female Pelvic Organs
Edited by E. K.Lang

Magnetic Resonance of the Heart and Great Vessels
Clinical Applications
Edited by J. Bogaert, A.J. Duerinckx, and F. E. Rademakers

Modern Head and Neck Imaging
Edited by S. K. Mukherji and J. A. Castelijns

Radiological Imaging of Endocrine Diseases
Edited by J. N. Bruneton in collaboration with B. Padovani and M.-Y. Mourou

Trends in Contrast Media
Edited by H. S. Thomsen, R. N. Muller, and R. F. Mattrey

Functional MRI
Edited by C. T. W. Moonen and P. A. Bandettini

Radiology of the Pancreas
2nd Revised Edition
Edited by A. L. Baert
Co-edited by G. Delorme and L. Van Hoe

Emergency Pediatric Radiology
Edited by H. Carty

Spiral CT of the Abdomen
Edited by F. Terrier, M. Grossholz,and C. D. Becker

Liver Malignancies
Diagnostic and Interventional Radiology
Edited by C. Bartolozzi and R. Lencioni

Medical Imaging of the Spleen
Edited by A. M. De Schepper and F. Vanhoenacker

Radiology of Peripheral Vascular Diseases
Edited by E. Zeitler

Diagnostic Nuclear Medicine
Edited by C. Schiepers

Radiology of Blunt Trauma of the Chest
P. Schnyder and M. Wintermark

Portal Hypertension
Diagnostic Imaging-Guided Therapy
Edited by P. Rossi
Co-edited by P. Ricci and L. Broglia

Recent Advances in Diagnostic Neuroradiology
Edited by Ph. Demaerel

Virtual Endoscopy and Related 3D Techniques
Edited by P. Rogalla, J. Terwisscha Van Scheltinga, and B. Hamm

Multislice CT
Edited by M. F. Reiser, M. Takahashi, M. Modic, and R. Bruening

Pediatric Uroradiology
Edited by R. Fotter

Transfontanellar Doppler Imaging in Neonates
A. Couture and C. Veyrac

Radiology of AIDS
A Practical Approach
Edited by J.W.A.J. Reeders and P.C. Goodman

CT of the Peritoneum
Armando Rossi and Giorgio Rossi

Magnetic Resonance Angiography
2nd Revised Edition
Edited by I. P. Arlart, G. M. Bongratz,and G. Marchal

Pediatric Chest Imaging
Edited by Javier Lucaya and Janet L. Strife

Applications of Sonography in Head and Neck Pathology
Edited by J. N. Bruneton in collaboration with C. Raffaelli and O. Dassonville

Imaging of the Larynx
Edited by R. Hermans

3D Image Processing
Techniques and Clinical Applications
Edited by D. Caramella and C. Bartolozzi

Imaging of Orbital and Visual Pathway Pathology
Edited by W. S. Müller-Forell

Pediatric ENT Radiology
Edited by S. J. King and A. E. Boothroyd

Radiological Imaging of the Small Intestine
Edited by N. C. Gourtsoyiannis

Imaging of the Knee
Techniques and Applications
Edited by A. M. Davies and V. N. Cassar-Pullicino

Perinatal Imaging
From Ultrasound to MR Imaging
Edited by Fred E. Avni

Radiological Imaging of the Neonatal Chest
Edited by V. Donoghue

Diagnostic and Interventional Radiology in Liver Transplantation
Edited by E. Bücheler, V. Nicolas, C. E. Broelsch, X. Rogiers, and G. Krupski

Radiology of Osteoporosis
Edited by S. Grampp

Imaging Pelvic Floor Disorders
Edited by C. I. Bartram and J. O. L. DeLancey
Associate Editors: S. Halligan, F. M. Kelvin, and J. Stoker

Imaging of the Pancreas
Cystic and Rare Tumors
Edited by C. Procassi and A. J. Megibow

High Resolution Sonography of the Peripheral Nervous System
Edited by S. Peer and G. Bodner

Imaging of the Foot and Ankle
Techniques and Applications
Edited by A. M. Davies, R. W. Whitehouse, and J. P. R. Jenkins

Radiology Imaging of the Ureter
Edited by F. Joffre, Ph. Otal, and M. Soulie

Imaging of the Shoulder
Techniques and Applications
Edited by A. M. Davies and J. Hodler

Radiology of the Petrous Bone
Edited by M. Lemmerling and S. S. Kollias

Interventional Radiology in Cancer
Edited by A. Adam, R. F. Dondelinger, and P. R. Mueller

Duplex and Color Doppler Imaging of the Venous System
Edited by G. H. Mostbeck

Multidetector-Row CT of the Thorax
Edited by U. J. Schoepf

Intracranial Vascular Malformations and Aneurysms
From Diagnostic Work-Up to Endovascular Therapy
Edited by M. Forsting

Functional Imaging of the Chest
Edited by H.-U. Kauczor

Radiology of the Pharynx and the Esophagus
Edited by O. Ekberg

Radiological Imaging in Hematological Malignancies
Edited by A. Guermazi

Imaging and Intervention in Abdominal Trauma
Edited by R. F. Dondelinger

Springer

MEDICAL RADIOLOGY Diagnostic Imaging and Radiation Oncology

Titles in the series already published

RADIATION ONCOLOGY

Lung Cancer
Edited by C.W. Scarantino

Innovations in Radiation Oncology
Edited by H. R. Withers and L. J. Peters

Radiation Therapy of Head and Neck Cancer
Edited by G. E. Laramore

Gastrointestinal Cancer – Radiation Therapy
Edited by R.R. Dobelbower, Jr.

Radiation Exposure and Occupational Risks
Edited by E. Scherer, C. Streffer, and K.-R. Trott

Radiation Therapy of Benign Diseases
A Clinical Guide
S. E. Order and S. S. Donaldson

Interventional Radiation Therapy Techniques – Brachytherapy
Edited by R. Sauer

Radiopathology of Organs and Tissues
Edited by E. Scherer, C. Streffer, and K.-R. Trott

Concomitant Continuous Infusion Chemotherapy and Radiation
Edited by M. Rotman and C. J. Rosenthal

Intraoperative Radiotherapy – Clinical Experiences and Results
Edited by F. A. Calvo, M. Santos, and L.W. Brady

Radiotherapy of Intraocular and Orbital Tumors
Edited by W. E. Alberti and R. H. Sagerman

Interstitial and Intracavitary Thermoradiotherapy
Edited by M. H. Seegenschmiedt and R. Sauer

Non-Disseminated Breast Cancer
Controversial Issues in Management
Edited by G. H. Fletcher and S.H. Levitt

Current Topics in Clinical Radiobiology of Tumors
Edited by H.-P. Beck-Bornholdt

Practical Approaches to Cancer Invasion and Metastases
A Compendium of Radiation Oncologists' Responses to 40 Histories
Edited by A. R. Kagan with the Assistance of R. J. Steckel

Radiation Therapy in Pediatric Oncology
Edited by J. R. Cassady

Radiation Therapy Physics
Edited by A. R. Smith

Late Sequelae in Oncology
Edited by J. Dunst and R. Sauer

Mediastinal Tumors. Update 1995
Edited by D. E. Wood and C. R. Thomas, Jr.

Thermoradiotherapy and Thermochemotherapy
Volume 1:
Biology, Physiology, and Physics
Volume 2:
Clinical Applications
Edited by M.H. Seegenschmiedt, P. Fessenden, and C.C. Vernon

Carcinoma of the Prostate
Innovations in Management
Edited by Z. Petrovich, L. Baert, and L.W. Brady

Radiation Oncology of Gynecological Cancers
Edited by H.W. Vahrson

Carcinoma of the Bladder
Innovations in Management
Edited by Z. Petrovich, L. Baert, and L.W. Brady

Blood Perfusion and Micro-environment of Human Tumors
Implications for Clinical Radiooncology
Edited by M. Molls and P. Vaupel

Radiation Therapy of Benign Diseases
A Clinical Guide
2nd Revised Edition
S. E. Order and S. S. Donaldson

Carcinoma of the Kidney and Testis, and Rare Urologic Malignancies
Innovations in Management
Edited by Z. Petrovich, L. Baert, and L.W. Brady

Progress and Perspectives in the Treatment of Lung Cancer
Edited by P. Van Houtte, J. Klastersky, and P. Rocmans

Combined Modality Therapy of Central Nervous System Tumors
Edited by Z. Petrovich, L. W. Brady, M. L. Apuzzo, and M. Bamberg

Age-Related Macular Degeneration
Current Treatment Concepts
Edited by W. A. Alberti, G. Richard, and R. H. Sagerman

Radiotherapy of Intraocular and Orbital Tumors
2nd Revised Edition
Edited by R. H. Sagerman, and W. E. Alberti

Biological Modification of Radiation Response
Edited by C. Nieder, L. Milas, and K. K. Ang

Palliative Radiation Oncology
R. G. Parker. N. A. Janjan, and M. T. Selch

Clinical Target Volumes in Conformal and Intensity Modulated Radiation Therapy
A Clinical Guide to Cancer Treatment
Edited by V. Grégoire, P. Scalliet, and K. K. Ang

Springer

Printing and Binding: Stürtz GmbH, Würzburg